The Diabetic Foot

Medical and Surgical Management

T0076272

Edited by

Aristidis Veves, MD, DSc

John M. Giurini, DPM

Frank W. LoGerfo, MD

Beth Israel Deaconess Medical Center

Boston, MA

Humana Press Totowa, New Jersey

The diabetic foot : medical and surgical management / edited by Aristidis Veves, John J. Giurini, Frank W. LoGerfo.
    p. ; cm.
Includes bibliographical references and index.
ISBN 978-1-61737-253-7
  1. Foot--Diseases. 2. Diabetes--Complications. I. Veves, Aristidis. II. Giurini, John M. III. LoGerfo, Frank W.
[DNLM: 1. Diabetic Foot--therapy. WK 835 D5318 2002]
RD563 .D495 2002
617.5'85--dc21

                                                                                    2001039365

Preface

It is estimated that diabetes mellitus afflicts 16 million people in the United States alone. Fifteen percent or nearly 2 million people will develop foot ulcerations in their lifetime. The consequences of these problems are not only important to the individual patient and their families, but to every healthcare system in the world. Diabetic foot ulcerations and infections are the main cause for hospitalization of the diabetic patient, thus placing a substantial financial burden on society. The direct and indirect costs for ulcer management and treatment may exceed $10 billion dollars. This is particularly disturbing since the incidence of diabetes worldwide is increasing at an alarming rate. It should therefore be expected that the practicing physician will see lower extremity problems more frequently over the next several decades.

The great tragedy of diabetic foot problems is that they are probably the most preventable of all long-term complications. Over the past 20 years, the establishment of multidisciplinary clinics that include the services of diabetologists, podiatrists, vascular surgeons, infectious disease specialists, plastic surgeons, orthopedic surgeons, diabetic nurse educators, and orthotists has clearly shown that the rate of foot ulceration and lower limb amputation can be dramatically reduced. Furthermore, substantial improvement can be expected as we capitalize on our recent understanding of wound healing pathophysiology and convert this knowledge into the development of new and more effective treatments. Recently introduced growth factors and living skin equivalents are examples of such developments.

In *The Diabetic Foot: Medical and Surgical Management,* we have tried to reflect these trends and present to the reader both established techniques that are effective in the treatment of foot ulcerations as well as upcoming developments that we believe may have an impact on diabetic foot care over the next few years. We have also tried to emphasize the multidisciplinary approach to diabetic foot problems drawing on the long tradition of the Joslin-Beth Israel Deaconess Foot Center, one of the oldest and most experienced of such clinics.

We hope that *The Diabetic Foot: Medical and Surgical Management* will appeal to all professionals involved in the care of the diabetic foot. We are very pleased and privileged to have secured the collaboration of a distinguished panel of authors from around the world and wish to offer them our most sincere gratitude and appreciation. Without their extraordinary efforts, this book would not have been possible. Finally, we would also like to express our gratitude to Paul Dolgert and Craig Adams of Humana Press for their expert guidance and professional handling of this publication. Most of all, we thank them for their unending patience.

Aristidis Veves, MD, DSc
John M. Giurini, DPM
Frank W. LoGerfo, MD

Contents

Contributors

CAMERON M. AKBARI, MD, *Attending Vascular Surgeon and Codirector, Noninvasive Vascular Lab, Beth Israel Deaconess Medical Center; Assistant Professor of Surgery, Harvard Medical School, Boston, MA*

DAVID G. ARMSTRONG, DPM, *Podiatry Section, Department of Surgery, Southern Arizona Veterans Affairs Medical Center, Tucson, AZ; Department of Medicine, Manchester Royal Infirmary, Manchester, UK*

PHILIP BASILE, DPM, *Division of Podiatry, Department of Surgery, Beth Israel Deaconess Medical Center, Boston, MA*

ANDREW J.M. BOULTON, MD, FRCP, *University Department of Medicine, Manchester Royal Infirmary, Manchester, UK*

DAVID P. BROPHY, MD, FFRRCSI, FRCR, MSCVIR, *Department of Radiology, Beth Israel Deaconess Medical Center; Assistant Professor of Radiology, Harvard Medical School, Boston, MA*

DAVID R. CAMPBELL, MD, *Division of Vascular Surgery, Department of Surgery, Beth Israel Deaconess Medical Center; Associate Clinical Professor of Surgery, Harvard Medical School, Boston, MA*

NANCY FALCO CHEDID, MD, *Division of Plastic Surgery, Department of Surgery, Beth Israel Deaconess Hospital; Instructor in Surgery, Harvard University School of Medicine, Boston, MA*

YVONNE CHEUNG, MD, *Department of Radiology, Beth Israel Deaconess Medical Center; Assistant Professor, Harvard Medical School, Boston, MA*

THANH L. DINH, DPM, *Division of Podiatry, Department of Surgery, Beth Israel Deaconess Medical Center, Boston, MA*

VINCENT FALANGA, MD, FACP, *Professor of Dermatology and Biochemistry, Boston University School of Medicine, Boston, MA; Chairman of Training Program, Roger Williams Medical Center, Providence, RI*

ROBERT G. FRYKBERG, DPM, MPH, *Associate Professor of Podiatric Medicine, College of Podiatric Medicine and Surgery, Des Moines University, Des Moines, IA*

JOHN M. GIURINI, DPM, *Chief, Division of Podiatry, Beth Israel Deaconess Medical Center; Associate Clinical Professor of Surgery, Harvard Medical School; Codirector, Joslin-Beth Israel Deaconess Diabetic Foot Center; Consultant, Joslin Diabetes Center; Chief, Section of Podiatry, New England Baptist Hospital, Boston, MA*

JOSEPH E. GREY, MB BCH, PhD, MRCP, *Wound Healing Research Unit, Cardiff Medicentre, University of Wales College of Medicine, Cardiff, UK*

ALLEN HAMDAN, MD, *Division of Vascular Surgery, Department of Surgery, Beth Israel Deaconess Medical Center; Assistant Professor of Surgery, Harvard Medical School, Boston, MA*

KEITH G. HARDING, MB ChB, MRCGP, FRCS, *Wound Healing Research Unit, Cardiff Medicentre, University of Wales College of Medicine, Cardiff, UK*

LAWRENCE B. HARKLESS, DPM, *Department of Orthopaedics, University of Texas Health Science Center, San Antonio, TX*

MARY HOCHMAN, MD, *Department of Radiology, Beth Israel Deaconess Medical Center, Boston, MA*

VANESSA JONES, MSc, RGN, NDN, RCNT, PGCE, *Wound Healing Research Unit, Cardiff Medicentre, University of Wales College of Medicine, Cardiff, UK*

EDWARD JUDE, MD, *Department of Medicine, Manchester Royal Infirmary, Manchester, UK*

NIKHIL KANSAL, MD, *Division of Vascular Surgery, Department of Surgery, Beth Israel Deaconess Medical Center; Clinical Fellow in Surgery, Harvard Medical School, Boston, MA*

ADOLF W. KARCHMER, MD, *Chief, Division of Infectious Diseases, Beth Israel Deaconess Medical Center; Professor of Medicine, Harvard Medical School, Boston, MA*

FRANK W. LoGERFO, MD, *Chairman, Department of Surgery; Chief, Division of Vascular Surgery, Beth Israel Deaconess Medical Center; William V. McDermott Professor of Surgery, Harvard Medical School, Boston, MA*

THOMAS E. LYONS, DPM, *Clinical Instructor of Surgery, Harvard Medical School; Department of Surgery, Beth Israel Deaconess Medical Center, Boston, MA*

COLEEN NAPOLITANO, DPM, *Assistant Professor, Department of Orthopaedic Surgery and Rehabilitation, Loyola University of Chicago Stritch School of Medicine, Maywood, IL*

HAU T. PHAM, DPM, *Division of Podiatry, Department of Surgery, Beth Israel Deaconess Medical Center, Boston, MA*

MICHAEL PINZUR, MD, *Professor, Department of Orthopaedic Surgery and Rehabilitation, Loyola University of Chicago Stritch School of Medicine, Maywood, IL*

FRANK B. POMPOSELLI, JR., MD, *Division of Vascular Surgery, Department of Surgery, Beth Israel Deaconess Medical Center; Associate Professor of Surgery, Harvard Medical School, Boston, MA*

GAYLE E. REIBER, MPH, PhD, *VA Career Scientist and Associate Professor, Health Services and Epidemiology, University of Washington, Seattle, WA*

JEREMY RICH, DPM, *Clinical Fellow in Surgery, Harvard Medical School; Department of Surgery, Beth Israel Deaconess Medical Center, Boston, MA*

BARRY I. ROSENBLUM, DPM, *Division of Podiatry, Department of Surgery, Beth Israel Deaconess Medical Center, Boston, MA*

RONALD A. SAGE, DPM, *Professor, Department of Orthopaedic Surgery and Rehabilitation, Loyola University of Chicago Stritch School of Medicine, Maywood, IL*

PETER SHEEHAN, MD, *Director, Diabetes Foot and Ankle Center, Hospital for Joint Diseases Orthopaedic Institute, New York, NY*

DAVID L. STEED, MD, *Professor of Surgery, Division of Vascular Surgery and Wound Healing, Department of Surgery, University of Pittsburgh School of Medicine, Pittsburgh, PA*

RODNEY STUCK, DPM, *Associate Professor, Department of Orthopaedic Surgery and Rehabilitation, Loyola University Stritch School of Medicine, Maywood, IL*

SOLOMON TESFAYE, MD, FRCP, *Consultant Physician and Honorary Senior Lecturer, Royal Hallamshire Hospital, Sheffield, UK*

LUIGI UCCIOLI, MD, *Department of Endocrinology, University of Rome 'Tor Vergata,' Rome, Italy*

CARINE H.M. VAN SCHIE, MSc, PhD, *University Department of Medicine, Manchester Royal Infirmary; Diabetes Foot Clinic Disablement Services Centre, Withington Hospital, Manchester, UK*

ARISTIDIS VEVES, MD, DSc, *Research Director, Joslin-Beth Israel Deaconess Diabetic Foot Center and Microcirculation Lab; Assistant Professor of Surgery, Harvard Medical School, Boston, MA*

Color Plates

Color plates follow page 178.

Color Plate 1. Diabetic foot with plantar callus. (*Fig. 1, Chapter 13*; *see* discussion on pp. 252–253.)

Color Plate 2. Diabetic foot post surgical debridement. (*Fig. 3, Chapter 13*; *see* discussion on pp. 254–255.)

Color Plate 3. Sharp debridement of diabetic foot ulcer. (*Fig. 4, Chapter 13*; *see* discussion on pp. 254–255.)

Color Plate 4. Grade 0 foot with callous formation is indicative of high foot pressures, requiring treatment and accommodation with orthotic devices. (*Fig. 2, Chapter 14*; *see* discussion on pp. 280–281.)

Color Plate 5. The presence of synovial drainage from an ulceration is indicative of joint involvement and requires resection of that joint. (*Fig. 3, Chapter 15*; *see* discussion on p. 297).

Color Plate 6. Osteomyelitis of the first metatarsophalangeal joint is best addressed by elliptical excision of the ulcer with resection of the joint. Adequate resection of the first metatarsal should be performed to ensure complete eradication of infected bone. (*Fig. 4, Chapter 15*; *see* discussion on pp. 297–299.)

Color Plate 7. **(A)** Infection of the midfoot with full-thickness necrosis of the skin, subcutaneous tissue, and plantar aponeurosis. **(B)** Intraoperative view showing excised plantar fascia and intact flexor digitorum brevis muscle. **(C)** Skin grafted directly to muscle provided stable coverage. (*Fig. 11, Chapter 17*; *see* discussion on p. 361.)

Color Plate 8. **(A)** Example of frequently encountered neuropathic ulcer, involving most of weight-bearing heel. **(C)** After debridement of bone and soft tissue, a thin skin flap was designed for rotation; the distal incision is at least 3 cm posterior to the metatarsal heads. **(D)** Skin flap elevated, and flexor brevis muscle transposed into ulcer. (*Fig. 16, Chapter 17*; *see* discussion on p. 366.)

Introduction to Diabetes

Principles of Care in the Surgical Patient with Diabetes

Peter Sheehan, MD

INTRODUCTION

The medical and surgical management of foot disorders in the patient with diabetes should have as its basis a thorough understanding of the complications and metabolic consequences of diabetes mellitus. This is especially true in the patient who is undergoing a surgical procedure. Diabetes is rapidly increasing in prevalence worldwide, and surgery in patients with diabetes is more common. Foot complications are a major cause of admissions for diabetes, and they cause a disproportionately high number of hospital days because of increased surgical procedures and prolonged length of stay.

With advances in surgical techniques and anesthesia, surgery has become safer for patients with diabetes; nonetheless, these patients are in a high-risk group for perioperative complications, such as infection and myocardial infarction. These may be avoided or minimized with proper anticipation and awareness of the patient's medical condition. Despite the increase in morbidity and mortality that has been observed in the surgical patient with diabetes, there are no widely accepted guidelines for the many clinical issues that present in the perioperative period.

The objective of this chapter is to present current concepts in the assessment and management of the surgical patient with diabetes, as well as the pathophysiologic basis upon which these concepts rest. To this end, an overview of diabetes mellitus and its complications also is presented, with the understanding that more thorough reviews exist elsewhere.

OVERVIEW OF DIABETES AND ITS COMPLICATIONS

Epidemiology

In the past few decades, there has been an alarming rise in the prevalence of diabetes, particularly type 2. In the well-studied town of Framingham, Massachusetts, the prevalence has risen from 0.9% in 1958 to 3% in 1995 *(1)*. Recently, the Centers for Disease Control and Prevention estimated the U.S. prevalence of diagnosed diabetes at 6.5% in 1998, compared with a similar study in 1990 reporting a rate of 4.9%; this represents a nearly 30% increase over the past decade *(2)*. The increased prevalence of diabetes in the United States correlates with the rising rates of obesity. Most disturbing was a 76%

From: *The Diabetic Foot: Medical and Surgical Management*
Edited by: A. Veves, J. M. Giurini, and F. W. LoGerfo © Humana Press Inc., Totowa, NJ

increase in the prevalence of diabetes among the 30–39-year age group. This portends a new wave of chronic diabetic complications in the coming decade. Furthermore, the undiagnosed population is nearly as large: the National Health and Nutrition Examination Survey (NHANES) II and III large-scale population screening studies revealed that only 50% of people found to have diabetes were previously diagnosed *(3)*.

The prevalence of diagnosed diabetes increases with age, affecting over 10% of those over 65 years of age in the United States. It is also slightly overrepresented in women compared with men. Some ethnic populations have a two- to five-fold increase in risk of developing diabetes. The highest incidence is seen in Native Americans, followed by Hispanics, African Americans, Asians, and Pacific Islanders. The risk of diabetes in all groups is associated with higher rates of obesity and, more specifically, with an increase in the waist-hip ratio, a measure of central adiposity. Clearly, the increasing prevalence of diabetes correlates with the increasing prevalence of obesity in the United States.

Worldwide, the rates of diagnosed diabetes are rising, especially in developing nations. Indigenous peoples of the Americas and Polynesia are those with the highest risk. The Pima tribe in Arizona has the highest prevalence of type 2 diabetes in the world, affecting nearly 50% of all adult members. Asians and Africans are of intermediate risk. People of European descent are actually among those with the lowest risk of developing diabetes *(4)*. Most epidemiologic studies suggest that lifestyle changes introduced with increasing industrialization and economic development may be responsible. A higher prevalence of diabetes can also be seen in urban dwellers vis-à-vis their rural counterparts. The obvious contributing factors are a more abundant and richer diet, a sedentary lifestyle, and higher rates of obesity.

One cohesive theory tying the genetic predisposition of type 2 diabetes seen in certain ethnic groups to a higher prevalence of obesity is the "thrifty phenotype" *(5)*. According to this hypothesis, first proposed by Neel in 1962, these high-risk ethnic groups, primarily indigenous peoples, have adapted over the millennia to survive conditions of scarcity and episodic "feast or famine." As a consequence, they have developed a degree of metabolic efficiency, or "thriftiness," that allows storage of ingested calories as fat with less energy expenditure or waste. This predisposes to a higher tendency to obesity, especially of the central type, when such people are placed in an environment of surfeit and rich foodstuffs. With the development of obesity, there is in turn a greater risk of diabetes.

At this time, approximately 1% of the population of China has diabetes. It is estimated that if that country assumes a more industrial, Western lifestyle the prevalence would rise to 8–10%. This alone would cause nearly a doubling of the world's population with diabetes. Similar projections are proposed for South Asians as well. Unfortunately, it is clear that we are presently in an epidemic of diabetes, which will constitute an even greater and more frequently encountered medical issue as chronic complications become manifest.

Diagnosis

An expert committee of the American Diabetes Association (ADA) amended the diagnostic criteria for diabetes mellitus in 1997 *(6)*. Previously, the diagnosis was made with the Fajans-Conn criteria as the standard. By that definition, a person was diagnosed with diabetes when 1) signs and symptoms of diabetes (polyuria, polydipsia, and so on) with glycosuria or a random blood glucose >200 mg%; 2) fasting blood glucose >140 mg% on two separate occasions; or 3) after an oral 75-g glucose load, a 2-h blood glucose and an interval blood glucose >200 mg%. The problem with the use of these criteria was the lack of sensitivity in the fasting blood glucose value in diagnosing diabetes compared with the 2-h glucose tolerance test. In addition, the Wisconsin Epidemiologic Study of Diabetic Retinopathy (WESDR) and NHANES III data suggested that retinopathy was associated with fasting blood glucose as low as 120 mg% *(7)*. It was concluded that use of a lower diagnostic value would improve correlation with the incidence and prevalence of microvascular complications, i.e., retinopathy, and would increase the sensitivity correlation to the oral glucose tolerance results. Therefore, the ADA expert consensus criteria are now as folllows:

1. Symptoms and a casual blood glucose >200 mg%
2. Fasting blood >126 mg% (7 mmol/dL) on two separate occasions or
3. A 2-h blood glucose >200 mg% after a 75-g oral glucose load.

The new criteria thus encourage use of the fasting blood glucose as an efficient and reliable measure in the diagnosis of diabetes. Persons with fasting values between normal (<110 mg%) and diabetes (>126 mg%) would be considered to have "impaired glucose tolerance" (IGT) and would carry a high risk of developing diabetes and its complications.

Classification

The classification of diabetes has also been revised. *Type 1 diabetes* previously called "juvenile" or "insulin-dependent" diabetes (IDDM), refers to beta cell destruction and absolute insulin deficiency. The typical patient is a 12-year-old child presenting with ketoacidosis. However, this type can be seen in older persons with a less dramatic, more insidious presentation. In the United Kingdom Prospective Diabetes Study (UKPDS), many adult patients had evidence of islet cell autoimmunity, especially the younger, less obese subgroups with diabetes *(8)*.

Over 90% of people with diabetes have *type 2 diabetes*, which typically affects an older population and is associated with a family history of diabetes, as well as obesity and sedentary lifestyle. In the past, type 2 diabetes was referred to as "adult-onset" and "non-insulin-dependent" diabetes (NIDDM). This labeling is less accurate in that many of these patients are treated with insulin and that the incidence is rising in the younger population, even in childhood. As will be discussed, type 2 diabetes is characterized by insulin resistance and an absolute or relative impairment in insulin secretion. As discussed, it is now reaching epidemic occurrence rates worldwide.

As already noted, individuals whose fasting plasma glucose falls between normal (<110 mg/dL) and diabetes (>126 mg/dL) are considered to have IGT. As will be discussed, there is a significant conversion rate over time of IGT to type 2 diabetes. In the past, terms like "prediabetes" and "chemical diabetes" have underscored the progressive aspect of the natural history of IGT.

Secondary causes of diabetes are uncommon, but they should be considered, especially if management of the patient is unusual or problematic. Pancreatic disease leads to insulin deficiency and diabetes, but it is also associated with marked insulin sensitivity because of exocrine insufficiency, malabsorption, and glucagon deficiency. Endocrine disorders may cause hyperglycemia that may be reversible; they and are usually recognized by their own stigmata. These include Cushing's disease, acromegaly, and hyperthyroidism. There are also rare hereditary and acquired disorders of extreme insulin resistance. These are often associated with an intertriginous dermopathy, acanthosis nigricans.

Finally, an increasingly more common presentation is diabetes during pregnancy, or *gestational diabetes mellitus* (GDM). Often occurring in the third trimester, it can lead to fetal wastage, macrosomia, and fetal malformation, especially neural crest and heart defects. The hyperglycemia typically resolves after delivery, implicating some placental factor as central to the pathogenesis. Nonetheless, these women are phenotypically insulin resistant and are at high risk for future development of diabetes, with a 10-year postpartum incidence of >30%.

PATHOPHYSIOLOGY

Type 1 Diabetes

Many studies over the past two decades have validated the characterization of type 1 diabetes as a chronic autoimmune disease *(9)*. The familiar pathologic finding of "insulitis," with lymphocytic infiltration of the pancreatic islets and loss of insulin-containing β-cells, suggests cell-mediated immune activation. In addition, 90% of individuals with type 1 diabetes at presentation have autoantibodies against islet cells and insulin. These include islet cell antibodies (ICAs), insulin autoantibodies (IAAs), and glutamic acid decarboxylase antibodies (GADAs). Whether these antibodies are the cause or result of β-cell destruction is not certain, but they serve as ancillary evidence of the autoimmune nature of this disorder.

Importantly, the presence of autoantibodies can be demonstrated years before the diagnosis of type 1 diabetes, underscoring the chronic, silent nature of its development. This belies the familiar, often dramatic clinical presentation of acute diabetic ketoacidosis in a young person. It is important to note that some older patients felt to have type 2 diabetes may in fact have type 1 diabetes, as suggested by the demonstration of circulating ICAs and GADAs. These patients tend to be leaner and younger at presentation, and they progress rapidly to a need for insulin treatment over 2 or 3 years *(8)*. The smoldering autoimmune destruction of the β-cells may also be arrested. These same autoantibodies are also highly predictive of future development of type 1 diabetes and serve as a screening mechanism in studies designed to prevent the onset of hyperglycemia with immune modulation *(10)*.

Type 1 diabetes has ethnic and geographic variations. The highest incidence, in contrast to type 2 diabetes, is found in Scandinavian and Northern European populations. Early-onset type 1 diabetes is associated with specific HLA phenotypes on chromosome 6 responsible for class II histocompatibility complexes, namely, DR3 and DR4. Other genes in the closely located DQ locus may confer increased risk or protection from clinical type 1 diabetes *(11)*. Since concordance rates in HLA-identical twins are <50%, and fewer than 15% of newly diagnosed patients have an affected first-degree relative, environmental factors are implicated in the pathogenesis of type 1 diabetes. Possible environmental triggers include viruses (mumps, Coxsackie B, and rubella) and dietary substances (bovine milk albumin and gluten) *(12)*.

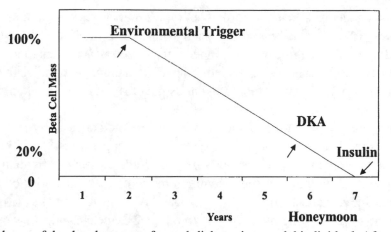

Fig. 1. Schema of the development of type 1 diabetes in a model individual. After activation by an environmental trigger, the autoimmune attack against pancreatic β-cells results in progressive loss of β-cell mass over several years. Clinical presentation often occurs with diabetic ketoacidosis (DKA) when the β-cell mass is approximately 20% of its original content. Over the next year or two, the autoimmune attack persists, resulting in complete loss of β-cell mass and true insulin dependence. The honeymoon period is the term for this temporary time when use of little or no insulin is required. (Adapted from: Eisenbarth GS. Type I diabetes mellitus—a chronic autoimmune disease. *N Engl J Med* 1986;314:1360–1368.)

The current model of the pathogenesis of type 1 diabetes is that an environmental factor triggers an autoimmune response against the pancreas, leading chronically over years to progressive loss of β-cell mass and impairment of insulin secretion (Fig. 1). When there is loss of 80–90% of β-cell mass, fasting hyperglycemia may develop. If there is also severe coincident or intercurrent illness, typically a viral infection, the initial presentation may be fulminant diabetic ketoacidosis (DKA). Indeed 20% of type 1 patients present with DKA. After stabilization, β–cell function may improve, and for a time the patient then requires little or no exogenous insulin. This is known as the "honeymoon period" of type 1 diabetes. However, months or years later, autoimmune β-cell destruction is complete. There is no odd endogenous insulin secretion, and the patient is rendered "insulin dependent."

Type 2 Diabetes

Type 2 diabetes can be best understood as heterogeneous, having both genetic and environmental causes. Although type 2 diabetes typically presents later in life than type 1 diabetes, there has been an increasing incidence in younger individuals. This is best explained by the association of type 2 diabetes with obesity, which is now more prevalent in the same population under 30 years of age. The recently reported increase in the prevalence of diabetes in the United States is highly correlated with a contemporaneous increase in the prevalence of obesity. Indeed, almost 90% of patients who present with type 2 diabetes are overweight. As will be discussed, increasing obesity leads to increasing insulin resistance in these individuals, causing insulin requirements that exceed the secretory capacity of the pancreas. A common clinical observation is that the presentation of type 2 diabetes is often at the time of the individual's lifetime maximum weight.

The strong genetic basis in the etiology of type 2 diabetes is substantiated by several observations. There is usually a family history of diabetes in affected individuals, typically involving a first-degree relative. Indeed, the concordance rates in identical twins approaches 100%. The clustering of diabetes in certain ethnic and racial groups, particularly Native Americans and other indigenous peoples, underscores the its hereditary nature.

One disturbing observation is the new increased incidence of type 2 diabetes in childhood in the United States. This is seen when strong expression of both primary risk factors, genetic predisposition and obesity, affect a young individual. Presently, type 2 diabetes in childhood is more common in members of high-risk ethnic populations in the United States, namely, Hispanics and African-Americans *(13)*. Therefore, young age no longer distinguishes type 1 from type 2 diabetes, and a new public health problem must now be addressed.

Insulin Resistance

Type 2 diabetes is unequivocally a genetic disorder; the exact nature of the inherited defect is not clear, and it may be complex and multigenic. Insulin resistance is the most likely factor. First, it is seen in almost all newly diagnosed individuals with type 2 diabetes and is only partially reversible with treatment. Second, studies in lean, nondiabetic, first-degree relatives of type 2 diabetic individuals and in patients with IGT have documented a state of insulin resistance *(14)*.

Insulin resistance has been most accurately quantified with the use of the euglycemic hyperinsulinemic clamp study *(15)*. In this procedure, a subject is infused with insulin in high concentrations, resulting in plasma levels of approximately 100 μIU/mL. To defend against hypoglycemia, the subject is also given a variable glucose infusion at a rate that preserves euglycemia. The amount of glucose infused is a quantitative reflection of the subject's insulin sensitivity: the higher the infusion rate, the more insulin-sensitive; the lower the infusion rate, the more insulin-resistant. Studies in subjects with type 2 diabetes have confirmed the presence of insulin resistance compared with normal control subjects. Insulin resistance is also found in those with IGT, suggesting that it precedes the development of type 2 diabetes. Studies of subjects with diabetes using glucose extraction studies over various organ beds have placed the site of insulin resistance overwhelmingly at the level of skeletal muscle uptake. This is important conceptually when considering the importance of exercise in the prevention and treatment of type 2 diabetes. In summary, insulin resistance is fundamental in the pathogenesis of type 2 diabetes and may be the primary inherited defect.

Insulin Secretion

It is important to note that not all insulin-resistant states result in hyperglycemia. This implies that a loss of β-cell function, either relative or absolute, is a prerequisite for the development of type 2 diabetes. Much of the impairment of insulin secretion is probably acquired, as β-cell loss in type 2 diabetes is approximately 20–40%. Some of the defect can be explained by the concept of "glucose toxicity," whereby hyperglycemia *per se* can impair insulin secretion and insulin action, thus becoming the cause and consequence of decompensated diabetes. The insulin secretory defect is partially reversible and may improve considerably with correction of the hyperglycemia. This suggests functional, rather than intrinsic cellular, abnormalities.

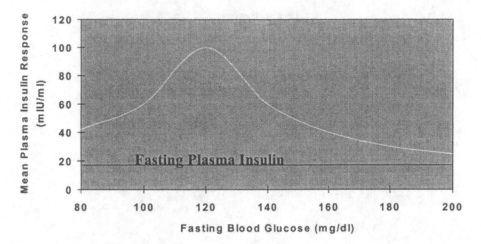

Fig. 2. Cross-sectional data from oral glucose tolerance testing in four different groups: normal fasting blood glucose, impaired glucose tolerance (IGT), type 2 diabetes, and uncontrolled type 2 diabetes. Curve is best fit to emphasize the compensatory increase and subsequent decrease in insulin secretion seen in IGT and diabetes. It is a model for the progression to type 2 diabetes observed in longitudinal studies. (From: DeFronzo RA. Lilly Lecture 1987. The triumvirate: beta-cell, muscle, liver. A collusion responsible for NIDDM. *Diabetes* 1988;37:667–687.)

The defects in insulin secretion are best conceptualized by the "Starling curve" proposed by DeFronzo *(16)* (Fig. 2). This model was drawn from cross-sectional studies of insulin secretion in response to an oral glucose load in four different clinical groups: normal fasting glucose, IGT, diabetes, and uncontrolled diabetes. The compensatory increase in insulin secretion seen in patients with IGT disappeared in the group with diabetes. However, insulin secretion may be relatively deficient in its ability to overcome the resistance. In those with uncontrolled diabetes, insulin secretion was significantly impaired. Although taken from cross-sectional data, this model proposes a mechanism for the observation of conversion of people with IGT to type 2 diabetes. In the Pima tribe, a longitudinal study of "progressors" from IGT to type 2 diabetes revealed that a lack of compensatory increase in insulin secretion in insulin-resistant subjects was predictive of the development of diabetes *(17)*. (Fig. 3)

A simplified model of the pathogenesis of type 2 diabetes is offered *(18)*. Insulin resistance is primary and is inherited in identifiable families and ethnic groups. This results in a compensatory increase in endogenous insulin secretion. Environmental factors, such as obesity and sedentary lifestyle, add to the insulin resistance, causing increased metabolic stresses. The individual may maintain normal blood glucose levels and progress to a state of impaired glucose tolerance. Over a period of time, the β-cell compensation fails. Defective insulin secretion can result from genetically determined limits, from aging, from senescent "β-cell exhaustion," or from the "glucose toxicity" of intermittent hyperglycemia. A marked decrease in β-cell function then leads to a conversion to fasting hyperglycemia and overt type 2 diabetes, as seen in the "progressors" in the Pima tribe.

Metabolic Abnormalities

The appropriate management of diabetes mellitus requires a basic understanding of the pathophysiologic mechanisms contributing to the development of hyperglycemia.

Insulin Resistance

↓

Hyperinsulinemia

↓

Compensated Insulin Resistance

↓

Normal Glucose Tolerance

↓

β-Cell Decompensation

↓

Impaired Glucose Tolerance

↓

β-Cell Exhaustion

↓

Type 2 Diabetes Mellitus

Fig. 3. Mechanism leading to type 2 diabetes. (Adapted from: Weyer C, Bogardus C, Mott DM, Pratley, RE. The natural history of insulin secretory dysfunction and insulin resistance in the pathogenesis of type 2 diabetes mellitus. *J Clin Invest* 1999;104:787-794.)

For the sake of brevity the discussion will focus on type 2 diabetes, since type 1 diabetes has a relatively less complex pathophysiology and is less commonly encountered. As defined by DeFronzo et al. *(18)*, three metabolic abnormalities (Fig. 4) have been identified in patients with type 2 diabetes that lead to the development and persistence of hyperglycemia:

1. Insulin resistance
2. Impaired insulin secretion
3. Increased hepatic glucose production.

In the fasting state, normal blood glucose is supported by the endogenous production of glucose, primarily by the liver, with some contribution from the kidneys. The rate of hepatic glucose production is approximately 2 mg/kg/min, or 125 g daily in an average individual. This production constitutes for the most part the fasting blood glucose that is commonly measured clinically. The purpose of this endogenous glucose production is to provide fuel to the brain and central nervous system.

With the ingestion of an oral glucose load, specific events must occur in concert to ensure the maintenance of normal glucose tolerance. First, insulin secretion is stimulated. The increased insulin secretion then prevents hyperglycemia by suppressing endogenous glucose production (primarily in the liver) and stimulating glucose uptake and disposal in the peripheral tissues (primarily in muscle).

In patients with type 2 diabetes who are in the fasting state, there is increased hepatic glucose production, despite increased ambient concentrations of plasma insulin. The increased glucose production rate is evidence of insulin resistance at the level of the liver but is suppressible with high concentrations of insulin. Second, the insulin secretory response to oral glucose is impaired. Initially, in early type 2 diabetes, there is a loss of the rapid or "first-phase" release of insulin and subsequently a relative or absolute deficiency in the total secretion, as discussed in the Starling curve model of

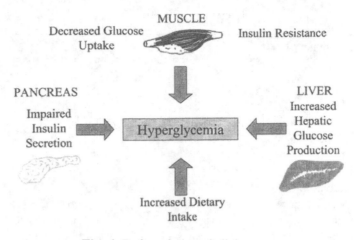

Fig. 4. Defects in type 2 diabetes.

insulin secretion. Third, muscle glucose uptake in response to oral glucose or exogenous insulin is reduced and is indeed the primary site of insulin resistance in type 2 diabetes. The earliest defect is in the nonoxidative muscle glucose uptake and storage as glycogen.

These events interplay to result in worsened hyperglycemia. According to the concept of *glucose toxicity*, hyperglycemia then in turn worsens insulin resistance and further impairs insulin secretion. The initiation of the vicious circle of glucose toxicity contributes to the progressive decline in insulin secretion and insulin action that characterizes type 2 diabetes, and provides a model to explain the "progressors," the individuals who convert from impaired glucose tolerance to type 2 diabetes *(19)*. In the management of uncontrolled diabetes, treating hyperglycemia may interrupt the vicious cycle of glucose toxicity and improve insulin secretion and insulin action.

The clinical characteristics of type 1 and type 2 diabetes are summarized in Table 1.

COMPLICATIONS

Acute Complications

Diabetic Ketoacidosis

Diabetic ketoacidosis (DKA) is a medical emergency in patients with diabetes, with an incidence of 4–8/1000 patient-years *(20)*. It affects type 1 patients almost exclusively, with approximately 25% manifesting clinical DKA at the time of onset of diabetes, but it may also occur in type 2 patients with severe intercurrent illness. Patients often require hospitalization, and mortality rates are 2–5%.

The pathogenesis of DKA begins with insulin deficiency in the face of abnormally high concentrations of counterregulatory hormones, usually in the setting of an intercurrent illness. The hormones involved are related to sympathoadrenal activation, specifically cortisol and epinephrine, as well as glucagon, growth hormone, and thyroxin. The underlying cause is usually infection, typically of viral etiology. Other provocative events include myocardial infarction, cerebrovascular accident, pulmonary embolus, pregnancy, and omission of insulin treatment.

Table 1
Clinical Features of Diabetes

Parameter	Type 1	Type 2
Age < 30 yr	Yes	No
Ketosis	Yes	No
Obesity	No	Yes (90%)
Family history	Possible	Usual
Ethnic groups	European	Indigenous peoples
Concordance twins	40%	90%
HLA type	DR3/4	None
Autoantibodies	90%	10%
Complications	Micro	Macro
Primary defects	↓ Insulin secretion	↑ Insulin resistance
Pathogenesis	Autoimmune	Heterogeneous

The metabolic condition of increased counterregulatory hormones in the state of deficient or absent insulin results in a marked increase in glucose production, primarily by the liver. This results in polyuria, free water loss, and eventual dehydration. Glucose uptake in muscle is impaired, and alterations in mitochondrial fatty acid oxidation result in excessive production of ketones, which are potent organic acids. Systemic acidosis results in anorexia, abdominal pain, nausea, and vomiting, further contributing to dehydration. The respiratory compensation for ketoacidosis is often characteristic deep, labored Kussmaul respirations. Treatment is urgent and consists of vigorous fluid and electrolyte replacement as well as high doses of insulin (0.1 U/kg/h) to inhibit ketone production. DKA is preventable with early recognition: it is most important to treat dehydration and to adjust—*but not omit*—insulin treatment during illness or surgery.

Hyperosmolar Hyperglycemic Nonketotic Syndrome

Hyperosmolar hyperglycemic nonketotic syndrome (HHNK) is an acute complication usually seen in older patients with type 2 diabetes. It results in more severe hyperglycemia and dehydration than in DKA, and with lesser or absent ketosis *(21)*. Unlike a viral infection causing DKA, it is usually a smoldering bacterial infection, typically of the respiratory or urinary tracts, that precipitates HHNK. The hyperglycemia causes polyuria and increased fluid losses. Patients affected often have underlying renal disease or are taking diuretics, further limiting urinary concentrating ability to prevent free water loss. The presence of a finite concentration of insulin in the patient with type 2 diabetes prevents the development of ketoacidosis but allows the progression of hyperglycemia and increasing dehydration. Patients present with marked hyperglycemia, often >700 mg%, after being ill for days to weeks. Neurologic manifestations, such as seizures or coma, are common. Fluid deficits are often 6–10 L, and potassium losses may approach 400 mEq. Mortality rates range from 10 to 50%, usually as a consequence of neurologic sequelae or concurrent bacterial infection and sepsis.

In contrast to DKA, treatment of HHNK should emphasize fluid replacement rather than insulin administration. Patients require gradual rehydration (approx 50% of estimated fluid deficit replaced in first 24 hr) to avoid induction of cerebral edema. Potassium replacement should be concomitant with administration of insulin, as uptake of glucose and potassium in muscle may precipitate hypokalemia and cardiac arrhythmias. A thorough search for the presence of a bacterial infection as well as empiric systemic therapy with antibiotics may decrease the mortality of HHNK from related sepsis. With the advent of home glucose monitoring and patient education, HHNK should be largely preventable, and incidence should be reduced from the current rate of 0.6/1000 patient-years *(22)*. Indeed, it is usually now seen only in patients who were not previously diagnosed with diabetes and are unaware of the meaning of the symptoms.

Hypoglycemia

Though it is rarely life threatening, hypoglycemia is an acute complication of the pharmacologic treatments of diabetes. It can result in mental status change, seizures, and coma if sustained and prolonged. Most episodes are mild to moderate. The causes are related to insulin excess that is absolute (from exogenous insulin or oral secretogogue) or relative (from exercise, alcohol, or lack of food). The earliest symptoms are a result of glucose counterregulation and sympathoadrenal activation—specifically epinephrine—that occur at a glycemic concentration of 55–70 mg%. Epinephrine is responsible for the characteristic symptoms, such as shakiness, palpitations, sweating, hunger, and irritability, which are accompanied by signs of pallor and diaphoresis. Neuroglycopenia usually occurs at glycemic concentrations <55 mg%. This often results in confusion and altered mental status. A severe episode of hypoglycemia is one that requires the assistance of another individual for correction. Of clinical importance is the observation that patients with frequent episodes of hypoglycemia may lose the early counterregulatory "warning" symptoms and sporadically develop severe episodes with neuroglycopenia and mental changes. This" hypoglycemic unawareness" is often seen in patients receiving intensive insulin therapy. Strict avoidance of hypoglycemic episodes can result in the restoration of the early counterregulatory response *(23)*.

The treatment of hypoglycemia should be prompt but not excessive, as overtreatment may result in marked hyperglycemia. Treatment during the elevation of the ambient counterregulatory hormones may cause a rebound from a low blood sugar to an excessively high blood sugar. The "rule of 15" is a treatment mnemonic: 15 g of glucose orally and retest in 15 min. This translates into 3 glucose tablets or 4 ounces of soda or juice. For a severe episode in which the patient's consciousness is impaired, glucagon (1 mg) should be administered parenterally, rather than risk aspiration with forced oral treatment.

Chronic Complications

Microvascular Complications

A unifying hypothesis of the pathogenesis of the microvascular complications of diabetes has not yet been reached, and a review of the possible candidate mechanisms is beyond the scope of this chapter. Epidemiologic studies, particularly of retinopathy, have strongly implicated hyperglycemia as a factor in the causal pathway. Retinopathy can be traced to the duration and the degree of hyperglycemia, which suggests a dose-response relationship. It is more prevalent in poorly controlled patients with diabetes, and in those with diabetes of longer duration. Conversely, achieving tight glycemic control and near normalization of blood glucose may prevent or postpone the development of complications *(24)*. Theories that incorporate hyperglycemia in their paradigm for the microvascular complications of diabetes include the hyperfiltration hypothesis *(25)*, increased polyol-sorbitol pathway activity *(26)*, accumulation of advanced glyco-sylation end products (AGEs) *(27)*, activation of cytokines through the receptor for AGEs (RAGE) *(28)*, and activation of protein kinase C (PKC) *(29)*. These are presently areas of intense scientific investigation.

The discussion of microvascular complications will be limited to retinopathy and neph-ropathy. Diabetic neuropathy, which includes elements of both microvascular and macro-vacular etiologies, is the subject of a more comprehensive discussion in Chapter 4.

Retinopathy

Although nearly 80% of patients with diabetes will have some retinopathy in their lifetime, most will be limited to background disease that carries little risk of loss of vision and blindness. Findings on fundoscopic exam include microaneurysms, small "dot and blot" hemorrhages, retinal ischemic lesions (cotton wool spots), and exudates that consist of lipid (hard) and plasma proteins (soft). Background retinopathy is a mani-festation of retinal ischemia (due to capillary loss and dropout), and increased capillary permeability to macromolecules. Visual disturbance and blurriness result from macula edema. This may occur if the central vision area of the macula is affected by excessive capillary leak. Macula edema may require treatment with laser photocoagulation to decrease local edema, with improvement in acuity over the ensuing months.

After 20 years of type 1 diabetes, the prevalence of proliferative retinopathy is approx-imately 20% *(30)*. It is hypothesized that in response to retinal ischemia and capillary dropout there is an increased production of angiogenic factors. These result in neovas-cularization of the retina, particularly around the more proximal vessels emerging from the optic disc. A likely candidate angiogenic factor is vascular endothelial growth fac-tor (VEGF), which has been shown to be in high concentrations in the vitreous humor of patients with retinopathy *(31)*. The neovascularization progresses in a dysregulated manner, creating adherent fronds and vessels growing out of the plane of the retina into the vitreous, characteristic of proliferative retinopathy. These frail vessels can sponta-neously bleed, initially causing vitreal hemorrhage and acute blurring of vision. With time, there is clot organization and retraction that may result in retinal detachment and loss of vision.

For almost 30 years, proliferative retinopathy has been successfully treated with panretinal laser photocoagulation. In this procedure, multiple laser burns are induced in the peripheral, ischemic areas of the retina. After treatment, there is regression of the more proximal neovascular vessels, presumably as a result of eliminating the produc-tion of angiogenic factors by now photocoagulated cells. Until there is active retinal hemorrhage, most patients are assymptomatic, making screening and prevention para-mount. Patients generally should begin yearly dilated eye examinations within 3–5 years of diagnosis; type 2 patients should be examined at the time of diagnosis *(32)*. Pre-vention and lack of progression may be achieved by tight glucose control, as reported in the Diabetes Control and Complication Trial (DCCT) *(33)*. The DCCT also showed elegantly that the risk of retinopathy increases with each incremental rise in the glyco-sylated hemoglobin (HbA_{1c}) In addition, aggressive blood pressure control, particularly with angiotensin-converting enzyme (ACE) inhibitors, has been shown to be effective.

Nephropathy

Nephropathy remains an all too common complication of diabetes, with a lifetime incidence of 30–50%. Approximately 35% of cases of end-stage renal disease in the United States are caused by diabetic nephropathy. Fortunately, better understanding of the pathophysiology has led to improved screening for and detection of early nephropathy, and interventional treatment with ACE inhibitors has improved the outlook for the individual and the entire population with diabetes.

The pathogenesis of nephropathy is best understood by the hemodynamic hypothesis, as advanced by Zatz and Brenner *(34)*. At the time of onset of hyperglycemia, the glomerular filtration rate (GFR) increases from 120 to >140 mL/min in the average-sized individual. With this hyperfiltration of the nephrons, there is the development of compensatory renal hypertrophy. Over several years, alterations in the renal vasculature occur, with loss of negatively charged heparan sulfate binding sites and increased capillary permeability. This allows for leak of macromolecules that deposit in the mesangium, causing expansion of the mesangial matrix and proliferation of cellular elements. Subsequent capillary and glomerular sclerosis causes loss of functioning nephrons; the remaining individual units are stressed, with more hyperfiltration and intraglomerular hypertension. Thus a vicious cycle is established. Inexorable and progressive loss of functioning nephrons leads to single nephron hyperfiltration and further nephon injury. The hemodynamic hypothesis is the model that best explains the clinical progression of diabetic nephropathy. In addition, excessive production of the inflammatory growth factor transforming growth factor-β_1, has been under intense study and may play a role in the progressive renal injury *(35)*.

Microalbuminuria is the first clinical manifestation of incipient nephropathy, preceding renal insufficiency and azotemia by 8–10 years. Systemic hypertension may also occur in incipient nephropathy and, in turn, accelerate its progression. Ultimately, clinical diabetic nephropathy may develop, characterized by decreasing GFR, rising serum creatinine, and overt proteinuria of >300 mg/24 hr. It should be emphasized that serum creatinine is often reduced in early nephropathy because of the supranormal GFR; a minimal elevation in serum creatinine may indicate that significant nephropathy has developed.

Along with hyperglycemia, hypertension plays a significant causal role in the development of diabetic nephropathy. Unlike retinopathy, nephropathy is only partly related to disease duration: after 15 years of diabetes, the incidence may start to decline *(30)*. This may be related to the requisite covariable of hypertension. Quite simply, systemic hypertension may exacerbate the established intraglomerular hypertension seen in diabetic nephropathy. The observed higher prevalence in certain ethnic groups, for example, African Americans, can be explained by the clinical link of diabetes with the tendency to hypertension in these populations *(36)*.

The management of nephropathy relies on early detection through screening for microalbuminuria. This should be performed yearly; acceptable ranges are <30 mg/24 hr, <30 µg/mg creatinine, or <20 µg/min (timed) *(37)*. Aggressive treatment of hypertension to <130/85 has a renal sparing effect, as demonstrated in the UKPDS *(40)* and also shown with tightly controlling blood glucose. Perhaps the most significant population-based intervention in altering the course of nephropathy has been the use of ACE inhibitors, which, in addition to lowering blood pressure, specifically reduce hyperfiltration and intraglomerular hypertension. If instituted in a timely period, ACE inhibition may forestall the development of overt nephropathy by more than a decade *(39)*.

Macrovascular Complications

Diabetes is a major factor for the development of cardiovascular disease (CVD), increasing the relative risk by three- to four-fold. The leading cause of death in patients with diabetes is coronary artery disease. Other clinical manifestations of macrovascular complications are congestive heart failure, peripheral vascular disease of the lower extremities, and stroke. The relative risk of these complications is greater in women, resulting in a more equal male/female distribution than is found in the nondiabetic population, where CVD is predominant in men.

Many patients, primarily those with type 2 diabetes, will exhibit significant macrovascular disease at the time of diagnosis of diabetes. Moreover, IGT *per se* is an identifiable risk factor. These observations have led to the conceptual model of the *multiple metabolic syndrome* as the basis for most CVD seen in the type 2 diabetes population *(40)*. The cornerstone of this paradigm is the presence of insulin resistance. Indeed, it has long been observed that the major cardiovascular risk factors—diabetes, obesity, and hypertension—are all conditions of insulin resistance. Insulin resistance is also associated with the clinical constellation of glucose intolerance, central adiposity, dyslipidemia, hyperuricemia and a procoagulant state—the so-called syndrome X as defined by Reaven *(41)*. This clinical syndrome has proved to be responsible for a large portion of CVD-related complications in developed nations. It is now clear that the macrovascular complications of diabetes have their origins in metabolic abnormalities that precede the onset of clinical diabetes by years, or even decades. Insulin resistance appears to play a pivotal role.

One plausible explanation is the clustering of known cardiovascular risk factors within this patient population. Glucose intolerance, hypertension, dyslipidemia, central obesity, and a sedentary lifestyle often occur coincidently in the same individuals. In addition, the same individuals have higher circulating levels of plasminogen activator inhibitor-1 (PAI-1), resulting in a procoagulant state *(42)*. The importance of insulin resistance in the pathogenesis of CVD is supported by the recent observation that insulin-resistant IGT is associated with coronary risk factors but not IGT with normal insulin sensitivity *(43)*.

Perhaps the most intriguing observation in the pathogenesis of CVD in diabetes is the endothelial dysfunction and impaired vascular reactivity associated with insulin resistance. These abnormalities are ultimately associated with defective activity of nitric oxide pathways of endothelial-mediated vasodilation and can be seen in individuals with diabetes, as well as in other subjects with insulin-resistant states such as those with IGT and first-degree relatives of type 2 diabetes *(44)*.

The conceptual model of the multiple metabolic syndrome gives primacy to insulin resistance in the pathogenesis of macrovascular complications. What is provocative is the concept that diabetes may be only one manifestation of this central metabolic disturbance that may also express itself clinically as hypertension, obesity, dyslipidemia, endothelial dysfunction, and/or a procoagulant state. Individuals may present with some, many, or none of these clinical findings but nonetheless share a common metabolic syndrome responsible for the development of atherosclerosis.

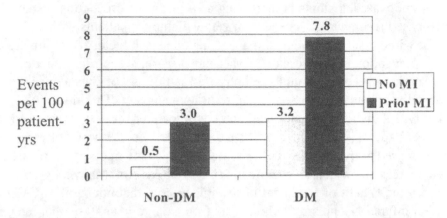

Fig. 5. Results of epidemiologic study comparing coronary event rates (fatal or nonfatal) in diabetic (DM) and nondiabetic (non-DM) cohorts. The striking observation is that the fatal and nonfatal occurrence rate of myocardial infarction (MI) for subjects with diabetes and no known history of MI is almost equal to the MI occurrence rate for nondiabetic individuals with a confirmed history of MI. This demonstrates the excess coronary risk imposed on individuals with diabetes. For patients with both diabetes and prior MI, the rate increases sharply to an even higher degree. (Adapted from: Haffner SM, Lehto S, Ronnemaa T, Pyorala K, Laakso M. Mortality from coronary heart disease in subjects with type 2 diabetes and in nondiabetic subjects with and without prior myocardial infarction. *N Engl J Med* 1998;339:229–234.)

Cardiovascular Disease and Diabetes

The macrovascular disease in diabetes has unique clinical characteristics. The atherosclerosis tends to be diffuse and more distal in location, affecting smaller sized vessels such as the coronary, the tibial trifurcation, and the internal carotid arteries. Patients may present with symptoms such as angina pectoris, claudication, or transient ischemic neurologic attacks. Unfortunately, many patients with vascular complications are relatively asymptomatic; this is often attributed to the coexistence of sensory neuropathy, which prevents full appreciation of pain and symptoms of ischemia. This is especially true for those individuals with coronary artery disease and "silent ischemia" of the myocardium. People with diabetes have a high prevalence of coronary disease. Haffner and colleagues *(45)* have strikingly observed that the risk of myocardial infarction in patients with diabetes alone is equal to that of nondiabetic patients with known coronary artery disease (Fig. 5). This makes screening and surveillance, especially for coronary disease, crucial in the long-term management of patients with diabetes.

Treatment of CVD in patients with diabetes is often surgical, because of the late presentation of patients and the significance of their underlying disease. Carotid endarterectomy, coronary artery bypass graft (CABG), and infrapopliteal bypass with saphenous vein are more frequently encountered in this population. Interventional procedures such as percutaneous balloon angioplasties of the coronary and iliofemoral arteries are performed but have an excessively high rate of restenosis within 1 year, making them less efficacious in the long-term management of coronary and vascular disease in diabetes. It has been unequivocally shown that CABG results in better long-term outcomes for patients with diabetes compared with percutaneous coronary angioplasty *(46)*. Presently, the use of endovascular stents is increasing as a means of preventing restenosis, but evidence-based recommendations are not yet available for patients with diabetes.

With or without surgery, medical management and risk factor reduction are essential in the prevention of progression of vascular disease. Weight loss, moderate exercise, and smoking cessation should be emphasized at the onset of diabetes and reinforced frequently throughout the course of long-term management. The impact of glycemic control in type 2 diabetes on macrovascular complications may be outweighed by that of control of hyperlipidemia and hypertension *(47)*. The lipid abnormalities in diabetes include increased triglyceride levels, decreased high-density lipoprotein (HDL) cholesterol, and increased low-density lipoprotein (LDL) cholesterol. Many long-term studies have shown the benefit of treatment of dyslipidemia in the reduction of CVD death, myocardial infarction, and stroke. It appears from subgroup analysis that the benefits of treatment of hyperlipidemia are greater for those patients with coexisting diabetes *(48)*. Because of the potential of prevention of cardiovascular events, optimal goals of treatment as recommended by the ADA are fairly stringent *(49)*. The ADA-recommended lipid levels are as follows:

1. LDL < 100 mg%
2. HDL: men > 45 mg%; women > 55 mg%
3. Triglycerides < 200 mg%.

Therapy should always include diet and lifestyle changes, but because most patients find it hard to achieve these goals, pharmacologic management with statins is usually required. Statins should be initiated promptly in any patient with known CVD. Hypertriglyceridemia can be managed with improved glycemic control, and if necessary, high-dose statins or fibrates *(48)*.

The beneficial impact of tight blood pressure control was recently found in the UKPDS *(50)*. A modest lowering of blood pressure (10 mmHg systolic) translated into significant reductions in deaths, congestive heart failure, and stroke. Patients were managed with either a β-blocker or an ACE inhibitor with equal efficacy. The results of the Heart Outcomes Prevention Evaluation (HOPE) study showed a 24% risk reduction in CVD end points in patients with diabetes receiving ramipril *(51)*. Because of these findings, as well as the known renal sparing effects of ACE inhibitors, they are often recommended for treating hypertension. It is the recommendation of the ADA to achieve a blood pressure of <130/80–85 mmHg *(52)*.

Because of the high prevalence of coronary artery disease (CAD) in patients with diabetes, screening recommendations are evolving to reduced thresholds for proceeding to exercise tolerance testing (ETT) or "stress test." These recommendations were derived at a consensus conference of the ADA on the evaluation of CAD in patients with diabetes *(53)*. Any typical or atypical symptom should serve as an indication for ETT. For asymptomatic patients, the presence of any other risk factors, an abnormal electrocardiogram, or any evidence of peripheral or carotid disease warrants an evaluation. Those patients with a high probability of significant CAD by ETT should proceed to coronary angiography. Those with low probability should be followed every 1–2 years. Intermediate- or moderate-risk patients may be better assessed with nuclear perfusion imaging with thallium for better specificity and risk stratification.

For those patients with diabetes who present with acute myocardial infarction, the use of β-blockers as an acute intervention to reduce mortality has been recommended. A long-term benefit has also been seen for use as a secondary intervention *(54)*. In addition, strict glycemic control may also be important. Interestingly, the Diabetes Mellitus Glucose Infusion in Acute Myocardial Infarction (DIGAMI) study showed a marked and significant reduction in deaths from myocardial infarction with the use of a glucose/insulin infusion to maintain glycemia between 126 and 196 mg% *(55)*. The initial infusion was followed by four subcutaneous insulin injections daily for 4 months. The benefit was seen over 5 years of follow-up observation. It is speculative but also possible that insulin *per se* has a cardioprotective effect through its action on endothelial-mediated vasodilatation.

Finally, the current understanding of an acute ischemic syndrome is that there is thrombus formation in an area of plaque disruption mediated by platelet aggregation. Diabetes may be viewed as a hypercoaguable state, part of the multiple metabolic syndrome. The benefits of daily intake of aspirin in reducing mortality in patients with diabetes and coronary artery disease have been observed, and in fact exceed those seen in nondiabetic patients *(56)*. Therefore, all patients with any risk should be placed on daily aspirin. For patients with CVD who fail or are intolerant of aspirin, antiplatelet treatment with ticlopidine or clopidrogrel should be considered.

MANAGEMENT OF DIABETES: GLYCEMIC CONTROL

Rationale and Goals of Treatment

Diabetes is a chronic metabolic disorder requiring long-term management and patient education to achieve an improved quality of life, to prevent acute complications, and to reduce the risk of chronic complications. The benefits of improved glycemic control are many. Correction of hyperglycemia reduces the likelihood of acute complications and decompensation into DKA or HHNK; it also relieves symptoms such as polyuria, polydipsia, blurry vision, and weight loss. The risks of developing microvascular complications (retinopathy, nephropathy, and neuropathy) are also reduced with improved glycemic control. For type 1 individuals, this was established by the Diabetes Control and Complications Trial (DCCT), in which the overall microvascular risk reduction was 50–75% *(57)*. There was no glycemic threshold for the development of microvascular complications, with benefit even at the lowest HbA_{1c}. Severe hypoglycemia limited the intensity of control. The UKPDS offers insight into treatment strategies for type 2 diabetes *(58)*. In this trial, 3867 patients with new-onset type 2 diabetes were randomized into intensive or standard treatment and followed for a median time of 10 years. In brief, the study showed a reduction in microvascular complications in the intensively treated group—a 35% risk reduction with a 1% drop in the HbA_{1c}. A trend toward a decrease in macrovascular complications was seen that reached significance only in the subgroup treated with metformin. As discussed previously, intensive treatment of hypertension significantly reduced macrovascular complications as well as microvascular end points.

Thus, it is clear that good glycemic control not only reduces acute complications of diabetes and improves the day-to-day life of the patient but also prevents the onset and

Table 2
Glycemic Guidelines of the American Diabetes Association

Biochemical index	Normal	Goal	Action suggested
Fasting blood glucose	<115 mg/dL	80–120 mg/dL	<80 or >140 mg/dL
Bedtime glucose	<120 mg/dL	100–140 mg/dL	<100 or >160 mg/dL
Hemoglobin A_{1c}	<6%	<7%	>8%

Data from ref. *59.*

progression of certain chronic complications. Because of these observations, the ADA presently recommends treatment goals of near normalization of blood glucose, with fasting glucose <120 mg% and HbA_{1c} 7%, and the additional action of pharmacologic treatment after diet and exercise if HbA_{1c} exceeds 8% *(59)* (Table 2). Some patients may be individualized to less stringent goals, such as the elderly, children, and those with comorbid conditions. For the prevention of macrovascular complications in type 2 diabetes, additional risk factor reduction and treatment of hypertension and dyslipidemia should be instituted as previously discussed.

Diet, exercise, and patient education are the fundamentals of the management of diabetes and should be emphasized in any and all treatment regimens. In the interest of parsimony, we will restrict our discussion to the pharmacologic management of diabetes. This should not be interpreted to mean that other therapies are subservient to pharmacology. In contrast, successful pharmacologic therapy depends on a foundation of a healthy lifestyle (diet and exercise) in a patient with good self-management skills.

Pharmacologic Treatment of Type 1 Diabetes

In type 1 diabetes, loss of β-cell mass renders the patient completely insulin dependent. There is no question as to whether to treat with insulin but only as to the choice of preparations and regimen. To achieve tight glycemic control, patients are generally required to use multidose regimens of intermediate- and short-acting insulin preparations in an attempt to mimic the fasting and postprandial blood glucose levels seen in normal individuals (Table 3).

The fundamental principle of insulin therapy is to attempt to recapitulate physiologic insulin secretion by providing a finite basal amount of insulin supplemented with mealtime bolus injections. Basal insulin is provided with long-acting insulin once daily (Ultralente, Glargine) or with twice daily injections of intermediate-acting insulin (NPH, Lente). When using twice daily intermediate-acting insulin, generally two-thirds of the total dose is given in the morning and one-third in the evening. Meal requirements are satisfied by short-acting insulin injections (Regular, Lispro, Aspart). Inhaled insulin may also provide rapid insulin coverage with meals. In general, with any insulin regimen used in type 1 diabetes, the average daily insulin requirement totals 0.6 U/kg (42 U for a 70-kg man). This provides a benchmark to guide the initiation and adjustment of insulin dosing.

Many patients benefit from the continuous subcutaneous insulin infusion (CSII) made possible with an insulin pump. CSII provides continuous basal insulin and allows for bolus amounts at mealtime. It predictably reduces daily insulin use by 25% because

Table 3
Action Timetable of Available Insulins

Insulin preparation	Onset (h)	Peak (h)	Duration (h)
Rapid-acting analog (Lispro)	5 min	45 min	4
Short-acting (regular)	30 min	2	5–8
Intermediate-acting (NPH or Lente)	1–3	6–12	16–24
Long-acting (Ultralente)	4–6	8–20	24–28
Long-acting analog (Glargine)	4–6	8–20	24–28
Mixtures (70/30 or 50/50)	30 min	6–12	16–24

of its efficiency and may reduce episodes of subclinical hypoglycemia (hypoglycemia unaware) seen with the multistick regimen (60).

Pharmacologic Treatment of Type 2 Diabetes

The principles of pharmacologic management of type 2 diabetes have been the subject of many reviews *(61)*, and they change with time as new concepts of treatment as well as new agents are introduced. Pharmacologic intervention is indicated when diet and exercise fail to attain desired goals of therapy, that is, $HbA_{1c} > 8\%$. Current treatment philosophy embraces polypharmacy to improve efficacy and reduce adverse effects of medications. The management should be flexible, with the understanding that correction of "glucose toxicity" results in a feedforward, positive feedback of improved insulin secretion and insulin action. Therefore, initial treatment is not binding, and adding and withdrawing treatments is typical.

The selection of pharmacologic agents is presently expanding. Because of this, the specific agents will not be addressed in detail, rather, the medications will be reviewed by class in terms of their clinical use. The observations of the UKPDS show benefits from intensive control of hyperglycemia but support no single pharmaceutical as superior to others, with the exception of the decrease in macrovascular end points seen in patients intensively treated with metformin *(62)*. It is important that treatment regimens then should be individualized and may not apply to all patients with type 2 diabetes.

Insulin

Insulin therapy is required in 10–30% of type 2 diabetes. The natural history is one of progressive loss of β-cell function and eventual failure of oral agents, making insulin treatment necessary after many years. In addition, there is heterogeneity in type 2 diabetes, with some patients actually demonstrating autoantibodies, suggesting type 1 β-cell destruction *(63)*. These patients are insulinopenic and have been shown to progress rapidly to insulin therapy.

Insulin can be used as monotherapy, or in combination with oral agents. Most commonly, nocturnal intermediate-acting insulin is used in combination with daytime oral agents. Insulin regimens may also be used to achieve tight glycemic control in type 2 diabetes, similar to regimens used in type 1. Another regimen for tight control would utilize rapid-acting insulin analogs solely to minimize postprandial hyperglycemia. Finally, in symptomatic patients in whom glycemia exceeds 300 mg% and glucose toxicity is present, temporary intervention with exogenous insulin may be necessary. This may reverse the defect in endogenous insulin secretion and action, restoring euglycemia. Afterwards, the patient may be safely withdrawn from therapy and placed on an oral agent.

Oral Agents

Oral agents have become the most common treatment modality for type 2 diabetes and are often used in combination. From the UKPDS we have learned that monotherapy for type 2 diabetes is unlikely to achieve tight control after a few years of treatment *(64)*. Therefore, combination regimens are necessary as well as desirable for many patients. When a two-drug regimen fails, often a third drug or insulin will be added. Combinations should capitalize on the synergy of using drugs with different mechanisms of action (Table 4). The three basic mechanisms are stimulation of insulin secretion, inhibition of hepatic glucose production, and improvement in insulin sensitivity. A list of oral agents and appropriate doses is also presented (Table 5).

SULFONYLUREAS

As a class, sulfonylureas have been in use for decades and remain the most potent oral hypoglycemics. The mechanism of action is stimulation of insulin secretion, which in turn inhibits hepatic glucose production and increases muscle glucose uptake. Earlier findings of improved insulin sensitivity were probably an indirect result of the improved glycemia and correction of glucose toxicity. Sulfonylureas are well tolerated but carry a risk of hypoglycemia, especially in elderly patients and those with renal disease.

METFORMIN

A second-generation biguanide, metformin, has less reported lactic acidosis than its predecessor, phenformin. Metformin lowers glycemia primarily by inhibiting hepatic glucose production and to a lesser extent by increasing insulin sensitivity in muscle *(65)*. This causes some decrease in plasma insulin. It has some salutary effects on lipids and may cause weight loss, making it the preferable agent for use in obese patients. As mentioned, the UKPDS suggested that metformin monotherapy may have added benefits in prevention of macrovascular end points. The major side effects are gastrointestinal disturbances, which are generally self-limited and transient.

THIAZOLIDINEDIONES: ROSIGLITAZONE AND PIOGLITAZONE

Since troglitazone was withdrawn from the marketplace because of hepatotoxic events, two thiazolidinediones have been introduced in the United States: rosiglitazone and pioglitazone. The mechanism of action is improvement of insulin sensitivity through the stimulation of peroxisome proliferator-activated receptor-γ (PPAR-γ), resulting in increased expression of glucose transporters *(66)*. These "insulin sensitizers" also have some effect in reducing hepatic glucose production. They are used in combination with other agents or as monotherapy. Thiazolidinediones are particularly useful in reducing insulin dose in poorly controlled patients. They are probably not as potent for monotherapy as sulfonylureas or metformin. Adverse effects on hepatic function are of potential concern.

MEGLITINIDES: REPAGLINIDE AND NATEGLINIDE

A non-sulfonylurea, repaglinide is a rapid acting insulin secretagogue that can be complimentary when used in combination with metformin and thiazolidinediones. It is

Table 4
Mechanism of Action and Metabolic Effects of Oral Agents for Type 2 Diabetes Therapy

	Sulfonylureas	Meglitinides	Metformin	Thiazolidinediones	Acarbose
Mechanism of action	Increase in insulin secretion	Increase in insulin secretion	Decrease in hepatic glucose production; increase in muscle insulin sensitivity	Increase in muscle insulin sensitivity; decrease in hepatic glucose production	Delayed absorption of dietary carbohydrates
Decrease in FPG (mg/dL)	60–70	60–70	60–70	35–40	20–30
Decrease in HbA$_{1c}$ (%)	1.5–2.0	1.5–2.0	1.5–2.0	1.0–1.2	0.7–1.0
LDL level	No effect	No effect	Decrease	Increase	No effect
HDL level	No effect	No effect	Increase	Increase	No effect
Triglycerides	No effect	No effect	Decrease	Decrease	No effect
Body weight	Increase	Increase	Decrease	Increase	No effect
Plasma insulin	Increase	Increase	Decrease	Decrease	No effect
Adverse events	Hypoglycemia	Hypoglycemia	GI disturbances; lactic acidosis	Anemia; hepatic toxicity	GI disturbances

FPG, fasting plasma glucose; LDL, low-density lipoprotein; HDL, high-density lipoprotein.
Adapted from ref. *61*.

Table 5
Oral Agents for Type 2 Diabetes Therapy

Oral agent	Starting dose (mg)	Maximum dose (mg)	Duration of action (h)
Sulfonylureas			
Chlorpropamide	250 qd	500 qd	60
Tolbutamide	250 bid	1000 tid	6–12
Tolazamide	100 qd	500 bid	12–24
Glyburide	2.5–5 qd	10 bid	16–24
Glipizide	5 qd	20 bid	12–24
Glimeperide	1–2 qd	8 qd	24
Thiazolidinediones			
Rosiglitazone	2 qd	8 qd	3–4 wk
Pioglitazone	15 qd	45 qd	3–4 wk
Meglitinides			
Repaglinide	1.5 tid	4 tid	4–6
Nateglinide	30 tid	180 tid	4
Metformin	500 bid	850 tid	3–4 wk
Acarbose	25 tid	100 tid	4

particularly helpful in reducing post-prandial hyperglycemia. It has more hypoglycemic potential when used in combination with metformin *(67)*. Nateglinide is a phenylalanine analogue that stimulates insulin secretion, but only in the presence of glucose *(68)*. It thus has little hypoglycemic potential. It is also short acting. Meglitinides are used increasingly as more attention is being directed towards the importance of postpradial hyperglycerimia in glycemic control and chronic complications.

Acarbose

The use of acarbose, an alpha-glycosidase inhibitor that delays the absorption of dietary carbohydrate, is limited by the frequency of gastrointestinal side effects of diarrhea and flatulence. Its effect is primarily on post-prandial hyperglycemia and dampening the swings in daytime glycemia. It has been used successfully in combination with other agents and insulin, but has received FDA approval only as monotherapy.

APPROACH TO THE SURGICAL PATIENT WITH DIABETES

The patient with diabetes poses a complex logistic management problem when hospitalized, especially in the event of surgery and anesthesia. Not only are there associated morbidities and complications of diabetes that require evaluation, there is also the unpredictable effect of the stress of surgery and intercurrent illness on glycemic control. The only treatment guideline that is universally accepted is that management allows for flexibility and feedback. After general considerations are reviewed, the focus of the remaining discussion will be on the unique issues of surgical patients with diabetes, in particular those with foot and lower extremity disease.

Preoperative Assessment

Evaluation of the patient with diabetes in anticipation of surgery should include the same principles of preoperative assessment used in all patients, with the expectation of frequent associated comorbidities. In the patients with neuropathy and foot disease, there are usually attendant microvascular and macrovascular complications. Although an attempt should be made to optimize the medical condition prior to surgery, this is often not feasible because of the extent of the comorbidities and the urgency of the procedure. Indeed, if the patient is medically unstable, with infection and altered hemodynamics, this is more often an indication than a contraindication for necessary surgery.

Microvascular Complications

Although most concern is directed toward macrovascular complications, as will be discussed, microvascular disease should be evaluated for its impact on the perioperative course. *Nephropathy* may result in abnormal fluid retention and electrolyte disturbances, especially hyperkalemia from type IV renal tubular acidosis (hyporeninemic hypoaldosteronism). Renal disease allows for a prolonged clearance of anesthetic drugs, and anemia can be a consequence of poor erythropoetin secretion. Proteinuria and subclinical nephropathy incur a risk of acute tubular necrosis after radiologic procedures utilizing contrast; patients should be well hydrated and volume replete prior to any angiography *(69)*. Patients with end-stage renal disease have impaired wound healing and are at high risk for limb amputation. They also pose difficulties for vascular surgery because of generalized arterial and soft tissue calcification from an increased calcium-phosphorous product.

In neuropathic patients, *autonomic neuropathy* contributes to more frequent cardiac arrhythmias and confers a risk of aspiration in those with gastroparesis. *Sensory neuropathy* is the primary cause of most foot ulcers and infections, but it may fortuitously permit less anesthesia, allowing more use of spinal, regional, and local methods. Patients with *retinopathy* should be assumed to have significant microvascular abnormalities ubiquitously. In addition, microalbuminuria has been found to be an independent cardiovascular risk factor and may be a marker of impaired vascular reactivity and endothelial dysfunction *(70)*. This has implications for impaired cutaneous microcirculation and healing.

Cardiovascular Risk: Assessment and Management

Perhaps the single most important preoperative assessment is that for coronary disease. Diabetes confers by itself an odds ratio of 2–4 for significant coronary disease compared with the nondiabetic population. As mentioned, the risk of fatal and nonfatal myocardial infarction in the general population with diabetes is equal to that of the nondiabetic population with known coronary disease that has had a prior myocardial infarction *(71)*. In the surgical group with peripheral vascular disease, approximately two-thirds will have concomitant coronary artery disease that should be addressed.

Several clinical guidelines and position papers have been drafted to assist in the assessment and perioperative management of patients with coronary disease *(72)*. Although none specifically addresses the issues of the patient with diabetes, certain common features can be gleaned that may be generalizeable. The noncardiac procedures that pose the greatest risk to the patient with coronary disease are emergency procedures and peripheral vascular surgery. For patients with diabetes, lower extremity vascular surgery has an associated death and cardiac complication rate of as high as 10%; for aortic procedures the rate increases to as high as 25% *(73).*

In addition to the type of procedure, the preoperative assessment of risk should include identification of potentially serious heart disease such as prior myocardial infarction or angina, prior coronary revascularization, congestive heart failure, and significant arrhythmia. Each of these conditions confers added risk of cardiac end points postoperatively. Advanced age (>70 years) is *per se* an added risk factor. When these historical features are considered, along with the general history of comorbid conditions (e.g., renal disease, chronic obstructive pulmonary disease), the physical exam, functional capacity, and the resting electrocardiogram, a fairly accurate assessment of low risk versus high risk can be made *(74).* This Bayesian approach to probability of coronary disease has been advocated as a simple and reliable method of risk stratification.

In patients of indeterminant or intermediate risk, further preoperative testing may be necessary. Echocardiography may identify patients with left ventricular dysfunction. A low ejection fraction (<35%) increases the risk of non-cardiac surgery *(75).* Both exercise and pharmacologic stress testing may assist in the evaluation, especially in stratifying patients of indeterminate or moderate risk. The most useful noninvasive evaluation is perfusion nuclear imaging with thallium. Patients increase their risk stratification if there are more than two reversible perfusion defects on thallium imaging. For patients with diabetes, the most important independent predictors of postoperative death are advanced age, resting electrocardiographic abnormalities, and thallium abnormalities *(76).* It should be noted that in patients with diabetes who are undergoing peripheral vascular surgery, the prevalence of thallium imaging abnormalities is high. In a study of patients with diabetes undergoing vascular surgery at the Deaconess Hospital in Boston, >90% of patients with clinical evidence of cardiac disease had abnormal dipyridimole thallium scans, whereas >50% of those without clinical disease had abnormalities *(77).* The clinical caveat is that all patients with diabetes undergoing vascular surgery should be managed with a high index of suspicion for significant coronary artery disease, whether or not noninvasive testing is performed.

The High-Risk Patient

A more complex decision tree presents when a patient is identified as high risk. Proceeding to invasive testing and coronary angiography rests on the decision of whether to commit the patient to CABG or percutaneous transluminal coronary angioplasty (PTCA). This decision is generally based on three probabilities: the prior Bayesian probability of CAD, the risks of the revascularization procedure, and the risks of the proposed surgery. It is generally felt that with close monitoring, the high-risk patient going directly to vascular surgery will fare better in terms of all outcomes than the same patient subjected to the potential morbidity and mortality of presurgical coronary angiography and revascularization followed by vascular surgery *(78).* This is even truer for less risky surgical procedures. Therefore, the short-term benefit of preoperative coronary revascularization is usually outweighed by the combined risks of both coronary revacularization and the intended operative procedure. Patients should not have coronary surgery solely in preparation for another noncardiac procedure.

It should be remembered, however, that coronary revascularization has evidence-based proof of benefit for long-term survival in selected patients. The American College of Cardiology/American Heart Association include in their recommendations for CABG patients with unstable angina, triple-vessel or left main CAD, and two-vessel with left anterior descending disease *(79)*. Patients should be evaluated for coronary revascularization by the clinical criteria for long-term prognosis independent of the preoperative evaluation. This also holds true for PTCA, which is less commonly advocated for patients with diabetes because of the high restenosis rate and less favorable outcomes compared with CABG *(80)*. The use of coronary stents is increasingly added to PTCA, but prospective data for short-term benefits of perioperative stent placement are lacking.

β-BLOCKERS

For the high-risk patient, use of β-blockers is becoming more routine. One recent study of perioperative β-blockade in high-risk patients undergoing vascular surgery showed a striking reduction in myocardial infarction and death *(81)*. In this prospective randomized trial, patients with abnormal thallium reperfusion imaging were randomized to bisoprolol or placebo prior to peripheral vascular surgery. There was a significant reduction in perioperative and inhospital mortality, which persisted throughout the treatment period of 6 months. A similar, although less dramatic, effect was previously reported with the use of atenolol *(82)*. Most observers consider that the beneficial results are class effects of β-blockers rather than specific drug effects.

If these clinical results are substantiated with more general use, the preoperative management of the high-risk patient, especially with diabetes, will be more simplified and will focus on vigilant perioperative monitoring and routine use of β-blockers. This philosophy of care has already been adopted at many centers with busy vascular surgery sections. The preoperative evaluation of coronary disease is evolving to a Bayesian evaluation of clinical risk and prior probability of disease, with or without noninvasive studies such as pharmacologic nuclear perfusion imaging or echocardiography *(83)*. The high-risk patient could then be initiated on β-blockade and followed closely during and after surgery. For low-risk patients or for those undergoing low-risk procedures, good medical support and vigilance should be sufficient. These simple clinical approaches require little ancillary testing, eliminate most invasive angiography, and should result in a substantial decrease in postoperative coronary events. One should realize, however, that even in the best circumstances, the mortality rates of vascular surgery in the high-risk patients with diabetes would most likely remain a finite quantity of 1–2%.

Glycemic Control in the Surgical Patient: Rationale

The most important consideration in the rationale for glycemic control in the perioperative period is to avoid the acute dangers of hypoglycemia, hyperglycemia, and ketoacidosis. After providing sound medical management, the question remains of how tight the glycemic control should be. Although the benefits of tight control have been documented in the prevention of long-term complications of diabetes by the DCCT and the UKPDS, the short-term benefits of near normal glycemia are not as clear in the perioperative period. The potential benefits versus demands of the increased resource utilization and risks of hypoglycemia with tight control should be assessed individually.

Infection

One concern is the increased risk of perioperative infection in patients with diabetes; however, this may be multifactorial and only partly a result of hyperglycemia. Many in vitro studies have demonstrated impaired chemotaxis of neutrophils, generally at glucose concentrations above 240 mg%. This concentration has thus been used as the high water mark for perioperative control. The clinical translation of an observed decrease in infection rates following surgery has been lacking. Hyperglycemia in the postoperative patient with diabetes has been associated with an increased risk of infection and this suggests that hyperglycemia *per se* is an independent risk factor for infection *(84)*. However, in a study in cardiac surgery patients, tighter control of hyperglycemia resulted only in a "trend" to fewer infections *(85)*.

The issue may be of less priority in patients hospitalized for foot disease, who are often already receiving systemic antibiotic therapy for infections and in whom surgery often treats infection rather than causes it. It should be underscored that hyperglycemia may also be a clinical sign of concurrent infection. Therefore, hyperglycemia should be considered as a factor associated with infection and may prove to be either a clear cause or a consequence.

Wound Healing

The effects of glycemic control on wound healing are even less well documented. Diabetes clearly contributes to faulty wound healing, but this may be attributed to associated factors such as infection, macrovascular disease, and microvascular disease *(86)*. Acute corrections in glycemia are likely to be of minor consequence in changing these impairments to healing. Animal models have shown impaired healing of acute wounds in diabetes, but these findings may not be generalizable as these animals are more moribund than their human counterparts.

Of interest and perhaps of more importance in impaired healing is the contribution of the low tissue oxygen tension that may be observed in the wounds of some patients with diabetes. This can be explained by poor oxygen delivery because of macrovascular and microvascular disease. Low oxygen tension has also been found to be a predictor of subsequent surgical wound infection *(87)*. Recently the use of supplemental perioperative oxygen has resulted in a decrease in abdominal surgical wound infections. In this study, patients who were breathing 80% oxygen during surgery and for 2 hr afterwards had nearly 60% less infections than those randomized to receiving 30% oxygen *(88)*. Supplemental oxygen may prove to be a useful adjunct in postoperative wound healing and prevention of infection. It is premature to recommend routine use, as no similar prospective data are yet available for surgical patients with diabetes.

Insulin Infusion

There is growing interest in the effects of insulin *per se* on operative outcomes independent of glycemic control. As mentioned previously, the DIGAMI study demonstrated a beneficial effect on cardiac events and death in diabetic patients with acute myocardial infarction who received glucose and insulin infusion acutely, followed by intensive insulin therapy for several months *(89)*. One hypothesis posed by observers is that insulin *per se* may account for some of this beneficial effect independent of the improved glycemia. Insulin has vasodilatory actions mediated through endothelial nitric oxide synthase *(90)*, and it is postulated that insulin infusion may have salutary effects on tissue hypoxia. In one study in diabetic patients undergoing coronary bypass, insulin infusion resulted in better glycemic control and less deep infections than in patients given subcutaneous insulin *(91)*. Insulin infusion may also have beneficial effects on neutrophil function *(92)*. A prospective study is needed to determine whether insulin infusion is beneficial in surgical patients with diabetes who are at high risk for infection and poor wound healing.

In summary, the benefits of tight glycemic control in the perioperative period in terms of infection and wound healing are only partly evidence based and must be considered in light of the risks of hypoglycemia and the costs of resource utilization and personnel to deliver the care. For most clinicians, it is acceptable to maintain the glucose level during surgery between 150 and 200 mg% to avoid hypoglycemia and to continue this into the postoperative period. For those desiring tight glycemic control, this is probably best achieved by intravenous insulin infusion, as will be discussed, but at this time, it can only be recommended for a minority of patients (outside of those with type 1 diabetes).

The Glucose Balancing Act

In approaching the surgical patient with diabetes, the attention is often initially directed to the issue of restriction of oral intake to prevent emesis and aspiration. Usually, the first intervention is the reduction of insulin and pharmacologic treatment to avoid hypoglycemia during and after surgery. It should be emphasized, however, that the stress and metabolic consequences of surgery often result in an increased insulin requirement *(93)*. In patients undergoing surgery, marked and significant increases in the levels of counterregulatory hormones are seen. These include growth hormone, glucagon, cortisol, epinephrine, and norepinephrine. In addition, gluconeogenic precursors such as lactate, amino acids, and free fatty acids are increased. In nondiabetic patients, this is accompanied by marked increases in insulin and C-peptide levels, reflecting an increased secretion of insulin to compensate for the metabolic changes. Insulin also prevents associated protein breakdown and catabolism and promotes protein synthesis. These metabolic changes are generally resolved and near normal by the day following surgery, provided no subsequent physiologic stress is superimposed.

In the patient with diabetes, the challenge of these metabolic changes may not be met adequately with increased insulin secretion. The most predictable consequence of the elevation in counterregulatory hormones is an increase in hepatic glucose output from both increased gluconeogenesis and release of stored glycogen. The gluconeogenesis is fueled by the increases in plasma lactate, amino acids, and free fatty acids and can result in hyperglycemia—*despite the restricted oral intake in the surgical patient.* Furthermore, the acute worsening of insulin resistance impairs glucose uptake and utilization by muscle. In the type 1 patient, these metabolic demands in the setting of little or absent insulin can result in increased ketogenesis and ketoacidosis.

Thus, it is not surprising that the most common error in the management of the patient with diabetes undergoing surgery is an excessive reduction of insulin dose for fear of hypoglycemia from food restriction. The endogenous glucose and ketone production during the stress of surgery may actually increase insulin requirements and acutely decompensate glycemic control. The net glycemic outcome is a balancing act between the counterregulatory hormones and stress, driving the glucose up, and the caloric restriction and medications, driving it down. Whatever treatment regimen is chosen, the lack of predictability makes the feedback of frequent glucose monitoring essential for glycemic control.

Treatment Regimens for Glycemic Control During Surgery

Intravenous Insulin Infusion

This regimen is generally reserved for insulin-requiring patients who are undergoing surgical procedures of long duration, or for patients who are unstable, with poor glycemic control *(94)*. In patients in whom tight glycemic control is desired, intravenous insulin infusion is usually preferable to subcutaneous insulin injection in that better glycemic control is achieved, usually with lesser insulin dosage *(95)*. This is especially true of the commonly prescribed "sliding scale" of subcutaneous dosing, which is inferior to intravenous infusion in terms of hyperglycemic and hypoglycemic episodes. Insulin infusion permits a more adjustable and dynamic treatment method.

The different infusion regimens have their advocates, but none has clearly been shown to be superior. The two most commonly utilized are the combined glucose-potassium-insulin infusion and the separate glucose and insulin infusion. The former is based on a 500-mL mixture of 10% dextrose, 10 mmol potassium, and 15 U crystalline zinc insulin. The infusion is initiated at 50 mL (1.5 U) hourly and then titrated to the blood glucose. Mean dosage is 3.2 U/h. Increased doses are required in infected patients, obese patients, and those on corticosteroids *(96)*. Glucose-potassium-insulin protocols are favored for their predictability and ease of use.

Separate glucose and insulin infusions are used to regulate each variable more specifically. Insulin is infused from 0.5 to 5 U each hour. It is useful and reassuring to recall from pathophysiology that the usual hepatic glucose production rate in the fasting state is 2 mg/kg/min, and that peripheral glucose uptake is maximized at an insulin infusion of 0.1 U/kg/h. In a 70-kg individual, one can be confident that a glucose infusion rate >8.4 g/h (84 mL of D10W/h) will prevent most hypoglycemia. The insulin dose in the same individual should not exceed 7 U/h. One practical issue is the adherence and nonspecific binding of insulin to the intravenous plastic tubing, so precise dosing is not feasible, and adaptability and responsiveness to frequent glucose monitoring are required.

Finally, there are advocates of intermittent insulin bolus of 10 U every 2 h and adjustment according to glycemic response *(97)*. This is simpler but less precise in achieving control. Again, much depends on the goals of therapy: to achieve a glycemic level between 150 and 200 mg% during surgery, bolus therapy should be sufficient.

Subcutaneous Insulin Regimens

All type 1 patients and many type 2 patients are insulin requiring, and subcutaneous insulin for these patients is appropriate in the setting of brief, less complicated procedures. This is especially true of a morning procedure with a prompt recovery time to allow the patient to resume meals. Generally, patients are given one-half to two-thirds of their usual morning dose in the form of intermediate-acting insulin (NPH or Lente). Patients should not receive short-acting insulin (Regular, Lispro, os Aspart) unless they are unstable, with hyperglycemia.

As previously stated, insulin requirements usually increase with the stress of surgery despite the absence of oral intake. Thus, patients are usually undertreated with insulin so as to avoid hypoglycemia and often require supplemental insulin immediately after surgery. If the procedure is delayed more than a few hours, intravenous glucose at 5–10 g/h (2 mg/kg/min) should prevent hypoglycemia. Patients who are receiving CSII pump therapy should be maintained on their usual basal infusion rate, with an anticipation of increasing the rate postoperatively to compensate for the metabolic stress of surgery.

Regimens for Type 2 Diabetes Control

For the type 2 patient who is on nonpharmacologic (diet, exercise) or pharmacologic therapy, insulin treatment during or after surgery may be required to correct hyperglycemia, and management should allow for that possibility. Patients are normally maintained on their usual regimens. Oral agents used to control glycemia have been reviewed previously. Generally, oral hypoglycemic drugs are not given on the morning of surgery and are safely resumed postoperatively. It should be noted that the hypoglycemic effect of sulfonylureas might persist after the drug is eliminated, and there is some hypoglycemic risk even if the dose is held. If medication is taken the day of surgery, close monitoring with or without glucose infusion is appropriate. Much effort has been expended to avoid use of metformin within 48 h of surgery or contrast injection because of concerns of precipitating lactic acidosis. Recently, an estimate of the incidence of lactic acidosis in metformin users was placed at 9/100,000 patient-years, suggesting that this concern is overstated *(98)*, and that surgery should not be postponed or delayed if a patient has been inadvertently given metformin.

Glycemic Regimens in the Postoperative Period

The maintenance of satisfactory glycemic control is highly individualized and is dependent on the rapidity of recovery, the stress of surgery and/or infection, and the ability to consume dietary regimens. If supplemental insulin is required, it is best to give intermediate-acting insulins that work physiologically to control endogenous glucose production. Bedtime dosing is especially useful in type 2 patients to normalize the fasting blood glucose and reversing the "glucose toxicity" of hyperglycemia in impairing insulin secretion. Short-acting insulins may be necessary but should not be used solely in sliding scale coverage schedules. Without the reservoir of longer acting insulin, the patient may be unprotected for 4–6 h with short-acting insulin regimens, allowing time for hyperglycemia and ketosis to develop. There is evidence that sliding scale insulin regimens, when utilized solely, frequently result in more episodes of hyperglycemia *(99)*. Sliding scale insulin regimens should be used on a base of long- or intermediate-acting insulin, or in combination with oral agents. The metabolic consequences of uncomplicated surgery should be normalized within 48 h, allowing a rapid return to the patient's preoperative regimen.

CONCLUSIONS

In conclusion, the management of the surgical patient with diabetes should be based on a knowledge of the pathophysiology of diabetes and on an assessment of its chronic complications. Of most concern in achieving satisfactory outcomes should be the presence of cardiovascular disease and avoidance of perioperative myocardial infection. In patients undergoing high-risk procedures, a clinical Bayesian approach of establishing prior probability of coronary artery disease, with or without ancillary noninvasive testing, can accurately assess risk. High-risk patients should be treated with β-blockers. All patients should be managed with a high index of suspicion for coronary disease and appropriate monitoring. Good glycemic control will prevent acute complications such as DKA and hypoglycemia, but there is no clear evidence that it will improve wound healing or prevent infection. There are no widely accepted guidelines for glycemic management in the perioperative period. What is agreed is that the treatment regimens employed must be flexible and adaptable to the feedback of frequent glucose monitoring. The benefits of tight glycemic control should be viewed with respect for the utilization of resources required to deliver the care. With proper awareness of expected consequences of surgery and with heightened vigilance for postoperative complications, surgical outcomes for patients with diabetes should continue to improve.

REFERENCES

1. Kenny SJ, Aubert RE, Geiss LS. Prevalence and incidence of non-insulin-dependent diabetes, in *Diabetes in America* (Harris MI, ed.), National Institutes of Health, Washington, DC, 1995, pp. 37–46.
2. Mokdad AH, Ford ES, Bowman BA, et al. Diabetes trends in the U.S.: 1990–1998. *Diabetes Care* 2000;23:1278–1283.
3. Harris MI, Flegal KM, Cowie CC, et al. Prevalence of diabetes, impaired glucose tolerance in U.S. adults. The third National Health and Nutrition Examination Survey, 1988–1994. *Diabetes Care* 1998;21:518–524.
4. Zimmet PZ. Kelly West Lecture 1991. Challenges in diabetes epidemiology—from the west to the rest. *Diabetes Care* 1992;15:232–252.
5. Neel JV. Diabetes mellitus: a thrifty genotype rendered detrimental by progress? *Am J Hum Genet* 1962;14:353–362.
6. Expert Committee for the Diagnosis and Classification of Diabetes Mellitus. *Diabetes Care* 1997;20:1183–1197.
7. Harris MI. Prevalence of retinopathy since time of diagnosis of type 2 Diabetes: WESDR Study, 1980–1988. *Consultant* 1997;37(Suppl):S9–S14.
8. Turner R, Stratton I, Horton V, et al. UKPDS 25: autoantibodies to islet-cell cytoplasm and glutamic acid decarboxylase for prediction of insulin requirement in type 2 diabetes. UK Prospective Diabetes Study Group. *Lancet* 1997;350:1288–1293.
9. Eisenbarth GS. Type I diabetes mellitus—a chronic autoimmune disease. *N Engl J Med* 1986;314:1360–1368.
10. Coutant R, Carel JC, Timsit J, Boitard C, Bougneres P. Insulin and the prevention of insulin-dependent diabetes mellitus. *Diabetes Metab* 1997;23(Suppl 3):25–28.
11. Eisenbarth GS. Lilly Lecture 1986. Genes, generator of diversity, glycoconjugates and autoimmune beta-cell insufficiency in type I diabetes. *Diabetes* 1987;36:355–364.
12. Dalhquist GG. Primary and secondary prevention strategies of pre-type 1 diabetes. Potentials and pitfalls. *Diabetes Care* 1999;22(Suppl 2):B4–B6.
13. Rosenbloom AL, Joe JR, Young RS, Winter WE. Emerging epidemic of type 2 diabetes in youth. *Diabetes Care* 1999;22:345–354.
14. Gulli G, Ferrannini E, Stern M, Haffner S, DeFonzo RA. The metabolic profile of NIDDM is fully established in glucose-tolerant offspring of two Mexican-American NIDDM parents. *Diabetes* 1992;41:1575–1586.

15. DeFronzo RA, Tobin JD, Andres R. Glucose clamp technique: a method for quantifying insulin secretion and resistance. *Am J Physiol* 1979;237:E214–E223.
16. DeFronzo RA. Lilly Lecture 1987. The triumvirate: beta-cell, muscle, liver. A collusion responsible for NIDDM. *Diabetes* 1988;37:667–687.
17. Weyer C, Bogardus C, Mott DM, Pratley, RE. The natural history of insulin secretory dysfunction and insulin resistance in the pathogenesis of type 2 diabetes mellitus. *J Clin Invest* 1999;104:787–794.
18. DeFronzo RA, Bonadonna RC, Ferrannini E. Pathogenesis of NIDDM. A balanced overview. *Diabetes Care* 1992;15:318–368.
19. Rossetti L. Glucose toxicity: the implications of hyperglycemia in the pathophysiology of diabetes mellitus. *Clin Invest Med* 1995;18:225–260.
20. Buse JB, Polonsky KS. Diabetic ketoacidosis, hyperglycemic hyperosmolar nonketotic coma, and hypoglycemia, in *Principles of Critical Care Medicine,* 2nd ed. (Hall JBM, Schmidt GA, Woods LDH, eds.), McGraw-Hill, New York, 1998, pp. 1183–1193.
21. Arieff AI, Carroll HJ. Nonketotic hyperosmolar coma with hyperglycemia: clinical features, pathohysiology, renal function, acid-base balance, plasma-cerebrospinal fluid equilibria and the effects of therapy in 37 cases. *Medicine* 1972;51:73–94.
22. Buse JB. The patient with diabetes, in *Management of Office Emergencies* (Barton CW, ed.), McGraw-Hill, New York, 1999, pp. 73–95.
23. Cranston I, Lomas J, Maran A, MacDonald I, Amiel SA. Restoration of hypoglycaemia awareness in patients with long-duration insulin-dependent diabetes. *Lancet* 1994;344: 283–287.
24. The Diabetes Control and Complications Trial Research Group. The effect of intensive treatment of diabetes on the development and progression of long-term complications in insulin-dependent diabetes mellitus. *N Engl J Med* 1993;329:977–986.
25. Zatz R, Brenner BM. Pathogenesis of diabetic microangiopathy. The hemodynamic view. *Am J Med* 1986;80:443–453.
26. Greene DA, Lattimer SA, Sima AA. Sorbitol, phosphoinositides, and sodium-potassium-ATPase in the pathogenesis of diabetic complications. *N Engl J Med* 1987;316:599–606.
27. Brownlee M. The pathological implications of protein glycation. *Clin Invest Med* 1995;18: 275–281.
28. Schmidt AM, Yan SD, Wautier JL, Stern D. Activation of receptor for advanced glycation end products: a mechanism for chronic vascular dysfunction in diabetic vasculopathy and atherosclerosis. *Circ Res* 1999;84:489–497.
29. Koya D, King GL. Protein kinase C activation and the development of diabetic complications. *Diabetes* 1998;47:859–866.
30. Krolewski AS, Warram JH, Rand Li, Kahn CR. Epidemiologic approach to the etiology of type I diabetes mellitus and its complications. *N Engl J Med* 1987;317:1390–1398.
31. Aiello LP, Avery RL, Arrigg PG, et al. Vascular endothelial growth factor in ocular fluid of patients with diabetic retinopathy and other retinal disorders. *N Engl J Med* 1994;331: 1480–1487.
32. Diabetic Retinopathy, ADA Position Statement. *Diabetes Care* 2000;23(Suppl 1):S73–S76.
33. The Diabetes Control and Complications Trial Research Group. The effect of intensive treatment of diabetes on the development and progression of long-term complications in insulin-dependent diabetes mellitus. *N Engl J Med* 1993;329:977–986.
34. Zatz R, Brenner BM. Pathogenesis of diabetic microangiopathy. The hemodynamic view. *Am J Med* 1986;80:443–453.
35. Border WA, Noble NA. Evidence that TGF-beta should be a therapeutic target in diabetic nephropathy. *Kidney Int* 1998;54:1390–1391.
36. Cowie CC, Port FK, Wolfe RA, et al. Disparities in incidence of diabetic end-stage renal disease according to race and diabetes. *N Engl J Med* 1989;321:1074–1079.

37. Diabetic Nephropathy, ADA Position Statement. *Diabetes Care* 2000;23(Suppl 1):S69–S72.
38. UK Prospective Diabetes Study. Tight blood pressure control and risk of macrosvacular and microvascular complications in type 2 diabetes: UKPDS 38. *BMJ* 1998;317:703–713.
39. Viberti G, Mogensen CE, Groop LC, Pauls JF. Effect of captopril on progression to clinical proteinuria in patients with insulin diabetes mellitus and microalbuminuria. European Microalbuminuria Captopril Study. *JAMA* 1994;271:275–279.
40. Zimmet P, Boyko EJ, Collier GR, de Courten M. Etiology of the metabolic syndrome: potential role of insulin resistance, leptin resistance, and other players. *Ann NY Acad Sci* 1999;892:25–44.
41. Reaven GM. Pathophysiology of insulin resistance in human disease. *Physiol Rev* 1995; 75:473–486.
42. Meigs JB, Mittleman MA, Nathan DM, et al. Hyperinsulinemia, hyperglycemia, and impaired hemostasis: the Framingham Offspring Study. *JAMA* 2000;283:221–228.
43. Haffner SM, Mykkanen L, Festa A, Burke JP, Stern MP. Insulin-resistant prediabetic subjects have more atherogenic risk factors than insulin-sensitive prediabetic subjects: implications for preventing coronary heart disease during the prediabetic state. *Circulation* 2000; 101:975–980.
44. Steinberg HO, Chaker H, Leaming R, et al. Obesity/insulin resistance is associated with endothelial dysfunction. Implications for the syndrome of insulin resistance. *J Clin Invest* 1996;97:2601–2610.
45. Haffner SM, Lehto S, Ronnemaa T, Pyorala K, Laakso M. Mortality from coronary heart disease in subjects with type 2 diabetes and in nondiabetic subjects with and without prior myocardial infarction. *N Engl J Med* 1998;339:229–234.
46. Comparison of coronary bypass surgery with angioplasty in patients with multivessel disease. The bypass angioplasty revascularization investigation (BARI) investigators. *N Engl J Med* 1996;335:217–225.
47. Turner RC. The U.K. Prospective Diabetes Study. A review. *Diabetes Care* 1998;21(Suppl): C35–C38.
48. Haffner SM. Management of dyslipidemia in adults with diabetes (technical review). *Diabetes Care* 1998;21:160–178.
49. Management of Dyslipidemia in Adults with diabetes, position statement, American Diabetes Association. *Diabetes Care* 2000;Suppl:S32–S42.
50. UK Prospective Diabetes Study Group. Efficacy of atenolol and captopril in reducing risk of macrovascular complications in type 2 diabetes, UKPDS 39. *BMJ* 1998;317:713–720.
51. Effects of ramipril on cardiovascular and microvascular outcomes in people with diabetes mellitus: results of the HOPE study and MICRO-HOPE substudy. Heart Outcomes Prevention Evaluation Study Investigators. *Lancet* 2000;355:253–259.
52. Standards of medical care for patients with diabetes mellitus, position statement, American Diabetes Association. *Diabetes Care* 2000;23(Suppl):S32–S42.
53. Consensus development conference on the diagnosis of coronary heart disease and diabetes: February 10–11, 1998, Miami, Florida, American Diabetes Association. *Diabetes Care* 1998;21:1551–1559.
54. Tse WY, Kendall M. Is there a role for beta-blockers in hypertensive diabetic patients? *Diabet Med* 1994;11:137–144.
55. Malmberg K. Prospective randomised study of intensive insulin treatment on long term survival myocardial infarction in patients with diabetes mellitus. DIGAMI (Diabetes Mellitus Glucose Infusion in Acute Myocardial Infarction) Study Group. *BMJ* 1997;314:1512–1515.
56. Harpaz D, Gottlieb S, Graff E, et al. Effects of aspirin treatment on survival in non-insulin-dependent diabetic patients with coronary artery disease. Israeli Bezafibrate Infarction Prevention Study Group. *Am J Med* 1998;105:494–499.
57. The absence of a glycemic threshold for the development of long-term complications: the perspective of the Diabetes Control and Complications Trial. *Diabetes* 1996;45:1289–1298.

58. UK Prospective Diabetes Study Group. Intensive blood-glucose control with sulphonyl-ureas or insulin compared with conventional treatment and risk of complications in patients with type 2 diabetes (UKPDS 33). *Lancet* 1998;352:857–853.

59. Standards of medical care for patients with diabetes mellitus, position statement, American Diabetes Association. *Diabetes Care* 2000;23(Suppl):S32–S42.

60. Bode BW, Steed RD, Davidson PC. Reduction in severe hypoglycemia with long-term continuous subcutaneous insulin infusion in type I diabetes. *Diabetes Care* 1996;19:324–327.

61. DeFronzo RA. Pharmacologic therapy for type 2 diabetes mellitus. *Ann Intern Med* 1999; 31:281–303.

62. UK Prospective Diabetes Study. Effect of intensive blood-glucose control with metformin on complications in overweight patient with type 2 diabetes (UKPDS 34). *Lancet* 1998;352: 854–865.

63. Turner R. Stratton I, Horton V, et al. UKPDS 25: autoantibodies to islet-cell cytoplasm and glutamic acid decarboxylase for prediction of insulin requirement in type 2 diabetes. UK Prospective Diabetes Study Group. *Lancet* 1997;350:1288–1293.

64. Turner RC, Cull CA, Frighi V, Holman RR. Glycemic control with diet, sulfonylurea, metformin, or insulin in patients with type 2 diabetes mellitus: progressive requirement for multiple therapies (UKPDS 49), UK Prospective Diabetes Study (UKPDS) Group. *JAMA* 1999;281:2005–2012.

65. DeFronzo RA, Barzilai N, Simonson DC. Mechanism of metformin action in obese and lean non-insulin-dependent diabetic subjects. *J Clin Endocrinol Metab* 1991;73:1294–1301.

66. Spiegelman BM. PPAR-[gamma]: adipogenic regulator and thiazolizinedione receptor. *Diabetes* 1998;47:507–514.

67. Moses R, Slobodniuk R, Boyages S, et al. Effect of repaglinide addition to metformin monotherapy on glycemic control in patients with type 2 diabetes. *Diabetes Care* 1999;22:119–124.

68. Dunn CJ, Faulds D. Nateglinide. *Drugs* 2000;60:607–615.

69. Manske CL, Spraka JM, Strony JT, Wang Y. Contrast nephropathy in azotemic diabetic patients undergoing coronary angiography. *Am J Med* 1990;89:615–620.

70. Tooke JE. Microvascular function in human diabetes: a physiological perspective. *Diabetes* 1995;44:721–726.

71. Haffner SM, Lehto S, Ronnemaa T, Pyorala K, Laakso M. Mortality from coronary heart disease in subjects with type 2 diabetes and in nondiabetic subjects with and without prior myocardial infarction. *N Engl J Med* 1998;339:229–234.

72. Palda VA, Detsky AS. Perioperative assessment and management of risk from coronary artery disease. *Ann Intern Med* 1997;127:313–328.

73. Hood DB, Weaver FA, Papnicolaou G, Wadhawani A, Yellin AE. Cardiac evaluation of the diabetic patient prior to peripheral vascular surgery. *Ann Vasc Surg* 1996;10:330–335.

74. Fleisher LA, Eagle KA. Screening for cardiac disease in patients having noncardiac surgery. *Ann Intern Med* 1996;124:767–772.

75. Eagle KA, Brundage BH, Chaitman BR, et al. Guidelines for perioperative cardiovascular evaluation for noncardiac surgery: an abridged version of the report of the American College of Cardiology/American Heart Association Task Force on Practice Guidelines. *Mayo Clin Proc* 1997;72:524–531.

76. Cohen MC, Curran PJ, L'Italien GJ, Mittleman MA, Zarich SW. Long-term prognostic value of preoperative dipyridamole thallium imaging and clinical indexes in patients with diabetes mellitus undergoing peripheral vascular surgery. *Am J Cardiol* 1999;83:1038–1042.

77. Zarich SW, Cohen MC, Lane SE, et al. Routine perioperative dipyridamole 201T1 imaging in diabetic patients undergoing vascular surgery. *Diabetes Care* 1996;19:355–360.

78. Mangano DT. Assessment of the patient with cardiac disease: an anesthesiologist's paradigm. *Anesthesiology* 1999;91:1521.

79. Guidelines and indicators for coronary artery bypass graft surgery: a report of the American College of Cardiology/American Heart Association Task Force on Assessment of Diagnostic and Therapeutic Cardiovascular Procedures (Subcommittee on Coronary Artery Bypass Graft Surgery). *J Am Coll Cardiol* 1991;17:543–589.

80. Comparison of coronary bypass surgery with angioplasty in patients with multivessel disease. The bypass angioplasty revascularization investigation (BARI) investigators. *N Engl J Med* 1996;335:217–225.

81. Poldermans D, Boersma E, Bax JJ, et al. The effect of bisoprolol on perioperative mortality and myocardial infarction in high-risk patients undergoing vascular surgery. Dutch echocardiographic cardiac risk evaluation applying stress echocardiography study group. *N Engl J Med* 1999;341:1789–1794.

82. Mangano DT, Layug EL, Wallace A, Tateo I. Effect of atenolol on mortality and cardiovascular morbidity after non cardiac surgery. *N Engl J Med* 1996;335:1713–1720.

83. Mehat RH, Bossone E, Eagle KA. Perioperative cardiac risk assessment for noncardiac surgery. *Cardiologia* 1999;44:409–418.

84. Pomposelli JJ, Baxter JK III, Babineau TJ, et al. Early postpoperative glucose control predicts nosocomial infection rate in diabetic patients. *JPEN J Parenter Enteral Nutr* 1998;22: 77–81.

85. Golden SH, Peart-Vigilance C, Kao L, Brancati FL. Perioperative glycemic control and the risk of infectious complications in a cohort of adults with diabetes. *Diabetes Care* 1999;22: 1408–1414.

86. Diabetic Foot Wound Care, consensus statement, American Diabetes Association. *Diabetes Care* 1999;22:1354–1360.

87. Hopf JW, Hunt TK, West JM, et al. Wound tissue oxygen tension predicts the risk of wound infection in surgical patients. *Arch Surg* 1997;132:997–1004.

88. Greif R, Akca O, Horn HP, Kurtz A, Sessler DI. Supplemental perioperative oxygen to reduce the incidence of surgical-wound infection. *N Engl J Med* 2000;342:161–167.

89. Malmberg K. Prospective randomised study of intensive insulin treatment on long term survival myocardial infarction in patients with diabetes mellitus. DIGAMI (Diabetes Mellitus Glucose Infusion in Acute Myocardial Infarction) Study Group. *BMJ* 1997;314:1512–1515.

90. Zeng G, Quon MJ. Insulin-stimulated production of nitric oxide is inhibited by wortmannin. Direct measurement in vascular endothelial cells. *J Clin Invest* 1996;98:894–898.

91. Furnary AP, Zerr KJ, Grunkemeier GL, Starr A. Continuous intravenous insulin infusion reduces the incidence of deep sternal wound infection in diabetic patients after cardiac surgical procedures. *Ann Thorac Surg* 1999;67:353–360.

92. Rassias AJ, Marrin CA, Arruda J, et al. Insulin infusion improves neutrophil function in diabetic cardiac surgery patients. *Anesth Analg* 1999;88:1011–1016.

93. Rümelin A, Nietgen M, Pirlich PT, et al. Postoperative pattern of various hormonal and metabolic variables. *Curr Med Res Opin* 1999;15:339–348.

94. Jacober SJ, Sowers JR. An update on perioperative management of diabetes. *Arch Intern Med* 1999;159:2405–2411.

95. Kaufman FR, Devgan S, Roe TF, Costin G. Perioperative management with prolonged intravenous insulin infusion versus subcutaneous insulin in children with type I diabetes mellitus. *J Diabetes Complications* 1996;10:6–11.

96. Alberti KG, Gill GV, Elliott MJ. Insulin delivery during surgery in the diabetic patient. *Diabetes Care* 1982;5(Suppl 1):65–77.

97. Husban DJ, Thai AC, Alberti KGMM. Management of diabetes during surgery with glucose-insulin-potassium infusion. *Diabetic Med* 1986;3:69–74.

98. Stang M, Wysowski DK, Butler-Jones D. Incidence of lactic acidosis in metformin users. *Diabetes Care* 1999;22:925–927.

99. Queale WS, Seidler AJ, Brancati FL. Glycemic control and sliding scale insulin use in medical inpatients with diabetes mellitus. *Arch Intern Med* 1997;157:545–552.

2

Epidemiology and Health Care Costs of Diabetic Foot Problems

Gayle E. Reiber, MPH, PhD

INTRODUCTION

The frequency of nontraumatic lower limb amputations in persons with diabetes has increased in the United States over the last decade. Currently two-thirds of all lower limb amputations occur in individuals with diagnosed diabetes. High geographic variation in age, sex, and race-adjusted amputation rates across U.S. populations suggest that important differences in practice patterns exist and that some patients may be receiving suboptimal care. Amputations reduce patient function and quality of life and place a heavy burden on individuals, families, and health care systems. In this chapter the epidemiology and risk factors for two major diabetic foot problems, ulcers and lower limb amputations, are described. Foot ulcer and amputation hospital discharge data are presented from two major U.S. surveys, the Nationwide Inpatient Sample (NIS), a database that also includes utilization and charge information, and the National Hospital Discharge Survey (NHDS) *(1,2)*. Comparisons between persons with and without diabetes are clearly specified. Findings from analytic and experimental studies that used multivariable modeling techniques to determine risk factors are presented. The chapter concludes with information on the economic impact of diabetic foot problems.

EPIDEMIOLOGY OF FOOT ULCERS

Foot ulcers result from various etiologic factors and are characterized by an inability to self-repair in a timely and orderly manner *(3)*. The 1997 U.S. NIS indicated that 3.2% of the hospital discharges in persons with diabetes were for chronic lower limb ulcers *(1)*.

Wide variation has been reported in incidence (new onset) and prevalence (history) of diabetic foot ulcers. Table 1 shows that the annual, population-based incidence of diabetic foot ulcers in different populations ranges from 1.0 to 4.1%, and the prevalence of foot ulcers ranges from 5.3 to 10.5% *(4–8)*. The lifetime risk for foot ulcers in persons with diabetes is estimated at 15% *(9)*.

The anatomic location of a foot lesion has both etiologic and treatment implications. Table 2 presents data from two large prospective studies showing that the most common ulcer sites were the toes (dorsal or plantar surface), followed by the plantar metatarsal heads *(10,11)*. The authors caution that ulcer severity is more important than

From: *The Diabetic Foot: Medical and Surgical Management*
Edited by: A. Veves, J. M. Giurini, and F. W. LoGerfo © Humana Press Inc., Totowa, NJ

Table 1
Population-Based Diabetic Foot Ulcer Incidence and Prevalence from Select Studies

Author	Population studied	Annual incidence/100	Prevalence/100
Borssen et al. *(4)*	375 patients, Umea County, Sweden; age 15–50 yr; type 1 = 298, type 2 = 77	2.0	10.0 IDDM 9.0 NIDDM
Kumar et al. *(5)*	Cross-sectional study of 811 type 2 patients from three UK cities	1.0	5.3
Moss et al. *(6)*	Cohort of 2990 patients with late- and early-onset diabetes	2.4 younger 2.6 older	9.5 younger 10.5 older
Ramsey et al. *(7)*	Nested case-control study in HMO, 8905 type 1, type 2	1.9	—
Walters et al. *(8)*	Cross-sectional study of 1077 type 1, 2 patients in 10 UK general medicine practices	4.1	7.4

Table 2
Anatomic Site and Outcome of Diabetic Foot Lesions in Two Prospective Studies

	All lesions (%) n = 314; Apelqvist et al. *(46)*[a]	Most severe lesion (%) n = 302; Reiber et al. *(11)*[b]
Lesion site, %		
Toes (dorsal and plantar surface)	51	52
Plantar metatarsal heads, midfoot and heel	28	37
Dorsum of foot	14	11
Multiple ulcers	7	NA
Total	100	100
Lesion outcomes, %		
Reepithelialization/primary healing	63	81
Amputation at any level	24	14
Death	13[c]	5
Total	100	100

[a]Study included consecutive patients whose lesions were characterized according to Wagner criteria from superficial nonnecrotic to major gangrene.
[b]Study patients were enrolled with a lesion through the dermis that could extend to deeper tissue.
[c]Includes eight amputees who had not yet met the 6-month healing criteria.

ulcer site in determining the final outcome *(10)*. Although foot ulcers healed in most of these patients, amputations occurred in 14% of the U.S. and 24% of the Swedish patients. The deaths in these study subjects were unrelated to the foot ulcer and were attributed to other comorbidity.

Diabetic foot ulcer conditions in the U.S. NIS include chronic ulcers, superficial and deep infections of the foot, and osteomyelitis. Figure 1 shows more foot ulcer hospital discharges in persons without diabetes than in those with diabetes. Even though there are approx 100,000 fewer hospital discharges annually in persons with diabetes, this group represents only about 5% of the U.S. population. Figure 2 shows the trend in hospital

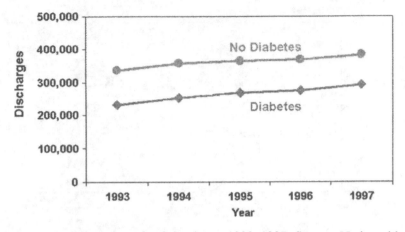

Fig. 1. U.S. hospital discharges for foot ulcers, 1993–1997. Source: Nationwide Inpatient Sample *(1)*.

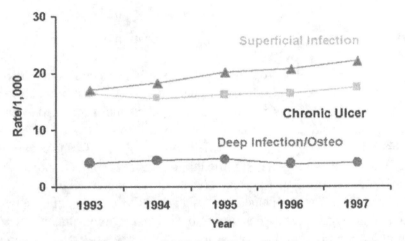

Fig. 2. U.S. hospital discharge rate/1000 for diabetic foot ulcers by condition, 1993–1997. Source: Nationwide Inpatient Sample *(1)*.

discharges for people with diabetes for the specified ulcer conditions. Increases were noted in superficial infections and chronic ulcers, whereas deep infections and osteomyelitis remained relatively constant over the interval. Figure 3 shows that NIS hospital discharge rates rose consistently from the youngest age group to the oldest age group. The second national data source, the NHDS, documented higher hospital ulcer discharge rates in males than females and year to year variation in discharges in rates for white and nonwhite individuals, with neither group consistently higher *(12)*.

Independent risk factors for diabetic foot ulcers from analytic and experimental studies using multivariable modeling techniques were identified. Results, summarized in Table 3, show that the most consistent independent foot ulcer risk factors were long diabetes duration, measures of peripheral neuropathy, measures of peripheral vascular disease, prior foot ulcer, and prior amputation. Long duration of diabetes, even after controlling for age, was a statistically significant finding in several studies *(5,8,13)*. In the study by Rith-Najarian et al. *(13)*, long duration of diabetes increased the risk of

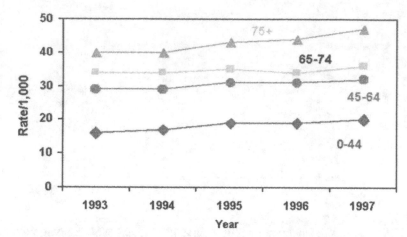

Fig. 3. U.S. hospital discharge rate/1000 for foot ulcers in people with diabetes by age, 1993–1997. Source: Nationwide Inpatient Sample *(1)*.

foot ulcers sixfold when persons with a diabetes duration of ≤9 years were compared with those with a duration of ≥20 years *(13)*.

Assessment of peripheral neuropathy is performed using several semiquantitative and quantitative measures and neurologic summary scores. Associations between peripheral neuropathy and foot ulcers are uniform across the studies reported in Table 3. In a randomized clinical trial using vibration perception threshold (VPT) ≥25 as an entry criteria, Abbott and colleagues *(14)* identified both baseline VPT and a combined score of reflexes and muscle strength as significant predictors of incident ulcers. Studies by Boyko et al. *(15)* and Rith-Najarian et al. *(13)* identified increased ulcer risk in patients unable to detect the 5.07 monofilament, a semiquantitative measure of light touch. There was no statistically significant association with ulcer risk in three other studies *(8,14,16)*.

Peripheral vascular function was measured as absent pulses, transcutaneous oxygen tension (TcPO$_2$), and low ankle-arm index (AAI). These variables appeared in the final ulcer prediction model in several studies. Low TcPO$_2$ indicating diminished skin oxygenation, and low ankle-arm index AAI, suggesting impaired large vessel perfusion, were both independent predictors of foot ulcers in the study by Boyko et al. *(15)*. However, in this study, laser Doppler flowmetry did not predictor foot ulcer. Kumar et al. *(5)* defined peripheral vascular involvement as the absence of two or more foot pulses or a history of previous peripheral revascularization. They reported that this variable was a significant predictor of foot ulcers. Walters et al. *(8)* found that an absent dorsalis pedis pulse was associated with a 6.3-fold increased risk of foot ulcer (95% CI 5.57–7.0).

Only one of three studies measuring HbA$_{1c}$ or blood glucose reported an association with foot ulcers. A cohort study by Moss et al. *(6)*, identified a statistically significant association between high levels of HbA$_{1c}$ and subsequent foot ulcers, odds ratio 1.6 (95% CI 1.3–2.0). Three of the studies reported in Table 3 address the relationship between foot deformity and subsequent foot ulcer. The study by Boyko et al. *(15)* found an independent association between Charcot deformity and foot ulcer, but other foot deformities were not independent ulcer predictors. Foot deformity did not enter the final analytic model in the studies by Litzelman et al. *(17)* and Rith-Najarian et al. *(13)*.

Table 3
Risk Factors for Foot Ulcers in Patients with Diabetes Mellitus from the Final Analysis Models of Select Studies

Author and type of analysis	Study design, diabetes type	Long DM duration	Neuropathy (monofilament, reflex, vibration, or neurologic summary score)	Low AAI, $TcPO_2$ or absent pulses	High HbA_{1c}	Deformity	Smoking	History Ulcer	History Amputation
Abbott et al. (14) Cox regression analysis	RCT, patients with VPT ≥ 25; (US, UK, Canada), type 1 = 255, type 2 = 780	0	0 Monofilament + VPT + Reflex	Exclusion criteria				Exclusion criteria	Exclusion criteria
Boyko et al. (15) Cox regression analysis	Cohort, veterans, type 1 = 48, type 2 = 701	0	+ Monofilament	+ AAI +$TcPO_2$	0	+ Charcot	0	+	+
Kumar et al. (5) Logistic regression	Cross-sectional, 811 type 2 from UK, general practices	+	+ NDS	+			0	0	+
Litzelman et al. (17) GEE	RTC, 352 type 2 patients	0	+ Monofilament		0	0		+	Exclusion criteria
Moss et al. (6) Logistic regression	Cohort, 2990 patients with early- and late-onset diabetes	Borderline older			+		Borderline older		
Pham et al. (16) Logistic regression	Cohort, 248 patients at three sites	Control variable	+ NDS + VPT + monofilament 0 Monofilament	Control variable					
Rith-Najarian et al. (13) Chi-square analysis	Cohort, 358 type 2 Chippewa Indians	+	+ Monofilament			0			
Walters et al. (8) Logistic regression	Cohort, 10 UK general practices, 1077 types 1, 2	+	+ Absent light touch + Impaired pain, perception 0 VPT	+ Absent pulses 0 Doppler			0		

blank, not studied;
+, statistically significant finding;
0, no statistically significant finding.
GEE, generalized estimating equations

AAI, ankle arm index;
DM, diabetes;
HbA_{1c}, hemoglobin A_{1c};
NDS, neuropathy disability score;

RCT, randomized controlled trial;
$TcPO_2$, transcutaneous oxygen tension;
VPT, vibration perception threshold;

The relationship between smoking and foot ulcers was assessed in four studies reported in Table 3; however, it was only of borderline significance in the younger population in the Wisconsin study *(6)*. The risk associated with a prior history of ulcers and amputations was assessed in three studies. Boyko et al. *(15)* and Litzelman et al. *(17)* reported that a prior history of ulcers significantly increased the likelihood of a subsequent ulcer. Kumar et al. *(5)* reported a relationship between prior amputation and subsequent ulcer. The cohort study of Boyko et al. *(15)* also identified higher body weight, insulin use, and history of poor vision as three additional independent predictors of foot ulcer.

Health care access and availability of diabetes education has been reported to influence development of foot ulcers. In the Litzelman et al. *(17)* randomized trial of a county hospital population, intervention patients were allocated to education, behavioral contracts, and reminders, while concurrently their providers received special education and chart prompts. The control population received usual care and education. After 1 year, patients in the intervention group reported more appropriate foot self-care behaviors, including inspection of feet and shoes, washing of feet, and drying between toes. Not all desirable behaviors were adopted. There was no significant difference between patient groups in testing bath water temperature and reporting foot problems. Patients in the intervention group developed fewer serious foot lesions including ulcers than did those in the control group *(17)*.

Foot ulcer recurrences were addressed in a U.K. study by Mantey and colleagues *(18)*. Diabetic patients with an initial foot ulcer and two ulcer recurrences were compared with diabetic patients who had only one ulcer and no recurrences over a 2-year interval. The authors' reported greater peripheral sensory neuropathy and poor diabetes control in the ulcer recurrence group. Members of the ulcer recurrence group waited longer after observing a serious foot problem until seeking care and consumed more alcohol than did the group without ulcer recurrences *(18)*.

In summary, foot ulcer frequency and rates increased in the United States between 1993 and 1997. Peripheral neuropathy and its sequelae, a long duration of diabetes and peripheral vascular disease, are the most consistent risk factors for predicting a foot ulcer. Reulceration occurred in about 60% of persons with prior ulcers and was more common accompanying severe peripheral neuropathy, high alcohol consumption, poor blood glucose control, and delays in seeking ulcer care.

EPIDEMIOLOGY OF LOWER LIMB AMPUTATION

The frequency of discharges for nontraumatic lower limb amputations in persons with and without diabetes according to the 1993–1997 NIS is shown in Figure 4. The combined NIS and Veterans Health Administration hospital discharges for persons with and without diabetes are presented in Table 4. In total, of the 134,677 discharges for nontraumatic lower extremity amputations in the United States in 1997, two-thirds were performed in persons with diabetes. Only 47% of amputations in persons with diabetes were major amputations (transtibial and transfemoral) compared with 70% in persons without diabetes. This suggests that amputations performed for vascular indications in persons without diabetes were performed at higher, more disabling levels. Figure 5 illustrates the frequency of lower limb amputation by level in persons with diabetes and

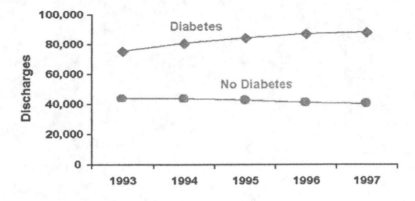

Fig. 4. U.S. hospital discharges for nontraumatic lower limb amputations, 1993–1997. Source: Nationwide Inpatient Sample *(1)*.

Table 4
Number and Percent of U.S. Amputation Discharges
by Diabetes Status and Amputation Level, 1997

	Nationwide Inpatient Survey	VA	Total	Percent
Diabetes				
Minor amputations	46,680	1987	48,667	53
Major amputations	41,661	1678	43,339	47
Subtotal	(88,341)	(3665)	(92,006)	(68)
No Diabetes				
Minor amputations	12,128	574	12,702	30
Major amputations	28,574	1405	29,979	70
Subtotal	(40,702)	(1997)	(42,681)	(32)
Total	129,043	5644	134,687	100

U.S. nationwide inpatient sample *(1)*; Veterans Health Administration Patient Treatment File *(61)*.

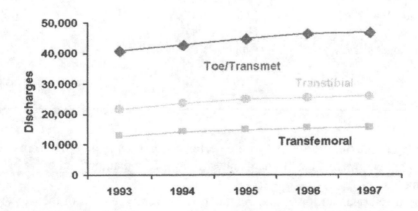

Fig. 5. U.S. hospital discharges for nontraumatic lower limb amputation by level for persons with diabetes, 1993–1997. Source: Nationwide Inpatient Sample *(1)*.

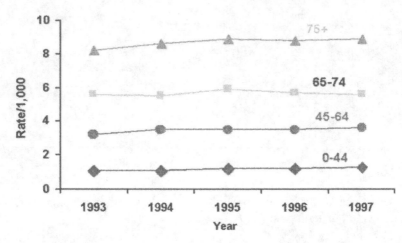

Fig. 6. U.S. hospital discharge rate/1000 for major diabetic nontraumatic lower limb amputations by age, 1993–1997. Source: Nationwide Inpatient Sample *(1)*.

Table 5
Age-Adjusted Population-Based Incident Amputation Rates
in Persons with Diabetes from Select Studies

Study	Population studied	Incidence rate/1000
Humphrey et al. *(19)*, ARG	Nauru	7.6
Humphrey et al. *(20)* LL	Rochester, MN, USA	3.8
Lehto et al. *(21)*	East and West Finland	8.0
Morris et al. *(22)*	Tayside, Scotland	2.5
Moss et al. *(40)*	Wisconsin, USA	
	Younger onset diabetes	5.1
	Older onset diabetes	7.1
Nelson et al. *(23)*	Pima Indians, USA	13.7
Siitonen et al. *(24)*	East Finland	3.4 Men
		2.4 Women
Trautner et al. *(25)*	Leverkusen, Germany	2.1
Van Houtum et al. *(26)*	California, USA	4.9
	Netherlands	3.6
Rith-Najarian et al. *(13)*	Chippewa Indians, USA	
	1986–89	21
	1990–93	12
	1994–96	6

documents that the majority (53%) were performed at the toe, ray, and transmetatarsal level. Figure 6 shows that the discharge rates for lower limb amputation were higher with advancing age.

Age-adjusted rates for lower limb amputations differ by regions of the world. Table 5 shows the variation across populations in age-adjusted incidence rates for nontraumatic lower limb amputations in persons with diabetes. The rates range from 2.1/1000 to 13.7/1000, a sixfold difference *(19–26)*.

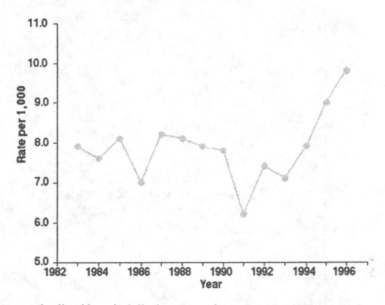

Fig. 7. Age-standardized hospital discharge rate for nontraumatic lower limb amputations in persons with diabetes, U.S., 1983–1996. (Source: National Hospital Discharge Survey, CDC.)

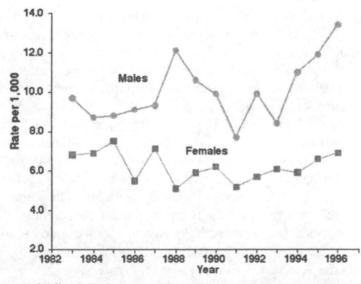

Fig. 8. Age-standardized discharge rate for nontraumatic lower limb amputation in persons with diabetes, by gender, U.S., 1983–1996. (Source: National Hospital Discharge Survey, CDC.)

Trends observed in National Hospital Discharge Survey data for nontraumatic lower limb diabetic amputation in the United States are provocative *(2)*. Figure 7 shows that the U.S. 1996 age-adjusted amputation rate in persons with diabetes was 9.8/1000, an increase of 26% from 1990 *(27)*. Figure 8 presents NHDS findings showing that age-standardized amputation rates were higher in males than females; Figure 9 shows that blacks had consistently higher amputation rates than whites *(2)*.

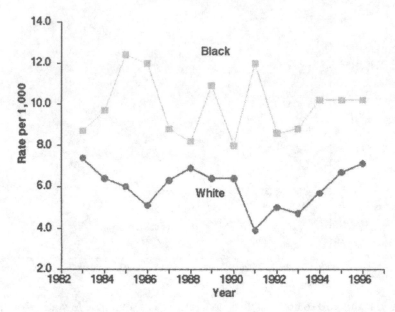

Fig. 9. Age-standardized hospital discharge rate for nontraumatic lower limb amputation in persons with diabetes, by race, U.S., 1983–1996. (Source: National Hospital Discharge Survey, CDC.)

Amputations in black and white Americans with and without diabetes were analyzed in the National Health and Nutrition Examination Survey Epidemiologic Follow-up Study. Black subjects constituted 15.2% of the cohort and accounted for 27.8% of the amputations. After controlling for the impact of education, hypertension, and smoking, incident and prevalent diabetes were statistically significant predictors of lower limb amputation, but race was not *(28)*.

In the United States there are 306 U.S. hospital referral regions which reflect geographic catchment areas served by major hospitals. Among Medicare recipients with diabetes who underwent a major (transtibial and transfemoral) amputation, there was an 8.6-fold variation in age, sex, and race-adjusted amputation rates, as shown in Figure 10 *(28)*. Only four surgical procedures exhibit higher variation than major amputation in persons with diabetes: lower extremity revascularization, carotid endarterectomy, back surgery, and radical prostatectomy *(29)*. Reasons for the wide variation in procedure rates include discipline-specific training, which may advocate for more or less aggressive limb salvage strategies. Some health care organizations have systems for prophylactic management of diabetic individuals with high-risk foot conditions. Providing this care over time may delay or prevent some foot ulcers and resultant amputations. Another factor is the experience and judgment of the surgeon is in selecting amputation level, surgical technique, and timing of the amputation. These decisions also influence the 10–15% of patients who require a subsequent amputation during the same hospitalization. Patient preferences are also important. Finally, the implication of twofold higher hospital reimbursement for amputation than limb salvage will be discussed later.

Variation in 1994 hospital discharge amputation rates, for people with diabetes in Wisconsin, shows blacks had 3.1 times, and American Indians had 4.4 times the ampu-

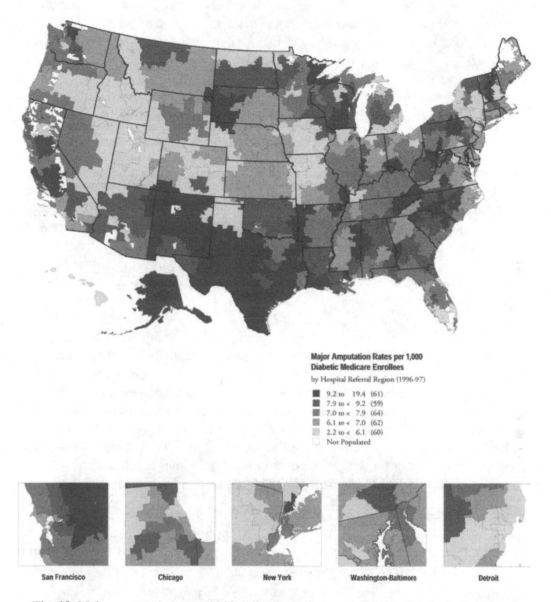

Fig. 10. Major amputation rates/1000 diabetic medicare enrollees by hospital referral region (1996–1997).

tation rates of whites *(31)*. Findings from a 1991 California hospital discharge survey indicated that the age-adjusted amputation rate was 4.4/1000 in Hispanics, 5.6 in non-Hispanic whites, and 9.5/1000 in African Americans *(32)*. In California, amputations in African-Americans were performed at higher levels than in persons from other ethnic and racial groups *(33)*. The importance of education, access to care, and socioeconomic status deserve consideration when assessing racial and ethnic differences and amputations. Both a case-control study performed on patients from a large California health maintenance organization and a prospective case-control study in veterans reported no difference in amputation rates by racial and ethnic status. Patients in these health care systems had access to HMO or VA health care *(34,35)*.

Risk factors for amputation from nine analytic studies that used multivariable analysis are summarized in Table 6. Major independent risk factors are long duration of diabetes, select measures of neuropathy and peripheral vascular disease, high levels of HbA_{1c} or fasting plasma glucose, and a history of ulcers, amputations, and retinopathy *(21,23,34–40)*. The two protective factors identified were provision of outpatient diabetes education *(34)* and use of aspirin *(40)*. Evidence for these risk factors follows.

Long duration of diabetes was a significant risk factor for amputation in five of the nine studies, and in one it was used as a risk adjuster. Risk for amputation increased with increasing duration of diabetes *(21,23,35,38,39)*.

Diminished or absent peripheral sensation decreases patients awareness of foot pressure, discomfort, and even pain and increases the risk of ulceration and amputation *(41)*. Several measures of peripheral neuropathy were identified as risk factors for amputation. Insensitivity to the 5.07 (10 g) Semmes-Weinstein monofilament was found to increase amputation risk in several studies. However, in the study by Adler et al. *(36)* this was only significant in the analysis model using $TcPO_2$. Other measures of peripheral neuropathy associated with amputation risk were absent or diminished bilateral vibration sensation or absent ankle reflexes *(21,34)*.

Measures of peripheral perfusion most commonly employed were AAI, which was associated with lower extremity arterial disease regardless of other symptoms, $TcPO_2$, and absent or diminished dorsalis pedis and posterior tibialis pulses. $TcPO_2$ measures cutaneous perfusion and is influenced by the underlying arterial circulation, as well as skin integrity, mechanical effects of repetitive pressure, and tissue edema. Table 6 presents findings from seven studies that directly assessed peripheral vascular function and its relationship to amputation. Adler et al. *(36)* found that AAI and $TcPO_2$ were independent predictors of amputation in the final reported models. Absence of peripheral pulses was a risk factor for amputation in three analytic studies *(21,36,39)*; however, in another study absent peripheral pulses were only significant for women in the univariate analysis *(38)*.

Intermittent claudication, absent peripheral pulses, and rest pain are symptoms of lower extremity arterial disease. Palumbo and Melton *(9)* reported on these variables in the Rochester, MN population. The incidence of lower extremity arterial disease was 8% at diabetes diagnosis, 15% at 10 years, and 45% at 29 years. Intermittent claudication, a fairly benign condition, progressed to rest pain or gangrene in only 1.6% and 1.8% of men and women, respectively, over 10 years *(9)*. In the Framingham Study, intermittent claudication was 3.8 and 6.5 times more common in diabetic than nondiabetic males and females, respectively *(42)*.

Rates of lower extremity arterial reconstruction in the United States were analyzed from 1979 to 1996. Feinglass and colleagues *(43)* reported that despite large numbers of bypass procedures, balloon angioplasties, endovascular stents, thrombolytic therapies, new imaging techniques, improved antibiotics, and provision of foot care, there was no evidence that major amputation rates had decreased during this decade.

In three analytic studies high blood pressure was an independent predictor of amputation. In two of these studies there was no direct measure of peripheral vascular function *(35,40)*. In the third study, Lee et al. *(38)* reported that systolic hypertension was significant only in the model for men and diastolic blood pressure was significant only

Table 6

Risk Factors for Lower Limb Amputations in Persons with Diabetes Identified in the Final Analysis Models of Select Studies

Author, type of analysis	Study design, diabetes type	Duration	Neuropathy (monofilament vibration, reflex)	PVD AAI, TcPO₂, pulses	HBP	High HbA1c, FPG	Smoking	History Ulcer	History Retinopathy	Pt Ed
Adler et al. (36) Multivariate proportional hazards	Cohort, 776 type 1, 2 veterans	0	+	+		0	0	+	+	
Hamalainen et al. (37) Logistic regression	733 type 1, 2, Finland	Control variable	+	+	0	0	0		+	0
Lee et al. (38) Cox regression	Cohort, 875 type 2 Oklahoma Indians	+			+SBP Male +DBP/Female	+ Male	0	0	+	
Lehto et al. (21) Cox regression	Cohort, 1044 type 2, Finland	+	+	+	0	+	0		+	
Mayfield et al. (39) Logistic regression	Retrospective case-control, 246 type 2 Pima Indians	+	+	+	0	+	0	+	+	
Moss et al. (40) Logistic regression	Cohort, 2990 early- and late-onset, S. WI, USA	0			+DBP	+	+ Younger	+	+	
Nelson et al. (23) Stratified	Cohort, 4399 Pima Indians, AZ, USA	+	+	+	0	+	0		+	
Reiber et al. (34) Logistic regression	Prospective case-control, 316 type 1, 2 veterans	Control variable	+	+	0	+	0	+	+	+
Selby and Zhang (35) Logistic regression	Nested retrospective case-control, 428 type 1, 2, HMO	+	+		+SBP	+	0		+	

blank cell, not studied;
+, statistically significant finding;
0, no statistically significant finding.

AAI, ankle-arm index;
DBP, diastolic blood pressure;
HbA1c, hemoglobin A1c;
HBP, high blood pressure;
FPG, fasting plasma glucose;

Pt Ed, outpatient education;
PVD, peripheral vascular disease;
SBP, systolic blood pressure;
TcPO₂, transcutaneous oxygen tension;

47

in the model for women. In this study peripheral vascular function, as measured by peripheral pulses, was not an independent predictor of amputation.

Poor glycemic control has been associated with an increased risk of amputation, primarily through neuropathy pathways. The Diabetes Control and Complications Trial randomized patients with type 1 diabetes to either the intensive blood glucose control group or conventional control. The intensively treated group achieved nearly normal blood glucose levels compared with the control group, whose blood glucose values remained in the conventional range. The intensively treated group had a 69% reduction in subclinical neuropathy, a 57% reduction in clinical neuropathy, and fewer peripheral vascular events than the control group. Elevated HbA_{1c} or plasma glucose was a statistically significant predictor of amputation in seven of the nine analytic studies reported in Table 9 *(21,23,34,35,38–40)*.

The modifiable risk factors for development of atherosclerosis in nondiabetic persons are cigarette smoking, lipoprotein abnormalities, and high blood pressure. These factors are assumed to be similarly atherogenic in diabetic individuals. Smoking was a risk factor in only one study, and only among persons with younger onset diabetes *(40)*. There are several possible explanations for the lack of statistically significant findings in persons with diabetes. Smoking was reported as an infrequent factor by several authors. Other measures of peripheral arterial disease, more proximal in time to the amputation, such as $TcPO_2$, AAI, or peripheral pulses, may better capture circulation on parameters in the multivariate analyses. An interesting protective association reported by Moss et al. *(40)* was the significant protective effect of aspirin on lower limb amputation in younger onset patients and a similar, although nonsignificant, trend in older onset patients. Aspirin has long been used as an agent to prevent cardiovascular disease.

Foot ulcer history was an independent predictor of amputation in three studies *(36, 39,40)*. Foot ulcers preceded approx 85% of nontraumatic lower limb amputations in two clinical epidemiology studies *(44,45)*. In studies by Boulton *(41)* in the United Kingdom and Reiber et al. *(46)* in the United States, 45–60% of patients with new-onset ulcers reported a prior history of foot ulcer.

Ulcer and amputation risk associated with footwear has been described in several studies. In a study by Edmonds et al. *(47)*, a specialized foot care team achieved high rates of ulcer healing and decreased amputations. Therapeutic footwear was provided to ulcer patients who were then monitored for ulcer recurrences for an average of 26 months. The authors report ulcer recurrences in 26% of persons who wore their special shoes compared with 83% who wore their own footwear. Uccioli et al. *(48)* randomized patients with a history of prior foot ulcer to therapeutic footwear or their own footwear for a 1-year period. He found a significant decrease in reulceration rates in the group randomized to therapeutic shoes and inserts.

Eight of the nine studies reported retinopathy as an independent predictor of amputation *(3,21,23,34,35,37,39,40)*. Retinopathy may reflect the extent of microvascular disease and may also be a proxy for diabetes severity.

In two studies, patient self-management education and self-care behaviors were linked to a decreased amputation risk. Veterans with high-risk foot conditions were randomized to "usual education" or a 1-hour lecture showing pictures of ulcers and amputations and a one-page instruction sheet. After a 1-year follow-up, persons receiving the special educational session had a threefold decrease in ulceration ($p < 0.005$) and amputation rates ($p < 0.0025$) *(49)*. A prospective case-control study also in veterans reported a strong protective effect comparing patients who had and had not received prior outpatient education *(34)*. Several foot care intervention programs reported decreases in amputations and reduced days of hospitalizations and costs. The interventions consisted of patient and professional education and changes in organization of foot care services. Given the multidimensional nature of these interventions, many components may have contributed to their success *(50–52)*.

National surveys indicate that only about 50% of patients with diabetes report a foot exam by their health care provider within the past 6 months. Foot exam frequency was lowest in type 2 patients on insulin where only 41% reported foot examinations *(12)*. The frequency of foot exams increased when there were chart reminders or clinician prompts or when the nurse removed the patient's shoes and stockings before the clinician entered the room. Provider foot examination frequency has not been associated with decreased ulcer or amputation rates.

SUBSEQUENT AMPUTATIONS AND MORTALITY

Higher level amputations on the same or the contralateral side are common in diabetic amputees. Table 7 displays the frequency of subsequent amputations by side and as available by year since amputation. Statewide hospital discharge data from California and New Jersey indicated that at 1 year post amputation, 9–13% of amputees experienced a new same-side or contralateral amputation *(53,54)*. Denmark maintains an amputation registry for surveillance purposes (excluding toe amputations). There are 27% of registrants with diabetes and 73% without *(55)*. The Danish Registry reported that 19% of all patients undergoing a major amputation for arteriosclerosis and gangrene had another same-side amputation within 6 months. This percentage increased to only 23% by 48 months following amputation, suggesting that most same-side amputations above the toe level are performed within 6 months of the initial amputation *(55)*.

The study by Braddeley and Fulford *(56)* reported that 12% of diabetic individuals had a contralateral amputation at 1 year, 23% at 3 years, and 28% at 5 years. According to the descriptive findings available, subsequent contralateral limb amputations occurred in persons with diabetes in 23–30% of amputees at 3 years and in 28–51% at 5 years *(56–58)*. The notable exception was the study from Newcastle-upon-Tyne: the 3-year ipsilateral amputation frequency was 6%, and the contralateral amputation frequency was 3%. This study did report high 3-year mortality rates of 50% *(59)*. Part of the variation in the frequency of ipsilateral and contralateral amputations reported in these studies is related to the age structure and health care of the study population.

Mortality among amputees with diabetes is rarely attributable to amputation and is usually related to concurrent comorbid conditions such as cardiac or renal disease. Table 8 presents amputation mortality data from nine select populations by interval—28 days (perioperative) and 1, 3, and 5 years.

US perioperative mortality from the National Hospital Discharge Survey for 1989 and 1992 was 5.8% *(60)*. Perioperative mortality was 10% in both the Newcastle study and in diabetic amputees in the Department of Veterans Affairs in 1998 *(59,61)*. Reports indicate that the 1-year mortality rates in diabetic amputees range from 13 to 40%, the 3-year mortality rates range from 35 to 65%, and the 5-year mortality rates span 39 to

Table 7
Percent of Individuals with Diabetes and Amputation Undergoing Subsequent Ipsilateral and Contralateral Amputation from Select Studies by Time Interval

Study	Population	1 Year		3 Years		5 Years	
		Ipsilateral	Contralateral	Ipsilateral	Contralateral	Ipsilateral	Contralateral
Braddeley et al. (56)	Birmingham, UK		12		23		28
Deerochanawong et al. (59)	Newcastle, UK			6	3		
Larsson et al. (44)	Lund, Sweden	14		30		49	
Miller et al. (53)	State of New Jersey, USA	9					
Silbert et al. (58)	New York, USA				30		51
Wright and Kaplan (54)	State of California, USA	13					

Table 8
Percent Mortality in Persons with Diabetes
and Amputation from Select Studies by Time Interval

Study	Population	% Perioperative (28 days)	Years (%)		
			1	3	5
Braddeley and Fulford *(56)*	Birmingham, UK		16	35	
Deerochanawong et al. *(59)*	Newcastle, UK	10	40	50	
Ebskov and Josephsen *(55)*	Denmark; excludes toe amputations[a]		32	55	72
Larsson et al. *(44)*	Lund, Sweden		15	38	68
Lee et al. *(38)*	Oklahoma Indians, USA			40	60
Mayfield et al. *(61)*	US Veterans	10	13	41	65
Nelson et al. *(23)*	Pima Indians				39
Pohjolainem and Alaranta *(62)*	S. Finland		38	65	80
Reiber et al. *(12)*	National Hospital Discharge Survey, USA	5.8			

[a]27% of individuals in the Danish Registry have diabetes.

80% *(12,23,38,40,44,55,56,59,62)*. Amputation mortality was also reported to vary by racial and ethnic status. In the 1991 Statewide California Hospital Discharge data, the age-adjusted amputation mortality rates were 1.6% among Hispanics, 2.7% among non-Hispanic whites, and 5.7% among African Americans *(32)*.

ECONOMIC CONSIDERATIONS

Studies on ulcers and amputations usually report only direct patient costs or charges (visits, hospitalizations, procedures, pharmaceuticals, dressings, referrals, and so on), because indirect cost (value of lost income from work, pain, suffering, and family burden, and so forth) is difficult to measure. In assessing the economic impact from ulcers and amputations, the studies by Apelqvist et al. *(63)* and Ramsey et al. *(7)* included the entire ulcer episode from lesion onset to final resolution. This methodology captures the many inpatient and outpatient costs/charges associated with foot ulcers and is preferable to reporting only the charges for a single hospitalization or limited time interval.

Table 9 shows the NIS findings for average hospital charges and length of stay in persons with diabetes in 1997. As can be seen, there are conditions in persons with diabetes that account for a higher proportion of hospitalizations and health care charges than do foot ulcers and amputations. Only 3.2% of discharges were for a chronic foot ulcer (ICD 707.1). Figure 11 shows that the average cost for common foot ulcer conditions (chronic ulcers, superficial infections, deep infections, and osteomyelitis) in 1997 was $16,580. The average length of stay was 8.9 days, 15% longer than in persons with diabetes and no foot ulcer.

Only 1.9% of diabetic discharges was for nontraumatic lower limb amputations. Figure 12 shows the average cost for lower limb amputations in persons with and without diabetes. The average charge for amputation in 1997 by level was toe/transmetatarsal amputation = $25,241, transtibial amputation = $31,436, and transfemoral amputation = $32,214.

Table 9
U.S. Hospital Discharges by Average and Median Charge
and Length of Stay (LOS) for Diabetes and Associated Conditions, 1997

	No.	Total charge ($)		Average LOS
		Average	Median	
Diabetes, total	4,548,246	14,742	8761	6.3
Foot ulcer (ICD 707.1)	147,110	16,919	10,831	8.9
Lower limb amputation	88,314	26,715	17,302	12.0
Myocardial infarction	256,502	24,500	15,354	6.9
Coronary artery bypass graft	116,759	51,630	42,728	9.9
Stroke	235,914	18,074	11,054	7.7

Data from the Nationwide Inpatient Sample (ref. *1*).

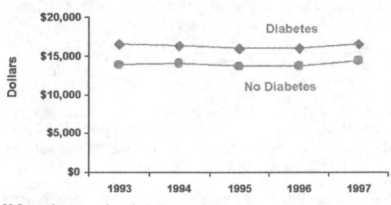

Fig. 11. U.S. total average hospital charges for any ulcer, 1993–1997. Source: Nationwide Inpatient Sample *(1)*.

Foot ulcer costs from three studies are presented in Table 10. The study by Apelqvist et al. *(63)* followed 314 patients across an entire ulcer episode, from ulcer presentation until final resolution. Healing was achieved in ≤2 months in 54% of patients, in 3–4 months in 19% of patients, and in ≥5 months in 27% of patients. The 63% of patients who healed without surgery had at an average cost of $6,664. Lower limb amputation was required for 24% of patients at an average cost of $44,790. The 13% of patients who died prior to final ulcer resolution were excluded from this analysis. The proportion of all costs related to hospitalization was 39% among ulcer patients and 82% among amputees *(63)*.

A nested case-control study was conducted by Ramsey et al. *(7)* in a large HMO involving 8905 patients with diabetes. In this group, 514 diabetic individuals developed one or more foot ulcers, and 11% of these patients required amputation. Costs were computed for the year prior to the ulcer and the 2 years following the ulcer for both cases and controls. The excess costs attributed to foot ulcers and their sequelae were $27,987 per patient for the 2-year period following ulcer presentation *(7)*.

Direct cost data on private insurance patients from the MEDSTAT Group, a large U.S. integrated administrative claims system affiliated with private health insurance plans, was analyzed by Holtzer et al. *(64)*. Utilization and cost for the entire ulcer episode may not have been captured from the administrative dataset for all patients in this

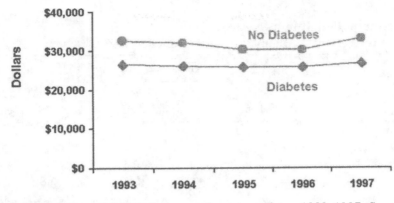

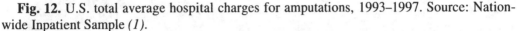

Fig. 12. U.S. total average hospital charges for amputations, 1993–1997. Source: Nationwide Inpatient Sample *(1)*.

Table 10
Direct Cost for Foot Ulcers in Persons with Diabetes from Three Studies

Study	No. of patients, study type	Outcome	Average Episode Cost (US $)	Inpatient cost (%)	Outpatient cost (%)
Apelqvist et al. *(63)*	Prospective, 314 general internal medicine patients	Primary healing, 63% Healed after amputation, 24%	$6,664 $44,790	61	39
Ramsey et al. *(7)*	Nested case-control study in HMO of 8905 type 1, 2	Primary healing, 84% Amputation, 16%	$27,987 total attributable cost	18	82
Holtzer et al. *(64)*	Retrospective, administrative records of 3013 patients and 3524 episodes	Primary healing, 52%	$1929	23	77
		Osteomyelitis, 33%	$3980	23	77
		Gangrene/amputation, 14%	$15,792	12	88

study. Study enrollment criteria were ages 18–64, employed, not on Medicare, and in this system during 1991–1992. Ulcer claims were submitted for 5.1% of diabetic patients. These 3013 patients had 3524 ulcer episodes costing an average of $4595 per episode. When ulcers were categorized by outcome, the costs were $1929 for ulcers that healed without complications, $3980 for those complicated with osteomyelitis, and $15,792 for patients whose ulcers were complicated with gangrene and required amputation. In this study over 70% of total costs were from hospital settings *(64)*. These direct costs are a conservative estimate for this cross section of persons under age 65, as they exclude amounts paid by the patient and by secondary insurance, episodes of less than 1 week, and individuals who failed to seek treatment.

Reimbursement to hospitals for patients with foot ulcers varies between public and private payers. Table 11 shows that in fiscal year 1998, under DRG reimbursement code 271 (skin ulcer), private insurance companies reimbursed hospitals on average $11,199

Table 11
Ulcer and Amputation Reimbursement
to Hospitals for Patients with and without Diabetes, 1998

Condition	DRG code no.	MEDSTAT (Private) *(66)*		Medicare *(65)*	
		LOS	Average $ reimbursement	LOS	Average $ reimbursement
Ulcers					
Osteomyelitis	238	14.1	11,193	8.4	6360
Skin ulcers	271	12.4	10,530	7.2	4567
Cellulitis > age 17 w/cc	277	4.9	5540	5.8	3554
Amputations					
Lower limb amputation, except toe	113	14.1	26,597	11.9	13,413
Toe and upper limb amputation	114	8.0	12,305	8.2	7390
Endocrine amputation	285	9.2	13,253	10.6	110,523

for an average 12.7-day length of stay, whereas Medicare reimbursed hospitals an average of $4855 (43% of the private reimbursement) for an average 7.9-day length of stay *(65,66)*. Payment for the health care provider is not included in these figures.

In 1998, the average reimbursement to private hospitals for DRG 113, a lower extremity amputation in persons with and without diabetes, was $26,126 for 14.3 days of hospitalization compared with $13,512 (51.7%) for an average 13.1 hospital day stay for Medicare patients *(65,66)*. Physician, rehabilitation, outpatient, and other follow-up care costs would be added to these figures for a complete estimate of the direct care costs.

The rise in U.S. amputation rates reported earlier may be influenced by the disparity in reimbursement between limb salvage and amputation in fee-for-service systems. Hospitals are reimbursed almost twice as much for a lower limb amputation as salvage *(65,66)*. Further information on financial impact to health care institutions is provided by the New England Deaconess Hospital. In 100 patients presenting with limb-threatening ischemia between 1984 and 1990, the frequency of diabetic amputation decreased from 44 to 7%, the frequency of popliteal and tibial bypass grafts remained constant, and the frequency of dorsalis pedis bypass grafts increased. The reported length of hospitalization decreased from 1984 levels of 44.1 days for amputees and 34.1 days for bypass grafts recipients to 22 days for both groups in 1990. The average bypass graft cost was $19,808 in 1984 and $15,981 in 1990; amputation costs were $20,248 in 1984 and $18,341 in 1990. Gibbons et al. *(67)* concluded that even though they were able to improve quality of care, maximize limb salvage, and reduce length of stay and overall cost, their Medicare reimbursement was insufficient and resulted in an average loss of $7480 per admission *(67)*.

The discharge status of diabetic amputees has been monitored in several populations. In Colorado the percentage of patients discharged to home or self-care gradually declined from 66% for those <age 45 years to 23% for those ages 75 and over. Conversely, as age increased, an increasing proportion required relocation from home or self-care settings to other acute, skilled, and intermediate care facilities for inpatient care *(68)*. In Larsson et al. *(44)* cohort in Sweden, 93% of patients living independently

before their minor index amputation were able to return to living independently compared with only 61% after a major amputation. Lavery et al. *(32)* reported that whereas 2.3% of amputees in South Texas were admitted from an institutional care facility, over 25% were discharged to one following amputation *(32)*.

SUMMARY

Persons with diabetes who develop foot ulcers and require lower limb amputations are an important and costly problem in the United States. The hospital amputation discharge rates have increased in the United States in recent years, particularly among males who are members of racial and ethnic minority groups. Many of the independent risk factors for ulcers and amputations identified from population-based, analytic, and experimental studies are similar. Several have the potential for modification by patients and their health care providers. Specific evidence is available demonstrating the benefit of better blood glucose control and self-care strategies learned through patient education. Widespread geographic variation in age, sex, and race-adjusted major amputations suggests that some patients are not receiving optimal care. Further study is needed to address this geographic area variation.

The risk of reulceration is high in persons with a prior foot ulcer. Similarly, once an individual has had an amputation, their risk of a subsequent amputation is approx 10–15% in the first year, approx 23–30% at 3 years, and approx 28–51% at 5 years. Mortality following amputation is about 6% in the first 28 days; thereafter, depending on the study population, mortality increases to an average of 15% at 1 year, 40% at 3 years, and up to 80% at 5 years.

The direct economic cost of foot ulcers and amputation is high and most of these costs are related to hospitalization. The NIS indicated that the average costs for ulcer and amputation, respectively, were $16,919 and $26,715. Hospital reimbursement for amputation was nearly double for patients covered by private insurance compared to those covered by Medicare. Hospital reimbursement for care of ulcers is less than half the reimbursement for a lower limb amputation. Patient benefit, quality of life, and rehabilitation potential must be carefully assessed before considering economic trade-offs in decisions regarding limb salvage and amputation.

REFERENCES

1. AHRQ. Nationwide Inpatient Sample, 2000. http://www.ahrq.gov/data/hcup/nisintro.htm.
2. Centers for Disease Control. Diabetes Surveillance. Atlanta, GA: U.S. Department of Health and Human Services, 1997.
3. Lazarus GS, Cooper DM, Knighton DR, et al. Definitions and guidelines for assessment of wounds and evaluation of healing. *Arch Dermatol* 1994;130:489–493.
4. Borssen B, Bergenheim T, Lithner F. The epidemiology of foot lesions in diabetic patients aged 15-50 years. *Diabet Med* 1990;7:438–444.
5. Kumar S, Ashe HA, Fernando DJS, et al. The prevalence of foot ulceration and its correlates in type 2 diabetic patients: a population-based study. *Diabet Med* 1994;11:480–484.
6. Moss SE, Klein R, Klein BEK. The prevalence and incidence of lower extremity amputation in a diabetic population. *Arch Intern Med* 1992;152:610–616.
7. Ramsey SD, Newton K, Blough D, et al. Incidence, outcomes, and cost of foot ulcers in patients with diabetes. *Diabetes Care* 1999;22:382–387.

8. Walters DP, Gatling W, Mullee MA, Hill RD. The distribution and severity of diabetic foot disease: a community study with comparison to a non-diabetic group. *Diabet Med* 1992;9: 354–358.
9. Palumbo PJ, Melton LJ, III. Peripheral vascular disease and diabetes. *Diabetes in America* (National Diabetes Data Group, ed.), DHHS, Washington, DC, 1995, pp. 401–407.
10. Apelqvist J, Castenfors J, Larsson J. Wound classification is more important than site of ulceration in the outcome of diabetic foot ulcers. *Diabet Med* 1989;6:526–530.
11. Reiber GE, Lipsky BA, Gibbons GW. The burden of diabetic foot ulcers. *Am J Surg* 1998; 176:5S–10S.
12. Reiber GE, Boyko EJ, Smith DG. Lower extremity foot ulcers and amputations in diabetes, in *Diabetes in America* (National Diabetes Data Group, ed.), DHHS, Washington, DC, 1995, pp. 409–428.
13. Rith-Najarian SJ, Stolusky T, Gohdes DM. Identifying diabetic patients at high risk for lower-extremity amputation in a primary health care setting. *Diabetes Care* 1992;15:1386–1389.
14. Abbott CA, Vileikyte L, Williamson S, Carrington AL, Boulton AJM. Multicenter study of the incidence of and predictive risk factors for diabetic neuropathic foot ulceration. *Diabetes Care* 1998;21:1071–1075.
15. Boyko E, Ahroni JH, Stensel V, et al. A prospective study of risk factors for diabetic foot ulcer: the Seattle Diabetic Foot Study. *Diabetes Care* 1999;22:1036–1042.
16. Pham H, Armstrong DG, Harvey C, et al. Screening techniques to identify people at high risk for diabetic foot ulceration: a prospective multicenter trial. *Diabetes Care* 2000;23: 606–611.
17. Litzelman DK, Slemenda CW, Langefeld CD, et al. Reduction of lower extremity clinical abnormalities in patients with non-insulin-dependent diabetes mellitus. *Ann Intern Med* 1993;119:36–41.
18. Mantey I, Foster AVM, Spencer S, Edmonds ME. Why do foot ulcers recur in diabetic patients. *Diabet Med* 1999;16:245–249.
19. Humphrey A, Dowse G, Thoma K, Zimmet P. Diabetes and nontraumatic lower extremity amputation: incidence, risk factors and prevention—a 12 year follow-up study in Nauru. *Diabetes Care* 1996;19:710–714.
20. Humphrey L, Palumbo P, Butters M, et al. The contribution of non-insulin dependent diabetes to lower extremity amputation in the community. *Arch Intern Med* 1994;154:885–892.
21. Lehto S, Pyorala K, Ronnemaa T, Laakso M. Risk factors predicting lower extremity amputations in patients with NIDDM. *Diabetes Care* 1996;19:607–612.
22. Morris AD, McAlpine R, Steinke D, et al. Diabetes and lower-limb amputations in the community. *Diabetes Care* 1998;21:738–743.
23. Nelson R, Gohdes D, Everhart J, et al. Lower-extremity amputations in NIDDM: 12-yr follow-up study in Pima Indians. *Diabetes Care* 1988;11:8–16.
24. Siitonen OL, Niskanen LK, Laakso M, Tiitonen J, Pyorala K. Lower extremity amputations in diabetic and nondiabetic patients. *Diabetes Care* 1993;16:16–20.
25. Trautner C, Giani G, Berger M. Incidence of lower limb amputations and diabetes. *Diabetes Care* 1996;19:1006–1009.
26. Van Houtum W, Lavery LA. Outcomes associated with diabetes-related amputations in the Netherlands and in the state of California. *J Intern Med* 1996;240:227–231.
27. Geiss LS. Personal communication. 1999.
28. Resnick HE, Valsania P, Phillips CL. Diabetes mellitus and nontraumatic lower extremity amputation in black and white Americans: The National Health and Nutrition Examination Survey epidemiologic follow-up study, 1971–1992. *Arch Intern Med* 1999;159:2470–2475.
29. Wrobel JS, Mayfield JA, Reiber GE. Geographic variation of lower-extremity major amputation in individuals with and without diabetes in the Medicare population. *Diabetes Care* 2001;24:1–5.

30. Birkmeyer JD, Sharp SM, Finlayson SRG, Fisher ES, Wennberg JE. Variation profiles of common surgical procedures. *Surgery* 1998;124:917–923.
31. Ford EJ, Remington PL, Sonnenberg GE. The burden of diabetes in Wisconsin: diabetes-related amputations, 1994. *Wis Med J* 1996;643.
32. Lavery LA, Ashry HR, van Houtum W, et al. Variation in the incidence and proportion of diabetes-related amputations in minorities. *Diabetes Care* 1996;19:48–52.
33. Lavery LA, van Houtum WH, Armstrong DG, et al. Mortality following lower extremity amputation in minorities with diabetes mellitus. *Diabetes Res Clin Pract* 1997;37:41–47.
34. Reiber GE, Pecoraro RE, Koepsell TD. Risk factors for amputation in patients with diabetes mellitus. *Ann Intern Med* 1992;117:97–105.
35. Selby JV, Zhang D. Risk factors for lower extremity amputation in persons with diabetes. *Diabetes Care* 1995;18:509–516.
36. Adler AL, Boyko EJ, Ahroni JH, Smith DG. Lower-extremity amputation in diabetes: the independent effects of peripheral vascular disease, sensory neuropathy, and foot ulcers. *Diabetes Care* 1999;22:1029–1035.
37. Hamalainen H, Ronnemma T, Halonen JP, Toikka T. Factors predicting lower extremity amputations in patients with type 1 or type 2 diabetes mellitus: a population-based 7-year follow-up study. *J Intern Med* 1999;246:97–103.
38. Lee J, Lu M, Lee V, et al. Lower extremity amputation. Incidence, risk factors, and mortality in the Oklahoma Indian Diabetes Study. *Diabetes* 1993;42:876–882.
39. Mayfield JA, Reiber GE, Nelson R, Greene T. A foot risk classification system to predict diabetic amputation in Pima Indians. *Diabetes Care* 1996;19:704–709.
40. Moss SE, Klein R, Klein BEK. The 14-year incidence of lower-extremity amputations in a diabetic population. *Diabetes Care* 1999;22:951–959.
41. Boulton AJM. Diabetic neuropathy. Marius Press, Carnforth, Lanshire, UK, 1997.
42. Kannel WB, McGee DL. Diabetes and cardiovascular disease: The Framingham Study. *JAMA* 1979;241:2035–2038.
43. Feinglass J, Brown JL, LoSasso A, et al. Rates of lower extremity amputation and arterial reconstruction in the United States, 1979 to 1996. *Am J Public Health* 1999;89:1222–1227.
44. Larsson J, Agardh CD, Apelqvist J, Stenstrom A. Long term prognosis after healed amputations in patients with diabetes. *Clin Orthop* 1998;350:149–158.
45. Pecoraro RE, Reiber GE, Burgess EM. Pathways to diabetic limb amputation: basis for prevention. *Diabetes Care* 1990;13:513–521.
46. Apelqvist J, Larsson J, Agard C. Long term prognosis for diabetic patients with foot ulcers. *J Int Med* 1993;233:485–491.
47. Edmonds M, Blundell M, Morris M, et al. Improved survival of the diabetic foot. *Q J Med* 1986;60:763–771.
48. Uccioli L, Faglia E, Monticone G, et al. Manufactured shoes in the prevention of diabetic foot ulcers. *Diabetes Care* 1995;18:1376–1378.
49. Malone JM, Snyder M, Anderson G, et al. Prevention of amputation by diabetic education. *Am J Surg* 1989;158:520–524.
50. Davidson JK, Alogna M, Goldsmith M. Assessment of program effectiveness at Grady Memorial Hospital, Atlanta, in *Educating Diabetic Patients* (Steiner G, Lawrence PA, eds.), Springer-Verlag, New York, 1981, pp. 329–350.
51. Miller LV. Evaluation of patient education: Los Angeles County Hospital experience: Report of National Commission on Diabetes, Volume 3, 1975: Part V.
52. Runyon J. The Memphis diabetes continuing care program. *JAMA* 1975;3:231–264.
53. Miller AE, Van Buskirk A, Verhoek W, Miller ER. Diabetes related lower extremity amputations in New Jersey, 1979–1981. *J Med Soc NJ* 1985;82:723–726.
54. Wright WE, Kaplan GA. Trends in lower extremity amputations, California, 1983–1987. Sacremento, CA: California Department of Health Services, 1989.

55. Ebskov B, Josephsen P. Incidence of reamputation and death after gangrene of the lower extremity. *Prosthet Orthot Int* 1980;4:77–80.
56. Braddeley RM, Fulford JC. A trial of conservative amputations for lesions of the feet in diabetes mellitus. *Br J Surg* 1965;52:38–43.
57. Larsson J. Lower extremity amputation in diabetic patients: Lund University, 1994.
58. Silbert S. Amputation of the lower extremity in diabetes mellitus. *Diabetes* 1952;1:297–299.
59. Deerochanawong C, Home PD, Alberti KGMM. A survey of lower limb amputation in diabetic patients. *Diabet Med* 1992;9:942–946.
60. Preston SD, Reiber GE, Koepsell TD. Lower extremity amputations and inpatient mortality in hospitalized persons with diabetes: national population risk factors and associations. University of Washington Thesis, 1993.
61. Mayfield J, Reiber G, Maynard C, Caps M, Sangeorzan B. Trends in lower extremity amputation in the Veterans Affairs Hospitals, 1989–1998. *J Rehabil Res Dev* 2000;37:23–30.
62. Pohjolainen T, Alaranta H. Ten-year survival of Finnish lower limb amputees. *Prosthet Orthot Int* 1998;22:10–16.
63. Apelqvist J, Ragnarson-Tennvall G, Persson U, Larson J. Diabetic foot ulcers in a multidisciplinary setting: an economic analysis of primary healing and healing with amputation. *J Intern Med* 1994;235:463–471.
64. Holzer SES, Camerota A, Martens L, et al. Costs and duration of care for lower extremity ulcers in patients with diabetes. *Clin Ther* 1998;20:169–181.
65. HCFA. DRG Inpatient Billing Data, 1998: Health Care Finance Administration, Bureau of Data Strategy and Management, 2000.
66. MEDSTAT. DRG Guide Descriptions and Normative Values. Ann Arbor, MI, 2000.
67. Gibbons GW, Marcaccio EJ Jr, Burgess AM, et al. Improved quality of diabetic foot care, 1984 vs 1990. *Arch Surg* 1993;128:576–581.
68. Colorado State Department of Health. Diabetes Prevalence and Morbidity in Colorado Residents, 1980–1991. 1993:119–136.

3

Physiology and Pathophysiology of Wound Healing

Vincent Falanga, MD, FACP

INTRODUCTION

The process of wound healing is characterized by a cascade of interrelated events involving inflammatory factors and pathways, resident cells, cells recruited to the site of injury, growth factors, and other signals. To make it more understandable, this process is generally viewed as occurring in three main phases: inflammation, proliferation and tissue formation, and tissue remodeling. Each phase is marked by series of complex interactions between many cell types, blood-borne elements, growth factors, and extracellular matrix. These phases do not represent separate and distinct events, however, and should be recognized as overlapping and continuous (Fig. 1).

INFLAMMATION (PHASE 1)

The first phase, that of inflammation, begins immediately after an acute injury. Disruption of blood vessels leads to local release of blood cells and blood-borne elements, resulting in clot formation. The inflammatory phase is dominated by the platelet, which directs clotting of the fresh wound by the intrinsic and extrinsic pathways. Platelets also release a number of chemotactic factors that attract other platelets, leukocytes, and fibroblasts to the site of injury. The inflammatory phase continues as leukocytes, specifically neutrophils and macrophages, enter the scene. Their key initial role is to debride the wound by phagocytosing and killing bacteria and scavenging cellular debris. However, it should be recognized that neutrophils and macrophages also release growth factors and other important mediators during this period.

Platelets

Platelets are essential components of the repair process, and thrombocytopenia may result in impaired wound healing. Tissue injury leads to blood vessel damage, platelet release, and activation of blood coagulation. Platelets at the wound site are exposed to thrombin and fibrillar collagen, which trigger their activation, adhesion, and aggregation *(1)*. Activated platelets release a number of mediators, including fibrinogen, fibronectin, thrombospondin, von Willibrand factor, adenosine diphosphate (ADP), thromboxane A_2, 5-hydroxy-tryptophan, and vitronectin. Fibrinogen, fibronectin, and thrombospondin, released in α-granules, act as ligands for platelet aggregation *(2)*. Platelet adhesion to fibrillar collagen is mediated by von Willebrand factor (VWF), whereas ADP and

From: *The Diabetic Foot: Medical and Surgical Management*
Edited by: A. Veves, J. M. Giurini, and F. W. LoGerfo © Humana Press Inc., Totowa, NJ

COMPONENTS OF WOUND HEALING

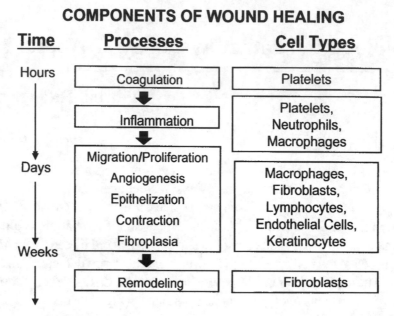

Fig. 1. Components of the wound healing process, in terms of time, events, and cell types involved. © Dr. V. Falanga 2000.

thrombin recruit additional platelets to the injury site. These activities result in the formation of a platelet plug. Fibrinogen, which is converted by thrombin to fibrin, adds to the developing clot, which will form the provisional extracellular matrix for later stages of wound healing. At the same time, endothelial cells produce several factors that control propagation of the clot, thereby limiting platelet aggregation and clot formation to the area of injury. These factors include the following: prostacyclin, which inhibits platelet aggregation; antithrombin III, which inhibits thrombin activity; protein C, which degrades coagulation factors V and VIII; and plasminogen activator, which initiates clot lysis by converting plasminogen to plasmin *(3)*.

Platelets also release a number of growth factors: platelet-derived growth factor (PDGF), transforming growth factor-β1 (TGF-β1), platelet factor-4, connective tissue-activating peptide III (CTAP-III), β-thromboglobulin, and neutrophil-activating peptide-2 (NAP-2). PDGF, for example, is mitogenic and chemotactic for fibroblasts *(4)*.

Coagulation

Leakage of plasma and other blood elements from injured blood vessels results in thrombus formation by both of the major clotting cascades. The intrinsic pathway, stimulated by exposure of blood to subendothelial tissue, leads to activation of factor X, the enzyme required for the formation of thrombin. The extrinsic pathway, beginning with factor VII activation by thromboplastin, also leads to the formation of thrombin. Thrombin cleaves fibrinopeptide A and B from fibrinogen, which allows polymerization of fribrinogen to fibrin. Later, factor XIII will provide crosslinking to the fibrin molecule and stabilization of the clot.

Several components of the formed thrombus are recognized by receptors present on such cells as monocytes, fibroblasts, endothelial cells, and keratinocytes, which migrate to the wound site. During the process of coagulation, other inflammatory mediators are produced and released. Activated Hageman factor, for example, leads to formation of bradykinin, C3a, and C5a. These inflammatory mediators cause enhanced vascular permeability, neutrophil and monocyte recruitment, and release of factors from the mast cells. The fibrinopeptides themselves, especially fibrinopeptide A, which is released very quickly upon cleavage from fibrinogen, probably contribute to the recruitment of fibroblasts to the wound site.

Leukocytes

There is a constant cascade of inflammatory molecules and recruitment of inflammatory cells during the early phases of wound healing. Neutrophils and monocytes arrive at the site of injury at about the same time. Initially, neutrophils are present in greater numbers because they constitute a larger fraction of peripheral white cells. Both neutrophils and monocytes are attracted to the wound by such chemotactic factors as kallikrein, fibrinopeptides released from fibrinogen, and fibrin degradation products. These chemotactic factors also stimulate the expression of CD11/CD18 complex on the surface of neutrophils, thereby enhancing the adherence of neutrophils to blood vessel endothelium and facilitating their diapedesis between adjacent endothelial cells *(5,6)*.

Neutrophils are important in tissue debridement and in bacterial killing, events that produce further products of complement activation with inflammatory and chemotactic properties. New evidence suggests that neutrophils are also a rich source of cytokines, such as PDGF-like molecules. Connective tissue growth factor (CTGF) is one such peptide. The action of neutrophils is enhanced by integrins, cell surface receptors that facilitate cell-matrix interactions *(7)*. However, neutrophils do not appear to be critical for wound healing, as neutropenia does not interfere with the healing process *(8)*.

As the inflammatory process continues, monocytes replace neutrophils and become the predominant leukocyte. They are attracted to the injury site by some of the same chemoattractants responsible for recruitment of neutrophils, such as kallikren, fibrinopeptides, and fibrin degradation products. Other more specific chemoattractants then take over in recruiting monocytes, including fragments of collagen, fibronectin, elastin, and TGF-β1. Monocytes undergo a phenotypic change to tissue macrophages and, unlike neutrophils, they are critical for the progression of wound healing. Macrophages phagocytose and kill bacteria and scavenge tissue debris *(9)*. They also release several growth factors, including PDGF, fibroblast growth factor (FGF), TGF-β, and TGF-α, thereby stimulating migration and proliferation of fibroblasts, as well as production and modulation of extracellular matrix. A few days after tissue injury, what remains of neutrophils is phagocytosed by tissue macrophages, and the first phase of wound healing comes to an end, while the second phase of proliferation and tissue formation is under way.

PROLIFERATION AND TISSUE FORMATION (PHASE 2)

In the second phase of wound healing, that of proliferation and tissue formation, keratinocytes undergo a remarkable change in morphology and function. They migrate to the wound bed, release a number of proteins and enzymes that help facilitate their migration and other cellular functions, and ultimately reconstitute the damaged epidermis and basement membrane. The later stages of the second phase of wound healing feature formation of granulation tissue, reconstitution of the dermal matrix (fibroplasia), and development of new blood vessels (angiogenesis). Fibroblasts and endothelial cells undergo activation, phenotypic alteration, and migration much like keratinocytes do.

Migration

The process of reepithelialization begins several hours after tissue injury. Keratinocyte migration, rather than proliferation, is actually responsible for most of the resurfacing of the epidermal defect. Phenotypic alteration of keratinocytes enables them to migrate both from the wound edge and from any adnexal structures remaining in the wound bed. One to 2 days after the initial injury, epidermal cells at the wound edge and within the wound begin to divide and proliferate, thereby contributing to the population of migrating cells.

Several studies have shown keratinocyte migration and proliferation to be two independent processes. In one such study *(10)*, investigators exposed keratincytes to a matrix of collagen that stimulated marked motility, and later to TGF-β, which resulted in marked inhibition of proliferation. Despite this effect, the keratinocytes continued to migrate. In fact, migration was enhanced by TGF-β *(10)*.

Keratinocyte migration begins and is associated with several morphologic changes, including retraction of tonofilaments, dissolution of intercellular desmosomes, and formation of peripheral cytoplasmic actin filaments *(11)*. These changes are accompanied by dissolution of hemidesmosomes, thereby diminishing the normal binding between the dermis and epidermis *(12)*. Keratinocytes also project pseudopodia from their basolateral side into the wound, thus facilitating migration. Factors responsible for initiating and directing these phenotypic changes are incompletely understood, although studies have shown a role for β1-integrin receptors (described below). It has also been shown that cultured keratinocytes exposed to low concentrations of calcium develop similar phenotypic changes.

Various cytokines and matrix proteins stimulate keratinocyte migration to the wound bed. Connective tissue promoters of migration include fibronectin and type IV collagen, both of which can be synthesized by keratinocytes *(13)*, and native denatured type I collagen *(14)*. Growth factors, such as TGF-β and epidermal growth factor (EGF), also stimulate keratinocytes to migrate. TGF-β also increases keratinocyte production of fibronectin.

A strong inhibitor of keratinocyte migration is laminin, a major component of the lamina lucida zone of the basement membrane. In normal skin this large glycoprotein helps prevent direct contact between keratinocytes and collagens contained within the basement membrane (types IV and VII) and dermis (types I, III, and VI) *(14)*. Acute injury, by disrupting the laminin component, brings the plasma membrane of basal keratinocytes in direct contact with underlying collagens, thereby stimulating migration. It has been shown that laminin reappears in the dermal-epidermal junction after keratinocytes have migrated and resurfaced the wound *(15)*. The presence of laminin in the wound therefore serves as a signal for keratinocytes that they are in contact with intact basement membrane, or undamaged skin, and should stop migrating. Interestingly, when laminin is added to keratinocyte cultures, it stimulates cell division and growth *(16)*. This observation serves as another example of the independence of the process of migration from that of proliferation.

The forces necessary for the sheet of keratinocytes to move over a defect are presumably generated by the coordinate action of basal layer keratinocytes at the wound margin. Two key components appear to be involved: use of lamellipodia for movement and development of an actin cable that acts as a drawstring to pull the migrating keratinocyte sheets together. Unlike adult wounds in which keratinocytes develop lamellipodia, the observation has been made that in embryonic wounds the advancing epidermis is smooth. A cable of filamentous actin appears around most of the wound margin and is confined to a single row of basal cells at the free edge of the epidermis. It has been hypothesized that the actin cable in these embryonic wounds acts as a contractile mechanism to close up the defect. Development of the actin filaments in adult keratinocytes would seem to indicate a similar function. Basal keratinocytes undergo a morphologic change from their normal cuboidal shape to a flattened cell with extended lamellipodia, which project into the wound bed *(14)*. Hemidesmisomes are retracted from the plasma membrane, and the number of gap junctions increases. Integrin receptor expression changes to facilitate keratinocyte movement on collagens, and keratinocytes begin to synthesize and release types I and IV collagenases.

In addition to migration and proliferation, keratinocytes must reconstitute the basement membrane. As pointed out earlier, some of the normal components of the basement membrane, laminin and type IV collagen, are absent under migrating keratinocytes *(17)*. Also absent is collagen VI, a component of anchoring fibrils. It has been shown that from the first day of wound healing keratinocytes migrating across the wound bed deposit kalinin, a component of anchoring filaments *(17)*. When keratinocytes have completed their migratory phase, they continue to proliferate and produce those components necessary to reconstitute the basement membrane fully. During this period there is regeneration of types IV and VII collagen and laminin in the basement membrane zone.

As observed with other cell types, adhesion of keratinocytes to the extracellular matrix is important in their migration and overall biologic behavior. Integrins, which are cell surface receptors expressed by many cell types, appear to play an important role in keratinocyte adhesion and movement. Each integrin has an α-chain and a β-chain that are noncovalently linked. Each chain has an intracellular, transmembrane, and extracellular domain.

A number of α- and β-integrin subunits have been identified, and multiple combinations of these subunits occur *(18)*. The specific combination determines to what ligand the integrin will bind. Some integrins, such as $\alpha5\beta1$, are known to bind to only one protein *(19)*, whereas others can bind multiple ligands *(20–22)*. Some cells display multiple integrins that bind to the same protein *(23–25)*, although at different regions of the ligand *(26)*. For example, $\alpha5\beta1$ and $\alpha4\beta1$ bind to separate regions of fibronectin, and $\alpha1\beta1$ and $\alpha6\beta1$ to different regions of laminin *(26)*. Multiple integrins have been shown to bind to the same region of a ligand; however, each may serve a different function *(27)*. Function specificity may be determined by the cytoplasmic domain of the integrin subunit *(22,28)*.

Two hypotheses, not mutually exclusive, may explain how integrin signal transduction occurs *(18)*. The first hypothesis suggests that integrins organize the cytoskeleton and can alter cell shape and internal cellular architecture. In the second hypothesis, integrins are true receptors that stimulate biochemical signals within the cell.

$\beta1$-integrin has been shown to complex with at least 10 different α-subunits, with the α-subunit affecting the specificity of the integrin complex: $\alpha2\beta1$ binds to several types of collagen and laminin; α3β1 binds to the arginine-glycine-aspartic acid (RGD) sequence of fibronectin and laminin; and α5β1 may be specific for the RGD sequence in fibronectin alone *(29)*.

A number of integrins have been shown to regulate keratinocyte mobility. Human keratinocytes migrate on fibronectin by using the α5β1 integrin receptor *(30)*. Along with α5β1, migrating keratinocytes also express high levels of αvβ5. Migration on collagen is mediated by the α2β1 receptor *(30)*. EGF, which stimulates migration of keratinocytes on collagen, may do so by upregulating the expression of α2β1 on the keratinocyte cell surface *(31)*. The α3β1 integrin has many ligands, including epiligrin, laminin, fibronectin, and collagen *(14)*. When the α3β1 receptor is blocked by specific antibodies, keratinocyte migration is enhanced on fibronectin and collagen matrices *(32)*.

Another important integrin subunit implicated in keratinocyte locomotion is β6, which is specific to epithelial cells and is upregulated by TGF-β *(33)*. The αvβ6 complex functions as a fibronectin and possibly tenascin receptor *(34)*. In one study, β6 was not expressed in unwounded epidermis but was strongly expressed by epithelial cells at the wound margin 2 days after an acute injury *(35)*. Seven days after the initial injury, once healing was completed, β6 was no longer detected. β6 was variably expressed during different stages of fetal tissue development in the skin, kidneys, and lungs. Interestingly, β6 integrins are strongly expressed by several types of malignant cells, such as those in oral squamous cell carcinoma and colon carcinoma and in epithelial cells of the lung and kidney at sites of inflammation. It has been reported that αvβ6 enhances invasive growth of carcinoma *(36)*. It would therefore appear that normal β6-integrin expression regulates cell-cell interaction during development and wound healing, and its abnormal expression may result in tumorigenesis.

As stated before, integrins also appear to be involved with other aspects of the migratory phase. Activation of keratinocytes that are removed from skin and placed into tissue culture involves altered β1-integrin subunit glycosylation and an increase in β1-integrin receptors. Of the two forms of β1-subunits contained in activated keratinocytes, the 93- and 113-kDa forms, only the 113-kDa subunit mature form is detected in cell surface integrin receptors. Experiments with endoglycosidase have shown that there are changes in keratinocyte α-subunits associated with changes in β1 expression. Moreover, keratinocytes maintained in low calcium proliferate, but their adhesiveness and potential to migrate are not increased, further evidence that migration and proliferation are regulated separately.

In addition to the cell-cell and cell matrix interactions described above, another level of integrin regulations is provided by growth factors. Some of the growth factors shown to have an important role in integrin expression in keratinocytes, fibroblasts, and other cell types include TGF-β, PDGF, and vascular endothelial growth factor (VEGF). Studies have shown that TGF-β1 upregulates α5β1 and αvβ3 expression in cultured fibroblasts, as well as β4 subunit expression in cultured keratinocytes *(37–39)*. Upregulation of keratinocyte α5β1 and αvβ5 in vivo is stimulated by TGF-β1 *(40)*. PDGF-BB upregulates β1 in cultured Swiss 3T3 cells, α5 and β3 in aortic smooth muscle cells, and α2 in human foreskin fibroblasts *(29)*.

The effect of cytokines and growth factors on the regulation of integrin expression must be viewed in context of the matrix surrounding the target cell. It has been shown that PDGF-BB, a prominent component of the early wound environment, upregulates α5β1 and α3β1 expression in fibroblasts grown in fibronectin-rich tissue culture of fibrin *(29)*. However, fibroblasts grown on collagen gels, thereby approximating the normal dermis or late wound environment, do not show upregulation of these integrins, even in the presence of PDGFF-BB. The vast array of cytokines affecting integrin expression are initially released by aggregating platelets in the early wound *(41)*. Later they are produced by fibroblasts, keratinocytes, monocytes, and macrophages *(40)*.

Fibroplasia

During the process of reepithelialization, the wound is also undergoing fibroplasia and angiogenesis (discussed below). Fibroplasia refers to formation of granulation tissue and reconstitution of the dermal matrix. The key cell in this aspect of wound repair is the fibroblast. It is generally accepted that fibroblasts migrate into the wound, produce large amounts of collagens, proteoglycans, elastin, and other matrix proteins, and participate in wound contraction. Fibroblasts, like keratinocytes, undergo phenotypic changes that modify their interactions with the extracellular matrix, allowing them to perform a number of functions *(42)*. There is evidence for the existence of subpopulations of fibroblasts, with each subpopulation responsible for a different aspect of healing *(43)*.

Immediately following acute injury, the wound is hypoxic owing to blood vessel disruption. Evidence points to low oxygen tension as an important early stimulus for fibroblast (and endothelial cell) activation. A number of growth factors, including TGF-β1, PDGF, VEGF, and endothelin-1 have been shown to be upregulated in hypoxia *(44)*. α_1-procollagen mRNA levels are also stimulated in low oxygen tension *(44)*. Because molecular oxygen is needed for procollagen hydroxylation and proper collagen formation, one hypothesis is that reoxygenation, brought about by revascularization, leads to enhanced collagenous protein synthesis in fibroblasts whose procollagen mRNA levels were stimulated by hypoxia *(44)*.

Soon after injury, the formation of a clot provides an appropriate early matrix for cell migration. Fibrin and fibronectin, components of that clot, act as the provisional matrix for fibroblast migration. An important relationship has been shown between this provisional matrix and PDGF *(29)*. Fibroblasts in unwounded skin are surrounded by a collagen-rich matrix, are biosynthetically inactive, and express high levels of collagen integrin receptor α2. In vitro studies have shown that the combination of fibrin/fibronectin and PDGF causes fibroblasts to express high mRNA levels of integrin receptors α3 and α5 *(29)*. These integrins facilitate fibroblast migration into the wound bed, where fibroblasts may be influenced by other growth factors and cytokines to proliferate or undergo further phenotypic changes. Ultimately, as the wound heals, the new collagen-rich extracellular matrix will cause downregulation of fibroblast integrins α3 and α5, while increasing levels of α2.

Just as it attracts monocytes and neutrophils to the wound area, TGF-β1 has also been implicated as an important chemoattractant for fibroblasts. As stated earlier, TGF-β1 upregulates the expression of provisional matrix integrins α5β1 and αvβ3. However, there are other mechanisms by which TGF-β1 might affect locomotion *(45)*. It has been shown that production of hyaluronan (HA) and RHAMM, a cell surface receptor for HA, is increased by TGF-β1 and is necessary for locomotion of tumor cells *(46)*.

Another HA receptor, CD44, has slightly different functions from the RHAMM receptor but ultimately mediates movement of fibroblasts on HA substrates *(47–49)*. Fibroblasts in hypertrophic scar tissue express greater amounts of CD44 and have decreased internalization of CD44 in the presence of HA *(50)*.

Fibroblasts begin to migrate into the wound 48 h after injury. They move along the fibrin/fibronectin matrix deposited in the initial clot, and they themselves produce fibronectin, which can facilitate their movement. Other extracellular matrix components, such as tenascin, are additional signals for fibroblast adhesion and movement. The Arg-Gly-Asp-Ser (RGDS) tetrapeptide that is common to these and other extracellular matrix proteins is important in the binding of these molecules to cell surface integrin receptors.

Fibroblasts produce other extracellular matrix components, including type I and III collagen, elastin, glycosaminoglycans, and proteoglycans. Type III collagen, which is present in large quantities in fetal dermis but not in adult dermis, is the predominant collagen type during early wound healing. Synthesis of type III collagen becomes maximal 5–7 days after injury. TGF-β has been shown to stimulate fibroblast production of types I and III collagen both in vitro and in vivo *(43)*. There is evidence that fibroblast clones with greater collagen synthetic phenotype are selected during the early stages of wound repair.

As the new connective tissue is formed, some fibroblasts undergo a further phenotypic change to actin-rich myofibroblasts. These cells display features characteristic of fibroblasts and smooth muscle cells. They contain an extensive network of rough endoplasmic reticulum, presumably needed to produce large amounts of matrix proteins *(43)*. Myofibroblasts are largely responsible for wound contraction and are very prominently present in granulation tissue *(51)*. Unlike other cells involved in the wound healing process, myofibroblasts undergo organized arrangements along the lines of contraction. Exposure to a number of mediators, including angiotensin, prostaglandins, bradykinins, and endothelins, leads to muscle-like contractions of the myofibroblasts. The amount of wound contraction that occurs depends in large part on the depth of the wound *(52)*. Skin wounds can be classified as full thickness or partial thickness. In full-thickness wounds the injury extends deeper than the adnexa. These wounds heal at least in part by contraction, which results in an approximately 40% decrease in wound size *(52)*. In full-thickness wounds epithelialization occurs from the wound edge alone. Partial-thickness wounds, in contrast, are not as deep, and parts of the adnexa remain in the wound bed. Partial-thickness wounds display less contraction, and epithelialization occurs from both the wound edge and from the adnexal structures with the wound bed *(52)*.

Angiogenesis

Antiogenesis describes the process by which new vessel growth, called neovascularization, takes place. Angiogenesis occurs at the same time as fibroplasia, and in fact the two are interdependent. As with other processes of wound healing, new vessel formation occurs in the context of the changing extracellular matrix. The chief cell of angiogenesis is the endothelial cell, which, like the keratinocyte and fibroblast, must undergo specific changes in order to migrate to the wound bed, proliferate, and direct new vessel formation. Migration of endothelial cells into the wound is dependent on chemotactic signals supplied by the extracellular matrix and neighboring cells. There is evidence that, like reepithelialization, cell migration is a more important component of angiogenesis than proliferation. However, many signals that are involved in endothelial cell migratin, such as fibronectin and heparin, may also stimulate proliferation.

Aside from its role in angiogenesis, endothelial cells play an active role in the inflammatory stage of wound healing. They produce several factors that control propagation of the initial clot, thereby limiting platelet aggregation and clot formation to the area of injury. These mediators include prostacyclin, which inhibits platelet aggregation; antithrombin III, which inhibits thrombin activity; protein C, which degrades coagulation factors V and VIII; and, most importantly, plasminogen activator, which initiates clot lysis by converting plasminogen to plasmin *(53)*.

Experiments with the avascular comea have shown that phenotypic alteration of endothelial cells during wound healing includes the development of pseudopodia that project through fragmented basement membranes. The stimulus for this phenotypic change is not as well known as those outlined for keratinocytes and fibroblasts. By the second day following acute injury, endothelial cells at the wound edge begin to migrate into the perivascular space, and those remaining in the blood vessel begin to proliferate *(42)*.

A number of factors have been implicated in stimulating angiogenesis. As described before, low oxygen tension in the early wound environment appears to potentiate angiogenesis and fibroplasia *(52)*. Low oxygen tension may also stimulate macrophages to produce and secrete angiogenic factors *(54)*. Growth factors shown to be angiogenic include TGF-β1 and FGF. Of interest is that TGF-β1 is a potent inhibitor of endothelial cell proliferation, yet it induces a dramatic angiogenic response when injected into the dermis. This is probably because TGF β leads to the recruitment of macrophages, which in turn secrete substances that stimulate endothelial cell ingrowth. This example underscores the complexities involved in this phase of wound healing and the difficulty in assigning definite effects to any particular factor or cell. However, it does appear that the FGF family is by far the most important in stimulating angiogenesis. These peptides are released by macrophages and interact with heparin, which enhances their biologic activity. As discussed before, macrophages are essential to the wound healing process.

As it does with other phases of wound healing, the extracellular matrix plays a critical role in angiogenesis. One component of the provisional matrix is secreted protein acidic and rich in cysteine (SPARC). Released from fibroblasts and macrophages, SPARC, or its proteolytic fragments, stimulate angiogenesis during formation of granulation tissue *(55)*. SPARC, tenascin, and thrombospondin are all components of the early provisional matrix and can also be found in tissues where cells are dividing or migrating *(56)*. They are considered antiadhesive proteins and have been shown to promote cell-rounding and partial detachment *(55)*. In addition to these effects, SPARC can also stimulate the production of collagenase, stromalysin, and gelatinase. Heparin and fibronectin, two other components of the provisional matrix stimulate endothelial cells to project pseudopodia through basement membrane defects at the site of injury *(42)*. FGF further stimulates cells to release procollagenase and plasminogen activator (PA) *(42)*. PA converts plasminogen to plasmin and activates collagenase. These enzymes help to break down the basement membrane and facilitate endothelial cell migration into the perivascular space.

Just as with other stages of wound healing, cell-to-cell and cell-to-matrix interactions play a key role in determining endothelial cell invasion, migration, and proliferation. During wound healing, a number of adhesive proteins are expressed in the basement membrane zone of blood vessels, including vWF, fibronectin, and fibrinogen. Studies have shown that several integrin receptors, especially $\alpha v \beta 3$, are upregulated on the surface of smooth muscle cells and endothelial cells during angiogenesis *(57)*. $\alpha v \beta 3$ is the endothelial cell receptor for vWF, fibrinogen/fibrin, and fibronectin. In one study, $\alpha v \beta 3$ was found to be expressed in newly formed blood vessels in granulation tissue but not in normal unwounded skin *(57)*. Exposure of cultured chick chorioallantoic membranes (CAMs) to several specific cytokines and tumor fragments stimulated angiogenesis and a fourfold increase in expression of $\alpha v \beta 3$. Exposure of CAMs to a monoclonal antibody to $\alpha v \beta 3$ resulted in a block in vessel formation, whereas no effect was seen on preexisting vessels. These studies suggest that $\alpha v \beta 3$ plays a key role in angiogenesis. One potential clinical application of these findings is that $\alpha v \beta 3$ may serve as a therapeutic target for diseases in which neovascularization plays a critical role, such as pyogenic granuloma and other vascular tumors, diabetic retinopathy, and rheumatoid arthritis.

TISSUE REMODELING (PHASE 3)

The third and final phase of wound healing is tissue remodeling. This phase begins at the same time as tissue formation and continues for months after injury. Over this time granulation tissue becomes mature scar tissue. This phase represents a very dynamic process that is not always homogeneous within the wound. Thus, there are quantitative and qualitative differences between the macromolecular makeup of the wound margin and its center. This is also a phase of wound healing that is less well studied and understood. We do know, however, that a number of enzymes are involved in breaking down matrix components, particularly collagen. Ultimately, the goal of this phase of wound healing is to restore the functional barrier of the skin and to increase the tensile strength of the scar.

Fibroblasts play a major role in the phase of wound healing. Fibroblasts produce fibronectin, HA, proteoglycans, and collagen, all of which play key roles in cellular migration of cells, as a linkage for myofibroblasts to cause wound contraction and as a template for collagen deposition. HA promotes cell migration and division *(58)*. Proteoglycans contribute to tissue resilience, modulate collagen deposition, and regulate cellular function. Collagen provides structural support, increases tensile strength of the tissue, and, like proteoglycans, has a number of important effects on cellular function.

Fibronectin

The initial extracellular matrix has a high concentration of fibronectin, which is produced by fibroblasts as they migrate into the wound area. It has been shown that the fibronectin matrix is established about 5 days after the initial injury *(59)*. Fibronectin is deposited along the same axis along which fibroblasts are aligned, and new collagen deposition will ultimately follow the same orientation *(59)*. Myofibroblasts link to and utilize the fibronectin network to cause wound contraction.

Growth factors, especially TGF-β, play an essential role in the formation of this early matrix. TGF-β is a chemoattractant for fibroblasts *(60)*, stimulates fibroblast proliferation *(61)*, and increases overall extracellular matrix formation *(58)*. TGF-β also stimulates fibroblasts to produce fibronectin and upregulates integrin receptors that bind to fibronectin *(58)*.

The mechanisms by which fibroblasts are able to modify their adhesion to the extra-cellular matrix (ECM), allowing for migration across the wound, are not completely understood. One possible mechanism is the process of controlled proteolysis, in which proteinases act on specific sites in some cells to modulate the assembly of their actin cytoskeleton *(56)*. Another mechanism by which cell adhesion may be altered is modification of the ECM by deposition or synthesis of ECM-associated molecules, including SPARC, thrombospondin, dermatan sulfate proteoglycans, and tenascin *(56)*. Thrombospondin and tenascin have both adhesive and antiadhesive properties, and it has been shown that SPARC upregulates fibroblast expression of metalloproteinases, especially collagenase *(62)*. The ability of SPARC to induce collagenase expression is at least in part regulated by the ECM to which fibroblasts are exposed. SPARC induces collagenase production in fibroblasts grown on collagen types I, II, III, and V, and on vitronectin, but not on collagen type IV.

The initial fibronectin matrix is slowly degraded by cell and plasma proteases. Over time, fibronectin is replaced by type III collagen and ultimately by type I collagen.

Hyaluronic Acid and Proteoglycans

Hyaluronan, a glycosaminoglycan (GAG), is another major component of early granulation tissue. Fibroblasts in the early wound produce substantially larger amounts of HA than fibroblasts in normal skin *(58)*. HA promotes cell motility, presumably by altering cell-matrix adhesion. It has been proposed that heparan sulfate and fibronectin mediate cell attachment to the ECM and that HA weakens this adhesion *(63)*. Another proposed mechanism by which HA may facilitate cell locomotion is based on its ability to become a highly hydrated structure, thereby causing tissue swelling and creating resilience but inhibit cell movement and proliferation *(58)*. Growth factors may play a role in the HA-induced cell locomotion. TGF-β1 has been shown to upregulate expression of HA and one of its receptors (RHAMM), thereby stimulating fibroblast motility *(64)*. Antibodies that block HA-RHAMM binding inhibit cell locomotion *(45)*.

As the wound matures, HA is slowly replaced by sulfated proteoglycans, which play a structural role in late granulation tissue formation and also regulate cell function. Two major proteoglycans, chondroitin-4-sulfate and dermatan sulfate, are produced by mature scar fibroblasts.

Collagen

There are at least three classes of collagen in normal connective tissue: fibrillar collagens (types I, III, and V); basement membrane collagen (type IV); and other interstitial collagens (types VI, VII, and VIII). The fibrillar collagens serve as the major structural collagens in all connective tissues *(58)*.

In the healing wound, granulation tissue is initially comprised of large amounts of type III collagen, which is found only in small amounts in the normal dermis. Over a period of a year or more, type III collagen is gradually replaced by type I collagen. This leads to increased tensile strength of the scar. However, the final tensile strength of a scar is only 70–80% of that of preinjured skin *(65)*. The process of converting the collagen content of the dermis from type III to type I collagen is controlled by interactions involving synthesis of new collagen with lysis of old collagen *(43)*. Key to this process of conversion are metalloproteinases, specifically the collagenases.

Matrix-degrading metalloproteinases (MMP) are proenzymes that need to be activated and are considered to be the physiologic mediators of matrix degradation. The prototypic MMP is interstitial collagenase, but there are at least 10 such enzymes that are secreted as zymogens. Three broad classes are recognized: collagenases, gelatinases, and stromelysins. The collagenases include interstitial collagenase (fibroblast collagenase, MMP-1), which acts on collagens I, II, III, VII, and X. Collagen type II is a particularly good substrate for MMP-1. MMP-1 also degrades type II and III collagens but is particularly active against type I collagen. MMP-1 collagenase cleaves α-chains of type I, II, and III collagens. Gelatinases are able to break down denatured collagen (gelatin). Of particular importance among the gelatinase class is gelatinase A (MMP-2), which is an established enzyme for the degradation of gelatins, collagen IV, and elastin. Another key gelatinase is gelatinase B (MMP-9), which was originally thought to be secreted mainly by macrophages but is now known to also be a product of other cell types, including neutrophils and keratinocytes. Stromelysins have a relatively broad substrate specificity. Both stromelysin 1 (MMP-3) and 2 (MMP-10) act on proteoglycans, fibronectin, laminin, gelatins, and collagens III, IV, and IX. Another member of the stromelysin family, matrilysin (MMP-7), degrades mainly fibronectin, gelatins, and elastin.

MMPs are stimulated not only by growth factors but also by ECM. They are single-chain proteins activated by trypsin, organomercurials, and sodium dodecyl sulfate (SDS), among others. Plasmin may also activate them. They are all zinc MMPs, with the zinc atom at the center of the molecule at a conserved sequence known as HEXGH. MMPs are stabilized by calcium and are inhibited by various chelators such as tissue inhibitor of metalloproteinase, which inhibits several members of the MMP family. MMPs have other inhibitors, such as α-2-macroglobulin, which entraps them. As stated, several cytokines, including interleukin-1 (IL-1), stimulate the synthesis of MMP. It should be noted that other enzymes and proteases play an important role in matrix degradation and in facilitating cellular migration. Urokinase is a good example of this. Interestingly, urokinase can stimulate the synthesis of plasminogen, which then leads to plasmin activation.

The remodeling phase is more than a breakdown of excess macromolecules formed during the proliferative phase of wound healing. Cells within the wound are returned to a stable phenotype, ECM material is altered (i.e., collagen type III to type I), and the graulation tissue that was so exuberant during the early phases of wound healing disappears.

ACKNOWLEDGMENTS

This work was supported by NIH grants AR42936 and AR46557, and by the Wound Biotechnology Foundation.

REFERENCES

1. Santaro SA. Identification of a 160,000 dalton platelet membrane protein that mediates the initial divalent cation-dependent adhesion of platelets to collagen. *Cell* 1986;46:913–920.
2. Moncada S, Gryglewski R, Bunting S, Vane JR. An enzyme isolated from arteries transforms prostaglandin endoperoxides to an unstable substance that inhibits platelet aggregation. *Nature* 1976;263:663–665.
3. Loskutoff DJ, Edgington TS. Synthesis of a fibrinolytic activator and inhibitor in endothelial cells. *Proc Natl Acad Sci USA* 1977;74:3903.

4. Katz MH, Alvarez AF, Kirsner RS, et al. Human wound fluid from acute wounds stimulates fibroblast and endothelial cell growth. *J Am Acad Dermatol* 1991;25:1054–1058.
5. Tonnesen MGT. Neutrophil endothelial cell interaction: mechanisms of neutrophil adherence to vascular endothelium. *J Invest Dermatol* 1989;93:53S–58S.
6. Doherty DE, Hasslet C, Tonnesen MG, Henson PM. Human monocyte adherence: a primary effect of chemotactic factors on the monocyte to stimulate adherence to human endothelium. *J Immunol* 1987;138:1762–1771.
7. Gresham HD, Goodwin JL, Allen PM, et al. A novel member of the integrin receptor family mediates Arg-Gly-Asp stimulated neutrophil phagocytosis. *J Cell Biol* 1989;108:1935–1943.
8. Simpson DM, Ross R. The neutrophilic leukocyte in wound repair. A study with antineutrophil serum. *J Clin Invest* 1972;51:2009–2023.
9. Newman SL, Henson JE, Henson PM. Phagocytosis of senescent neutrophils by human monocyte derived macrophages and rabbit inflammatory macrophages. *J Exp Med* 1982;156:430–442.
10. Sarret Y, Woodley DT, Grigsby K, et al. Human kerotinocyte locomotion: the effect of selected cytokines. *J Invest Dermatol* 1992;98:12–16.
11. Gabbiani G, Chapponnier C, Huttner I. Cytoplasmic filaments and gap junctions in epithelial cells and myofibroblasts during wound healing. *J Cell Biol* 1978;76:561–568.
12. Krawczyk WS, Wilgram GF. Hemidesmosome and desmosome morphogenesis during epidermal wound healing. *J Ultrastruct Res* 1973;45:93–101.
13. O'Keefe EJ, Payne RE, Russell N, et al. Spreading and enhanced motility of human keratinocytes on fibronectin. *J Invest Dermatol* 1985;85:125–130.
14. Woodley DT, Chen JD, Kim JP, Sarret Y, et al. Re-epithelialization. Human keratinocyte locomotion. *Dermatol Clin* 1993;11:641–646.
15. Clark RAF, Lanigan JM, Dellpella P, et al. Fibronectin and fibrin provide a provisional matrix for epidermal cell migration during wound reepithelialization. *J Invest Dermatol* 1982;79:264–269.
16. Woodley DT, Bachmann PM, O'Keefe EJ. Laminin inhibits human keratinocyte migration. *J Cell Physiol* 1988;136:140–146.
17. Larjava H, Salo T, Haapasalmi, K, et al. Expression of integrins and basement membrane components by wound keratinocytes. *J Clin Invest* 1993;92:1425–1435.
18. Juliano RL, Haskill S. Signal transduction from the extracellular matrix. *J Cell Biol* 1993;120(3):577–585.
19. Brown PJ, Juliano RL. Selective inhibition of fibronectin-mediated adhesion by monoclonal antibodies to a cell surface glycoprotein. *Science* 1985;228:1448–1451.
20. Carter WG, Ryan MC, Gahr PF. Epiligrin, a new cell adhesion ligand for integrin $\alpha3\beta1$ in epithelial basement membranes. *Cell* 1991;65:599–610.
21. Phillips DR, Charo IF, Parise LA, Fitzgerald LA. The platelet membrane glycoprotein IIb-IIIa complex. *Blood* 1988;71:831–843.
22. Takada Y, Murphy E, Pil P, et al. Molecular cloning and expression of the cDNA for alpha 3 subunit of human alpha3/beta1 (VLA3) an integrin receptor for fibronectin laminin and collagen. *J Cell Biol* 1991;115:257–266.
23. Albelda SM, Buck CA. Integrins and other cell adhesion molecules. *Fed Am Soc Exp Biol J* 1990;4:2868–2880.
24. Defilippi P, Truffa G, Stefanuto G, et al. Tumor necrosis factor α and interferon gamma modulate the expression of the vitronectin receptor (integrin$\alpha3$) in human endothelial cells. *J Biol Chem* 1991;266:7638–7645.
25. Hemler ME. VLA proteins in the integrin family: structures, functions, and their role in leukocytes. *Annu Rev Immunol* 1990;8:365–400.
26. Guan JL, Hynes RO. Lymphoid cells recognize an alternatively spliced segment of fibronectin via the integrin receptor alpha4/beta1. *Cell* 1990;60:53–61.

27. Elices MJ, Urry LA, Hemler ME. Receptor functions for the integrin VLA-3: fibronectin, collagen, and laminin binding are differentially influenced by ARG-GLY-ASP peptide and by divalent cations. *J Cell Biol* 1991;112:169–181.

28. Takada Y, Elices MJ, Crouse C, Hemler ME. Primary structure of the alpha 4 subunit of VLA4; homology to other integrins and a possible cell-cell adhesion function. *Eur Mol Biol Organ* 1989;8:1361–1368.

29. Xu J, Clark RA. Extracellular matrix alters PDGF regulation of fibroblast integrins. *J Cell Biol* 1996;132:239–249.

30. Kim JP, Zhang K, Chen JD, et al. Mechanism of human keratinocyte migration on fibronectin: unique roles of RGD site and integrins. *J Cell Physiol* 1992;151:443–450.

31. Chen JD, Kim JP, Sarret Y, et al. Recombinant human epidermal growth factor (rEGF) promotes human keratinocyte locomotion. *J Invest Dermatol* 1992;98:614.

32. Kim JP, Zhang K, Kramer RH, et al. Integrin receptors and RGD sequences in human keratinocyte migration: unique anti-migratory function of $\alpha 3\beta 1$ epiligrin receptor. *J Invest Dermatol* 1992;98:764–770.

33. Sheppard D, Cohen DS, Wang A, Busk M. Transforming growth factor beta differentially regulates expression of integrin subunits in guinea pig airway epithelial cells. *J Biol Chem* 1992;267:17,409–17,414.

34. Prieto AL, Edelman GM, Crossin KL. Multiple integrins mediate cell attachment to cytotactin/tenascin. *Proc Natl Acad Sci USA* 1993;90:10,154–10,158.

35. Breuss JM, Gallo J, DeLisser HM, et al. Expression of the $\alpha 6$ subunit in development. Neoplasia and tissue repair suggests a role in epithelial remodeling. *J Cell Sci* 1995;108: 2241–2251.

36. Agrez M, Chen RI, Cone RI, et al. The alpha-v beta-6 integrin promotes proliferation of colon carcinoma cells through a unique region of the beta-6 cytoplasmic domain. *J Cell Biol* 1994;27:547–556.

37. Roberts CJ, Birkenmeier TM, McQuillan JJ, et al. Transforming growth factor-β stimulates the expression of fibronectin and of both subunits of the human fibronectin receptor by cultured human lung fibroblasts. *J Biol Chem* 1988;263:4586–4592.

38. Heino J, Ignotz RA, Hemler ME, Crouse C, Massague J. Regulation of cell adhesion receptors by transforming growth factor-β: concomitant regulation of integrins that share a common $\beta 1$ subunit. *J Biol Chem* 1989;264:380–388.

39. Ignotz RA, Heino J, Massague J. Regulation of cell adhesion receptors by transforming growth factor-β regulation of vitronectin receptor and LFA-1. *J Biol Chem* 1989;264:389–392.

40. Gailit J, Welch MP, Clark RA. TGF-$\beta 1$ stimulates expression of keratinocyte integrins during re-epithelialization of cutaneous wounds. *J Invest Dermatol* 1994;103:221–227.

41. Assoian RK, Komoriya A, Meyers CA, et al. Transforming growth factor-β in human platelets: identification of a major storage site, purification, and characterization. *J Biol Chem* 1983;258:7150–7160.

42. Singer AJ, Clark RAF. Cutaneous wound healing. *N Engl J Med* 1999;341:738–746.

43. Yamaguchi Y, Crane S, Zhou L, Ochoa S, Falanga V. Lack of coordinate expression of the $\alpha 1(I)$ and $\beta 1(III)$ procollagen genes in fibroblast clonal cultures. *Br J Dermatol* 2000;143: 1149–1153.

44. Falanga V, Martin TA, Tagaki H, et al. Low oxygen tension increases mRNA levels of alpha 1 (I) procollagen in human dermal fibroblasts. *J Cell Physiol* 1993;157:408–412.

45. Samuel SK, Hurta RAR, Spearman MA, et al. TGF-$\beta 1$ stimulation of cell locomotion utilizes the hyaluronan receptor RHAMM and hyaluronan. *J Cell Biol* 1993;123:749–758.

46. Hardwick C, Hoare K, Owens R, et al. Molecular cloning of a novel hyaluronan receptor that mediates tumor cell motility. *J Cell Biol* 1992;117:1343–1350.

47. Estes JM, Adzick NS, Harrison MR, et al. Hyaluronate metabolism undergoes an ontogenic transition during fetal development: implications for scar-free wound healing. *J Pediatr Surg* 1993;28:1227–1231.

48. Undersell C. CD44: the hyaluronan receptor. *J Cell Sci* 1992;103:293–298.
49. Thomas L, Byers HR, Vink J, Stamenkovic I. CD44H regulates tumor cell migration on hyaluronate-coated substrate. *J Cell Biol* 1992;118:971–977.
50. Messadi DV, Bertolami CN. CD44 and hyaluronan expression in human cutaneous scar fibroblasts. *Am J Pathol* 1993;142:1041–1049.
51. Skalli O, Gabbiana G. The biology of the myofibroblast relationship in wound contraction and fibrocontractive disease, in *Molecular and Cellular Biology of Wound Repair* (Clark RAF, Henson PM, eds.), Plenum Press, New York, 1988, pp. 373–402.
52. Falanga V. Growth factors and wound healing. *Dermatol Clin* 1993;11:667–675.
53. Loskutoff DJ, Edgington TS. Synthesis of a fibrinolytic activator and inhibitor by endothelial cells. *Proc Natl Acad Sci USA* 1977;74:3903.
54. Knighton DR, Hunt TK, Scheuenstuhl H, et al. Oxygen tension regulates the expression of angiogenesis factor by macrophages. *Science* 1983;221:1283–1285.
55. Gailit J, Clark RAF. Wound repair in the context of the extracellular matrix. *Curr Opin Cell Biol* 1994;6:717–725.
56. Tremble PM, Lane TF, Sage EH, Werb Z. SPARC, a secreted protein associated with morphogenesis and tissue remodeling, induces expression of metalloproteinases in fibroblasts through a novel extracellular matrix-dependent pathway. *J Cell Biol* 1993;121:1433–1444.
57. Brooks PC, Clark RAF, Cheresh DA. Requirement of vascular integrin $\alpha v \beta 3$ for angiogenesis. *Science* 1994;264:569–571.
58. Lawrence TW. Physiology of the acute wound. *Clin Plast Surg* 1998;25:321–340.
59. Welch MP, Odland GF, Clark RA. Temporal relationships of F-actin bundle formation, collagen and fibronectin matrix assembly, and fibronectin receptor expression to wound contraction. *J Cell Biol* 1990;110–133.
60. Postlethwaite AE, Kcski-Oja J, Moscs HL, Kang AH. Stimulation of the chemotactic migration of human fibroblasts by transforming growth factor-beta. *J Exp Med* 1987;165–251.
61. Loef EB, et al. Induction of c-six RNA and activity similar to platelet derived growth factor by transforming growth factor-beta: a proposed model for indirect mitogenesis involving autocrine activity. *Proc Natl Acad Sci USA* 1986;83:2453.
62. Lawler J, Weinstein R, Hynes RO. Cell attachment to thromobospondin: the role of ARG-GLY-ASP, calcium and integrin receptors. *J Cell Biol* 1988;107:2351–2361.
63. Lark MW, Laterra J, Culp LA. Close and focal contact adhesions of fibroblasts to fibronectin-containing matrix. *Fed Proc* 1985;44:394.
64. Yang B, Zhang L, Turley EA. Identification of two hyaluronan-binding domains in the hyaluronan receptor RHAMM. *J Biol Chem* 1993;268:8617–8623.
65. Abercrombie M, Flint MH, James DW. Wound contraction in relation to collagen formation in scorbutic guinea pigs. *J Embryol Exp Morphol* 1956;4:167–175.

4

Diabetic Polyneuropathy

Solomon Tesfaye, MD, FRCP

INTRODUCTION

Polyneuropathy is one of the commonest complications of diabetes and the commonest form of neuropathy in the developed world. Diabetic polyneuropathy encompasses several neuropathic syndromes, the commonest of which is distal symmetrical neuropathy, the main initiating factor for foot ulceration. The epidemiology of diabetic neuropathy has recently been reviewed in reasonable detail *(1)*. Several clinic- *(2,3)* and population-based studies *(4,5)* show surprisingly similar prevalence rates for distal symmetrical neuropathy, affecting about 30% of all diabetic people. The EURODIAB Prospective Complications Study, which involved the examination of 3250 type 1 patients from 16 European countries, found a prevalence rate of 28% for distal symmetrical neuropathy *(2)*. After excluding those with neuropathy at baseline, the study showed that over a 7-year period, about one-fourth of type 1 diabetic patients developed distal symmetrical neuropathy, age, duration of diabetes, and poor glycemic control being major determinants *(6)*. The development of neuropathy was also associated with potentially modifiable cardiovascular risk factors such as serum lipids, blood pressure, body mass index, and albumin excretion rate *(6)*. Based on recent epidemiologic studies, established correlates of diabetic neuropathy include increasing age, increasing duration of diabetes, poor glycemic control, retinopathy, and albuminuria *(1,2,4)*. Less well-established correlates of diabetic neuropathy include increasing height, hypertension, and cardiovascular risk factors *(1,2,4)*.

CLASSIFICATION

Clinical classification of the various syndromes of diabetic peripheral neuropathy has proved difficult. The variation and overlap in etiology, clinical features, natural history, and prognosis have meant that most classifications are necessarily oversimplified, and none has proved capable of accounting for all these factors. Nevertheless, attempts at classification stimulate thought as to the etiology of the various syndromes and also assist in the planning of management strategies for the patient.

Clinical manifestations *(7)* and measurements *(8)* of somatic neuropathy have recently been reviewed, and there are a number of classifications. Based on the various distinct clinical presentations to the physician, Ward *(9)* recommended the classification depicted in Table 1. This practical approach provides the clinician with workable, crude definitions for the various neuropathic syndromes and also assists in management of the patient.

From: *The Diabetic Foot: Medical and Surgical Management*
Edited by: A. Veves, J. M. Giurini, and F. W. LoGerfo © Humana Press Inc., Totowa, NJ

Table 1
Presentations of the Neuropathic
Syndromes Associated with Diabetes

Chronic insidious sensory neuropathy
Acute painful neuropathy
Proximal motor neuropathy
Diffuse symmetric motor neuropathy
The neuropathic foot
Pressure neuropathy
Focal vascular neuropathy
Neuropathy present at diagnosis
Treatment-induced neuropathy
Hypoglycemic neuropathy

Adapted from ref. *9.*

More recently, Watkins and Edmonds *(10)* have suggested a classification based on the natural history of the various syndromes, which clearly separates them into three distinct groups:

1. *Progressive neuropathies.* These are associated with increasing duration of diabetes and with other microvascular complications. Sensory disturbance predominates, and autonomic involvement is common. The onset is gradual, and there is no recovery.
2. *Reversible neuropathies.* These have an acute onset, often occurring at the presentation of diabetes itself, and are not related to the duration of diabetes or other microvascular complications. There is spontaneous recovery.
3. *Pressure palsies.* Although these are not specific to diabetes only, they tend to occur more frequently in diabetic patients than the general population. There is no association with duration of diabetes or other microvascular complications of diabetes.

Another method of classifying diabetic polyneuropathy is by considering whether the clinical involvement is symmetrical or assymetrical. However, such a separation, although useful in identifying distinct entities and perhaps providing clues to the varied etiologies, is an oversimplification, as the overlap of the syndromes is great. This method was originally suggested by by Bruyn and Garland *(11)* and was later modified by Thomas *(12).* More recently, Low and Suarez *(13)* have modified it further (Table 2).

SYMMETRICAL NEUROPATHIES

Distal Symmetrical Neuropathy

This is the commonest neuropathic syndrome and what is meant in clinical practice by the phrase *diabetic neuropathy.* There is a "length-related" pattern of sensory loss, with sensory symptoms starting in the toes and then extending to involve the feet and legs in a stocking distribution. In more severe cases, there is often upper limb involvement, with a similar progression proximally starting in the fingers. Although the nerve damage can extend over the entire body including the head and face, this is exceptional. Subclinical neuropathy detectable by autonomic function tests is usually present. However, clinical autonomic neuropathy is less common. As the disease advances, overt motor manifestations such as wasting of the small muscles of the hands and limb weak-

Table 2
Classification of Diabetic Neuropathy

Symmetric neuropathies
    Distal sensory and and sensorimotor neuropathy
    Large-fiber type of diabetic neuropathy
    Small-fiber type of diabetic neuropathy
    Distal small-fiber neuropathy
    "Insulin neuropathy"
    Chronic inflammatory demyelinating polyradiculoneuropathy (CIDP)

Asymmetric neuropathies
    Mononeuropathy
    Mononeuropathy multiplex
    Radiculopathies
    Lumbar plexopathy or radiculoplexopathy
    Chronic inflammatory demyelinating polyradiculoneuropathy

Adapted from ref. *13*.

ness become apparent. However, subclinical motor involvement detected by magnetic resonance imaging appears to be common, and thus motor disturbance is clearly part of the functional impairment caused by distal symmetrical neuropathy *(14)*.

The main clinical presentation of distal symmetrical neuropathy is sensory loss, which the patient may not be aware of, or may describe as "numbness" or "dead feeling." However, some may experience a progressive buildup of unpleasant sensory symptoms including tingling (paresthesiae); burning pain; shooting pains down the legs; lancinating pains; contact pain, often with daytime clothes and bedclothes (allodynia); pain on walking, often described as "walking barefoot on marbles" or "walking barefoot on hot sand"; sensations of heat or cold in the feet; and persistent achy feeling in the feet and cramp-like sensations in the legs. Occasionally pain can extend above the feet and may involve the whole of the legs; when this is the case there is usually upper limb involvement also. There is a large spectrum of severity of these symptoms. Some may have minor complaints such as tingling in one or two toes; others may be affected with such devastating complications as "the numb diabetic foot" or severe painful neuropathy that does not respond to drug therapy.

Diabetic neuropathic pain is characteristically more severe at night and often prevents sleep *(15,16)*. Some patients may be in a constant state of tiredness because of sleep deprivation *(15)*. Others are unable to maintain full employment *(15–17)*. Severe painful neuropathy can occasionally cause marked reduction in exercise threshold so as interfere with daily activities *(17)*. This is particularly the case when there is an associated disabling, severe postural hypotension due to autonomic involvement *(10)*. Not surprisingly therefore, depressive and symptoms are not uncommon *(15)*. Although subclinical autonomic neuropathy is commonly found in patients with distal symmetrical neuropathy *(18)*, symptomatic autonomic neuropathy is uncommon.

It is important to appreciate that many subjects with distal symmetrical neuropathy may not have any of the above symptoms, and their first presentation may be with a foot ulcer *(19)*. This underpins the need for careful examination and screening of the feet of all diabetic people, to identify those at risk of developing foot ulceration. The insensate foot is at risk of developing mechanical and thermal injuries, and patients must therefore be warned about these and given appropriate advice with regard to foot care *(19,20)*. A curious feature of the neuropathic foot is that both numbness and pain may occur, the so-called painful, painless leg *(20)*. It is indeed a paradox that the patient with a large foot ulcer may also have severe neuropathic pain. In those with advanced neuropathy, there may be sensory ataxia. The unfortunate sufferer is affected by unsteadiness on walking, or even falls, particularly if there is associated visual impairment owing to retinopathy.

Neuropathy is usually easily detected by simple clinical examination *(21)*. Shoes and socks should be removed and the feet examined at least annually and more often if neuropathy is present. The most common presenting abnormality is a reduction or absence of vibration sense in the toes. As the disease progresses, there is sensory loss in a "stocking" and sometimes in a "glove" distribution involving all modalities. When there is severe sensory loss, proprioception may also be impaired, leading to a positive Romberg's sign. Ankle tendon reflexes are lost, and with more advanced neuropathy, knee reflexes are often reduced or absent.

Muscle strength is usually normal early during the course of the disease, although mild weakness may be found in toe extensors. However, with progressive disease there is significant generalized muscular wasting, particularly in the small muscles of the hand and feet. The fine movements of the fingers are then affected, and there is difficulty in handling small objects. Wasting of dorsal interossei is, however, usually caused by entrapment of the ulnar nerve at the elbow. The clawing of the toes is believed to be caused by unopposed (because of wasting of the small muscles of the foot) pulling of the long extensor and flexor tendons. This scenario results in elevated plantar pressure points at the metatarsal heads that are prone to callus formation and foot ulceration *(19)*. Deformities such as a bunion can form the focus of ulceration; with more extreme deformities, such as those associated with Charcot arthropathy, the risk is further increased. As one of the most common precipitants to foot ulceration is inappropriate footwear, a thorough assessment should also include examination of shoes for poor fit, abnormal wear, and internal pressure areas or foreign bodies.

Autonomic neuropathy affecting the feet can cause a reduction in sweating and consequently dry skin that is likely to crack easily, predisposing the patient to the risk of infection *(19)*. The "purely" neuropathic foot is also warm, owing to the arterio/venous shunting first described by Ward et al. *(21)*. This results in the distension of foot veins that fail to collapse even when the foot is elevated. It is not unusual to observe a gangrenous toe in a foot that has bounding arterial pulses, as there is impairment of the nutritive capillary circulation caused by arteriovenous shunting. The oxygen tension of the blood in these veins is typically raised *(22)*. The increasing blood flow brought about by autonomic neuropathy can sometimes result in neuropathic edema, which is resistant to treatment with diuretics but may respond to treatment with ephedrine *(23)*.

Small-Fiber Neuropathy

The existence of "small-fiber neuropathy" as a distinct entity has been advocated by some authorities *(24,25)*, usually within the context of young type 1 patients. A prominent feature of this syndrome is neuropathic pain, which may be very severe, with relative sparing of large-fiber functions (vibration and proprioception). The pain is described as burning, deep, and aching. The sensation of pins and needles (paresthesiae) is also often experienced. Contact hypersensitivity may be present. However, rarely, patients with small-fiber neuropathy may not have neuropathic pain, and some may occasionally have foot ulceration. Autonomic involvement is common, and severely affected patients may be disabled by postural hypotension and/or gastrointestinal symptoms. The syndrome tends to develop within a few years of diabetes as a relatively early complication.

On clinical examination there is little evidence of objective signs of nerve damage, apart from a reduction in pinprick and temperature sensation, which are reduced in a "stocking" and "glove" distribution. There is relative sparing of vibration and position sense (due to relative sparing of the large-diameter Aβ fibers). Muscle strength is usually normal, and reflexes are also usually normal. However, autonomic function tests are frequently abnormal, and affected male patients usually have erectile dysfunction. Electrophysiologic tests support small-fiber dysfunction. Sural sensory conduction velocity may be normal, although the amplitude may be reduced. Motor nerves appear to be less affected. Controversy still exists as to whether small-fiber neuropathy is a distinct entity or an earlier manifestation of chronic sensory motor neuropathy *(24,25)*. Said et al. *(24)* studied a small series of subjects with this syndrome and showed that small-fiber degeneration predominated morphometrically. Veves et al. *(26)* found a varying degree of early small-fiber involvement in all diabetic polyneuropathies, which was confirmed by detailed sensory and autonomic function tests. It is unclear, therefore, whether this syndrome is in fact distinct or merely represents the early stages of distal symmetrical neuropathy that has been detected by the prominence of early symptoms.

Differential Diagnosis

Diabetic peripheral neuropathy presents in a similar way to neuropathies of other causes, and thus the physician needs to carefully exclude other common causes before attributing the neuropathy to diabetes. Absence of other complications of diabetes, rapid weight loss, excessive alcohol intake, and other atypical features in either the history or clinical examination should alert the physician to search for other causes of neuropathy. Table 3 shows the differential diagnoses.

Natural History

Although distal symmetrical neuropathy is common in clinical practice, few prospective studies have looked at its natural history, which remains poorly understood, partly because of our inadequate knowledge of the pathogenesis. Several mechanisms have been suggested *(27–30)*, however, and the list is growing. Unlike in diabetic retinopathy and nephropathy, the scarcity of simple, accurate, and readily reproducible methods of measuring neuropathy further complicates the problem *(8)*. One study *(31)* reported that neuropathic symptoms remain or get worse over a 5-year period in patients with chronic distal symmetrical neuropathy. A major drawback of this study was that it involved highly selected patients from a hospital base. A more recent study reported improvements in painful symptoms over 3½ years *(32)*. Neuropathic pain was assessed using a visual analog scale, and small-fiber function by thermal limen, heat pain threshold, and weighted pinprick threshold. At follow-up 3½ years later, one-third of the 50 patients at baseline had died or were lost to follow-up. Clearly this is a major drawback. There

Table 3
Differential Diagnosis of Distal Symmetrical Neuropathy

Metabolic disorders
  Diabetes
  Amyloidosis
  Uremia
  Myxedema
  Porphyria
  Vitamin deficiency (thiamin, B_{12}, B_6, pyridoxine)

Drugs and chemicals
  Alcohol
  Cytotoxic drugs, e.g., vincristine
  Chlorambucil
  Nitrofurantoin
  Isoniazid

Neoplastic disorders
  Bronchial or gastric carcinoma
  Lymphoma

Infective or inflammatory conditions
  Leprosy
  Guillain-Barré syndrome
  Lyme borreliosis
  Chronic inflammatory demyelinating polyneuropathy
  Polyarteritis nodosa

Genetic conditions
  Charcot-Marie-Tooth disease
  Hereditary sensory neuropathies

was symptomatic improvement in painful neuropathy in most of the remaining patients. Despite this symptomatic improvement, however, small-fiber function as measured by the above tests deteriorated significantly. Thus, there was a dichotomy in the evolution of neuropathic symptoms and neurophysiologic measures.

Are Painful and Painless Neuropathies Distinct Entities?

One of the complexities of distal symmetrical neuropathy is the its variety of presentation to the clinician. A relative minority present with pain as the predominant symptom *(33)*. There is controversy as to whether the clinical, neurophysiologic, peripheral nerve hemodynamic/morphometric findings are distinctly different in subjects with painful and painless diabetic neuropathy. Young et al. *(34)* reported that patients with painful neuropathy had a higher ratio of autonomic (small-fiber) abnormality to electrophysiologic (large-fiber) abnormality. In contrast, they found that electrophysiologic parameters were significantly worse in patients with foot ulceration compared with those who had painful neuropathy. They concluded that in distal symmetrical neuropathy, the relationship between large- and small-fiber damage is not uniform and that there may be different etiologic influences on large- and small-fiber neuropathy in diabetic subjects, with the predominant type of fiber damage determining the form of the presenting clinical syndrome *(34)*. This view is supported by the study of Tsigos et al. *(35)*, who also suggested that painful and painless neuropathies represent two distinct clinical entities with little overlap. However, a contarary view was expressed by Veves et al. *(36)*, who found that painful symptoms were frequent in diabetic neuropathy, irrespective of the presence or absence of foot ulceration and that these symptoms may occur at any stage of the disease. They concluded that there is a spectrum of presentations from varying degrees of painful neuropathy to predominantly painless neuropathy associated with foot ulceration and that much overlap is present *(36)*. The author's clinical observations support this view, as painful symptoms are often similarly present in patients with and without foot ulceration, suggesting that painless and painful neuropathies represent extreme forms of the same syndrome. Thus, an important clinical point is that the neuropathic foot with painful symptoms is just as valnerable to foot ulceration as the foot with absence of painful neuropathic symptoms. The crucial determining factor is elevation of vibration perception threshold *(37)* and not the presence or absence of painful symptoms. Indeed, the "painful-painless" foot with ulceration is frequently observed in the diabetic foot clinic, a phenomenon first described by Ward *(20)*.

Acute Painful Neuropathies

These are transient neuropathic syndromes characterized by an acute onset of pain in the lower limbs. Acute neuropathies present in a symmetrical fashion and are relatively uncommon. Pain is invariably present, is usually distressing to the patient, and can sometimes be incapacitating. There are two distinct syndromes, the first of which occurs within the context of poor glycemic control and the second with rapid improvements in metabolic control.

Acute Painful Neuropathy of Poor Glycemic Control

This phenomenon usually occurs in type 1 or 2 diabetic subjects with poor glycemic control. There is no relationship to the presence of other chronic diabetic complications. There is often an associated severe weight loss *(38)*. Ellenberg *(39)* termed this condition *neuropathic cachexia (39)*. Patients typically develop persistent burning pain associated with allodynia (contact pain). The pain is most marked in the feet but often affects the whole of the lower extremities. As in chronic distal symmetrical neuropathy, the pain is typically worse at night, although persistent pain during the day is also common. The pain is likened to "walking on burning sand," and there may be a subjective feeling of the feet being "swollen." Patients also describe intermittent bouts of stabbing pain that shoot up the legs from the feet ("peak pain"), superimposed on the background of burning pain ("background pain"). Not surprisingly, therefore, these disabling symptoms often lead to depression.

On examination, sensory loss is usually surprisingly mild or even absent. There are usually no motor signs, although ankle jerks may be absent. Nerve conduction studies are also usually normal or mildly abnormal. Temperature discrimination threshold (small-fiber function) is, however, affected more commonly than vibration perception threshold (large-fiber function) *(40)*. There is complete resolution of symptoms within 10 months, and weight gain is usual, with continued improvement in glycemic control with the use of insulin. The lack of objective signs should not raise the doubt that these painful symptoms are not real. Many patients feel that people (including health care professionals) don't fully appreciate their predicament.

Acute Painful Neuropathy of Rapid Glycemic Control (Insulin Neuritis)

The term "insulin neuritis" was coined by Caravati *(41)*, who first described the syndrome of acute painful neuropathy of rapid glycemic control. The term is a misnomer, as the condition can follow rapid improvement in glycemic control with oral hypoglycemic agents, and "neuritis" implies a neural inflammatory process for which there is no evidence. The author has therefore recommended that the term *acute painful neuropathy of rapid glycemic control* be used to describe this condition *(42)*.

The natural history of acute painful neuropathies is an almost guaranteed improvement *(38)*, in contrast to chronic distal symmetrical neuropathy *(31,32)*. The patient presents with burning pain, paresthesiae, and allodynia, often with a nocturnal exacerbation of symptoms; depression may be a feature. There is no associated weight loss, unlike acute painful neuropathy of poor glycemic control. Sensory loss is often mild or absent, and no motor signs are present. There is little or no abnormality on nerve conduction studies, but there is impaired exercise-induced conduction velocity increment *(42,43)*. Symptoms resolve completely within 10 months.

On sural nerve biopsy, typical morphometric changes of chronic distal symmetrical neuropathy but with active regeneration, were observed *(44)* (Fig. 1). In contrast, degeneration of both myelinated and unmyelinated fibers was found in acute painful neuropathy of poor glycemic control *(38)*. A recent study looking into the epineurial vessels of sural nerves in patients with this condition demonstrated marked arteriovenous abnormality including the presence of proliferating new vessels, similar to those found in the retina *(42)*. The study suggested that the presence of this fine network of epineural vessels may lead to a "steal" effect, rendering the endoneurium ischemic, and the authors also suggested that this process may be important in the genesis of neuropathic pain *(42)*. These findings were also supported by studies in experimental diabetes demonstrating that insulin administration led to acute endoneurial hypoxia by increasing nerve arteriovenous flow and reducing the nutritive flow of normal nerves *(45)*. Further work needs to address whether these observed sural nerve vessel changes resolve with the resolution of painful symptoms.

ASYMMETRICAL NEUROPATHIES

Asymmetrical or focal neuropathies are well-recognized complications of diabetes. They have a relatively rapid onset, and complete recovery is usual. This contrasts with chronic distal symmetrical neuropathy, where there is usually no improvement in symptoms 5 years after onset *(31)*. Unlike chronic distal symmetrical neuropathy, symptoms are often unrelated to the presence of other diabetic complications *(8,10)*. Asymmetrical neuropathies are more common in men and tend to predominantly affect older patients *(46,47)*. A careful history is therefore mandatory in order to identify any associated symptoms that might point to another cause for the neuropathy. A vascular etiology has been suggested by virtue of the rapid onset of symptoms and the focal nature of the neuropathic syndromes *(48)*.

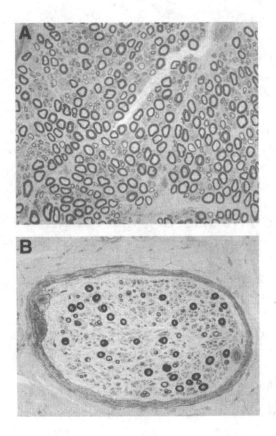

Fig. 1. Sural nerve biopsies from a healthy control (**A**) and a neuropathic patient (**B**). A considerable loss of myelinated nerve fibers can be seen in the neuropathic patient.

Proximal Motor Neuropathy
(Femoral Neuropathy, Amyotrophy, Plexopathy)

The syndrome of progressive asymmetrical proximal leg weakness and atrophy was first described by Garland *(49)*, who coined the term "diabetic amyotrophy." This condition has also been termed "proximal motor neuropathy," "femoral neuropathy," or "plexopathy." The patient presents with severe pain that is felt deep in the thigh but can sometimes be of a burning quality and extend below the knee. The pain is usually continuous and often causes insomnia and depression *(50)*. Both type 1 and type 2 patients over the age of 50 years are affected *(49–52)*. The associated weight loss which can sometimes be very severe and can raise the possibility of an occult malignancy.

Examination reveals profound wasting of the quadriceps with marked weakness in these muscle groups, although hip flexors and hip abductors can also be affected *(53)*. Thigh adductors, glutei, and hamstring muscles may also be involved. The knee jerk is usually reduced or absent. The profound weakness can lead to difficulty in getting out of a low chair or climbing stairs. Sensory loss is unusual, and if present indicates a coexistent distal sensory neuropathy.

It is important to carefully exclude other causes of quadriceps wasting such as nerve root and cauda equina lesions, as well as occult malignancy causing proximal myopathy syndromes such as polymyocytis. An erythrocyte sedimentation rate (ESR), an x-ray of the lumbar/sacral spine, a chest x-ray, and ultrasound of the abdomen may be required. Electrophysiologic studies may demonstrate increased femoral nerve latency and active denervation of affected muscles. Occasionally more detailed investigation with magnetic resonance imaging of the lumbar/sacral spine may be required to exclude focal nerve root intrapment.

The cause of diabetic proximal motor neuropathy is not known. It tends to occur within the background of diabetic distal symmetrical neuropathy *(54)*. Some have suggested that the combination of focal features superimposed on diffuse peripheral neuropathy may suggest vascular damage to the femoral nerve roots as a cause of this condition *(55)*.

As in distal symmetrical neuropathy, prospective studies that have looked at the natural history of proximal motor neuropathy are few. Coppack and Watkins *(50)* have reported that pain usually starts to settle after about 3 months and usually settles by 1 year; the knee jerk is restored in 50% of the patients after 2 years. Recurrence on the other side is a rare event. Management is largely symptomatic and supportive. Patients should be encouraged and reassured that this condition is likely to resolve. There is still controversy as to whether the use of insulin therapy influences the natural history of this syndrome *(58)*. Some patients benefit from physiotherapy that involves extension exercises aimed at strengthening the quadriceps. The management of pain in proximal motor neuropathy is similar to that of the chronic or acute distal symmetrical neuropathies (see below).

Cranial Mononeuropathies

The commonest cranial mononeuropathy is the third cranial nerve palsy. The patient presents with pain in the orbit, or sometimes with a frontal headache *(48,56)*. There is typically ptosis and ophthalmoplegia, although the pupil is usually spared *(57,58)*. Recovery occurs usually over 3 months. The clinical onset and time scale for recovery, as well as the focal nature of the lesions on the third cranial nerve, suggested an ischemic etiology on postmortem studies *(48,59)*. It is important to exclude any other cause of third cranial nerve palsy (aneurysm or tumor) by computed tomography or magnetic resonance scanning, when the diagnosis is in doubt. Fourth, sixth, and seventh cranial nerve palsies have also been described in diabetic subjects, but the association with diabetes is not as strong as that with third cranial nerve palsy.

Truncal Radiculopathy

Truncal radiculopathy is well recognized to occur in diabetes. It is characterized by an acute-onset pain in a dermatomal distribution over the thorax or the abdomen *(60)*. The pain is usually asymmetrical and can cause local bulging of the muscle *(61)*. There may be patchy sensory loss, and other causes of nerve root compression should be excluded. Some patients presenting with abdominal pain have undergone unnecessary investigations such as barium enema, colonoscopy, and even laparotomy, when the diagnosis could easily have been made by careful clinical history and examination. Recovery is usually the rule within several months, although symptoms can sometimes persist for a few years.

Pressure Palsies

Carpal Tunnel Syndrome

A number of nerves are vulnerable to pressure damage in diabetes. In the Rochester Diabetic Neuropathy Study, which was a population-based epidemiologic study, Dyck et al. *(62)* found electrophysiologic evidence of median nerve lesions at the wrist in about 30% of diabetic subjects, although the typical symptoms of carpel tunnel syndrome occurred in less than 10%. The patient typically has pain and paresthesia in the hands, which sometimes radiate to the forearm and are particularly marked at night. In severe cases clinical examination may reveal a reduction in sensation in the median territory in the hands and wasting of the muscle bulk in the thenar eminence. The clinical diagnosis is easily confirmed by median nerve conduction studies, and treatment involves surgical decompression at the carpel tunnel in the wrist. There is generally good response to surgery, although painful symptoms appear to relapse more commonly than in the nondiabetic population *(63)*.

Ulnar Nerve and Other Isolated Nerve Entrapments

The ulnar nerve is also vulnerable to pressure damage at the elbow in the ulnar groove. This results in wasting of the dorsal interossei, particularly the first dorsal interosseus. This is easily confirmed by ulnar electrophysiologic studies that localize the lesion to the elbow. Rarely, the patients may present with wrist drop caused by radial nerve palsy after prolonged sitting (with pressure over the radial nerve in the back of the arms) while unconscious during hypoglycemia or asleep after an alcohol binge.

In the lower limbs the common peroneal (lateral popliteal) is the most commonly affected nerve. The compression is at the level of the head of the fibula and causes foot drop. Unfortunately, complete recovery is not usual. The lateral cutaneous nerve of the thigh is also occasionally affected by entrapment neuropathy in diabetes. Phrenic nerve involvement in association with diabetes has also been described, although the possibility of a pressure lesion could not be excluded *(64)*.

PATHOGENESIS OF DISTAL SYMMETRICAL NEUROPATHY

Despite considerable research, the pathogenesis of diabetic neuropathy remains undetermined *(27)*. Morphometric studies have demonstrated that distal symmetrical neuropathy is characterized by pathologic changes including 1) axonal loss distally, with a "dying back" phenomenon *(24)*; 2) a reduction in myelinated fiber density *(65)*; and 3) focal areas of demyelination on teased fiber preparations *(24)*. Nerve regenerative activity may also be seen with the emergence of "regenerative clusters" *(66)*, containing groups of myelinated axons and nonmyelinated axon sprouts. However, the small and unmyelinated fibers that make up around 80% of all nerve fibers have proved more difficult to assess.

Historically, there have been two distinct views with regard to the pathogenesis of distal symmetrical neuropathy: 1) that metabolic factors *(67)* are of primary importance; and 2) that vascular factors *(29)* are the major cause (Table 4). However, most authorities now agree that the truth is probably in the middle and that both metabolic and vascular factors are important (Fig. 2). Evidence for this comes from recent work that has demonstrated an interaction between some of the proposed metabolic hypotheses of peripheral nerve damage and the vascular endothelium *(27)*.

Table 4
Proposed Hypotheses for the Pathogenesis
of Diabetic Peripheral Nerve Damage

Chronic hyperglycemia
Nerve microvascular dysfunction
Increased free radical formation
Polyol pathway hyperactivity
Protein kinase C hyperactivity
Nonenzymatic glycation
Abnormalities of nerve growth

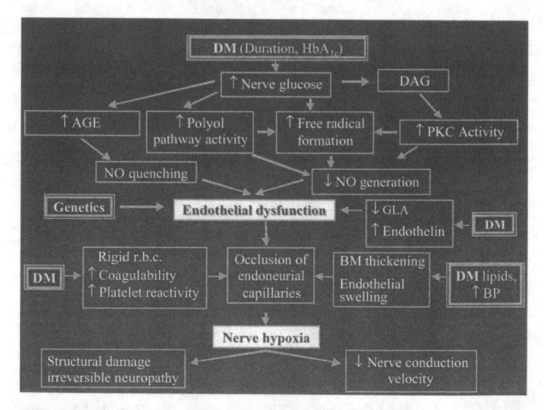

Fig. 2. Metabolic and vascular factors in the pathogenesis of diabetic distal symmetrical neuropathy. AGE, advanced glycation endproducts; BP, blood pressure; DAG, diacyl glycerol; DM, diabetes mellitus; GLA, γ-linoleneic acid; NO, nitric oxide; PKC, protein kinase C; RBC, red blood cells.

Chronic Hyperglycemia

Over the past decade, at least three large prospective studies have conclusively demonstrated that chronic hyperglycemia is implicated in the pathogenesis of diabetic neuropathy. The EURODIAB Prospective Study *(6)*, The Diabetes Control and Complications Trial *(68)*, and more recently the United Kingdom Prospective Diabetes Study *(69)* have demonstrated that poor glycemic control is related to the increased prevalence of neuropathy in diabetic patients and that improved glycemic control may prevent/reverse distal symmetrical neuropathy. However, there are major gaps in our understanding of exactly how the effects of chronic hyperglycemia result in nerve damage.

Oxidative Stress

Hyperglycemia leads to an increase in free radical generation as a result of several metabolic derangements, including nonenzymatic glycation and polyol pathway hyperactivity. Moreover, the capacity to neutralize free radicals is also reduced, owing to several metabolic abnormalities including NADPH depletion as a result of polyol pathway hyperactivity *(70)*. Thus, oxidative stress may impair nerve function by a direct toxic effect or by reducing nitric oxide and hence nerve blood flow. Recent studies in rats with experimental diabetes have shown that free radical scavengers may improve nerve conduction velocity abnormalities *(71)*, although these findings need to be proved in human diabetic neuropathy. Future studies may also explore an alternative to free radical scavenging, i.e., preventing free radical formation in the first place.

Increased Polyol Pathway Flux

In 1966 Gabbay et al. *(72)* postulated that polyol pathway hyperactivity could be mechanism linking hyperglycemia to neuropathy. It was proposed that hyperglycemia led to sorbitol accumulation in the peripheral nerve due to increased conversion from glucose, via the enzyme aldose reductase. This is supported by the demonstration of elevated sorbitol levels in diabetic nerves *(73,74)*. Elevated sorbitol levels are associated with depletion of myoinositol, which is important in phosphoinositide metabolism, and reduction in Na^+-K^+-ATPase, which plays an important role in intra- and extracellular sodium balance and hence nerve membrane potential *(73,74)*. Indeed, aldose reductase inhibitors (ARIs) administered either to animals *(75)* or to humans *(76)* cause improvement in nerve conduction velocity. Some improvement in nerve fiber count has also been reported *(77)*, but there is no unequivocal demonstration of amelioration of symptoms and clinical signs in humans. Thus no convincing evidence yet exists for the use of these agents in routine clinical practice, particularly when one considers the possibility of side effects in the long term. A number of studies are currently exploring newer and possibly more potent ARIs, in early neuropathy. (In advanced neuropathy, the nerve is highly disorganized and is unlikely to respond to treatment.) The long-term safety of these drugs remains an important issue of concern for many clinicians.

Nonenzymatic Glycation

Glucose is highly reactive, and free amino groups on proteins may be nonenzymatically glycated. From this reversible step there follows a series of reactions that are progressively irreversible: the production of Amadori products and then advanced glycation end products (AGEs). Nonenzymatic glycosylation of proteins has been demonstrated in brain tubulin and peripheral nerve *(78,79)*. This process may be an important initiating factor for nerve demyelination *(66)* by interfering with axonal transport. AGEs can also absorb ("quench") nitric oxide, a potent vasodilator, and hence lead to impaired nerve blood flow *(80)*. Aminoguanidine, which inhibits AGE formation, has been demonstrated to improve nerve conduction deficits and blood flow in experimental diabetes *(81)*, although its role in human diabetic neuropathy is still undetermined.

Neurotrophic Factors

Various neurotrophic factors support the growth and differentiation of neurons such as insulin-like growth factors (IGF-I and IGF-II) and the neurotrophin (NT) family.

The NT family includes nerve growth factor (NGF), the levels of which are found to be reduced in experimental diabetes *(82)*. NGF treatment corrects some aspects of sensory neuropathy related to small-fiber dysfunction in diabetic rats. A recent clinical trial looking into the effect of parental NGF in human diabetic neuropathy was stopped because of lack of effect, and therefore the precise role of neurotrophic factors in human diabetic neuropathy and the potential use of trophic intervention in diabetic neuropathy remain undetermined.

Protein Kinase C Activation

Diabetes results in hyperactivity of vascular protein kinase C (PKC), in particular for the β-isoform *(83)*. Increased synthesis of diacylglycerol (DAG) from glucose activates PKC. PKC activation is associated with abnormalities in vascular function seen in preclinical models of diabetes. In rats with streptozotocin diabetes, retinal blood flow is decreased in parallel with an increase in retinal PKC activity. PKC inhibitor treatment corrected deficits in retinal perfusion and prevented early glomerular hyperfiltration and increased urinary albumin excretion in diabetic rats *(83)*. Moreover, a PKC inhibitor has recently been shown to correct nerve conduction velocity and perfusion deficits and to protect endothelial-dependent relaxation in diabetic rats *(84)*. A clinical trial of a PKC inhibitor in subjects with early distal symmetrical neuropathy is currently taking place, and the results are awaited.

Vascular Factors

The view that microvessel disease may be central to the pathogenesis of diabetic neuropathy is not new *(85)*. Severe neural microvascular disease has been demonstrated in subjects with clinical diabetic neuropathy *(86)*. Several workers have reported basal membrane thickening of endoneurial capillaries, degeneration of pericytes, hypoplasia and swelling of endothelial cells, and sometimes vessel closure. The degree of microvascular disease has been correlated with the severity of neuropathy by Malik and colleagues *(87)*.

In vivo studies looking at the exposed sural nerve in human subjects have demonstrated epineural arteriovenous shunting, which appears to result in a steal phenomenon, by which blood is diverted from the nutritive endoneurial circulation *(29,42)*. The consequent impairment of nerve blood flow causes a fall in endoneural oxygen tension *(88)*. In addition, several other studies provide indirect evidence supporting a vascular etiology for diabetic neuropathy. Strenuous exercise increases nerve blood flow and thereby increases nerve conduction velocity by an average of 4 m/s in nonneuropathic diabetic subjects *(43)*. However, this significant increase in nerve conduction velocity, with exercise, is absent in neuropathic subjects, as the nerve microvasculature is severely diseased *(43)*. Moreover, there is a strong correlation between nerve conduction velocity and lower limb transcutaneous oxygenation measurements in diabetes; macrovascular disease appears to exacerbate neuropathy, and surgical restoration of perfusion improves nerve conduction velocity *(89)*. A recent epidemiologic study has also found a strong correlation between diabetic neuropathy and cardiovascular risk factors including body weight, hypertension, smoking, and reduced high-density lipoprotein cholesterol *(1,2,4,6)*.

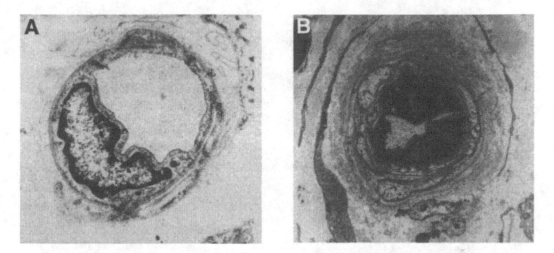

Fig. 3. Photomicrographs of endoneurial capillaries from sural nerve biopsies. (**A**) A normal capillary from a diabetic subject without neuropathy. (**B**) A closed capillary from a subject with chronic diabetic neuropathy showing endothelial cell proliferation and basement membrane (BM) thickening. (Courtesy of Dr. R.A. Malik, Department of Medicine, Manchester Royal Infirmary, Manchester, UK.)

Impairment of blood flow has also been found to be an early feature in rats with streptozotocin diabetes. Several vasodilators have also been found to enhance nerve blood flow and nerve function in diabetic animals *(70)*. In human diabetic neuropathy, angiotensin-converting enzyme inhibitors have been found to improve nerve function *(90,91)*. The presence of severe microvascular changes in subjects with acute painful neuropathy of rapid glycemic control (insulin neuritis), hitherto thought to be purely metabolic in origin, provides even more compelling evidence for the importance of microvascular factors in the pathogenesis of distal symmetric neuropathy *(42)*.

A number of metabolic derangements brought about by the diabetic state (mentioned above; Table 4) have an impact on nerve perfusion, the vascular endothelium being a major target *(70)*. Oxidative stress, activation of the PKC system, and nonenzymatic glycation lead to reduced nerve nitric oxide. Occlusion of endoneural capillaries and the presence of hemorrheologic abnormalities associated with diabetes further exacerbate the impairment of nerve blood flow (Fig. 3), leading to nerve hypoxia and hence nerve structural and functional abnormalities (Fig. 1).

AUTONOMIC NEUROPATHY

Abnormalities of autonomic function are very common in subjects with long-standing diabetes; however, clinically significant autonomic dysfunction is uncommon. Several systems are affected (Table 5). Autonomic neuropathy has a gradual onset and is slowly progressive. The prevalence of diabetic autonomic neuropathy depends on the type of population studied, and a number of tests of autonomic function are employed. In the EURODIAB study the prevalence of autonomic neuropathy (defined as the presence of two abnormal cardiovascular autonomic function tests), was 24%, and the

Table 5
Autonomic Neuropathy

Cardiovascular	Gastrointestinal
Resting tachycardia	Gastroparesis
Heart rate abnormalities	Diarrhea
Edema	Constipation
Postural hypotension	Dermatological
Arrhythmias	Gustatory sweating
Sudden death	Dry skin
Genitourinary	Sudomotor dysfunction
Erectile Dysfunction	Arteriovenous shunting
Retrograde ejaculation	Neurological
Atonic bladder	Pupillary dysfunction
Bladder infection	Respiratory
Abnormal renal sodium handling	Bronchoconstrictor dysfunction
Nephropathy	

prevalence increased with age, duration of diabetes, glycemic control, and presence of cardiovascular risk factors *(92)*.

Cardiovascular Autonomic Neuropathy

Cardiovascular autonomic neuropathy cases postural hypotension and change in peripheral blood flow and may be a cause of sudden death.

Postural Hypotension

It is now generally accepted that a fall in systolic blood pressure of >20 mmHg is considered abnormal. Coincidental treatment with both tricyclic antidepressants for neuropathic pain and diuretics may exacerbate postural hypotension, the chief symptom of which is dizziness on standing. The symptoms of postural hypotension can be disabling for some patients, who may not be able to walk for more than a few minutes. In clinical practice the severity of dizziness does not correlate with the postural drop in blood pressure. There is increased mortality in subjects with postural hypotension, although the reasons for this are not clear. The management of subjects with postural hypotension poses major problems, and for some patients there may not be any satisfactory treatment. Current treatment includes improving glycemic control, advising patients to get up from the sitting or lying position slowly, treatment with fludrocortisone while carefully monitoring urea and electrolytes, and the use of support stockings. In severe cases, antigravity (or space) suits, which may compress the lower limbs, or the α-1-adrenal receptor agonist midodrine or occasionally octreotide may be effective.

Changes in Peripheral Blood Flow

Autonomic neuropathy can cause arteriovenus shunting, with prominent veins in the neuropathic leg *(21)*. Leg vein oxygen tension *(22)* and capillary pressure *(93)* are increased in the neuropathic leg owing to sympathetic denervation. Thus, in the absence of peripheral vascular disease, the neuropathic foot is warm, which may be one of the factors that causes osteopenia associated with the development of Charcot neuroarthropathy.

Table 6
Reference Values for Cardiovascular Function Tests

Parameter	Normal	Borderline	Abnormal
Heart rate tests			
Heart rate response to standing up (30:15 ratio)	≥1.04	1.01–1.03	≤1.00
Heart rate response to deep breathing (maximum minus minimum heart rate)	≥15 beats/min	11–14 beats/min	≤10 beats/min
Heart rate response to Valsalva maneuver (Valsalva ratio)	≥1.21	—	≤1.20
Blood pressure tests			
Blood pressure response to standing up (fall in systolic BP)	≤10 mmHg	11–29 mmHg	≥30 mmHg
Blood pressure response to sustained handgrip (increase in diastolic BP)	≥16 mmHg	11–15 mmHg	≤10 mmHg

Cardiovascular Autonomic Function Tests

Five cardiovascular autonomic function tests are now widely used for the assessment of autonomic function. These tests are noninvasive, and do not require sophisticated equipment. (All that is required is an electrocardiogram machine, an aneroid pressure gauge attached to a mouthpiece, a hand grip dynamometer, and a sphygmomanometer.) Table 6 shows a reference list for cardiovascular autonomic function testing *(94)*.

Gastrointestinal Autonomic Neuropathy

Gastroparesis

Autonomic neuropathy can affect the upper gastrointestinal system by reducing esophageal motility (dysphagia and heartburn) and gastroparesis (reduced gastric emptying, vomiting, swings in blood sugar) *(95)*.

Management of diabetic gastroparesis includes optimization of glycemic control, the use of antiemetics (metoclopramide and domperidone) and the use of a cholinergic agent to stimulate esophageal motility (erythromycin, which may enhance the activity of the gut peptide motilin).

The diagnosis of gastroparesis is often made on clinical grounds by the evaluation of symptoms and sometimes the presence of succusion splash; barium swallow and follow-through as well as gastroscopy may reveal a large food residue in the stomach. Gastric motility and emptying studies can sometimes be performed in specialized units and may help with diagnosis.

Severe gastroparesis causing recurrent vomiting is associated with dehydration, swings in blood sugar, and weight loss; it is therefore an indication for hospital admission. The patient should be adequately hydrated with intravenous fluids, and blood sugar should be stabilized by intravenous insulin; antiemetics may be given intravenously, and if the course of the gastroparesis is prolonged, total parentral nutrition or feeding through a gastrostomy tube may be required.

Autonomic Diarrhea

The patient may present with diarrhea that tends to be worse at night; alternatively, some patients may present with constipation. Both the diarrhea and constipation respond to conventional treatment. Diarrhea associated with bacterial overgrowth may respond to treatment with a broad-spectrum antibiotic such as erythromycin, tetracycline, or ampicillin.

Abnormal Sweating

Increased sweating, usually affecting the face and often brought about by eating (gustatory sweating), can be very embarrassing to patients. There may also be reduced sweating in the feet of affected patients, which can cause dry feet that are at risk of fissuring and hence infection. Unfortunately, there is no totally satisfactory treatment for gustatory sweating, although the anticholinergic drug poldine may be useful in a minority of patients.

Abnormalities of Bladder Function

Bladder dysfunction is a rare complication of autonomic neuropathy involving the sacral nerves. The patient presents with hesitancy of micturition, increased frequency of micturition, and (in serious cases) urinary retention associated with overflow incontinence. Such a patient is prone to urinary tract infections. Ultrasound scan of the urinary tract, intravenous urography, and urodynamic studies may be required. Treatment maneuvers include mechanical methods of bladder emptying by applying suprapubic pressure, or the use of intermittent self-catheterization. Anticholinesterase drugs such as neostigmine or peridostigmine may be useful. Long-term indwelling catheterization may be required in some, but this unfortunately predisposes the patient to urinary tract infections, and long-term antibiotic prophylaxis may be required.

MANAGEMENT OF DIABETIC NEUROPATHY

The two chief presentations of diabetic neuropathy are pain and the numb foot, which predisposes the patient to foot ulceration. The problems associated with the numb foot are discussed in detail elsewhere in this book. The treatment scenario for painful neuropathy is less than satisfactory, as currently available treatment approaches are highly symptomatic and often ineffective. As the pathologic processes leading to diabetic nerve damage become clear, potential therapeutic agents that have the capacity to prevent or reverse the neuropathic process will emerge.

A careful history and examination of the patient is essential to exclude other possible causes of leg pain such as peripheral vascular disease, prolapsed intervertebral discs, spinal canal stenosis, and corda aquina lesions. Unilateral leg pain should arouse a suspicion that the pain may be due to lumbar-sacral nerve root compression. These patients may well need to be investigated with lumbar-sacral magnetic resonance imaging. Other causes of peripheral neuropathy are excessive alcohol intake and B_{12} deficiency. When pain is the predominant symptom, the quality and severity should be assessed. Neuropathic pain can be disabling in some patients, and an empathic approach is essential. In general, patients should be allowed to express their symptoms freely without too many interruptions. Psychological support of the patient's painful neuropathy is an important aspect of the overall management of the pain.

Glycemic Control

There is now little doubt that good blood sugar control prevents/delays the onset of diabetic neuropathy *(6,68,69)*. In addition, painful neuropathic symptoms are also improved by improving metabolic control, if necessary with the use of insulin in type 2 diabetes *(96)*. The first step in the management of painful neuropathy is a concerted effort aimed at improving glycemic control.

Tricyclic Compounds

Tricyclic compounds are now regarded as the first-line treatment for painful diabetic neuropathy *(16)*. A number of double-blind clinical trials have confirmed their effectiveness beyond any doubt. As these drugs do have unwanted side effects such as drowsiness, anticholinergic side effects such as dry mouth, and dizziness due to postural hypotension in those that have autonomic neuropathy, patients should be started on imipramine or amitriptyline at a low dose (25–50 mg taken before bed); the dose should be gradually titrated if necessary up to 150 mg/day. The mechanism of action of tricyclic compounds in improving neuropathic pain is not known, but their effect does not appear through their antidepressant property, as they appear to be effective even in those with a depressed mood *(97)*.

Anticonvulsants

Anticonvulsants, including carbamazepine, phenytoin, and (more recently) gabapentin *(98)*, have also been effective in the relief of more severe neuropathic pain. Unfortunately, treatment with anticonvulsants is often complicated with troublesome side effects such as sedation, dizziness, and ataxia, and therefore treatment should be started at a relatively low dose and gradually increased to a maintenance dose, while carefully looking for side effects.

Topical Capsaicin

Topical capsaicin (0.075%) applied sparingly 3–4 times/day to the affected area has also been found to relieve neuropathic pain. Topical capsaicin works by depleting substance P from nerve terminals, and there may be worsening of neuropathic symptoms for the first 2–4 weeks of application *(99)*.

Intravenous Lignocaine and Oral Mexiletine

Intravenous lignocaine at a dose of 5 mg/kg body weight, with another 30 min with a cardiac monitor *in situ*, has also been found to be effective in relieving neuropathic pain for up to 2 weeks *(100)*. This form of treatment is useful in subjects who are having severe pain that is not responding to the above agents, although it does necessitate bringing the patient into hospital for a few hours. Oral mexiletine, which has a similar structure to lignocaine, may have a beneficial effect in reducing neuropathic pain, although in the author's experience treatment is disappointing.

α-Lipoic Acid

Infusion of the antioxidant α-lipoic acid, at a dose of 600 mg intravenously per day over a 3-week period, has also been useful in reducing neuropathic pain *(101)*.

Management of Disabling Painful Neuropathy Not Responding to Pharmacological Treatment

Neuropathic pain can sometimes be extremely severe, interfering significantly with sleep and daily activities. Unfortunately, some patients are not helped by conventional pharmacologic treatment. Such patients pose a major challenge; they are severely distressed and sometimes wheelchair bound. A recent study has demonstrated that such patients may respond to electrical spinal cord stimulation, which relieves both background and peak neuropathic pain *(17)*. This form of treatment is particularly advantageous, as the patient does not have to take any other pain-relieving medications, with all their side effects. A recent follow-up of patients fitted with electrical spinal cord stimulators found that stimulators continued to be effective 5 years after implantation. Transcutaneous electrical nerve stimulation may also be beneficial for the relief of localized neuropathic pain in one limb.

REFERENCES

1. Shaw JE, Zimmet PZ. The epidemiology of diabetic neuropathy. *Diabetes Rev* 1999;7: 245–252.
2. Tesfaye S, Stephens L, Stephenson J, et al. The prevalence of diabetic neuropathy and its relation to glycaemic control and potential risk factors: the EURODIAB IDDM Complications Study. *Diabetologia* 1996;39:1377–1384.
3. Young MJ, Boulton AJM, Macleod AF, Williams DRR, Sonksen PH. A multicentre study of the prevalence of diabetic peripheral neuropathy in the United Kingdom hospital clinic population. *Diabetologia* 1993;36:150–154.
4. Maser RE, Steenkiste AR, Dorman JS, et al. Epidemiological correlates of diabetic neuropathy. Report from Pittsburgh Epidemiology of Diabetes Complications Study. *Diabetes* 1989;38:1456–1461.
5. Ziegler D. Diagnosis, staging and epidemiology of diabetic peripheral neuropathy. *Diabetes Nutr Metab* 1994;7:342–348.
6. Tesfaye S, Chaturvedi N, Eaton SEM, Ward JD, Fuller J. Cardiovascular risk factors predict the development of diabetic neuropathy. *Diabetic Med* 2000;17(Suppl 1):P153.
7. Tesfaye S, Ward JD. Clinical features of diabetic polyneuropathy, in *Clinical Management of Diabetic Neuropathy* (Veves A, ed.), Humana Press, Totowa, NJ, 1998, pp. 49–60.
8. Eaton SEM, Tesfaye S. Clinical manifestations and measurement of somatic neuropathy. *Diabetes Rev* 1999;7:312–325.
9. Ward JD. Clinical features of diabetic neuropathy, in *Diabetic Neuropathy* (Ward JD, Goto Y, eds.), John Wiley, New York, 1990, pp. 281–296.
10. Watkins PJ, Edmonds ME. Clinical features of diabetic neuropathy, in *Textbook of Diabetes*, vol 2 (Pickup J, Williams G, eds.), Blackwell Science, Oxford, UK, 1997, pp. 50.1–50.20.
11. Bruyn GW, Garland H. Neuropathies of endocrine origin, in *Handbook of Clinical Neurology,* vol 8 (Vinken PJ, Bruyn GW, eds.), Amsterdam, North-Holland, 1970, p. 29.
12. Thomas PK. Metabolic neuropathy. *J R Coll Phys* (Lond) 1973;7:154–174.
13. Low PA, Suarez GA. Diabetic neuropathies. *Baillieres Clin Neurol* 1995;4:401–425.
14. Andersen H, Jakobsen J. Motor function in diabetes. *Diabetes Rev* 1999;7:326–341.

15. Watkins PJ. Pain and diabetic neuropathy. *BMJ* 1984;288:168–169.
16. Tesfaye S, Price D. Therapeutic approaches in diabetic neuropathy and neuropathic pain, in *Diabetic Neuropathy* (Boulton AJM, ed.), Marius Press, Carnforth, Lancashire, UK, 1997, pp. 159–181.
17. Tesfaye S, Watt J, Benbow SJ, et al. Electrical spinal cord stimulation for painful diabetic peripheral neuropathy. *Lancet* 1996;348:1696–1701.
18. Ewing DJ, Borsey DQ, Bellavere F, Clarke BF. Cardiac autonomic neuropathy in diabetes: comparison of measures of R-R interval variation. *Diabetologia* 1981;21:18–24.
19. Boulton AJM. Foot problems in patients with diabetes mellitus, in *Textbook of Diabetes,* vol 2 (Pickup J, Williams G, eds.), Blackwell Science, Oxford, UK, 1997, pp. 58.1–58.20.
20. Ward JD. The diabetic leg. *Diabetologia* 1982;22:141–147.
21. Ward JD, Simms JM, Knight G, Boulton AJM, Sandler DA. Venous distension in the diabetic neuropathic foot (physical sign of arterio-venous shunting). *J R Soc Med* 1983;76:1011–1014.
22. Boulton AJM, Scarpello JHB, Ward JD. Venous oxygenation in the diabetic neuropathic foot: evidence of arterial venous shunting? *Diabetologia* 1982;22:6–8.
23. Edmonds ME, Archer AG, Watkins PJ. Ephedrine: a new treatment for diabetic neuropathic oedema. *Lancet* 1983;i:548–551.
24. Said G, Slama G, Selva J. Progressive centripital degeneration of of axons in small-fibre type diabetic polyneuropathy. A clinical and pathological study. *Brain* 1983;106:791.
25. Vinik AI, Park TS, Stansberry KB, Pittenger GL. Diabetic neuropathies. *Diabetologia* 2000;43:957–973.
26. Veves A, Young MJ, Manes C, et al. Differences in peripheral and autonomic nerve function measurements in painful and painless neuropathy: a clinical study. *Diabetes Care* 1994;17:1200–1202.
27. Ward JD, Tesfaye S. Pathogenesis of diabetic neuropathy, in *Textbook of Diabetes,* vol 2 (Pickup J, Williams G, eds.), Blackwell Science, Oxford, UK, 1997, pp. 49.1–49.19.
28. Tesfaye S, Malik R, Ward JD. Vascular factors in diabetic neuropathy. *Diabetologia* 1994;37:847–854.
29. Tesfaye S, Harris N, Jakubowski J, et al. Impaired blood flow and arterio-venous shunting in human diabetic neuropathy: a novel technique of nerve photography and fluorescein angiography. *Diabetologia* 36:1266–1274.
30. Malik RA. Pathology and pathogenesis of diabetic neuropathy. *Diabetes Rev* 1999;7:253–260.
31. Boulton AJM, Armstrong WD, Scarpello JHB, Ward JD. The natural history of painful diabetic neuropathy—a 4 year study. *Postgrad Med J* 1983;59:556–559.
32. Benbow SJ, Chan AW, Bowsher D, McFarlane IA, Williams G. A prospective study of painful symptoms, small fibre function and peripheral vascular disease in chronic painful diabetic neuropathy. *Diabetic Med* 1994;11:17–21.
33. Chan AW, MacFarlane IA, Bowsher DR, et al. Chronic pain in patients with diabetes mellitus: comparison with non-diabetic population. *Pain Clin* 1990;3:147–159.
34. Young RJ, Zhou YQ, Rodriguez E, et al. Variable relationship between peripheral somatic and autonomic neuropathy in patients with different syndromes of diabetic polyneuropathy. *Diabetes* 1986;35:192–197.
35. Tsigos C, White A, Young RJ. Discrimination between painful and painless diabetic neuropathy based on testing of large somatic nerve and sympathetic nerve function. *Diabet Med* 1992;9:359–365.
36. Veves A, Manes C, Murray HJ, Young MJ, Boulton AJM. Painful neuropathy and foot ulceration in diabetic patients. *Diabetes Care* 1993;16:1187–1189.
37. Young MJ, Manes C, Boulton AJM. Vibration perception threshold predicts foot ulceration: a prospective study (abstract). *Diabet Med* 1992;9(Suppl 2):1992;542.

38. Archer AG, Watkins PJ, Thomas PJ, Sharma AK, Payan J. The natural history of acute painful neuropathy in diabetes mellitus. *J Neurol Neuorosurg Psychiatr* 1983;46:491–496.
39. Ellenberg M. Diabetic neuropathic cachexia. *Diabetes* 1974;23:418–423.
40. Guy RJC, Clark CA, Malcolm PN, Watkins PJ. Evaluation of thermal and vibration sensation in diabetic neuropathy. *Diabetologia* 1985;28:131.
41. Caravati CM. Insulin neuritis: a case report. *Va Med Mon* 1933;59:745–746.
42. Tesfaye S, Malik R, Harris N, et al. Arteriovenous shunting and proliferating new vessels in acute painful neuropathy of rapid glycaemic control (insulin neuritis). *Diabetologia* 1996;39:329–335.
43. Tesfaye S, Harris N, Wilson RM, Ward JD. Exercise induced conduction veolcity increment: a marker of impaired nerve blood flow in diabetic neuropathy. *Diabetologia* 1992; 35:155–159.
44. Llewelyn JG, Thomas PK, Fonseca V, King RHM, Dandona P. Acute painful diabetic neuropathy precipitated by strict glycaemic control. *Acta Neuropathol (Berl)* 1986;72: 157–163.
45. Kihara M, Zollman PJ, Smithson IL, et al. Hypoxic effect of endogenous insulin on normal and diabetic peripheral nerve. *Am J Physiol* 1994;266:E980–E985.
46. Clements RS, Bell DSH. Diagnostic, pathogenic and therapeutic aspects of diabetic neuropathy. *Special Top Endocrinol Metab* 1982;3:1–43.
47. Matikainen E, Juntunen J. Diabetic neuropathy: epidemiological, pathogenetic, and clinical aspects with special emphasis on type 2 diabetes mellitus. *Acta Endocrinol Suppl (Copenh)* 1984;262:89–94.
48. Asbury AK. Aldredge H, Hershberg R, Fisher CM. Oculomotor palsy in diabetes mellitus: a clinicopathological study. *Brain* 1970;93:555–557.
49. Garland H. Diabetic amyotrophy. *BMJ* 1955;2:1287–1290.
50. Coppack SW, Watkins PJ. The natural history of femoral neuropathy. *QJ Med* 1991;79: 307–313.
51. Casey EB, Harrison MJG. Diabetic amyotrophy: a follow-up study. *BMJ* 1972;1:656.
52. Garland H, Taverner D. Diabetic myelopathy. *BMJ* 1953;1:1405.
53. Subramony SH, Willbourn AJ. Diabetic proximal neuropathy. Clinical and electromyographic studies. *J Neurol Sci* 1982;53:293–304.
54. Bastron JA, Thomas JE. Diabetic polyradiculoneuropathy: clinical and electromyographic findings in 105 patients. *Mayo Clin Proc* 1981;56:725–732.
55. Said G, Goulon-Goeau C, Lacroix C, Moulonguet A. Nerve biopsy findings in different patterns of proximal diabetic neuropathy. *Ann Neurol* 1994;33:559–569.
56. Zorilla E, Kozak GP. Ophthalmoplegia in diabetes mellitus. *Ann Intern Med* 1967;67: 968–976.
57. Goldstein JE, Cogan DG. Diabetic ophthalmoplegia with special reference to the pupil. *Arch Ophthalmol* 1960;64:592–600.
58. Leslie RDG, Ellis C. Clinical course following diabetic ocular palsy. *Postgrad Med J* 1978; 54:791–792.
59. Dreyfuss PM, Hakim S, Adams RD. Diabetic ophthalmoplegia. *Arch Neurol Psychiatry* 1957;77:337–349.
60. Ellenberg M. Diabetic truncal mononeuropathy—a new clincal syndrome. *Diabetes Care* 1978;1:10–13.
61. Boulton AJM, Angus E, Ayyar DR, Weiss R. Diabetic thoracic polyradiculopathy presenting as abdominal swelling. *BMJ* 1984;289:798–799.
62. Dyck PJ, Kratz KM, Karnes JL, et al. The prevalence by staged severity of various types of diabetic neuropathy, retinopathy, and nephropathy in a population-based cohort: the Rochester Diabetic Neuropathy Study. *Neurology* 1993;43:817–824.
63. Clayburgh RH, Beckenbaugh RD, Dobyns JH, Carpal tunnel release in patients with diffuse peripheral neuropathy. *J Hand Surg* 1987;12A:380–383.

64. White JES, Bullock RF, Hudgson P, Home PD, Gibson GJ. Phrenic neuropathy in association with diabetes. *Diabet Med* 1992;9:954–956.
65. Malik RA. The pathology of diabetic neuropathy. *Diabetes* 1997;46(Suppl 2):S50–S53.
66. Bradley JL, Thomas PK, King RH, et al. Myelinated nerve fibre regeneration in diabetic sensory polyneuropathy: correlation with type of diabetes. *Acta Neuropathol Berl* 1995; 90:403–410.
67. Stevens MJ, Feldman EL, Thomas T, Greene DA. Pathogenesis of diabetic neuropathy, in *Contemporary Endocrinology: Clinical Management of Diabetic Neuropathy* (Veves A, ed.), Humana, Totowa, NJ, 1998, pp. 13–48.
68. Diabetes Control and Complications Trial Research Group: The effect of intensive diabetes therapy on the development and progression of neuropathy. *Ann Intern Med* 1995;122: 561–568.
69. United Kingdom Prospective Diabetes Study Group: Intensive blood glucose control with sulphonylureas or insulin compared with conventional treatment and risk of complications in patients with type 2 diabetes. *Lancet* 1998;352:837–853.
70. Cameron NE, Cotter MA. The relationship of vascular changes to metabolic factors in diabetes mellitus and their role in the development of peripheral nerve complications. *Diabetes Metab Rev* 1994;10:189–224.
71. Cameron NE, Cotter MA, Archbald V, Dines KC, Maxfield EK. Anti-oxidant and pro-oxidant effects on nerve conduction velocity, endoneurial blood flow and oxygen tension in non-diabetic and streptozotocin-diabetic rats. *Diabetologia* 1994;37:449–459.
72. Gabbay KH, Merola LO, Field RA. Sorbitol pathway: presence in nerve and cord with substrate accumulation in diabetes. *Science* 1966;151:209–210.
73. Dyck PJ, Zimmerman BR, Vilan TH, et al. Nerve glucose, fructose, sorbitol, myo-inositol, and fiber degeneration in diabetic neuropathy. *N Engl J Med* 1988;319:542–548.
74. Ward JD, Baker RWR, Davis B. Effect of blood sugar control on the accumulation of sorbitol and fructose in nervous tissue. *Diabetes* 1972;21:1173–1178.
75. Tomlinson DR, Moriarty RJ, Mayer H. Prevention and reversal of defective axonal transport and motor nerve conduction velocity in rats with experimental diabetes by treatment with addose reductase inhibitor sorbinil. *Diabetes* 1984;33:470–476.
76. Judzewitsch RG, Jaspan JB, Polonsky KS, et al. Aldose reductase inhibition improves nerve conduction velocity in diabetic patients. *N Engl J Med* 1983;308:119–125.
77. Sima AAF, Bril V, Nathaniel V, McEwen TAG, Greene DA. Regeneration and repair of myelinated fibres in sural nerve biopsy specimens from patients with diabetic neuropathy treated with sorbinil. *N Engl J Med* 1988;319:548–555.
78. Williams SK, Howarth NL, Devenny JJ, Bitensky MW. Structural and functional consequences of increased tubulin glycosylation in diabetes mellitus. *Proct Natl Acad Sci USA* 1982;79:6546–6550.
79. Vlassara H, Brownlee M, Cerami A. Accumulation of diabetic rat peripheral nerve myelin by macrophages increases with the presence of advanced glycosylation end products. *J Exp Med* 1984;160:197.
80. Bucala R, Cerami A, Vlassara H. Advanced glycosylation end products in diabetic complications. Biochemical basis and prospects for therapeutic intervention. *Diabetes Rev* 1995;3:258–268.
81. Kihara J, Schmelzer JD, Poduslo JF, et al. Aminoguanidine effects on nerve blood flow, vascular permeability, electrophysiology and oxygen free radicals. *Proc Natl Acad Sci USA* 1991;88:6107–6111.
82. Hellweg R, Hartung HD. Endogenous levels of nerve growth factor (NGF) are altered in experimental diabetes mellitus: a possible role for NGF in the pathogenesis of diabetic neuropathy. *J Neurosci Res* 1990;26:258–267.
83. Koya D, King GL. Protein kinase C activation and the development of diabetic complications. *Diabetes* 1998;47:859–866.

84. Cameron NE, Cotter MA, Lai K, Hohman TC. Effects of protein kinase C inhibition on nerve function, blood flow and Na$^+$, K$^+$ ATPase defects in diabetic rats. *Diabetes* 1997; 46(Suppl 1):31A.

85. Fagerberg SE. Diabetic neuropathy: a clinical and histological study on the significance of vascular affections. *Acta Med Scand* 1959;164(Suppl 345):5–81.

86. Giannini C, Dyck PJ. Ultrastructural morphometric abnormalities of sural nerve endoneurial microvessels in diabetes mellitus. *Ann Neurol* 1994;36:408–415.

87. Malik RA, Newrick PG, Sharma AK, et al. Microangiopathy in human diabetic neuropathy: relationship between capillary abnormalities and the severity of neuropathy. *Diabetologia* 1998;32:92–102.

88. Newrick PG, Wilson AJ, Jakubowski J, Boulton AJM, Ward JD. Sural nerve oxygen tension in diabetes. *BMJ* 1985;193:1053–1054.

89. Young MJ, Veves A, Smith JV, Walker MG, Boulton AJM. Restoring lower limb blood flow improves conduction velocity in diabetic patients. *Diabetologia* 1995;38:1051–1054.

90. Reja A, Tesfaye S, Harris ND, Ward JD. Is ACE inhibition with lisinopril helpful in diabetic neuropathy? *Diabet Med* 1995;12:307–309.

91. Malik RA, Williamson S, Abbott CA, et al. Effect of the angiotensin converting enzyme inhibitor trandalopril on human diabetic neuropathy: a randomised controlled trial. *Lancet* 1998;352:1978–1981.

92. Tesfaye S, Kempler P, Stevens L, et al. Prevalence of autonomic neuropathy and potential risk factors in type 1 diabetes in Europe. *Diabetes* 1998;47(Suppl 1):A132.

93. Rayman G. Diabetic neuropathy and microcirculation. *Diabetes Rev* 1999;7:261–274.

94. Ewing DJ, Martyn CN, Young RJ, Clarke BF. The value of cardiovascular autonomic function tests: ten years experience in diabetes. *Diabetes Care* 1985;8:491–498.

95. Horowitz M, Fraser R. Disordered gastric motor function in diabetes mellitus. *Diabetologia* 1994;37:543–551.

96. Boulton AJM, Drury J, Clarke B, Ward JD. Continuous subcutaneous insulin infusion in the management of painful diabetic neuropathy. *Diabetes Care* 1982;5:386–390.

97. Max MB, Culnane M, Schafer SC, et al. Amitriptyline relieves diabetic neuropathy pain in patients with normal or despressed mood. *Neurology* 1987;37:598–596.

98. Backonja M, Beydoun A, Edwards KR, et al. Gabapentin for the symptomatic treatment of painful neuropathy in patients with diabetes mellitus: a randomised controlled trial. *JAMA* 1998;280:1831–1836.

99. Capsaicin Study Group. The effect of treatment with capsaicin on daily activities of patients with painful diabetic neuropathy. *Diabetes Care* 1992;15:159–165.

100. Kastrup J, Angelo H, Peterson P, Deigard A, Hilsted J, et al. Treatment of chronic painful neuropathy with intravenous lidocaine infusion. *BMJ* 1986;292:173.

101. Zeigler D, Hanefeld M, Ruhnau KJ, et al. Treatment of symptomatic diabetic peripheral neuropathy with anti-oxidant alpha-lipoic acid: a 3-week multicentre randomised controlled trial (ALADIN Study). *Diabetologia* 1995;38:1425–1433.

5

Microvascular Changes in the Diabetic Foot

Cameron M. Akbari, MD and Frank W. LoGerfo, MD

INTRODUCTION

Problems of the diabetic foot are the most common cause for hospitalization in diabetic patients, with an annual health care cost of over $1 billion (1). Diabetes is a contributing factor in half of all lower extremity amputations in the United States, and the relative risk for amputation is 40 times greater in people with diabetes (2). Diabetic foot ulceration will affect 15% of all diabetic individuals during their lifetime and is clearly a significant risk factor in the pathway to limb loss (3). The main etiologic factors in foot ulceration are diabetic neuropathy and vascular disease, the latter being further classified into macrovascular (i.e., atherosclerosis) and microvascular disease. Ultimately, all efforts at prevention and treatment of the diabetic foot should be focused on an understanding of these disease entities. Both neuropathy and peripheral vascular disease have been discussed thoroughly elsewhere in this book. In this chapter, the fundamental alterations in the microcirculation of the diabetic foot are addressed, with particular attention to endothelial dysfunction and its contribution to ulceration of the diabetic foot.

OVERVIEW OF DIABETIC MICROVASCULAR DISEASE

The complications of diabetes may best be characterized as alterations in vascular structure and function, with subsequent end-organ damage and death (4). Specifically, two types of vascular disease are seen in patients with diabetes: a nonocclusive microcirculatory dysfunction involving the capillaries and arterioles of the kidneys, retina, and peripheral nerves, and a macroangiopathy characterized by atherosclerotic lesions of the coronary and peripheral arterial circulation (5–8). The former is relatively unique to diabetes, whereas the latter lesions are morphologically and functionally similar in both nondiabetic and diabetic patients.

Retinopathy is the most characteristic microvascular complication of diabetes, and population-based studies have identified a correlation between its development and the duration of diabetes (9). Similar correlations have been found with nephropathy and neuropathy (10), with perhaps the strongest evidence coming from the Diabetes Control and Complications Trial (DCCT). The results from the DCCT clearly showed a delay in the

From: *The Diabetic Foot: Medical and Surgical Management*
Edited by: A. Veves, J. M. Giurini, and F. W. LoGerfo © Humana Press Inc., Totowa, NJ

development and progression of these microvascular complications with intensive glycemic control, thus supporting the direct causal relationship among hyperglycemia, diabetes, and its microvascular sequelae *(11)*. These and other clinical trials have provided
the rationale for experimental studies investigating the fundamental pathophysiology
of micro- and macrovascular disease in diabetes mellitus.

In simplest terms, microvascular dysfunction in diabetes may be described by an
increased vascular permeability and impaired autoregulation of blood flow and vascular
tone. These changes predominate at (though are not limited to) the capillary and arteriolar
level and culminate in nephropathy, retinopathy, and neuropathy. Although multiple
theories have been postulated as to the etiology of accelerated microangiopathy, it is
likely that several biochemical derangements exist in the presence of hyperglycemia and
diabetes and that these mechanisms work synergistically to cause microvascular dysfunction. Consequently, these metabolic alterations produce functional and structural changes
at multiple areas within the arteriolar and capillary level, including the basement membrane *(9)*, the smooth muscle cell *(12)*, and (in particular) the endothelial cell *(13)*.

MORPHOLOGIC CHANGES
IN THE MICROCIRCULATION OF THE DIABETIC FOOT

Perhaps the greatest obstacle to understanding the diabetic foot is the misconception
of an untreatable occlusive lesion in the microcirculation. This idea originated from a
retrospective histologic study demonstrating the presence of periodic acid-Schiff (PAS)-
positive material occluding the arterioles in amputated limb specimens from diabetic
patients *(14)*. However, subsequent prospective anatomic staining and arterial casting
studies *(15,16)* have demonstrated the *absence* of an arteriolar occlusive lesion. Further
evidence comes from physiologic studies of femoropopliteal bypass grafts in diabetic
and nondiabetic patients in which direct vasodilator administration into these grafts demonstrates a comparable fall in peripheral resistance between the two groups *(17)*. These
data, coupled with the vast clinical experience of nearly three decades of successful
arterial reconstruction in diabetic patients, have thoroughly dispelled the hopeless notion
of diabetic "small-vessel disease."

Although there is no occlusive lesion in the diabetic microcirculation, other structural changes do exist, most notably thickening of the capillary basement membrane.
This alteration in extracellular matrix may represent a response to the metabolic changes
related to diabetes and hyperglycemia. However, this does not lead to narrowing of
the capillary lumen, and arteriolar blood flow may be normal or even increased despite
these changes *(18)*. Capillary basement membrane thickening is the dominant structural
change in both diabetic retinopathy and neuropathy. In the kidney, nonenzymatic glycosylation reduces the charge on the basement membrane, which may account for trans-
udation of albumin, an expanded mesangium, and albuminuria *(19)*. Similar increases
in vascular permeability occur in the eye and probably contribute to macular exudate
formation and retinopathy.

In the diabetic foot, basement membrane thickening is found in muscle capillaries
and may increase the susceptibility of the diabetic foot to infection *(20)*. This thickening
may act as a barrier to the exchange of nutrients and activated leukocyte migration

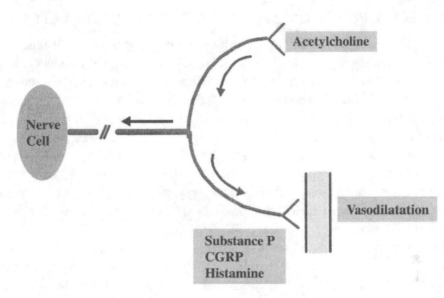

Fig. 1. Graphic illustration of the axon reflex, whereby nociceptive fibers cause vasodilation by release of active substances such as histamine, substance P, and calcitonin gene-related peptide (CGRP).

between the capillary and interstitium. However, there does not appear to be an impairment of oxygen diffusion (again emphasizing the nonocclusive nature of the disease), and in fact, transcutaneous pO_2 measurements are higher in diabetic patients with foot ulcers compared with the nondiabetic population *(21)*. In addition, increased rigidity of the thickened basement membrane encasing the microcirculation may limit compensatory arteriolar dilatation in response to local injury, thereby further reducing the hyperemic response *(22)*.

Although resting total skin microcirculatory flow is similar in both diabetic and nondiabetic patients, the capillary blood flow is reduced in diabetes, indicating a maldistribution and functional ischemia of the skin *(23)*. Moreover, studies of skin microvascular flow have demonstrated reduced maximal hyperemic response to heat in diabetic patients, suggesting that a *functional* microvascular impairment is a major contributing factor for diabetic foot problems. All these changes result in an inability to vasodilate and achieve maximal blood flow following injury.

Diabetes also affects the axon reflex (Fig. 1). Injury directly stimulates nociceptive C fibers, which results in both orthodromic conduction to the spinal cord and antidromic conduction to adjacent C fibers and other axon branches. One function of this axon reflex is the secretion of several active peptides, such as substance P and calcitonin gene-related peptide, which directly and indirectly (through mast cell release of histamine) cause vasodilation and increased permeability. This protective mechanism, in which blood flow is increased to an area of injury, is impaired in diabetes, thus further reducing the hyperemic response when it is most needed *(24)*. Impairment of the axon reflex, although most marked in patients with overt neuropathy, is also seen in diabetic patients without clinically evident neuropathy, thus suggesting that other mechanisms, possibly related to the microcirculation, may be contributory.

ENDOTHELIAL FUNCTION AND DYSFUNCTION IN DIABETES

The normal endothelium plays an important role in blood vessel wall function and homeostasis by synthesizing and releasing substances such as prostacyclin, endothelin, prostaglandins, and nitric oxide that modulate vasomotor tone and prevent thrombosis *(25)*. There is substantial evidence that endothelial function is abnormal in animal models of diabetes mellitus *(26–28)* and in patients with both insulin-dependent and non-insulin-dependent diabetes mellitus *(29,30)*, thus directly implicating either hyperglycemia or hyperinsulinemia as possible mediators of abnormal endothelium-dependent responses. A variety of mechanisms responsible for endothelial dysfunction have been proposed, principally abnormalities in the nitric oxide pathway, abnormal production of vasoconstrictor prostanoids, intracellular signaling, reduction in Na^+-K^+ ATPase activity, and advanced glycosylated end products (AGEs) *(31–33)*.

In 1980, Furchgott and Zawadzki *(34)* discovered that arterial vasodilation was dependent on an intact endothelium and its release of a substance they called endothelium-derived relaxing factor (EDRF), which causes arterial smooth muscle relaxation in response to acetylcholine and other vasodilators. Later identified as endothelial-derived nitric oxide (EDNO), it activates vascular smooth muscle guanylate cyclase, elevates cGMP levels, and may increase Na^+-K^+ ATPase activity *(35)*. A variety of substances other than acetylcholine may cause EDNO-mediated vasodilation. Notably, it appears that the vasodilatory effects of insulin are nitric oxide dependent *(36,37)*, and that insulin mediates vasodilation by modulating the synthesis and release of EDNO.

Hyperglycemia, Hyperinsulinemia, and Diabetes

Although hyperglycemia with hyperinsulinemia impairs endothelial-dependent vasodilation, hyperinsulinemia with euglycemia actually potentiates endothelium-dependent vasodilation via enhanced EDNO release, suggesting that hyperglycemia, independent of hyperinsulinemia, contributes to endothelial dysfunction. Studies from our laboratory have corroborated these findings *(38)*. Twenty healthy subjects were examined fasting and 1 hour after the ingestion of 75 g of glucose. The endothelium-dependent vasodilation of the brachial artery, a conduit vessel, was evaluated by employing high-resolution ultrasonography to measure the changes in vessel diameter induced by reactive hyperemia. In the microcirculation the endothelial function was assessed by measuring changes in erythrocyte flux after acetylcholine iontophoresis. The brachial artery endothelium-dependent dilation was greater during fasting compared with the response after the glucose load, and fasting microcirculatory endothelial-dependent vasodilation was also significantly greater than the response after the glucose load.

Impaired endothelial-dependent vasodilation in certain insulin-resistant states may be instrumental in the pathogenesis of atherosclerosis and hypertension and is postulated to be caused by diminished insulin-mediated EDNO production and release *(39)*. Patients with insulin-dependent and non-insulin-dependent diabetes demonstrate impaired endothelium-dependent responses to acetylcholine, but the response to exogenous nitric oxide donors (i.e., sodium nitroprusside) remains intact in insulin-dependent diabetes only *(29,30)*. It thus appears that abnormal nitric oxide release and/or synthesis predominates in insulin-dependent diabetes, whereas non-insulin-dependent diabetes may be characterized by either a diminished response of smooth muscle to EDNO or increased inactivation of nitric oxide.

Although there is considerable controversy regarding the role of free radicals in diabetic vascular disease *(40)*, an increased production of oxygen-derived free radicals has been described in diabetes and may contribute to endothelial dysfunction *(41)*. Superoxide anions and other oxygen-derived free radicals directly inactivate endothelium-derived nitric oxide *(42)*. In animal models, endothelium-derived free radicals impair EDNO-mediated vasodilation, and administration of superoxide dismutase and other free radical scavengers normalizes EDNO-dependent relaxation in diabetic arteries *(43)*. Defective endothelium-dependent relaxation in the diabetic rat aorta is significantly attenuated by vitamin E, a potent free radical scavenger *(44)*. In human studies, administration of vitamin C restores and improves endothelium-dependent vasodilation, but not endothelium-independent responses, in patients with both insulin-dependent and non-insulin-dependent diabetes mellitus, thus further suggesting that oxygen-derived free radicals may decrease the bioavailability of EDNO *(45)*.

A potentially treatable source of oxygen-derived free radicals is hyperlipidemia. Increased levels of low-density lipoprotein (LDL) and very low-density lipoprotein (VLDL) are common in diabetic patients. Hyperglycemia promotes the oxidation and nonenzymatic glycation of LDL, which has been strongly implicated in atherogenesis by a variety of mechanisms *(46)*. In animal models of hypercholesterolemia, the vascular endothelium produces several free radicals, presumably through xanthine oxidase activation, and these endothelial derived free radicals inactivate EDNO *(47)*. Moreover, flow-mediated vasodilation and reactive hyperemia (endothelium-dependent) is more impaired in patients with insulin-dependent diabetes and elevated LDL cholesterol levels, which further supports the relationship of hypercholesterolemia, free radicals, and EDNO *(48)*.

AGEs have also been implicated in the pathogenesis of diabetic microvascular complications. These are formed from a reversible reaction between glucose and protein to form Schiff bases, which then rearrange to form stable Amadori-type early glycosylation products. Some of these reversible early glycosylation products may undergo complex rearrangements to form irreversible AGEs. In experimental diabetes, AGEs impair the actions of EDNO and cause an impaired endothelium-dependent response, which is ameliorated by administration of an AGE inhibitor *(49)*. AGEs also displace disulfide crosslinkages in collagen and scleral proteins, accounting for the diminished charge in the capillary basement membrane. This may contribute to the increased vascular permeability of diabetes, since blockade of a specific receptor for AGE reverses diabetes-mediated vascular hyperpermeability *(50)*. Moreover, the presence of AGE receptors on both endothelial cells and monocytes, along with AGE deposition in the subendothelium, suggests monocyte deposition into the subendothelial space and secondary complications *(51)*. Higher AGE levels have been found in patients with diabetes as compared to nondiabetic controls, with the highest levels occurring among diabetic patients with nephropathy *(52)*. Since at least part of AGE-induced cellular dysfunction is caused by an oxidant-sensitive mechanism, which is inhibited by antioxidants, it is likely that both oxygen-derived free radicals and AGEs each contribute to cause impaired EDNO-dependent vasodilation in diabetes. Taken together, the effects of AGEs on vascular permeability, subendothelial protein deposition, inactivation of nitric oxide, and modification of LDL provide strong evidence for their important role in diabetic vascular disease.

Experimental studies in diabetic animals have also indicated that abnormal endothelial production of vasoconstrictor prostanoids, notably thromboxane $(TX)A_2$ and prostaglandin $(PG)H_2$ may be a cause of endothelial cell dysfunction. Increased levels of TXA_2 have been isolated only from segments of diabetic aortic tissue with an intact endothelium, suggesting that the endothelium is responsible for the increased release and that impaired relaxation to acetylcholine in these segments is restored by treatment with cyclooxygenase inhibitors. In humans, however, the role of vasoconstrictor prostanoids is less clear. Flow-dependent vasodilation in healthy subjects, which may be used as an index of endothelial function is unaffected by aspirin, thus demonstrating that it is entirely mediated by EDNO and independent of vasoactive prostanoids *(53)*. Moreover, the attenuated endothelium-dependent vasodilation following acetylcholine administration seen in diabetic patients is not affected by pretreatment with cyclooxygenase inhibitors *(29,30)*.

MICROVASCULAR DISEASE
AND NEUROPATHY IN THE DIABETIC FOOT

It therefore appears that dysfunction of the microcirculation strongly contributes to the renal, eye, and macrovascular complications of diabetes. Several lines of evidence have indicated that the microcirculation is also implicated in the pathogenesis of diabetic neuropathy, and the etiology of diabetic neuropathy may be a complex interplay between metabolic and microvascular defects involving aldose reductase, Na^+-K^+ ATPase activity, and nitric oxide. Some of these may include EDNO stimulation of Na^+-K^+ ATPase activity, decreased Na^+-K^+ ATPase activity by EDNO inhibitors, and hyperglycemic inhibition of Na^+-K^+ ATPase activity in normal rabbit aorta, which is preventable by administering aldose reductase inhibitors or by raising plasma myoinositol levels *(54,55)*.

Recent studies from our laboratory have helped to further define the relationship among the microcirculation, diabetes, and neuropathy *(56)*. To determine the effect of neuropathy and hypoxia on the foot microcirculation, we studied five groups of patients: diabetic neuropathic patients, patients with diabetes and Charcot osteoarthropathy, diabetic patients with neuropathy and clinically evident lower extremity peripheral vascular disease, diabetic patients without complications, and healthy controls. The microcirculation was studied in vivo by employing laser Doppler imaging to measure the vasodilatory response to iontophoresis (a noninvasive method of introducing soluble ions into skin) of acetylcholine (endothelium-dependent) and sodium nitroprusside (an exogenous nitric oxide donor, endothelium independent). Both the direct and indirect (which depends on a normal axon reflex) vasodilatory response were measured. The direct response to acetylcholine, which stimulates the production of nitric oxide, was similarly reduced in the groups with neuropathy, Charcot osteoarthropathy, and vascular disease compared with the remaining two groups ($p < 0.001$), whereas the direct response to nitroprusside was lowest in diabetic patients with vascular disease (Fig. 2). The indirect vasodilation during acetylcholine iontophoresis was also reduced in the neuropathy,

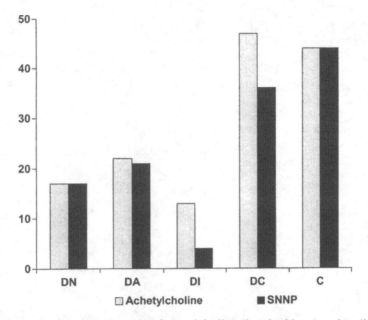

Fig. 2. Response to the iontophoresis of acetylcholine (hatched bars) and sodium nitroprusside (SNNP, black bars) expressed as percentage of increase over baseline flow and measured by a laser scanner imager. The response to acetylcholine was equally reduced in the diabetic neuropathic patients with a history of foot ulceration (DN group), the patients with both neuropathy and peripheral vascular disease (DI), and the patients with Charcot neuroarthropathy (DA) when compared with nonneuropathic diabetic patients (D) and healthy controls (C) ($p < 0.0001$). The response to SNNP was more pronounced in the DI group and was also reduced in the DN and DA groups compared with the D and C groups ($p < 0.0001$). (From: Veves A, Akbari CM, Primavera J, et al. Endothelial dysfunction and the expression of endothelial nitric oxide synthetase in diabetic neuropathy, vascular disease, and foot ulceration. *Diabetes* 1997;47:457–463. Copyright American Diabetes Association)

Charcot, and vascular disease groups but not in healthy controls or diabetic patients without complications ($p < 0.0001$; Fig. 3). The data suggest that the endothelium-dependent vasodilation and the axon reflex are impaired in the presence of diabetes and neuropathy, but the endothelium-independent response is spared, and that this dysfunction may be attributed to an impaired production of nitric oxide. In addition, the nerve axon reflex is reduced in diabetic neuropathic patients with and without vascular disease, whereas it is intact in diabetic patients without neuropathy.

Because of these findings, we also studied the expression of endogenous endothelial nitric oxide synthetase (eNOS) activity in skin taken from the foot of patients with diabetic neuropathy, diabetic lower extremity vascular disease, and healthy controls *(57)*. Full-thickness skin biopsies from the dorsum of the foot were obtained and immunostained with antiserum to human eNOS, glucose transporter I (GLUT I), and von Willebrand factor, which is an anatomic marker of the endothelium. No differences were found among the three groups in the staining intensity of von Willebrand factor and GLUT I. In contrast, the staining intensity of eNOS was reduced in both diabetic groups

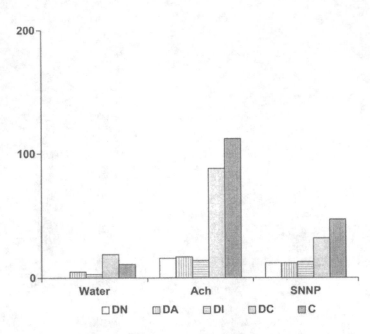

Fig. 3. Response of blood flow (percentage of increase over baseline, measured by a single-point laser probe) in a skin area adjacent to but not in direct contact with the iontophoresis solution. During the iontophoresis of deionized water, a mild response was observed in all groups. In contrast, during the iontophoresis of acetylcholine, the response was reduced in the diabetic neuropathic patients with a history of foot ulceration (DN group), the patients with both neuropathy and peripheral vascular disease (DI), and the patients with Charcot neuroarthropathy (DA) compared with nonneuropathic diabetic patients (D) and healthy controls (C) ($p < 0.0001$). A similar response was observed during the iontophoresis of sodium nitroprusside (SNNP), but it was less than half compared with the response achieved with acetylcholine. (From: Veves A, Akbari CM, Primavera J, et al. Endothelial dysfunction and the expression of endothelial nitric oxide synthetase in diabetic neuropathy, vascular disease, and foot ulceration. *Diabetes* 1997; 47:457–463. Copyright American Diabetes Association)

compared with controls (Fig. 4). Therefore, it appears that in diabetic neuropathic patients, with or without lower extremity ischemia, the eNOS activity is reduced, even though the endothelium is anatomically present and endothelial functional changes may be related to the development of neuropathy.

Current hypotheses regarding the etiology of diabetic neuropathy are centered on a combination of metabolic defects secondary to hyperglycemia and vascular changes that result in nerve hypoxia *(58)*. Evidence for a hypoxic etiology is considerable and includes reduced endoneurial blood flow, increased vascular resistance, and decreased endothelial production of nitric oxide *(59,60)*. Although microvascular dysfunction has been mainly implicated, the role of peripheral vascular disease remains considerable, as it appears likely that a decrease in total limb blood flow would potentiate nerve ischemia. This concept has been supported by clinical trials, which have demonstrated a more severe neuropathy in diabetic patients with lower limb ischemia compared with nonischemic diabetic and ischemic nondiabetic patients, and an improvement of the nerve function a short time after the revascularization *(60,61)*.

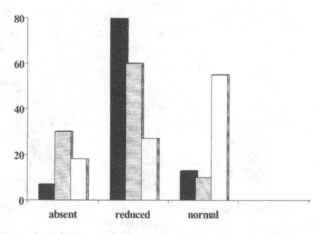

Fig. 4. Expression of eNOS in patients with diabetic neuropathy (black column), patients with both neuropathy and peripheral vascular disease (hatched column), and healthy subjects (white column). The expression of eNOS was reduced in both the diabetic groups compared with the healthy subjects. (Data from ref. 57).

Clinical studies from our laboratory have focused on the effect of arterial reconstruction on the natural history of diabetic neuropathy *(62)*. Fifty-five patients with diabetes and peripheral vascular disease requiring revascularization were studied. Peroneal nerve conduction velocity was measured prior to arterial bypass and then again at a mean follow-up of 19 months. In the operated leg, the peroneal nerve conduction velocity remained unchanged during the follow-up period (preoperative 35.79 ± 6.02 vs. postoperative 35.33 ± 7.51 m/s, $p = NS$), but deteriorated in the nonoperated leg (36.68 ± 6.22 vs. 33.64 ± 7.30, $p < 0.05$). The data suggest that reversal of hypoxia in diabetic patients halts the progression of neuropathy, lending further support to the role of localized ischemia, and possibly endothelial dysfunction, in the pathogenesis of diabetic sensorimotor neuropathy *(63)*.

In addition, increased lower extremity capillary pressure upon assuming the erect posture, owing to early loss of postural vasoconstriction, has recently been proposed as an additional contributing factor in the pathogenesis of diabetic neuropathy *(64)*. Based on this, a recent study has hypothesized that the vasodilatory response of the cutaneous microcirculation of the foot is reduced when compared with the forearm in diabetic patients with peripheral neuropathy, and that the development of neuropathy will further impair the microcirculation owing to the involvement of the C nociceptive fibers *(65)* (Fig. 5). The authors compared endothelium-dependent and hyperemic responses between the dorsum of the foot and the forearm in diabetic neuropathic and nonneuropathic patients and healthy control subjects. Significant differences were found between foot and forearm level in both endothelium-dependent and endothelium-independent vasodilation. Thus, the percent increase in vasodilation over baseline during the iontophoresis of acetylcholine was lower in the foot compared with the forearm in the neuropathic group, the nonneuropathic group, and the controls. Similar results were observed during the iontophoresis of sodium nitroprusside in the neuropathic group, the nonneuropathic group, and the controls. No differences were found among the three groups when the ratio of the forearm/foot response was calculated for both the endothelium-dependent

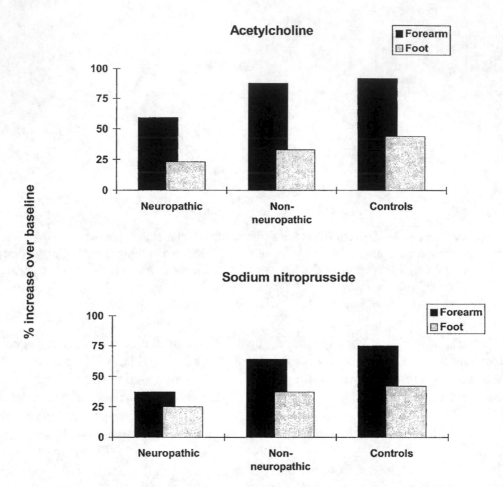

Fig. 5. Results of iontophoresis of acetylcholine (endothelium dependent) and sodium nitro-prusside (endothelium independent) at the forearm (black bars) and foot (white bars). The response at the foot was significantly lower than that of the forearm in all three groups ($p < 0.01$). In addition, the responses at the foot and forearm level were lower in the neuropathic group compared with the control subjects ($p < 0.05$). (From: Arora S, Smakowski P, Frykberg RG, et al. Differences in foot and forearm skin microcirculation in diabetic patients with and without neuropathy. *Diabetes Care* 1998;21:1339. Copyright American Diabetes Association)

and endothelium-independent vasodilation. The authors concluded that in healthy subjects, the endothelium-dependent and -independent vasodilation is lower at the foot level when compared with the forearm and that a generalized impairment of the microcirculation in diabetic patients with neuropathy preserves this forearm-foot gradient. These changes may be a contributing factor for the early involvement of the foot with neuropathy when compared with the forearm.

CONCLUSIONS

The association of microvascular disease and diabetic retinopathy, neuropathy, and nephropathy is well established, and more recent data have suggested a link between endothelial dysfunction and many of the metabolic consequences of diabetes (*66*). The diabetic foot is unique in that it manifests virtually all the microvascular abnormalities seen in the other organ systems. Preventive and treatment efforts are directed toward these abnormalities and should be considered when evaluating a patient with diabetic foot ulceration. At our institution, knowledge of the altered pathophysiology of the diabetic foot has resulted in an aggressive approach toward treatment, incorporating our understanding of the pattern of macrovascular (atherosclerotic) and microvascular disease. The results of such a plan are reflected in two recent reports from our institution *(67,68)*. There has been a significant decrease in every category of major amputation since 1984, concomitant with a greater number of patients undergoing distal arterial reconstruction. However, given the complexity of the microcirculation in diabetes, this is truly only the tip of the iceberg, as our understanding of diabetic vascular disease and its effects on all organ systems is still in its infancy.

REFERENCES

1. Grunfeld C. Diabetic foot ulcers: etiology, treatment, and prevention. *Adv Intern Med* 1991; 37:103–132.
2. Nathan DM. Long-term complications of diabetes mellitus. *N Engl J Med* 1993;328:1676–1685.
3. Reiber GE, Boyko EJ, Smith DG. Lower extremity foot ulcers and amputations in diabetes, in *Diabetes in America,* 2nd ed. (National Diabetes Data Group, ed.), National Institutes of Health, Washington, 1995, pp. 409–428.
4. Akbari CM, LoGerfo FW. Diabetes and peripheral vascular disease. *J Vasc Surg* 1999;30: 373–384.
5. Cameron NE, Cotter MA. The relationship of vascular changes to metabolic factors in diabetes mellitus and their role in the development of peripheral nerve complications. *Diabetes Metab Rev* 1994;10:189–224.
6. LoGerfo FW, Coffman JD. Vascular and microvascular disease of the foot in diabetes. *N Engl J Med* 1984;311:1615–1619.
7. Williamson JR, Titlon RG, Chang K, Kilo C. Basement membrane abnormalities in diabetes mellitus: relationship to clinical microangiopathy. *Diabetes Metab Rev* 1988;4:339–370.
8. LoGerfo FW. Vascular disease, matrix abnormalities, and neuropathy: implications for limb salvage in diabetes mellitus. *J Vasc Surg* 1987;5:793–796.
9. Palmberg P, Smith M, Waltman S, et al. The natural history of retinopathy in insulin-dependent juvenile-onset diabetes. *Ophthalmology* 1981;88:613–618.
10. Pirart J. Diabetes mellitus and its degenerative complications: a prospective study of 4400 patients observed between 1947 and 1973. *Diabetes Care* 1978;1:168–188, 252–261.
11. DCCT Research Group. The effect of intensive treatment of diabetes on the development and progression of long-term complications in insulin-dependent diabetes mellitus. *N Engl J Med* 1993;329:977–986.
12. Vanhoutte PM. The endothelium—modulator of vascular smooth-muscle tone. *N Engl J Med* 1988;319:512–513.
13. Cohen RA. Dysfunction of vascular endothelium in diabetes mellitus. *Circulation* 1993;87: V67–V76.
14. Goldenberg SG, Alex M, Joshi RA, Blumenthal HT. Nonatheromatous peripheral vascular disease of the lower extremity in diabetes mellitus. *Diabetes* 1959;8:261–273.
15. Strandness DE Jr, Priest RE, Gibbons GE. Combined clinical and pathologic study of diabetic and nondiabetic peripheral arterial disease. *Diabetes* 1964;13:366–372.
16. Conrad MC. Large and small artery occlusion in diabetics and nondiabetics with severe vascular disease. *Circulation* 1967;36:83–91.

17. Barner HB, Kaiser GC, Willman VL. Blood flow in the diabetic leg. *Circulation* 1971;43: 391–394.
18. Parving HH, Viberti GC, Keen H, Christiansen JS, Lassen NA. Hemodynamic factors in the genesis of diabetic microangiopathy. *Metabolism* 1983;32:943–949.
19. Morgensen CE, Schmitz A, Christensen CR. Comparative renal pathophysiology relevant to IDDM and NIDDM patients. *Diabetes Metab Rev* 1988;4:453–483.
20. Rayman G, Williams SA, Spencer PD, et al. Impaired microvascular hyperaemic response to minor skin trauma in type I diabetes. *BMJ* 1986;292:1295–1298.
21. Wyss CR, Matsen FA III, Simmons CW, et al. Transcutaneous oxygen tension measurements on limbs of diabetic and nondiabetic patients with peripheral vascular disease. *Surgery* 1984;95:339–346.
22. Flynn MD, Tooke JE. Aetiology of diabetic foot ulceration: a role for the microcirculation? *Diabet Med* 1992;8:320–329.
23. Jorneskog G, Brismar K, Fagrell B. Skin capillary circulation severely impaired in toes of patients with IDDM, with and without late diabetic complications. *Diabetologia* 1995;38: 474–480.
24. Parkhouse N, LeQueen PM. Impaired neurogenic vascular response in patients with diabetes and neuropathic foot lesions. *N Engl J Med* 1988;318:1306–1309.
25. Vane JR, Anggard EE, Botting RM. Regulatory functions of the vascular endothelium. *N Engl J Med* 1990;323:27–36.
26. Gupta S, Sussman I, McArthur CS, et al. Endothelium-dependent inhibition of Na+-K+ ATPase activity in rabbit aorta by hyperglycemia. Possible role of endothelium-derived nitric oxide. *J Clin Invest* 1992;90:727–732.
27. Pieper GM, Meier DA, Hager SR. Endothelial dysfunction in a model of hyperglycemia and hyperinsulinemia. *Am J Physiol* 1995;269:H845–H850.
28. Tesfamarian B, Brown ML, Cohen RA. Elevated glucose impairs endothelium-dependent relaxation by activating protein kinase C. *J Clin Invest* 1991;87:1643–1648.
29. Williams SB, Cusco JA, Roddy M, Johnstone MY, Creager MA. Impaired nitric oxide-mediated vasodilation in patients with non-insulin-dependent diabetes mellitus. *J Am Coll Cardiol* 1996;27:567–574.
30. Johnstone MT, Creager SJ, Scales KM, et al. Impaired endothelium-dependent vasodilation in patients with insulin-dependent diabetes mellitus. *Circulation* 1993;88:2510–2516.
31. Tesfamarian B, Brown ML, Deykin D, Cohen RA. Elevated glucose promotes generation of endothelium-derived vasoconstrictor prostanoids in rabbit aorta. *J Clin Invest* 1990;85: 929–932.
32. Simmons DA, Winegrad AI. Elevated extracellular glucose inhibits an adenosine-Na+-K+ ATPase regulatory system in rabbit aortic wall. *Diabetologia* 1991;34:157–163.
33. Brownlee M, Cerami A, Vlassare H. Advanced glycosylation end products in tissue and the biochemical basis of diabetic complications. *N Engl J Med* 1988;318:1315–1321.
34. Furchgott RF, Zawadzki JV. The obligatory role of endothelial cells in the relaxation of arterial smooth muscle by acetylcholine. *Nature* 1980;288:373–376.
35. Palmer RM, Ferrige AG, Moncada S. Nitric oxide release accounts for the biologic activity of endothelium-derived relaxing factor. *Nature* 1987;327:524–526.
36. Scherrer U, Randin D, Vollenweider P, Vollenweider L, Nicod P. Nitric oxide release accounts for insulin's vascular effects in humans. *J Clin Invest* 1994;94:2511–2515.
37. Taddei S, Virdis A, Mattei P, et al. Effect of insulin on acetylcholine-induced vasodilation in normotensive subjects and patients with essential hypertension. *Circulation* 1995;92: 2911–2918.
38. Akbari CM, Saouaf R, Barnhill DF, et al. Endothelium-dependent vasodilatation is impaired in both microcirculation and macrocirculation during acute hyperglycemia. *J Vasc Surg* 1998;28:687–694.

39. Baron AD. The coupling of glucose metabolism and perfusion in human skeletal muscle. The potential role of endothelium-derived nitric oxide. *Diabetes* 1996;45:S105–S109.
40. Oberly LW. Free radicals in diabetes. *Free Radic Biol Med* 1988;5:113–124.
41. Wolff SP, Dean RT. Glucose autoxidation and protein modification: the role of oxidative glycosylation in diabetes. *Biochem J* 1987;245:234–250.
42. Gryglewski RJ, Palmer RM, Moncada S. Superoxide anion is involved in the breakdown of endothelium-derived vascular relaxing factor. *Nature* 1986;320:454–456.
43. Diederich D, Skopec J, Diederich A, Dai FX. Endothelial dysfunction in mesenteric resistance arteries of diabetic rats: role of free radicals. *Am J Physiol* 1994;266:H1153–H1161.
44. Keegan A, Walbank H, Cotter MA, Cameron NE. Chronic vitamin E treatment prevents defective endothelium-dependent relaxation in diabetic rat aorta. *Diabetologia* 1995;38: 1475–1478.
45. Timimi FK, Ting HH, Haley EA, et al. Vitamin C improves endothelium-dependent vasodilation in patients with insulin-dependent diabetes mellitus. *J Am Coll Cardiol* 1998;31: 552–557.
46. Witzum JL. The oxidation hypothesis of atherosclerosis. *Lancet* 1994;344:793–795.
47. Ohara Y, Peterson TE, Harrison DG. Hypercholesterolemia increases endothelial superoxide anion production. *J Clin Invest* 1993;91:2546–2551.
48. Clarkson P, Celermajer DS, Donald AE, et al. Impaired vascular reactivity in insulin-dependent diabetes mellitus is related to disease duration and low density lipoprotein cholesterol levels. *J Am Coll Cardiol* 1996;28:573–579.
49. Bucala R, Tracey KJ, Cerami A. Advanced glycosylation end products quench nitric oxide and mediate defective endothelium-dependent vasodilatation in experimental diabetes. *J Clin Invest* 1991;87:432–438.
50. Wautier JL, Zoukourian C, Chappey O. Receptor-mediated endothelial cell dysfunction in diabetic vasculopathy. Soluble receptor for advanced glycation end products blocks hyperpermeability in diabetic rats. *J Clin Invest* 1996;97:238–243.
51. Schmidt AM, Hori O, Brett J, et al. Cellular receptors for advanced glycation end products. Implications for induction of oxidant stress and cellular dysfunction in the pathogenesis of vascular lesions. *Arterioscler Thromb* 1994;14:1521–1528.
52. Makita Z, Radoff S, Rayfield EJ. Advanced glycosylation end products in patients with diabetic nephropathy. *N Engl J Med* 1991;325:836–842.
53. Joannides R, Haefeli WE, Linder L, et al. Nitric oxide is responsible for flow-dependent dilatation of human peripheral conduit arteries in vivo. *Circulation* 1995;91:1314–1319.
54. Simmons DA, Winegrad AI. Mechanism of glucose-induced Na+-K+ ATPase inhibition in aortic wall of rabbits. *Diabetologia* 1989;32:402–408.
55. Stevens MJ, Dananberg J, Feldman EL, et al. The linked roles of nitric oxide, aldose reductase and Na+-K+ ATPase in the slowing of nerve conduction in the streptozotocin diabetic rat. *J Clin Invest* 1994;94:853–859.
56. Veves A, Akbari CM, Donaghue VM, et al. The effect of diabetes, neuropathy, Charcot arthropathy, and arterial disease on the foot microcirculation. *Diabetologia* 1996;39(Suppl 1):A3.
57. Veves A, Akbari CM, Primavera J, et al. Endothelial dysfunction and the expression of endothelial nitric oxide synthetase in diabetic neuropathy, vascular disease, and foot ulceration. *Diabetes* 1997;47:457–463.
58. Stevens MJ, Feldman EL, Greene DA. The aetiology of diabetic neuropathy: the combined roles of metabolic and vascular defects. *Diabet Med* 1995;12:566–579.
59. Tuck RR, Schmelzer JD, Low PA. Endoneurial blood flow and oxygen tension in the sciatic nerves of rats with experimental diabetic neuropathy. *Brain* 1984;107:935–950.
60. Tesfaye S, Harris N, Jakubowski JJ, et al. Impaired blood flow and arterio-venous shunting in human diabetic neuropathy: a novel technique of nerve photography and fluorescin angiography. *Diabetologia* 1993;36:1266–1274.

61. Ram Z, Sadeh M, Walden R, Adar R. Vascular insufficiency quantitatively aggravates diabetic neuropathy. *Arch Neurol* 1991;48:1239–1242.
62. Akbari CM, Gibbons GW, Habershaw GM, LoGerfo FW, Veves A. The effect of arterial reconstruction on the natural history of diabetic neuropathy. *Arch Surg* 1997;132:148–152.
63. Akbari CM, LoGerfo FW. The micro- and macrocirculation in diabetes mellitus, in *A Clinical Approach to Diabetic Neuropathy*, 1st ed. (Veves A, ed.), Humana, New York, 1998, pp. 319–331.
64. Flynn MD, Tooke JE. Diabetic neuropathy and the microcirculation. *Diabet Med* 1995;12: 298–301.
65. Arora S, Smakowski P, Frykberg RG, et al. Differences in foot and forearm skin microcirculation in diabetic patients with and without neuropathy. *Diabetes Care* 1998;21:1339.
66. Pinckney JH, Stehouwer CDA, Coppack SW, Yudkin JS. Endothelial dysfunction: cause of the insulin resistance syndrome. *Diabetes* 1997;46:S9–S13.
67. LoGerfo FW, Gibbons GW, Pomposelli FB Jr, et al. Trends in the care of the diabetic foot: expanded role of arterial reconstruction. *Arch Surg* 1992;127:617–621.
68. Akbari CM, Pomposelli FB Jr, Gibbons GW, et al. Lower extremity revascularization in diabetes: late observations. *Arch Surg* 2000;135:452–456.

6

Clinical Features and Diagnosis of Macrovascular Disease

Nikhil Kansal, MD and Allen Hamdan, MD

INTRODUCTION

The concomitant occurrence of atherosclerotic peripheral vascular disease in patients with diabetes is a major factor in the progression of diabetic foot pathology. The rate of lower extremity amputation in the diabetic population is 15 times that seen in the nondiabetic population *(1)*. This rate is secondary to a number of factors present in the diabetic that lead to the foot pathology in a synergistic fashion. These factors include 1) peripheral neuropathy, which leads to structural and sensory changes within the foot; 2) microvascular changes, nonocclusive changes in the microcirculation leading to impairment of normal cellular exchange; 3) infection, often aggressive and polymicrobial; and 4) macrovascular disease, atherosclerosis of the peripheral arteries. Although the underlying pathogenesis of atherosclerotic disease in diabetics is similar to that noted in nondiabetics, there are significant differences. It is important to realize that the diabetic foot is more susceptible to moderate changes in perfusion than in nondiabetic patients, resulting in a greater sensitivity to atherosclerotic occlusive disease. Compounding this scenario is the fact that diabetics are noted to have a fourfold increase in the prevalence of atherosclerosis as well as a propensity for accelerated atherosclerosis. This chapter reviews the pathobiology and anatomic distribution of the occlusive disease, the clinical presentation, and the various diagnostic modalities. It concludes with a diagnostic and treatment protocol that can be used in patients presenting with this multifactorial disease process.

PATHOLOGY OF ATHEROSCLEROSIS IN DIABETES

The understanding of the basic pathology of atherosclerosis in diabetics has evolved considerably over the last 15 years. The commonly held belief that diabetics are prone to small vessel disease has been refuted by a number of studies detailed below. This popular misconception, in which the arterioles of the ankle and foot are thought to be preferentially affected by atherosclerotic occlusive disease, originated from a paper by Goldenberg et al. *(2)*. In their retrospective review of amputation specimens from diabetics and nondiabetics, they used periodic acid-Schiff staining to examine the peripheral vasculature histologically. Deposits that stained positive in the arterioles of the foot

From: *The Diabetic Foot: Medical and Surgical Management*
Edited by: A. Veves, J. M. Giurini, and F. W. LoGerfo © Humana Press Inc., Totowa, NJ

and ankle were noted to be unique to the diabetic specimens. These deposits were considered atherosclerotic lesions and were felt to be the principle cause of the worsened prognosis in patients with diabetes. It is important to realize that this assumption led (partly) to the prevailing idea that, because the small vessels (arterioles) were somehow preferentially involved in the occlusive process, diabetics were not candidates for distal revascularization. This label of unreconstructable disease has in the past led to unnecessary amputation in the diabetic population.

A number of research studies attempted to determine whether a diffuse and unique type of atherosclerosis existed in diabetics. In a prospective analysis of amputation specimens, this time with a blinded histologic review, Strandness and co-workers *(3)* used periodic acid-Schiff staining and showed no difference between diabetics and nondiabetics: both groups had similar patterns of atherosclerosis, namely, a paucity of occlusive disease at the arteriolar level. In another prospective study, using a sophisticated casting technique for evaluating the peripheral vasculature, Conrad *(4)* confirmed the similar characteristics of arteriolar atherosclerosis in both groups of patients. To dispel the theory that the peripheral vascular bed in diabetics was less reactive, Barner et al. *(5)* measured the flow rate in femoropopliteal bypass grafts in the two groups. By infusing papavarine into the outflow vascular bed, they were able to assess differences in vessel reactivity; again, no difference was noted between diabetics and nondiabetics. It is clear from these studies that a unique small vessel occlusive pattern does not exist in diabetic patients.

Some aspects of atherosclerotic peripheral vascular disease are in fact different from those of the nondiabetic population. As has already been mentioned, diabetics have a fourfold higher prevalence of atherosclerosis, which progresses at a more rapid rate. It is also noteworthy that diabetic patients with the sequelae of atherosclerotic disease often present at an earlier age than their nondiabetic counterparts. In addition, diabetics often have a unique distribution of atherosclerosis at the arterial level: occlusive disease in diabetics has a distinct propensity to occur in the infrageniculate vessels in the calf. The affected arteries (the anterior tibial, posterior tibial, and peroneal arteries) are more severely affected and are more likely to present with occlusion in diabetics (Figs. 1 and 2). The proximal arteries, to the level of the popliteal artery, are often spared in diabetics. Equally important is the observation that the arteries of the foot, namely, the dorsalis pedis arteries, are spared from the occlusive disease (Fig. 3). These patterns are generalizations, and it is important to mention that some diabetics present with atherosclerotic lesions very similar to those seen in nondiabetics.

These observations have had a crucial impact in the way that peripheral vascular disease in diabetics is approached. Based in part on the expected presence of small vessel disease, diabetics were not treated as aggressively as is now standard. Because diabetics were thought to have occlusive disease at the arteriolar level, bypass to patent vessels proximal to the foot was thought to be futile. Now, as our understanding of the disease process has evolved, so has our treatment protocol. Through our current understanding that calf vessels are more severely affected by atherosclerosis while the pedal vessels are spared, we have been able to modify our approach to the evaluation and treatment of diabetic patients. A more aggressive approach to identifying pedal arteries suitable for bypass along with aggressive measures to control local infection has radically changed the prognosis of peripheral vascular disease in the diabetic foot.

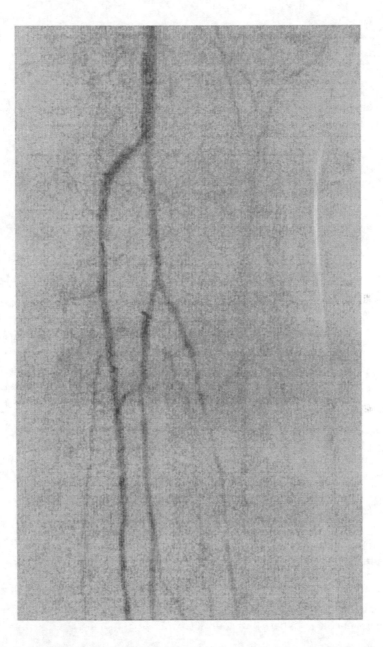

Fig. 1. Digital subtraction angiogram showing the below-knee popliteal artery and tibial arteries in a diabetic patient. The diffuse pattern of atherosclerotic disease is typical of this population.

CLINICAL PRESENTATION

To appreciate the differences in the presentation of peripheral vascular disease in patients with diabetes, it is important to understand its presentation in nondiabetics. Atherosclerotic disease is manifest by a continuum of signs and symptoms that can be divided into three categories, as follows (in order of increasing severity): (1) claudication, (2) rest pain, and (3) tissue loss. These categories represent the normal evolution

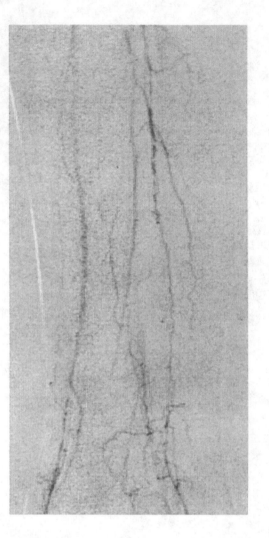

Fig. 2. A more distal view of the same patient as in Fig. 1. It is evident that there are no patent tibial arteries. The blood flow to the foot in this patient is entirely dependent on the small collateral vessels visible. In the past, a patient with this angiogram would not have been considered a candidate for bypass. Now, however, it is known that the pedal arteries in diabetic patients with this type of disease should also be visualized; many of these patients are found to have pedal arteries amenable to bypass procedures. (See Figs. 3, 6, and 7.)

of symptoms in the nondiabetic population with peripheral vascular disease. It is important to note that because of the effects of diabetic neuropathy, this progression of symptoms (from mild to severe) may be absent in diabetics. This topic is further detailed in another chapter.

Claudication is defined as ischemic muscle pain that occurs as the result of inadequate blood flow. This lack of tissue perfusion is due to proximal arterial occlusive disease, resulting in diminished blood flow to large muscle groups. Claudication of the thigh and buttocks can occur and is a result of occlusive disease of the aortoiliac system. More commonly, claudication of the calf is the initial presenting symptom. The pain is

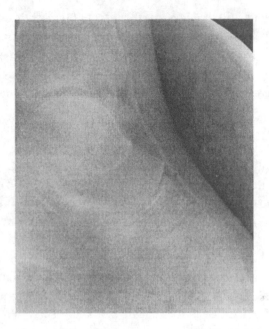

Fig. 3. Lateral view of the foot (nonsubtraction) of a diabetic patient with severe tibial artery occlusive disease. This patient had no patent tibial vessels to which bypass could be performed. Note the location and patency of the artery on the dorsum of the foot. This is the dorsalis pedis artery and is an excellent target artery for bypass.

characteristic, involving the calf muscles, and is described as cramping in nature. It is often aggravated by exercise and is often relieved by several minutes of rest. The patient's ability to quantify the distance (termed the "initial claudication distance") he or she is able to walk before becoming symptomatic is helpful in tracking the progression of claudication. This assessment is extremely valuable in clinical practice for the follow-up of patients with peripheral vascular disease. As a result of the rich collateral network of blood supply to the lower extremity, occlusive disease at two levels is usually required to cause claudication. This does not hold true for diabetics, however, since they are more susceptible than nondiabetics to small changes in tissue perfusion. Therefore, it is not uncommon for diabetics to present with symptoms owing to vascular occlusive disease localized to one level, whereas nondiabetics will often have multi-level disease at presentation.

Claudication is an important early sign of peripheral vascular disease that should always be elicited in a patient's history. Careful follow-up and monitoring of claudication can identify patients with worsening occlusive disease before the progression to more severe pathology. Most patients, about 75%, will remain stable with regard to their claudication. Operative treatment or amputations are required in only 1% of diabetic patients per year.

Rest pain is another symptom of peripheral vascular disease and is an indication of severe occlusive disease. It is characterized as a burning pain involving either the forefoot or the region of the metatarsal heads. Unlike claudication, rest pain is constant, occurs even at rest (most commonly at night), and is relieved only by dependant hanging of the extremity. Patients will often dangle the affected leg off the side of the bed at night to gain relief. Rest pain is often an ominous sign of severely progressive occlusive disease. Unfortunately, secondary to peripheral neuropathy, diabetics may not develop rest pain, or it may be confused with the pain of neuropathy. The absence of this hallmark clinical sign may lead to a delay in the diagnosis of severe ischemia of the foot in diabetics.

Tissue loss is the most severe presentation of vascular disease. Two separate types can be distinguished: foot ulceration and gangrene. Foot ulceration is the most common presentation of peripheral vascular disease in diabetic patients. The increased incidence of foot ulceration in diabetics is caused by the synergistic effects of the various other contributing factors. It is important to realize that ulceration in diabetics is rarely owing to ischemia alone, a fact that should be kept in mind when devising treatment strategies. All diabetics presenting with foot ulceration should be evaluated for peripheral vascular disease.

Gangrene seen in diabetics and nondiabetics is quite similar. The gangrenous extremity is a hallmark of severe vascular occlusive disease. The diagnosis is established at clinical exam. The affected extremity appears black and shriveled, is insensate, and has no motor function. Gangrene as defined does not include the presence of infection and thus, is of little systemic consequence in the affected patient. This is not the case when the gangrenous tissue is secondarily infected, so-called wet gangrene. This separate clinical entity is characterized by the classical findings of gangrene, with the additional signs of invasive infection: fever, chills, leukocytosis, erythema, cellulitis, pus, abscess, or osteomyelitis. In contrast to uninfected or dry gangrene, wet gangrene poses a surgical emergency.

Any discussion regarding the presentation of peripheral vascular disease would not be complete without the mention of infection as a presenting symptom. Although less common in the nondiabetic population, infection can be the first sign of peripheral ischemia in diabetics. In addition, infection associated with ulceration and gangrene is also more common in diabetics. These infections are often aggressive and polymicrobial, cause significant tissue destruction, and are the most common cause of amputation in the diabetic foot. In terms of presentation, it is crucial to realize that the signs of infection may be subtle. Because the normal immune response to infection is altered in diabetics, patients with massive invasive infection may not have fever, chills, leukocytosis, or even cellulitis. In fact, many diabetic patients with foot infection may present merely with hyperglycemia, or simply an increase in the insulin requirement. Because of these factors the index of suspicion of foot infection in diabetics should always be high.

DIAGNOSIS AND EVALUATION

The cornerstone in the evaluation of patients with diabetes and peripheral vascular disease remains the physical exam. Our experience has shown that the absence of pedal pulses, either dorsalis pedis or posterior tibial, is an indication of advanced occlusive disease. Beyond the physical exam, a myriad of noninvasive and invasive diagnostic modalities are available to the clinician. Noninvasive modalities are preferred for screening and initial workup and include ankle-brachial indexes, pulse volume recordings, segmental pressures, toe pressures, and transcutaneous oxygen measurements. There are many conflicting arguments regarding the efficacy and reproducibility of these methods. This continued controversy, along with the inapplicability of many of these tests in diabetics, has hampered their usefulness. The only invasive diagnostic test in the evaluation of vascular disease is digital subtraction angiography. This is currently considered the gold standard in the assessment of occlusive disease. In addition, magnetic resonance angiography (MRA) and computed tomography angiography (CTA) are also relatively noninvasive; they are being considered as alternatives to the more invasive digital subtraction angiography. They have significant limitations and have yet to be accepted as replacements for conventional angiography.

Noninvasive measurements in patients with peripheral vascular disease can often yield a large amount of information regarding the location and severity of occlusive lesions. Unfortunately, many of these modalities are either altered by the diabetic process or simply cannot be performed consistently on the diabetic foot. Ankle-brachial index is an easily measurable way to compare the systolic pressure of the upper extremity with that of the affected lower extremity. Using a Doppler probe and a blood pressure cuff, the systolic pressure in the pedal arteries (dorsalis pedis or posterior tibial) is taken. The higher of these two measurements is compared with a similarly taken brachial artery systolic pressure. (Again, the highest brachial pressure is used.) A ratio (ankle/brachial) of less than 1 is considered a sign of impaired flow to the extremity. Because of the arterial wall medial calcification that occurs in diabetics, the arteries are often less compressible than similar arteries at the same pressure. As a result, this measurement is often falsely elevated and unreliable (Fig. 5). In some diabetics, this process is so severe that the cuff pressure cannot occlude the arteries, which are termed noncompressible. For this reason this measurement can have limited clinical applicability in diabetic patients.

The technique of measuring segmental pressures from the high thigh down to the foot is a popular method for assessing the location of occlusive lesions. The test is performed by placing a series of pressure cuffs at various levels along the affected extremity. The systolic pressure measurements at each level are an indication of the amount of tissue perfusion at that level. A drop in the pressure from one level to the next is predictive of an occlusive lesion within the arterial system between those two levels (Figs. 4 and 5). Unfortunately, this measurement is also affected by the arterial wall calcification in diabetics and as a result is often not reliable in this population.

Pulse volume recordings (PVR) assess the flow characteristics within the arterial system. A series of air plethysmography cuffs is placed at different levels of the extremity in question. These cuffs detect the small change in diameter of the leg during systole and diastole. This change with each heartbeat is recorded as a waveform (Figs. 4 and 5). A progression from a triphasic to a monphasic or dampened waveform would be indicative of occlusive disease. The advantage of this method is the fact that it is not hampered by arterial wall calcification (Fig. 4). Although this technique does give some information, it is mostly a qualitative rather than quantitative examination and is difficult to use as an absolute or objective determinent of disease severity.

Transcutaneous oxygen measurements have also been used to evaluate the amount of tissue perfusion in patients with vascular disease. This method had been used to predict the healing potential of a diseased extremity, i.e., to determine whether the patient

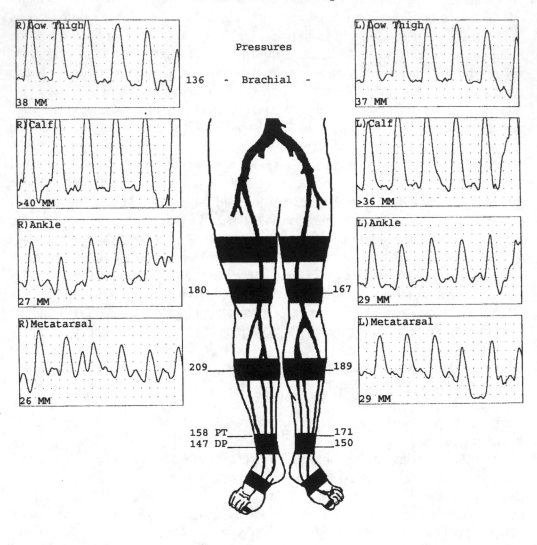

Fig. 4. Example of a pulse-volume recording (PVR) data sheet. Included are the segmental pressures (alongside the diagram) and the ankle/brachial indices (ABIs; bottom of diagram). Patient is diabetic and was noted to have elevated segmental pressures (the absolute pressure increases distally) and elevated ABIs. (Both ABIs are greater than 1.) Because medial wall calcification often causes elevation of these two measurements, PVRs are utilized to assess the presence or absence of true occlusive disease. Note that the amplitude of the waveforms is maintained from the thigh to the metatarsal level. This indicates that this patient does not have significant vascular occlusive disease.

would be able to heal a wound that either exists or would be created by performing a surgical procedure. The test is performed by placing a probe over the metatarsal region of the affected foot. After equilibrating to a specific temperature, the oxygen level is determined. Enthusiasm for this measurement has been hampered by the large degree of variability noted in the measurements. Many different factors, including the site of

Pulse Volume Recording

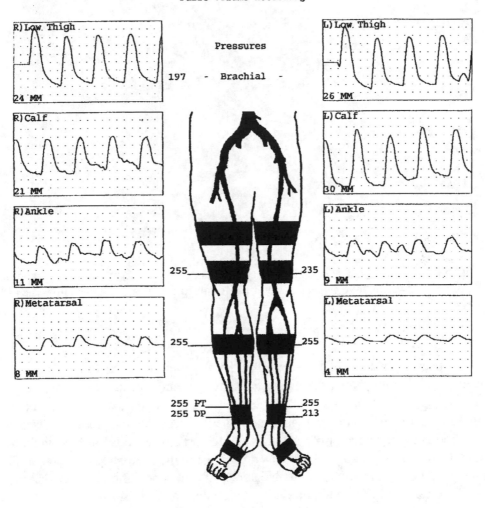

Fig. 5. PVR recording also taken from a diabetic patient. As in Fig. 6, the patient is noted to have elevated segmental pressures and ankle/brachial indices. The difference is that this patient clearly has dampening of the waveforms on both extremities beginning at the level of the ankle. This decrease in amplitude of the tracing suggests that an occlusive vascular lesion exists between the level of the calf and ankle. As you can see, the results of this test are merely qualitative and do not provide an objective quantification of the extent of vascular disease present.

measurement and the temperature, affect the oxygen reading, but in a review of multiple factors, no one factor could account for the variability *(6)*. Another review noted that the $TcPO_2$ was lower in diabetics than nondiabetics when comparing groups with similar disease severity *(7)*. Although there is some literature supporting the use of $TcPO_2$ in the evaluation of the diabetic foot *(8)*, results are difficult to interpret. This has lead to a gray zone of values without a significantly predictive value. The continued evaluation of this modality may lead to a better understanding of its importance.

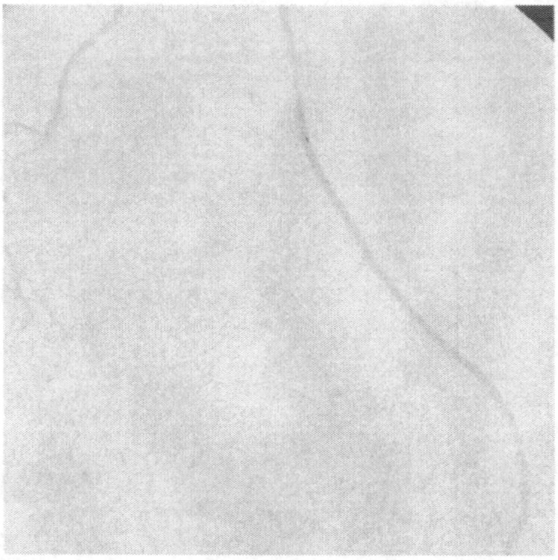

Fig. 6. The same patient as in Fig. 3 viewed here using digital subtraction angiography. This technology allows improved visualization of difficult to see arteries, especially when blood flow is diminished.

As it became increasingly evident that the vasculature of the foot was spared the changes noted in the more proximal vessels, measurement of digital toe pressures was initiated. Subsequent study has confirmed that toe pressures are not hampered by the coexistence of diabetes. In fact, Vincent et al. *(9)* showed that toe pressure was an accurate hemodynamic indicator of total peripheral arterial obstructive disease in diabetics. Although this methodology can be a useful adjunct in the evaluation of vascular disease in the diabetic foot, its use is often obviated by the presence of ulceration, gangrene or amputation of the toe, and unfamiliarity with its use at some hospitals.

The gold standard in the evaluation of diabetic patients with peripheral vascular disease is digital subtraction angiography. The results of conventional angiography have been greatly enhanced with the advent of this technique (Figs. 3 and 6). This technology, by subtracting the bone and soft tissue to visualize the contrast column better, allows the radiographer to follow the contrast bolus over a greater period and select the optimal images, which has resulted in greater visualization of the distal and pedal vessels. The most important point for a radiographer to understand, especially in diabetics, is that even in the presence of tibial vessel occlusion, priority must be given to visualizing the pedal anatomy. Angiograms are often terminated prematurely in these situations with the misconception that tibial occlusion represents unreconstructable disease. Two views (anteroposterior and lateral) of the foot should be obtained, and care should be taken to avoid excessive plantar flexion of the foot during the exam (as this may impede flow to the dorsalis pedis artery) (Fig. 7). The prevailing concern with the use of angiography has to do with the risk of renal failure in diabetic patients with preexisting renal insufficiency. The most important factor in the prevention of renal failure in these patients has been the use of hydration prior to obtaining the angiogram *(10)*. When renal failure does occur, it is almost always reversible *(11)*, but it may delay the arterial reconstructive surgery for several days before the creatinine returns to baseline.

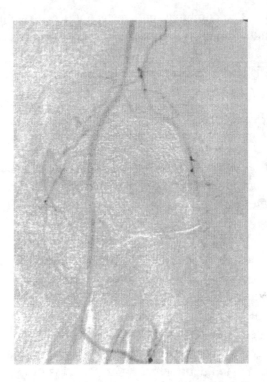

Fig. 7. Anteroposterior view of the foot of the patient seen in Figures 3 and 6. The widely patent dorsalis pedis artery is well visualized and can be seen feeding the pedal arch. It is mandatory to obtain lateral and anteroposterior angiograms of the foot when evaluating the pedal vasculature.

MRA and spiral CTA have been investigated as alternatives to conventional angiography. MRA with two-dimensional time of flight was used to assess the distal lower extremity vasculature in diabetics in comparison with digital subtraction angiography *(12)*. Although MRA was shown to have acceptable sensitivity and specificity in the evaluation of the tibial vessels, it was not sufficiently capable of identifying patent pedal vessels. The three areas that are prone to error by MRA were 1) the bifurcation of the peroneal artery; 2) the plantar arch; and 3) retrograde flow into the lateral plantar artery. These shortcomings are especially significant in the diabetic population, in whom the pedal vessels are often a target for revascularization. The role of CTA in the evaluation of peripheral vascular disease has also been investigated. Some reviews *(13)* have reported an accuracy of 95%. Reading of CTA is inaccurate in instances of overlapping leg veins and in the setting of vessel wall calcification. It is also limited by the amount of contrast required to image the length of the distal aorta to the foot. For this reason, studies evaluating CTA have not included the pedal vessels in their evaluation, and to do so would likely require prohibitively high contrast levels. The combination of inaccuracy with calcification and the inability to visualize the pedal vessels makes CTA an ineffective means of evaluating vascular disease in the diabetic.

Noninvasive diagnostic tests are quite useful in the evaluation of nondiabetic patients with peripheral vascular disease. Unfortunately, these tests are easy to misinterpret in patients with diabetes. The combination of peripheral neuropathy and medial arterial wall calcification limits the ability to diagnose and predict accurately the location or severity of occlusive disease. Because the traditional approach to the workup of peripheral vascular disease is not adequate in the diabetic patient, a separate algorithm in the management of these patients is required.

TREATMENT PROTOCOL

The approach to the diabetic with signs and symptoms of vascular occlusive disease is separate from that in the nondiabetic population. Patients being evaluated with diabetic foot complications should be considered at high risk for both the development and progression of atherosclerotic occlusive disease. In lieu of the previously discussed shortcomings of noninvasive testing, we place emphasis on the presence or absence of pedal pulses. As a general rule, a patient with a diabetic foot ulcer and nonpalpable pulses is considered to have a significant component of ischemia. If the ulcer does not heal with conservative measures, or if bone, joint, or tendon is involved, digital subtraction arteriography should be performed.

The management of a patient presenting with an ischemic diabetic foot should be approached in a premeditated and stepwise fashion. The initial priority is the prompt and thorough drainage of any infected or necrotic tissue. This can be accomplished either by simple incision and debridement of an abscess or by more extensive procedures. The goal of these procedures, whether extensive soft tissue debridement or partial amputation, is the complete eradication of an ongoing site of sepsis. This can often require multiple daily trips to the operating suite to ensure adequate results. Again, one must keep in mind that the signs of continued infection in diabetics are often blunted and their diagnosis requires a high level of suspicion. The next step in the treatment of the diabetic foot is the evaluation of the level of ischemia. This step should not be delayed and can be pursued even in the presence of active infection. As was previously mentioned, the absence of pedal pulses is a good predictor of the need for angiography, especially in the setting of tissue loss, poor healing, or gangrene. Once angiography is complete, planning for revascularization is undertaken. Even in the face of tibial and peroneal occlusion, the pedal vessels should be evaluated for patency. The fundamental goal of any revascularization in the diabetic foot should be restoration of pulsatile blood flow to the foot. Bypass surgery should preferentially be to those arteries with direct runoff into the foot (anterior and posterior tibial arteries); however, results of bypass to the peroneal artery are also excellent. Once revascularization has been accomplished, attention can then again be turned to the repair of the initial foot lesion. Secondary revisions or closure may be required and may be carried out as a separate procedure.

The care and management of the diabetic patient presenting with the sequelae of peripheral vascular disease is a complex undertaking. A thorough knowledge of the pathobiology associated with this disease is essential. All aspects of the care of these patients, from presentation to diagnosis to treatment, must be approached differently than in nondiabetics. As the evolution of our understanding of this disease process has evolved, so has our ability to affect improvement in outcome. Patients presenting with diabetic foot complications exacerbated by atherosclerotic occlusive disease are now treated very aggressively. This approach has led to improved results and an optimistic prognosis in the diabetic population.

REFERENCES

1. Armstrong DG, Lavery LA. Diabetic foot ulcers: prevention, diagnosis and classification. *Am Fam Physician* 1998;57:1325–1332.
2. Goldenberg SG, Alex M, Joshi RA, et al. Nonatheromatous peripheral vascular disease of the lower extremity in diabetes mellitus. *Diabetes* 1959;8:261–273.
3. Strandness DE, Priest RE, Gibbons GE. Combined clinical and pathologic study of diabetic and nondiabetic peripheral arterial disease. *Diabetes* 1964;13:366–372.
4. Conrad MC. Large and small artery occlusion in diabetics and nondiabetics with severe vascular disease. *Circulation* 1967;36:83–91.
5. Barner HB, Kaiser GC, Willman VL. Blood flow in the diabetic leg. *Circulation* 1971;43: 391–394.
6. Boyko EJ, Afroni JF. Predictors of transcutaneous oxygen tension in the lower limbs of diabetic subjects. *Diabet Med* 1996;13:549–554.
7. Rooke TW, Osmundson PJ. The influence of age, sex, smoking, and diabetes on lower limb transcutaneous oxygen tension in patients with arterial occlusive disease. *Arch Intern Med* 1990;150:129–132.
8. Ballard JL, Ede CC, Bunt TJ, Killeen JD. A prospective evaluation of transcutaneous oxygen measurements in the management of diabetic foot problems. *J Vasc Surg* 1995;22: 485–490.
9. Vincent DG, Salles-Cunha SX, Bernhard VM, Towne JB. Noninvasive assessment of toe systolic pressures with special reference to diabetes mellitus. *J Cardiovasc Surg* 1983;24: 22–28.
10. Solomon R, Werner C, Mann D, D'Elia J, Silva P. Effects of saline, mannitol, and furosemide on acute decreases in renal function by radiocontrast agents. *N Engl J Med* 1994; 331:1416–1420.
11. Parfrey PS, Griffiths SM, Barret BJ, et al. Contrast material-induced renal failure in patients with diabetes mellitus, renal insufficiency, or both: a prospective controlled study. *N Engl J Med* 1989;320:143.
12. McDermott VG, Meakem TJ, Carpenter JP, et al. Magnetic resonance angiography of the distal lower extremity. *Clin Radiol* 1995;50:747–746.
13. Lawrence JA, Kim D, Kent KC, Stehling MK, Rosen MP, Raptopoulos V. Lower extremity spiral CT angiography versus catheter angiography. *Radiology* 1995;194:903–908.

7

Foot Pressure Abnormalities in the Diabetic Foot

Thomas E. Lyons, DPM, Jeremy Rich, DPM, and Aristidis Veves, MD, DSc

INTRODUCTION

For over 50 years, foot pressure measurements have been used to evaluate many medical conditions. Early techniques to assess plantar foot pressure were simple, innovative methods that provided investigators with semiquantitative data. The introduction of the optical pedobarograph significantly improved the accuracy of foot pressure measurements. Furthermore, computer technologies have allowed accurate and reproducible measurements that can be used not only for research purposes, but also for treating patients with diabetes mellitus.

Foot pressure measurements and plantar ulceration have been extensively researched in the insensate foot (1–19). In Western societies, the principal cause of the insensate foot is diabetes mellitus; in other regions of the world, leprosy remains an important contributing factor (19). In fact, the study of patients with Hansen's disease has allowed an understanding of the pathophysiology of the insensate foot and its principles of treatment (19). Moreover, foot pressure measurements can be clinically valuable in other settings such as rheumatoid arthritis, hallux valgus, and sports medicine.

METHODS OF MEASURING FOOT PRESSURES

Out-of-Shoe Methods

One of the earliest studies to examine foot pressures was that of Beely in 1882 (20). Subjects ambulated over a cloth sack filled with plaster of Paris to produce a footprint. Beely postulated that the plaster would capture the plantar aspect of the foot with the highest load, representing the deepest impression. However, this technique was limited because it principally measured the total force rather than the dynamic pressures underneath the foot during gait. Moreover, this method was strictly qualitative and therefore susceptible to both inter- and intraobserver unreliability.

In 1930, Morton (21) described a ridged, deformable rubber pad, termed the *kinetograph*. This pad made contact with an inked paper placed underneath the foot while the subject ambulated over the pad. The kinetograph examined the relationship between static and rigid foot deformity and was the first documented attempt to measure foot pressures rather than forces. Elftman (22) further developed a system that allowed the observation of dynamic changes in pressure distribution as the subject ambulated. This

From: *The Diabetic Foot: Medical and Surgical Management*
Edited by: A. Veves, J. M. Giurini, and F. W. LoGerfo © Humana Press Inc., Totowa, NJ

device was called the *barograph* and consisted of a rubber mat that was smooth on top yet studded with pyramidal projections on the bottom. The mat was placed on a glass plate, and as subjects ambulated over the mat, the area of contact of the projections increased according to changes in pressures under the foot. A video camera recorded the deformation pattern of the mat from below as the subject walked on the mat.

Harris-Beath Mat

Similarly, in 1947, Harris and Beath *(23)* used a similar method to study foot problems and related foot pressure changes in a large group of Canadian soldiers. Their device used a multilayered inked rubber mat that allowed contact with a piece of paper below. When pressure was applied to the mat from ambulation, the ink escaped from it, thereby staining the paper. Thus, the density of the inked impression was dependent on the applied pressure. By using this technique, Barrett and Mooney *(24)* found high loading under the feet of diabetic subjects. The major problem with this device, however, is that it saturates at a level within the normal limits of foot pressures. Furthermore, the amount of ink placed onto the mat cannot be standardized. Silvino and associates *(25)*, however, calibrated the Harris-Beath mat by using a contact area of known size and weight, thereby producing both qualitative and semiquantitative data.

Podotrack

A similar device to the Harris-Beath mat is the Podotrack system (Medical Gait Technology, The Netherlands) *(26–28)*. This system is based on the principles of the Harris-Beath mat. However, the footprint impression is produced by a chemical reaction with carbon paper instead of ink. The Podotrack system has a few advantages over the Harris-Beath mat. For example, there is a standard ink layer that is carbon paper. Furthermore, the system can be calibrated with a scale representing shades of colors corresponding to foot pressures. In 1994, a study reported that the Podotrack system provided reproducible results in 61% of the foot pressure values when compared with those obtained from the pedobarograph *(29)*. Furthermore, the Podotrack and pedo-baraograph systems were comparatively examined. By placing the Podotrack system on top of the pedobarograph, one could obtain real-time data as subjects ambulated over both systems.

In 1974, Arcan and Brull *(30)* described a system that had the capability of providing more detailed, albeit semiquantitative, information regarding foot pressure distribution. The apparatus consisted of a rigid transparent platform with optical filters. An optically sensitive elastic material and reflective layer were combined together. Foot pressure measurements were performed either statically or dynamically, and the changes in motion of the foot were recorded using a video camera.

An earlier quantitative technique to measure foot pressures was described by Hutton and Drabble in 1972 *(31)*. Their device consisted of a force plate in which 12 beams were suspended from two load cells. These load cells were attached to several sets of wired strain gauges that permitted the measurement of longitudinal tension. The apparatus was placed onto the walkway because subjects could step on and off the plate during their gait cycle. By using this technique, Stott and colleagues *(32)* scrutinized the load distribution in subjects with and without pes planus (flatfeet) and hallux valgus deformities. The distribution of peak loads was expressed as a percentage of body weight, and the results demonstrated that the load of the control subjects was low in the midfoot and high in the forefoot. However, there was considerable variation in loads across the ball of the foot. Conversely, in subjects with pes planus, an increased load was appreciated. In addition, their study reported that subjects who had greater body weight tended to have higher peak loads on the lateral aspect of the foot.

In a later study by Stokes and associates *(18)*, foot pressures, body weight, and foot ulceration in diabetic patients were examined. Their study was remarkable in that it demonstrated that foot ulcers occurred at sites of maximal load. Furthermore, increased loads in patients with foot ulceration were related to their body weight when they were compared to healthy controls and diabetic patients without ulcerations.

Subsequently, Ctercteko and colleagues *(17)* developed a computer system that measured vertical foot pressures of the sole on the foot in diabetic patients with and without ulceration and in subjects during ambulation. The system consisted of a load-sensitive device divided into 128 strain gauge load cells with a 15×15-mm surface area that was built into a 8-m walkway. The foot was divided into eight areas, and the output from each load cell was processed and transmitted into a microcomputer. An evaluation of the data provided quantitative values for the sites of peak force and pressure under the foot and duration of contact time. It was demonstrated that in both groups of diabetic subjects, with and without ulceration, a similar pattern of reduced toe loading was noted when compared with control subjects. This resulted in a higher loading at the metatarsal head region, where the majority of ulcerations were present. These results confirmed that foot ulceration occurred at sites of maximal load under the foot.

Optical Pedobarograph

The optical pedobarograph is a device that measures dynamic plantar pressures. This device is based on an earlier system described by Chodera in 1957. The optical pedobaragraph consists of an elevated walkway with a glass plate that is illuminated along the edge and is covered with a thin sheet of soft plastic *(33)*. The light is then reflected internally within the plate when no pressure is applied. However, when a subject stands or ambulates across the surface, light escapes from the glass at these pressure points and is scattered by the plastic sheet, producing an image of the foot that can be seen from below.

A monochromatic camera detects the image, and the pressure at any given point can be determined automatically by measuring the intensity of that image at that specific point. This system has high spatial resolution and thereby allows an accurate measurement of high foot pressures under small areas of the foot with satisfactory precision. The optical barograph is used widely in the examination of high foot pressures such as in the diabetic foot. Additionally, this system has been used for interventional trials that study the effectiveness of off-loading high pressure areas. However, this system is limited to measurements of barefoot pressures and therefore does not allow the evaluation of in-shoe pressures. Moreover, this system requires substantial space and is not easily portable.

In-Shoe Methods

Over the last two decades, developments in computer technology have enabled microprocessor-like recording devices to measure in-shoe foot pressures. In 1963, Bauman and Brand *(34)* recognized the limitations of barefoot pressure measurements in the insensate and deformed foot. The apparatus they devised was composed of thin, pressure-sensitive transducers that were attached to suspected areas of high pressure underneath the foot. Although this method was expensive and elaborate in design, it proved that in-shoe foot pressures were both feasible and indeed useful. In essence, Bauman and Brand laid the foundation for the design of less expensive devices to become available for general use.

Electrodynogram

The aforementioned principles were used in the mid-1970s to develop the electrodynogram system (EDG System, Langer Biomechanics Group, Deer Park, NY). Although not commercially available, it is currently used in both clinical and research settings *(35,36)*. This apparatus is a computer-assisted system that uses seven small, separate sensors that adhere to the plantar aspect of the foot. They are attached by cable and relay information into a computer pack carried by the subject. In-shoe and out-of-shoe walking pressures can be evaluated. However, the system is limited because only peak pressures can be measured where the sensors are placed. Hence, this system cannot provide pressure information pertaining to the entire plantar aspect of the foot.

EMED System

The EMED system is another computer-assisted and image-generating device that can record both in-shoe and out-of-shoe dynamic foot pressures. Its design is continually updated regularly and permits the examination of the entire plantar aspect of the foot. The system consists of a mat based on the principle that a change in the presure on a wire causes a similar change on its electrical capacitance, thereby allowing foot pressures to be measured by recording electrical flow though the mat. The device incorporates a sensor area 445×225 mm that has a resolution of 5 mm^2 and can provide measurements with satisfactory reliability. This system has wide clinical appeal and has been used to scrutinize the asymmetry of plantar pressure distribution in young adults with ankle fractures and diabetic patients with foot ulcerations or Charcot neuroarthropathy *(37)*.

FSCAN System

At the authors' unit, much study has been conducted using the FSCAN system. This system is a high-resolution, computerized gait analysis program that was designed according to the principles described previously *(38,39)*. The hardware system collects both static and dynamic plantar pressure data by using either the mat or sensor. The mat measures foot pressures as the subject freely ambulates over the mat without sensor cables that may potentially influence an individual's gait pattern (Figs. 1A,B).

The FSCAN system uses a sensor that is ultrathin (0.007 inch/0.15 mm) and flexible. It consists of 960 sensing locations that are distributed uniformly across the entire plantar surface *(39,40)*. These sensing locations provide the spatial resolution required for detecting differential pressures exerted over relatively small areas. This unique sensor can be trimmed to any size and inserted into the subjects' footwear. The sensor does not interfere with the subject's gait or reduce the true pressures by accommodating to existing deformities (Fig. 1C).

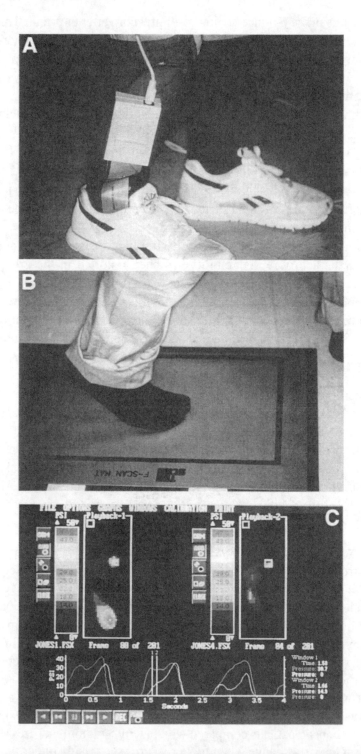

Fig. 1. (**A**) A subject walking with the FSCAN sensor inserted in his shoes. Changes in the electrical capacitance, which are related to the applied pressures on the sensors during walking, are transmitted via the cable to an IBM-compatible computer, where they are analyzed using the FSCAN software. (**B**) The FSCAN mat, which is based on the same principles used to design the FSCAN sensors, can be used to measure pressures of bare feet. The mat is compatible and is connected to the same apparatus used for in-shoe measurements. (**C**) Computer-assisted analysis of a foot step. The highest foot pressures in this subject are seen underneath the heel and the first metatarsal area. (From ref. *12*.)

The sensor plugs into a 6-ounce analog-to-digital converter cuff unit. This is attached to one or both of the subject's legs. A cable connects the cuff unit to the receiver card placed in the computer. For clinical use, the calibration method entails applying a known load, which is commonly the subject's weight, over the sensing cells. By using the prescribed calibration method, an accuracy of ±10% may be obtained.

For research use, the scanner system uses an additional calibration technique called *equilibration*. Equilibration assigns a unique calibration curve to each sensing cell. It is used to increase the uniformity of sensing cells within a given sensor. Therefore, this dampens the effect of cell-to-cell variation without reducing the spatial resolution. If these additional calibration techniques are followed, the accuracy of the pressure measurement system is within 5%. The system has been upgraded to include a sensor mat that can measure out-of-shoe foot pressures.

This system is advantageous because of its simplicity, easy storage, and reproducibility of data. Satisfactory reproducibility has been reported in the great majority of studies that have used this system. No significant differences in peak pressure were found in eight neuropathic diabetic patients who had foot pressures measured three times over a short duration, whereas in another study, the coefficient of variation in healthy subjects was 7.8% among separate studies and 2.6% among different steps during the same study *(40,58)*.

The FSCAN system, however, has potential limitations. For example, the FSCAN mat system has decreased resolution compared with the in-shoe technique. Furthermore, because the sensor is very thin, the mat may fail from wrinkling and breakage and thereby yield inaccurate data *(38)*. Rose and colleagues *(38)* found that two insole sensors gave different results when used on the same subject. Additionally, there was a decline in sensitivity if the sensor was used 12 times. Altering the shoe insole can also affect foot pressure measurement.

NATURAL HISTORY OF FOOT PRESSURE ABNORMALITIES IN DIABETES MELLITUS

Foot pressure measurements in diabetic patients have been attempted for over 30 years. Stokes et al. *(18)* used a segmental force platform to study 37 feet of 22 diabetic patients. High loads were found at the sites of ulcers. Patients with high loads under the feet were also heavier in weight than those with lower loads. Toe loads in patients with ulcers were found to be reduced. A shift of maximum loads to the lateral foot in neuropathic patients was also reported. In a subsequent study, Ctercteko and colleagues *(17)* confirmed all these findings, except for the lateral shift of maximum loads. Conversely, a medial shift was discovered in their study. In another study, neither a medial nor a lateral shift was found. However, peak pressures under the heel occurred with a lower frequency in all diabetic patients compared with patients without diabetes *(9)*. This finding may suggest an early change when foot pressures start rising under the forefoot but still remain within normal limits, as in patients without neuropathy.

In previous studies, we have shown that in diabetic neuropathic patients, there is a transfer of high pressures from the heel and the toes to the metatarsal head *(9)*. The main reasons for this transfer are neuropathy and limited joint mobility *(8,9)*. Neuropathy leads to atrophy of the intrinsic musculature of the foot and clawing of the toes, which may cause prominent metatarsal heads under which high pressures occur. Moreover, a transfer of peak pressures from the rearfoot to the metatarsal heads was noted in patients with diabetic neuropathy *(13)*. This further indicates the inability of the neuropathic foot to distribute foot pressure and avoid the development of high foot pressures. Additionally, limited joint mobility impairs the ability of the foot to absorb and redistribute the forces related to impact on the ground while walking. Consequently, this contributes to the development of high foot pressures and subsequent ulceration *(9,14)*.

FOOT PRESSURES AND FOOT ULCERATION

Foot ulceration is a significant cause of morbidity in patients with diabetes mellitus and can lead to prolonged lengths of hospital stay. Numerous risk factors for foot ulceration in diabetes have been ascertained. Among others, limited joint mobility, peripheral neuropathy, vascular disease, and high plantar pressures have been implicated as significant predisposing factors leading to ulceration in population-based and clinical studies seeking to quantify such relationships.

Boulton and associates *(5)* were the first group to employ the optical pedobaragraph for research purposes to examine the relationship between high foot pressures and ulceration. In their study, diabetic patients with and without neuropathy and individuals without diabetes were examined to evaluate the relationships among foot pressures, neuropathy, and foot ulceration. Their results demonstrated that a significantly larger number of patients with diabetic neuropathy had abnormally high foot pressures compared with controls. Furthermore, patients with a previous history of foot ulceration had high pressures at ulcerative sites. Because ulceration occurred at sites of high plantar foot pressures, foot pressure reduction, therefore, should lead to a reduced incidence of foot ulceration in neuropathic diabetic patients.

In a subsequent study performed by the same group, sorbothane shoe inserts were employed in an attempt to evaluate pressure reduction in diabetic patients *(41)*. Abnormally high foot pressures were measured in 33% of feet without insoles and in 6% of feet when using the insoles, thereby indicating that special accommodative insoles may help reduce plantar foot pressures in diabetic neuropathic patients.

In a prospective study that lasted 3 years and included diabetic patients with longstanding diabetes and neuropathy, Kelly and Coventry *(42)* also examined the long-term changes in plantar foot pressure. Their results demonstrated that important alterations of foot pressure distribution had occurred in a significant number of these subjects, some of whom had developed recurrent ulcerations at these sites of high pressure. Moreover, it was again confirmed that patients with neuropathy and the characteristic intrinsic-minus foot had abnormally high pressures measured at the metatarsal heads *(15)*.

Definite proof that abnormally high foot pressures in diabetic patients were related to the development of plantar foot ulceration can be derived from a pivotal prospective study that followed a large number of patients for a mean period of 30 months *(15)*. During this study, plantar ulcers developed in 17% of all feet and in 45% of feet with diabetic neuropathy. All these ulcerations occurred in patients with high foot pressures at baseline, thereby suggesting that high foot pressures, especially in neuropathic patients, are highly predictive for the development of foot ulceration and may be useful for identifying at-risk patients (Fig. 2).

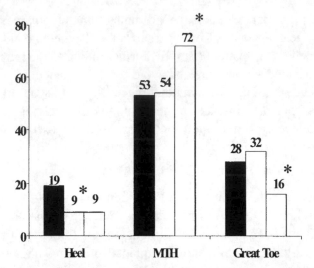

Fig. 2. Histogram demonstrating the distribution of peak pressures under the foot of healthy subjects (black columns), diabetic nonneuropathic patients (gray columns), and neuropathic diabetic patients (white columns). Peak pressures were more often under the metatarsal heads (MTH) of the neuropathic patients and less often under the heel and great toe. It is also of interest that peak pressures under the heel were less frequent in the nonneuropathic patients *, $p < 0.05$. (From ref. *15*.)

Given the correlation between foot pressures and foot ulceration, a study to evaluate the role between joint mobility and racial affinity in the development of high foot pressures was performed. This study demonstrated that black subjects without diabetes and patients with diabetes have increased joint mobility compared with Caucasian healthy subjects and patients with diabetes (*16*). An increase in joint mobility results in lower peak plantar pressures and therefore a lower risk of foot ulceration.

Similarly, the role of neuropathy and high foot pressures in diabetic foot ulceration was evaluated (*43*). In a cross-sectional multicenter study, the magnitude of association of several different risk factors for foot ulceration in patients with diabetes was determined. A cross-sectional group of 251 subjects consisting of Caucasian, black, and Hispanic races were studied. There was an equal distribution of men and women across the entire the study population. All patients underwent a complete medical history and lower extremity evaluation for neuropathy and foot pressures. Neuropathic factors were dichotomized (0/1) into two high-risk variables: patients with a vibration perception threshold (VPT) ≥25 V were categorized as HiVPT ($n = 132$) and those with Semmes-Weinstein monofilament tests ≥5.07 were classified as HiSWF ($n = 190$). The mean dynamic foot pressures of three footsteps were measured using the FSCAN mat system with patients walking in stockings but without shoewear. Maximum plantar pressures were dichotomized into a high-pressure variable (P_{max6}) indicating those subjects with pressures ≥6 kg/cm^2 ($n = 96$). The total of 99 patients had a current or prior history of ulceration at baseline.

The sensor was used in a floor mat system designed to measure barefoot or stocking-foot dynamic pressures. Maximum peak pressures for the entire foot were obtained without regard for specific location by averaging those obtained for three midgait footsteps and were then dichotomized into a high-pressure variable indicating those subjects with pressures ≥ 6 kg/cm^2.

With a specific focus on plantar foot pressures, joint mobility, and neuropathic parameters consistent with ulceration, this study demonstrated that patients with foot pressures ≥ 6 kg/cm^2 were twice as likely to have ulcerations than those without high pressures, even after adjustment for age, gender, diabetes duration, and racial affinity. In the black and Hispanic groups, significantly lower plantar pressures were demonstrated compared with the Caucasian group. High plantar pressures were relatively infrequent and were not found to be significant predictors of ulceration. Foot pressures ≥ 6 kg/cm^2 were independently associated with ulceration, but to a lesser extent than the neuropathy variables (Tables 1 and 2).

This study demonstrated that the association of high foot pressures, high vibration pressure threshold, and insensitivity to a 5.07 monofilament contributed to the development of foot ulceration. Furthermore, their group demonstrated significant racial differences in joint mobility, associated foot pressures, and the prevalence of ulceration among Caucasian, black, and Hispanic patients. These findings have guided efforts at detecting diabetic patients at risk of ulceration by incorporating such parameters into screening programs. Foot pressures should be evaluated to detect those neuropathic individuals at risk of ulceration from excessive callous formation or repetitive stress *(9,10)*. Although the two measures of neuropathy have the greater magnitude of effect, foot pressures should still be evaluated to detect those neuropathic individuals at risk of ulceration from excessive plantar callous formation or repetitive stress.

THE ROLE OF FOOT PRESSURES
AS A SCREENING METHOD TO IDENTIFY AT-RISK PATIENTS

Because diabetic foot ulceration is a preventable long-term complication of diabetes mellitus, screening techniques to identify the at-risk patient are probably the most important step in reducing the rate of foot ulceration and lower limb amputation. To this end, various screening techniques have been proposed and are currently in use. These include the evaluation of VPT, foot pressure measurements, joint mobility, and 5.07 SWF testing. Furthermore, a history of previous foot ulceration, TcPO$_2$ level of <30 mmHg and the existence of foot deformities have been shown to be risk factors for the development of diabetic foot ulceration. In our unit, a study evaluated plantar pressures and screening techniques to identify people at high risk for diabetic foot ulceration *(44)*. The objective of this study was to compare the specificity, sensitivity, and prospective predictive value of the most commonly used screening techniques for the identification of high risk for foot ulceration in a prospective multicenter fashion. Furthermore, this study aimed to identify as many risk factors as possible and to develop a screening strategy that, by combining the detection of two or more risk factors, would provide the best tool for identifying the at-risk patient.

Two hundred forty eight patients from three large diabetic foot centers including our own unit were evaluated in a prospective study. Neuropathy symptom score, neuropathy disability score (NDS), VPT, SWF, joint mobility, peak plantar foot pressures, and vascular status were evaluated in each of the subjects. Patients were followed up every

Table 1
Logistic Regression Results for Risk of Ulceration

	OR	95% CI	p value
Univariate results			
Age[a]	1.02	1.00–1.03	0.019
Sex[b]	0.26	0.18–0.38	0.000
BMI	0.97	0.94–0.99	0.048
Diabetes duration[a]	1.04	1.02–1.06	0.000
Pulses	0.31	0.18–0.52	0.000
P_{max6}	3.9	2.6–5.7	0.000
HiVPT	11.77	7.4–18.4	0.000
HiSWF	9.6	5.02–18.5	0.000
HiRisk	7.4	4.8–11.6	0.000
Multivariate results[d]			
P_{max6}	2.1	1.32–3.39	0.002
HiVPT	4.4	2.58–7.54	0.000
HiSWF	4.1	1.89–8.87	0.000
HiRisk[c]	4.1	2.48–6.63	0.000

BMI, body mass index; VPT, vibration perception threshold; SWF, Semmes-Weinstein monofilament test; P_{max6}, pressure $\geq$6 kg/cm^2.

[a]Indicates OR per year of increase.

[b]Indicates reduced risk of ulceration in females relative to males.

[c]Indicates multivariate OR for interaction term without other neuropathic or pressure variables in model.

[d]Controlling for age, sex, duration, and race.

6 months for a mean period of 30 months, and all new foot ulcers were recorded. The sensitivity, specificity, and positive predictive value of each risk factor were evaluated.

Foot ulcers developed in 73 patients during the study. Patients who developed foot ulcers were more frequently men, had diabetes for a longer duration, and had an inability to detect a 5.07 monofilament. NDS alone had the best sensitivity, whereas the combination of the NDS and the inability to detect a 5.07 monofilament reached a sensitivity of 99%. However, foot pressures had the best specificity, and the best combination was that of NDS and foot pressures.

This study prospectively evaluated the association of several risk factors for foot ulceration. The results demonstrated that a high NDS obtained during a simple stratified clinical examination provided the best sensitivity in identifying patients at risk for foot ulceration, whereas high VPT, the inability to feel a 5.07 SWF, and high foot pressures were independent risk factors. Furthermore, the combination of NDS and a 5.07 (10-g) SWF could identify all but 1 of the 95 ulcerated feet. The use of these two simple methods in clinical practice can assist in identifying the at-risk patient, which is the first step in the prevention of foot ulceration. Hence, foot pressure measurements offered a substantially higher specificity and may be used as a valuable postscreening test in conjunction with providing appropriate footwear.

Although several studies exist evaluating whole foot pressures, there is a paucity of research examining forefoot and rearfoot plantar pressures. In our unit, we measured

Table 2
Multivariate Logistic Regression for Ulceration
by Race, Controlling for Age, Sex, and Diabetes Duration

	OR	95% CI	p value
Caucasian			
P_{max6}	7.7	2.07–28.4	0.002
HiVPT	7.4	2.4–22.9	0.001
HiSWF	3.7	1.3–10.3	0.013
Black			
P_{max6}	0.53	0.05–5.8	0.608
HiVPT	7.2	1.2–43.7	0.032
HiSWF	19.8	1.1–344.2	0.041
Hispanic			
P_{max6}	2.1	0.38–11.5	0.395
HiVPT	6.6	2.3–18.5	0.000
HiSWF[a]	—	—	—

[a]Dropped owing to perfect prediction of outcome.
For abbreviations, *see* Table 1 footnote.

forefoot and rearfoot pressures separately and examined their validity in predicting foot ulceration *(13)*. Ninety patients with diabetes mellitus were examined, and peak pressures under the rearfoot and forefoot were evaluated using the FSCAN mat system with subjects ambulating without footwear *(13)*. Significant correlations were found between forefoot peak pressures and age, height, neuropathy disability score, VPT, and force applied on the ground while walking. In contrast, reverse correlations were found between rearfoot peak pressures and measurements of neuropathic severity.

Binary regression analysis demonstrated a higher risk of foot ulceration in patients with high foot pressures. However, no association was found for rearfoot pressure. Thus, peak foot pressure measurements of the forefoot, but not the rearfoot, correlate with neuropathy measurements and can also predict foot ulceration over 36 months. Moreover, forefoot pressure correlated with the severity of diabetic neuropathy and limited joint mobility. It is also of interest that a negative correlation was found between rearfoot and forefoot pressures. This finding confirms that there is a transfer of peak pressures from the rearfoot to the metatarsal heads in diabetic neuropathy. Additionally, it indicates an inability of the neuropathic foot to distribute pressure and avoid the development of high pressures that eventually leads to the production of foot ulceration under these areas. Therefore, measurement of forefoot peak pressures rather than the whole foot may be more useful for identifying at-risk patients *(13)*.

OFF-LOADING THE DIABETIC FOOT:
THE ROLE OF FOOTWEAR

Given the high rate of foot ulceration in at-risk diabetic patients, the need for better preventive methods to off-load the foot cannot be more apparent. The effectiveness of footwear in reducing high plantar pressures has been scrutinized using the optical pedobarograph *(5,45–47)*. Several foot pressure studies have examined hosiery and insole materials in the diabetic at-risk population and in patients with rheumatoid arthritis and neuropathy *(12,15,16,45–47)*. Currently available footwear products are constantly evolving. Thus, the lack of uniform data can make the interpretation of pressure reduction studies challenging in both clinical and research settings.

Hosiery

The use of padded hosiery to reduce foot pressures has been evaluated in the literature *(41,46–48)*. In an initial study, the pressure-relieving capacity of specially designed hosiery with padding at the heel and forefoot was tested *(46)*. A significant reduction in peak plantar pressure, up to 31%, was obtained from diabetic patients who were at risk for ulceration. In a subsequent study, commercially available hosiery, experimental hosiery, and padded socks were evaluated for foot pressure reduction *(47)*. Ten patients who wore experimental padded hosiery for 6 months were tested with an optical pedobarograph. The experimental hosiery continued to provide a significant reduction in forefoot pressures at 3 months and 6 months, although the level of reduction was less than that seen at baseline.

Furthermore, commercial hosiery designed as sportswear was examined and compared with experimental hosiery. Although these socks (medium or high-density padding) provided a substantial pressure reduction versus barefoot, this was not as great as that seen with experimental hosiery *(47)*. Thus, the use of socks designed to reduce pressures on diabetic neuropathic feet may be an effective adjunctive measure for the reduction of foot pressures. While development of fiber technology and padding distribution continues, the currently available high-density socks are perhaps the best choice of hosiery for protection of the insensate foot.

In another study, in-shoe foot pressures of patients with at-risk feet were compared with healthy subject foot pressures without shoes using the FSCAN system *(14)*. Foot pressures were measured under three conditions in each subject. First, subjects were placed directly in the shoes (S) to measure the pressure between the footwear and sock. Second, the sensor was taped directly to the bare foot (B), and the subject ambulated wearing both footwear and socks. Finally, the footwear was removed, and each subject ambulated wearing only socks (H). The total force and peak pressure under each foot was measured for each condition.

The results demonstrated that the diabetic group had greater peak pressures compared with the controls and that in both groups a significant pressure reduction was found when subjects ambulated with footwear *(14)*. The study concluded that footwear can offer a cushioning effect and that this property may be further incorporated to design shoewear that can protect against the development of high foot pressures and foot ulceration (Fig. 3).

Following this study, the authors prospectively examined the effect of using specially padded hosiery in combination with specially fit footwear on providing in-shoe pressure relief *(48)*. Fifty patients at risk for foot ulceration were recruited for the study. All the patients were provided with three pairs of specially padded hosiery and with two pairs of extra-depth footwear or extra-width running shoes. Dynamic foot pressures were measured at baseline with the patients wearing their regular socks alone, regular footwear and socks, the padded socks, and the new footwear and padded socks.

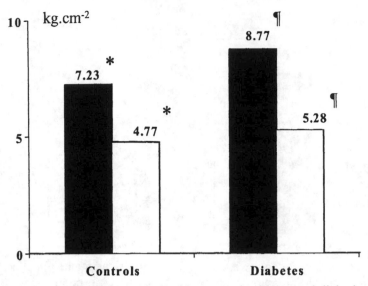

Fig. 3. Foot pressure measurement in healthy control subjects and diabetic patients while wearing either their socks alone (black column) or both shoes and socks (white columns). Foot pressures with socks alone were significantly lower than the ones measured when ambulating with both shoes and socks in both diabetic and healthy subjects *, ¶, $p < 0.02$. (From ref. *14*.)

Foot pressures were measured at baseline and subsequent visits over a period of 30 months (Fig. 4).

An initial pressure relief was provided by the new footwear at baseline compared with the patients' own footwear, yet very few differences in peak forces were found among the baseline, interim, and final visits. Moreover, no significant changes in foot pressures were found over a period of 6 months of continuous usage using specially designed footwear in a group of diabetic patients at risk for foot ulceration. Hence, further prospective studies are required to evaluate the impact of specially designed footwear for reducing foot pressures.

Shoewear

Given the potential of shoes and associated modalities to reduce foot pressures in neuropathic feet and healthy subjects, a discussion of the associated off-loading capabilities is warranted. It is anticipated that the use of modern technology may be helpful in designing shoes and insoles that will redistribute and reduce foot pressures from areas prone to ulceration.

Shoes are an important consideration for patients at risk for ulceration. They provide protection as a covering for the feet and function as a barrier against toxic substances and thermal extremes. Shoes can also function to decrease plantar foot pressures. For example, noncustom footwear worn by healthy nondiabetic subjects decreased foot pressures by 30–35% *(18)*. Moreover, greater foot pressure reductions may be observed in patients with elevated foot pressures wearing shoes compared with walking barefoot.

Healing sandals have been employed to decrease plantar pressures in the diabetic foot *(49)*. These sandals consist of a postoperative shoe with a thick, soft insole that can be further modified by making the sole rigid with a rocker bottom. The rocker sole

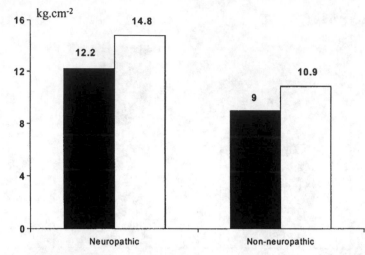

Fig. 4. Changes in the peak foot pressures in neuropathic and nonneuropathic patients over a period of 30 months. The pressures at the end of the study (white columns) were higher compared with the baseline measurements (black columns) in both the neuropathic and nonneuropathic patients. (From ref. *15*.)

is important for the reduction of plantar pressures underneath the forefoot *(2,50)*. The soft sole allows for greater pressure distribution beneath the metatarsal heads while the rocker sole alters the mechanics of the forefoot just prior to toe-off, both of which lead to reduced forefoot pressures *(50)*.

The postoperative shoe is another modality used in the treatment of plantar foot ulcerations. This shoe is used quite frequently because of its availability; it provides the patient with a gait-modifying device. Although it does decrease foot pressures, the postoperative shoe is only minimally effective in the treatment of foot ulcers compared with other modalities *(49)* and is slightly more effective than a canvas shoe *(51)*. Modifications to the sole and insole may further enhance the effectiveness of the postoperative shoe.

Additionally, half-shoes have been used with success for plantar pressure reduction *(49–51)*. These shoes consist of a postoperative shoe with a large wedged heel that extends just behind the forefoot. The forefoot in the postoperative shoe with a heel of this configuration is kept off the ground. Pressure reduction can be as high as 66% compared with pressures in a baseline canvas shoe *(51)*. Because of the configuration of the heel, instability when ambulating can be a problem. This instability is even more significant with neuropathic patients. Therefore, an ambulatory aid such as a cane or crutches may assist with walking.

Not all shoes relieve foot pressures equally; however, employing materials that significantly reduce foot pressures may prevent the recurrence of ulceration in patients with a prior history of ulceration *(51)*. Shoes that provide a cushion effect reduce plantar foot pressures *(49,51)*. Leather oxford shoes may decrease plantar pressures in some areas and yet increase pressures in other regions, particularly underneath the lateral metatarsal heads and great toe *(51)*. Therefore, when purchasing a dress shoe, patients should select a softer sole as opposed to a harder sole, which may not afford as much pressure relief. A dress shoe with a rigid sole can be replaced with a much softer sole

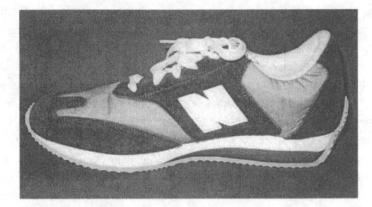

Fig. 5. Running shoes can reduce foot pressures. They are readily available, lightweight, and affordable. The material of the shoe upper is soft and padded on the inside where it interfaces with the foot. A soft sole will reduce foot pressures along with a soft insole that should be removable to allow for frequent replacement.

without dramatically altering the appearance of the shoe. Also, selection of a shoe with a removable insole allows for frequent replacement of worn insoles with a new insole and results in a greater cushioning effect.

Running shoes are an option for patients with elevated foot pressures and at-risk feet *(51–53)* (Fig. 5). Also, running shoes are less expensive than extra-depth and custom footwear. They provide a readily available option for obtaining protective shoewear for patients with a reasonably shaped foot. Moreover, running shoes may provide a more cosmetically acceptable alternative to extra-depth or custom shoes. Significant pressure reduction can be expected with running shoes. Thirty nine subjects were studied to evaluate the pressure-reducing effects of running shoewear *(53)*. Three groups of 13 subjects were categorized as having diabetes with neuropathy, diabetes without neuropathy, and those with neither diabetes nor neuropathy. Foot pressures were evaluated while subjects were wearing thin socks and compared with those of subjects wearing leather oxfords and running shoes. A mean decrease in foot pressures of 31% was noted for all three groups while wearing running shoes compared with wearing the socks alone *(53)*.

In another study, 13 patients with diabetes and neuropathy were evaluated in various types of footwear, including the patient's own leather oxfords and extra-depth and running shoes *(54)*. Running shoes were found to decrease mean plantar foot pressures in comparison with the patient's own leather oxfords by 47% at the second and third metatarsal phalangeal joint (MTPJ), 29% at the first MTPJ, and 32% at the great toe *(54)*. Running shoes are therefore a viable option for patients at risk for ulceration. For patients with significant foot deformities and prominences, other options such as custom footwear must be considered.

Different types of shoes provide various levels of plantar pressure relief. A recent study using a running shoe product found a decrease of between 27 and 38% in plantar pressures compared with a leather oxford product *(55)*. Similarly, another study employing a running shoe demonstrated a reduction of between 29 and 47% in foot pressures compared with leather oxford footwear *(56)*.

Note that athletic shoes may not provide the same pressure relief compared with running shoes. For example, cross-trainer-style footwear may not decrease foot pressures compared with running shoes *(57)*. Foot pressures in 32 diabetic patients with neuropathy and histories of recently healed ulcerations were examined. Foot pressures were measured in a canvas oxford and compared with those using an extra-depth shoe, an SAS comfort shoe, and athletic cross-trainer shoes. Measurements were obtained with the manufacturers' insoles and with a viscoelastic insole for each shoe type. For patients with a history of ulcerations underneath the metatarsal heads, pressure reductions in all three shoe types were relatively similar to those of the canvas shoe *(57)*.

However, for those patients with a history of great toe ulcers, the extra-depth and comfort SAS shoes decreased foot pressures under the great toe, whereas the cross-trainer shoewear actually increased foot pressures in this area compared with the canvas oxfords. One may surmise that foot pressure reductions of running shoes and cross-training shoes may be different, particularly underneath the great toe. Therefore, patient counseling on the selection and purchase of specific footwear is vital, especially in a marketplace where the vast choices of footwear available may easily overwhelm a patient not familiar with athletic shoes.

Extra-depth footwear is another option for the patient with at-risk feet. The extra space in the toe box is particularly useful for patients with forefoot deformities. Extra-depth footwear also decreases foot pressures significantly *(51–53)*. The pressure reduction ability of extra-depth shoewear can be further augmented with the use of specially padded socks, as discussed previously *(54,55)*, and insoles *(55)*. It is the authors' experience that many extra-depth shoes contain a flat insole with minimal cushioning quality. A study evaluating extra-depth shoes demonstrated pressure reductions with the factory insole of 16, 27, 19, and 34% at the great toe, first MTPJ, second MTPJ, third MTPJ, and heel, respectively *(50)*. With a custom accommodative insole, the pressure reductions were increased to 33, 50, 48, and 49%, respectively *(50)*. In a subsequent study, 32 patients with diabetes and a history of ulceration noted a significant reduction in foot pressures using extra-depth shoes compared with a baseline of the patient's own canvas oxford. When the factory-constructed insole was replaced with a commercially available insole, a further pressure reduction of 4–15% was observed. Therefore, pressure reduction using extra-depth shoes can easily be augmented with the use of a readily available insole. The pressure-reducing ability of extra-depth footwear can be further augmented with specially padded socks *(42)*.

In another study, diabetic patients who exercised and those who did not were evaluated to determine what effect aerobic exercise might have on foot pressures with and without shoes *(55)*. When participants ambulated without their shoes, the peak pressures were highest in group DNE (diabetic nonexercisers). Foot pressures were also higher in groups CE (healthy exercisers), CS (healthy nonexercisers), and DE (diabetic exercisers), probably as a result of the increased stress on the foot skin and subsequent callous formation.

However, when foot pressures were measured wearing shoes, a different picture emerged. The foot pressures were highest in groups CS and DS, intermediate in group DNE, and lowest in groups CE and DE (Fig. 6). Those who consistently exercised achieved the highest pressure relief. These differences may reflect the ability of regularly exercising individuals to choose comfortable and good quality shoewear. In sum-

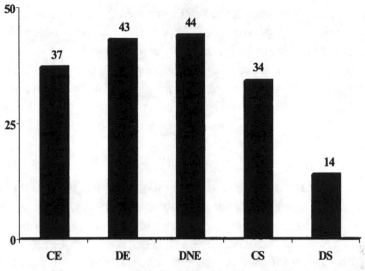

Fig. 6. Percentage of foot pressure relief achieved by the athletic shoes in healthy controls who exercised regularly (CE group), type 1 nonneuropathic diabetic patients who exercised regularly (DE), type 1 diabetic neuropathic patients who exercised regularly (DNE), healthy controls who did not exercise regularly (CS), and diabetic patients who did not exercise regularly (DS). The highest pressure relief was achieved in the first three groups (regularly exercising subjects). These data indicate that proper selection of footwear can result in considerable pressure relief. (From ref. *55.*)

mary, these results indicate that proper selection of footwear can result in considerable pressure relief.

Insoles and Orthotics

Insoles and orthotics are recommended for the prevention of ulcerations in at-risk feet *(56–60)*. The addition of a material to cushion the plantar aspect of the foot can decrease foot pressures significantly *(5)*. By using a 5-mm-thick viscoelastic polymer insole, reduced foot pressures in approximately 50% have been reported *(56)*. In another study, 4-mm-thick viscoelastic insoles were noted to decrease foot pressures from 5 to 20% above what was observed with stock insoles of extra-depth, comfort, and athletic shoes *(33)*.

Custom orthotics of both the soft and rigid variety are used to decrease foot pressures *(56–60)*. Heat-pressed Plastizote insoles decrease foot pressures for diabetic patients by 40–50% *(58)*. Modifications to these insoles by adding arch or metatarsal pads do not increase the pressure reduction significantly *(58)*. However, rigid materials such as polyurethane foot orthoses may reduce plantar pressures by approximately 50% *(59)*. Rigid orthotics composed of graphite materials decrease pressures underneath the first metatarsal head and medial heel by approximately 30–40% *(59,60)*.

The FSCAN system was employed to measure dynamic pressures at the shoe-foot interface during normal walking with different orthotics *(61)*. This study evaluated the efficacy of pressure redistribution with Plastizote, Spenco, cork, and plastic foot orthoses compared with a control (no orthotic). Measurements varied upwards to 18% between sensors, and changes in stance time of up to 5% occurred between the orthotics and the control conditions. These results demonstrated the inherent measurement variances of the FSCAN system using numerous orthoses.

Although these variances hindered reliability among the orthoses, statistically significant differences in peak pressure between the orthotics were noted. Plastizote, cork, and plastic foot orthoses were beneficial for decreasing pressure in the forefoot, heel, and second through fifth metatarsal regions. However, these orthotics had the potential to increase the plantar pressures in the midfoot region. In conclusion, the results demonstrated that using an orthotic to relieve pressures in one region of the shoe-foot interface may increase pressures over another region of the plantar surface *(61)*.

SUMMARY

Several methods of measuring and reducing foot pressures including their advantages and limitations have been discussed. Extra-depth footwear, jogging shoes, hosiery, insoles, and orthoses have been shown to decrease plantar foot pressures. Furthermore, these devices can prevent the occurrence and recurrence of foot ulceration. However, when using orthoses or other inserts, care must be taken not to increase pressures over another region of the foot.

In the last two decades, the development of intricate computerized systems has revolutionized diabetic foot pressure measurements and made their application possible for daily clinical practice. Foot pressure measurements obtained from out-of-shoe and in-shoe methods may have far-reaching consequences for both research and clinical applications. Moreover, these systems can potentially identify at-risk patients and provide a basis for the implementation of either footwear modifications or surgical intervention. Foot pressure measurement systems are still being developed. In the future, computer systems will become more widely available and may be employed routinely for diabetic foot management and a variety of foot conditions.

REFERENCES

1. Wagner FW. The diabetic foot. *Orthopedics* 1987;10:163–172.
2. Pollard JP, LeQuesne IP, Tappin JW. Forces under the foot. *J Biomed Eng* 1983;5:37–41.
3. Lang-Stevenson AI, Sharrad WJ, Betts RP, et al. Neuropathic ulcers of the foot. *J Bone Joint Surg [Br]* 1985:67B:438–442.
4. Boulton AJ, Betts RP, Franks CI, et al. The natural history of foot pressure abnormalities in neuropathic diabetic subjects. *Diabetes Care* 1987;7:73–77.
5. Boulton AJ, Hardisty CA, Betts RP, et al. Dynamic foot pressure and other studies as diagnostic and management aids in diabetic neuropathy. *Diabetes Care* 1983;6:26–33.
6. Betts RP, Duckworth TJ. Plantar pressure measurements and prevention of ulceration in the diabetic foot. *J Bone Joint Surg* 1985;67:79–85.
7. Boulton AJ, Veves A, Young MJ. Etiopathogenesis and management of abnormal foot pressures, in *The Diabetic Foot*, 5th ed. (Levin ME, O'Neal LW, Bowker JH, eds.), Mosby, St. Louis, 1993, pp. 233–246.
8. Fernando DJ, Masson EA, Veves A, et al. Limited joint mobility: relationship to abnormal foot pressures and diabetic foot ulceration. *Diabetes Care* 1991;14:8–11.
9. Veves A, Fernando DJ, Walewski P, et al. A study of plantar pressures in a diabetic clinic population. *Foot* 1991;2:89–92.
10. Young MJ, Cavanagh P, Thomas G, et al. The effect of callus removal on dynamic plantar foot pressures in diabetic patients. *Diabet Med* 1992;5:55–57.
11. Cavanagh PR, Sims DS, Sander LJ. Body mass is a poor predictor of peak plantar pressure in diabetic men. *Diabetes Care* 1991;14:750–755.

12. Donaghue VM, Veves A. Foot pressure measurement. *Orthop Phys Ther Clin North Am* 1997;6:1–16.
13. Rich J, Veves A. Forefoot and rearfoot plantar pressures in diabetic patients: correlation to foot ulceration. *Wounds* 2000:12;82–87.
14. Sarnow MR, Veves A, Giurini JM, et al. In-shoe foot pressure measurements in diabetic patients with at-risk feet and in healthy subjects. *Diabetes Care* 1994:17;1002–1006.
15. Veves A, Murray HJ, Young MJ, et al. The risk of foot ulceration in diabetic patients with high foot pressure: a prospective study. *Diabetologia* 1992;35:660–663.
16. Veves A, Sarnow MR, Giurini JM, et al. Differences in joint mobility and foot pressures between black and white diabetic patients. *Diabet Med* 1995;12:585–589.
17. Ctercteko G, Dhanendran M, Hutton WC, et al. Vertical forces acting on the feet of diabetic patients with neuropathic ulceration. *Br J Surg* 1981;68:608–614.
18. Stokes IA, Furis IB, Hutton WC. The neuropathic ulcer and loads on the foot in diabetic patients. *Acta Orthop Scand* 1975;46:839–847.
19. Brand PW. *Insensitive Feet, a Practical Handbook of Foot Problems in Leprosy*. The Leprosy Mission, London, 1984.
20. Beely F. Zur mechanik des Stehens uber die Bedentung des Fussgewolbes beim Stehen Langenbecks. *Arch Klini Chir* 1882;27:47.
21. Morton DJ. Structural factors in static disorders of the foot. *Am J Surg* 1930;19:315.
22. Elftman H. A cinematic study of the distribution of pressure in the human foot. *Anat Rec* 1934;59:481.
23. Harris RI, Beath T. *Army foot survey. Report of National Research Council of Canada.* NRC, OH. 1947.
24. Barrett JP, Mooney V. Neuropathy and diabetic pressure lesions. *Orthop Clin North Am* 1973;4:43.
25. Silvino N, Evanski PM, Waugh TR. The Harris and Beath footprinting mat: diagnostic validity and clinical use. *Clin Orthop* 1980;265–269.
26. Welton EA. The Harris and Beath footprint: interpretation and clinical value. *Foot Ankle* 1992;13:462–468.
27. van Schie CH, Abbott CA, Vileikyte L, et al. A comparative study of Podotrack, a simple semiquantitative plantar pressure measuring device and the optical pedobarograph on the assessment of pressure under the diabetic foot. *Diabet Med* 1999;16:154–159.
28. van Ijzer M. The Podotrack, a new generation Harris mat. *Podopost* 1993, pp. 39–41.
29. Barnes D. A comparative study of two barefoot pressure measuring systems. BMSc thesis, University of Dundee, 1994.
30. Arcan M, Brull MA. Fundamental characteristics of the human body and foot: the foot-ground pressure pattern. *J Biomech* 1976;9:453–457.
31. Hutton WC, Drabble GE. An apparatus to give the distribution of vertical load under the foot. *Rheum Phys Med* 1972;11:313–317.
32. Stott JR, Hutton WC, Stokes IA. Forces under the foot. *J Bone Joint Surg [Br]* 1973;55B: 335–344.
33. Holmes GB, Willits NH. Practical considerations for the use of the pedobarograph. *Foot Ankle* 1991;12:105–108.
34. Bauman JH, Brand PW. Measurement of pressure between the foot and shoe. *Lancet* 1963; 1:629–632.
35. Duckworth T, Betts RP, Franks CI, et al. The measurement of pressures under the foot. *Foot Ankle* 1992;3:130–141.
36. Feehery RV. Clinical applications of the electrodynogram. *Clin Podiatr Med Surg* 1986;3: 609–612.
37. Wolf L, Stess R, Graf P. Dynamic foot pressure analysis of the diabetic Charcot foot. *J Am Podiatr Med Assoc* 1991;81:281.

38. Rose N, Feiwell LA, Cracchiolo AC. A method for measuring foot pressure using a high resolution, computerized insole sensor: the effect of heel wedges on plantar pressure distribution and center of force. *Foot Ankle* 1992;13:263–270.

39. Pitei D, Edmonds M, Lord M, et al. FSCAN: a new method of in-shoe dynamic measurement of foot pressure (abstract). *Diabet Med* 1993;7:(Suppl 2):S39.

40. Young CR. The FSCAN system of foot pressure analysis. *Clin Podiatr Med Surg* 1993;10:455–461.

41. Boulton AJ, Franks CI, Betts RP, et al. Reduction of abnormal foot pressures in diabetes neuropathy using a new polymer insole material. *Diabetes Care* 1984;7:42–46.

42. Kelly PJ, Coventry MB. Neurotrophic ulcers of the feet: review of 47 cases. *JAMA* 1958;168:388.

43. Frykberg RG, Lavery LA, Pham H, et al. Role of neuropathy and high foot pressures in diabetic foot ulceration. *Diabetes Care* 1998:21;1714–1719.

44. Pham H, Armstrong DG, Harvey C, et al. Screening techniques to identify people at high risk for diabetic foot ulceration: a prospective multicenter trial. *Diabetes Care* 2000;23:606–611.

45. Veves A, Boulton AJM. The optical pedobaragraph. *Clin Podiatr Med Surg* 1993;10:463–470.

46. Veves A, Masson EA, Fernando DJ, et al. The use of experimental padded hosiery to reduce abnormal foot pressures in diabetic neuropathy. *Diabetes Care* 1989;12:653–655

47. Veves A, Masson EA, Fernando DJ, et al. Studies of experimental hosiery in diabetic neuropathic patients with high foot pressures. *Diabet Med* 1990;7:324–326.

48. Donaghue VM, Sarnow MR, Giurini JM, et al. Longitudinal in-shoe foot pressure relief achieved by specially designed footwear in high risk diabetic patients. *Diabetes Res Clin Pract* 1996;31:109–114.

49. Giacalone VF, Armstrong DG, Ashry HR, et al. A quantitative assessment of healing sandals and postoperative shoes in offloading the neuropathic diabetic foot. *J Foot Ankle Surg* 1997;36:28–30.

50. Nawoczenski DA, Birke JA, Coleman WC. Effect of rocker sole design on plantar forefoot pressures. *J Am Podiatr Med Assoc* 1988;78:450–455.

51. Fleischli JG, Lavery LA, Vela SA, et al. Comparison of strategies for reducing pressure at the site of neuropathic ulcers. *J Am Podiatr Med Assoc* 1997;87:466–472.

52. Chanteleau E, Kushner T, Spraul M. How effective is cushioned therapeutic footwear in protecting diabetic feet. *Diabet Med* 1990;7:355–359.

53. Perry JE, Ulbrecht JS, Derr JA, et al. The use of running shoes to reduce plantar pressures in patients who have diabetes. *J Bone J Surg [Br]* 1995;77A:1819–1827.

54. Kastenbauer T, Sokol G, Auiuger M, et al. Running shoes for relief of plantar pressure in diabetic patients. *Diabet Med* 1998;15:518–522.

55. Veves A, Saouaf R, Donaghue VM, et al. Aerobic exercise capacity remains normal despite impaired endothelial function in the micro- and macrocirculation of physically active IDDM patients. *Diabetes* 1997:46;1846–1852.

56. Lavery LA, Vela SA, Lavery DC, et al. Reducing dynamic foot pressures in high risk diabetic subjects with foot ulcerations. *Diabetes Care* 1996;19:818–821.

57. Lavery LA, Vela S, Fleischli JG, et al. Reducing plantar pressures in the neuropathic foot. *Diabetes Care* 1997;20:1706–1710.

58. Ashry HR, Lavery LA, Murdoch DP, et al. Effectiveness of diabetic insoles to reduce foot pressures. *J Foot Ankle Surg* 1997;36:268–271.

59. Albert S, Rinoie C. Effect of custom orthotics on plantar pressure distribution in the pronated diabetic foot. *J Foot Ankle Surg* 1994;33:598–604.

60. Kato H, Takada T, Kawamura T, et al. The reduction and redistribution of plantar pressures using foot orthoses in diabetic patients. *Diabetes Res Clin Pract* 1996;31:115–118.

61. Brown M, Rudicel S, Esquenazi A. Measurement of dynamic pressures at the shoe-foot interface during normal walking with various foot orthoses using the FSCAN system. *Foot Ankle Int* 1996:17;152–156.

8

Biomechanics of the Diabetic Foot:
The Road to Foot Ulceration

Carine H. M. van Schie, MSc, PhD and Andrew J. M. Boulton, MD, FRCP

FOOT FUNCTION

One of the principal functions of the foot is to absorb shock during heel strike and adapt to the uneven surface of the ground during gait. In this function the subtalar joint plays a basic role. The subtalar joint allows motion in three planes and is described as pronation (a combination of eversion, abduction, and dorsiflexion) and supination (a combination of inversion, adduction, and plantar flexion) *(1,2)*. The ankle joint is the major point for controlling sagittal plane movements of the leg relative to the foot, which is essential for bipedal ambulation over flat or uneven terrain *(3)*. The midtarsal joint represents the functional articulation between the hindfoot and midfoot. The inter-relationship of the subtalar and midtarsal joint provides full pronation and supination motions throughout the foot. The first metatarsophalangeal joint (MTPJ) incorporates the first metatarsal head, the base of the proximal phalanx, and the superior surfaces of the medial and lateral sesamoid bones within a single joint capsule. The main motion of the first MTPJ and the lesser MTPJs is in the sagittal plane (dorsiflexion and plantar flexion). During propulsion, the body weight is moving forward over the hallux, creating relative dorsiflexion of the first MTPJ. This occurs with the hallux planted firmly on the ground and with the heel lifting for propulsion. It has previously been reported that the force acting across the first MTPJ approximates body weight, whereas the force across other MTPJs is considerably less *(4)*. In addition, maximum loading of the first metatarsal head and hallux is around the same time during stance in normal gait, highlighting the importance of the load-bearing function of the hallux and first metatarsal head.

During gait, the foot is required to be unstable at first for shock absorption and to adapt to the terrain, whereas during the propulsive phase the foot has to be stable to function as a lever. Foot flexibility and rigidity are mainly controlled with pronation and supination of the subtalar and midtarsal joints. As subtalar joint pronation after heel strike is a major shock-absorbing mechanism, limited joint mobility or structural abnormality could compromise flexibility and shock absorption, thereby placing increased stress on the plantar skin surface *(5,6)*. In addition, limited ankle dorsiflexion could result in increased pressure on the forefoot, particularly during the late stance phase of gait, caused by an early heel rise or compensatory pronation *(5,7,8)*.

From: *The Diabetic Foot: Medical and Surgical Management*
Edited by: A. Veves, J. M. Giurini, and F. W. LoGerfo © Humana Press Inc., Totowa, NJ

GAIT CYCLE

The gait cycle consists of two parts: the stance and the swing phase. The stance or weight-bearing phase can be divided into three parts; the first one is the contact phase initiated by initial contact to toe-off of the opposite limb. Normally, the first area of the foot in contact with the ground is the heel; however, in many cases initial foot contact is with a flat foot, or sometimes even with the forefoot. In cases of a midfoot deformity, such as a Charcot joint, the midfoot could be the site of initial contact. The midstance phase begins with opposite-side toe-off and full forefoot loading and terminates with heel-lift. The third phase, the propulsion phase, can be further subdivided into two phases: active propulsion and passive lift-off. Active propulsion begins with heel-lift of the support side and ends with opposite-side heel strike. During this stage the greatest horizontal and vertical forces are directed against the foot, and weight bearing is over a relatively small area (forefoot). It is therefore not surprising to find that the highest pressures are usually observed during this part of the stance phase. The passive lift-off begins with opposite heel contact and terminates with support-side toe-off.

Each part of the stance phase is characterized by a rocker action of the foot and ankle. During the contact phase, the heel (heel rocker) serves as an axis to allow smooth plantar flexion and to make full contact with the ground. During midstance, the ankle (ankle rocker) allows the tibia to advance forward over the foot, causing relative dorsiflexion of the ankle. This advances the center of pressure from the heel and midfoot to the forefoot. During active propulsion and passive lift-off, the first MTPJ (the forefoot rocker) allows progression of the limb over the forefoot and accelerates heel-lift.

CHANGES IN THE FOOT CAUSED BY DIABETES

Diabetic foot ulceration occurs as a consequence of the interaction of several contributory factors. Peripheral neuropathy is believed to cause changes in foot function and structure (prominent metatarsal heads), as well as dryness of the skin, which can lead to excessive callus formation *(9–11)*. Another important predictive risk factor for the development of diabetic foot ulceration is high plantar foot pressure *(12,13)*. High foot pressures usually occur at sites with bony prominence and have been strongly associated with reduced plantar tissue thickness *(14,15)*. In addition, several authors have reported that foot deformities are strongly associated with and predictive of increased plantar pressures and foot ulceration *(11,16,17)*. Prominent metatarsal heads have been ascribed to weakness of the intrinsic muscles of the foot, which causes an imbalance of toe flexors and extensors, causing the toes to claw, thereby pulling the fat padding away from the metatarsal heads and leaving them unprotected *(18,19)*. Evidence of atrophy of these muscles was recently demonstrated as fatty infiltration in plantar muscles of diabetic patients with a history of foot ulceration *(20)*. Loss of hallux function due to clawing of the toes could severely alter pressure distribution in the forefoot during the second half of the stance phase, as it was previously described that the hallux shares a significant proportion of the load on the first ray *(4,21,22)*.

Charcot arthropathy usually causes gross deformation of the foot, thereby severely affecting functional use of the foot and causing abnormal pressure loading during walking. Peak plantar pressure in patients with Charcot arthropathy were shown to be higher compared with those in patients with a neuropathic ulcer *(23)*. Patients with partially amputated feet have also been shown to exhibit abnormal pressure loading *(24)*, and amputation of the hallux greatly increases pressure under the metatarsal heads *(25,26)*.

Callus has also been reported to be highly predictive for foot ulceration *(27)*. Callus acts as a foreign body, and its removal leads to reduced plantar pressure in most cases *(28,29)*. Furthermore, neuropathic ulcers are commonly found beneath plantar calluses; therefore frequent removal of callus is strongly recommended in diabetic patients.

Thus, foot deformity appears to be a strong indicator of abnormal foot loading during walking, thereby causing high plantar foot pressures. Alleviation of these high-pressure areas is best achieved with accommodative footwear, including insoles and shoes. It is extremely important to ensure that the altered foot shape is properly fitted and accommodated in the footwear. For many patients, normal street footwear will not meet these criteria.

Limited Joint Mobility

Limited joint mobility (LJM) of the foot and ankle has also been suggested to increase plantar pressure in diabetic patients *(30–32)* and to be related to foot ulceration *(33,34)*. Subtalar joint mobility was reported significantly less in the ulcerated foot compared with the contralateral nonulcerated foot in diabetic neuropathic patients *(33)*. In this same study, the authors also reported a significant association between mobility of joints of the hand and foot, indicating that stiffening of joints appears to be a general feature in diabetic patients. Similarly, another study reported on reduced ankle dorsiflexion and subtalar range of motion in diabetic patients with a history of plantar ulceration compared with patients without a history of ulceration and nondiabetic controls *(34)*. Furthermore, a relationship has been demonstrated between reduced range of motion of the first MTPJ and ulceration of the great toe *(8)*. Figure 1 illustrates the relationship between reduced first ray range of motion (first metatarsal head [MTH] dorsiflexion) and increased pressure variables at the first MTH in patients with a history of ulceration at the first MTH as opposed to no apparent relationship for patients with a history of plantar forefoot ulceration not at the first MTH *(8)*.

Joint mobility is defined as the range of motion and is related to age, sex, and ethnic background *(35–37)*. The etiology of LJM is unknown, although most evidence favors a relationship with the collagen abnormalities that occur in diabetes, resulting in thickening of skin, tendons, ligaments, and joint capsules, thereby reducing tissue flexibility *(38,39)*. The prevalence of LJM (diagnosed with a positive "prayer sign") has been reported to vary between 49 and 58% for type 1 diabetic patients and between 45 and 52% for type 2 patients *(40–42)*.

Increased foot pressures have been shown to be related to decreased (passive) joint mobility of the subtalar joint in a group of diabetic patients *(30)*. Another study has reported on reduced dynamic ankle range of motion during walking and when measured passively in diabetic neuropathic patients compared with nondiabetic controls *(43)*. Similarly, Andersen and Mogensen *(44)* reported that maximum movements at the ankle were delayed and slowed using an isokinetic dynamometer in long-term type 1 diabetic patients.

In contrast to the above studies, it was recently reported that joint mobility of the foot (i.e., subtalar, ankle, and first MTPJ) was not related to plantar pressures. The only joint mobility measurement related to plantar pressure was the measurement in

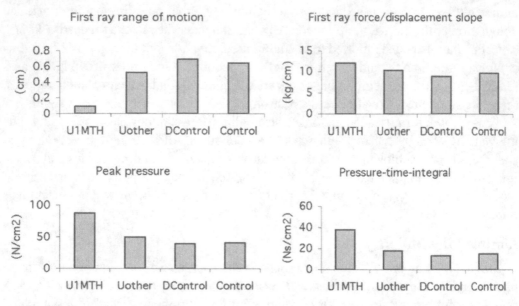

Fig. 1. Range of motion and plantar pressure of first metatarsal head (MTH). First ray dorsi-flexion was measured as vertical displacement of the first MTH, while the second through the fifth MTH were stabilized. The force (up to 8 kg) applied to and the vertical displacement of the first MTH were measured simultaneously. Pressure under the first MTH was measured during barefoot walking at standardized walking velocity. U1MTH, patients with history of ulceration at first MTH; Uother, patients with history of plantar forefoot ulceration not at the first MTH; DControl, diabetic patients without history of foot ulceration; Control, nondiabetic controls. The U1MTH group had a significant stiffer first MTH and higher pressure under the first MTH compared with the other three groups ($p < 0.05$). (Adapted from ref. *8*.)

the hand (extension of the fifth MPTJ) *(45)*. It was suggested that joint mobility of the hand may be a surrogate marker for diabetic complications in general and is therefore associated with peak pressure of the foot. In addition, it was shown that dynamic range of motion (measured during walking) of the subtalar and ankle joint was not related to peak pressures.

Thus, although joint mobility appears to be reduced in diabetic patients, the effect of reduced joint mobility on plantar pressure and foot ulceration remains a controversial area. The relationship with foot ulceration has only been studied retrospectively; thus this could possibly indicate that foot ulceration causes stiffening of the joints as opposed to LJM causing foot ulceration. Foot ulcers are frequently healed using casts for off-loading; in addition, patients are advised to minimize their level of activity while heal-ing the ulcer. These two factors are quite likely to compromise joint mobility. In addition, the reduced joint mobility may not be the causative factor but may just be related to other diabetic complications and/or diabetes duration and therefore related to increased foot pressures and foot ulceration.

DEVELOPMENT OF DIABETIC FOOT ULCERATION

Foot ulcers in diabetes result from multiple pathophysiologic mechanisms, including roles for neuropathy, peripheral vascular disease, foot deformity, higher foot pressures, and diabetes severity *(46)*. Diabetic neuropathy and peripheral vascular disease are the main etiologic factors predisposing to foot ulceration; they may act alone, together, or in combination with other factors, such as microvascular disease, biomechanical abnormalities, and an increased susceptibility to infection *(46–49)*. Trauma is needed in addition to neuropathy and vascular disease to cause tissue breakdown. Trauma could be intrinsic, such as repetitive stress from high pressure and/or callus, or extrinsic, such as from ill-fitting footwear rubbing on the skin or an object inside the shoe (e.g., drawing pin, pebble).

As trauma, and therefore foot ulceration can be minimized, it is extremely important to identify insensitive feet at risk of ulceration in order to implement preventative care such as the provision of appropriate foot care, education, and referral for podiatry treatment.

Biomechanical Aspects of Foot Ulceration

Ulcer sites are predominantly under the plantar surface of the toes, forefoot, and midfoot, followed by the dorsal surface of the toes and heel *(11)*. As high plantar foot pressures are an important factor in the pathogenesis of diabetic foot ulceration, the proposed mechanism of pressure-induced ulcers is discussed next.

Skin is the mechanical link through which intrinsic forces are transmitted to the outside world and environmental forces to the skin and subcutaneous tissue. Ulceration seems to be caused by repetitive and/or excessive pressure on the surface of the insensitive skin, leading to tissue damage. If the same pressures occurred in a person with adequate sensation, the person would experience pain and avoid the offending pressures. However, in a person with loss of protective sensation, there is no warning of excessive pressures or tissue damage, and persistent localized pressures can lead to skin breakdown or ulceration. Foot deformities are usually responsible for these excessive pressures. In addition, healing of plantar ulcers is prevented as long as patients keep walking on their foot wounds, highlighting the key issue of mechanical offloading.

Thus, excessive and/or repetitive pressures appear to be the main causative factor for development of skin breakdown. There are three mechanisms that account for the occurrence of these pressures: 1) increased duration of pressures; 2) increased magnitude of pressures; and 3) increased number of pressures *(50)*. The first mechanism includes relatively low pressures applied for a long period, causing ischemia. Prolonged ischemia leads to cell death and wound formation, as has been demonstrated in a classic experiment by Kosiak *(51)*, who showed an inverse time-pressure relationship (Fig. 2). High pressures took a relatively short time to cause ulceration, and low pressures took a relatively long time. Thus, ulceration can develop at very low pressures but may take a few days to occur. This type of offending pressure and resulting ulcers can occur with ill-fitting footwear, improperly fitted orthotics, or prolonged resting of a heel on a bed or footrest.

The second mechanism of tissue injury includes high pressures acting for a short time period. This injury only occurs if a large force is applied to a relatively small area of skin. This happens, for example, if a person steps on a nail or piece of glass, which is not unusual for diabetic neuropathic patients. Alternatively, a foot slap may also conform to this mechanism. A foot slap indicates a reduced deceleration of the forefoot after heel strike caused by weak dorsiflexion muscles. It has previously been demon-

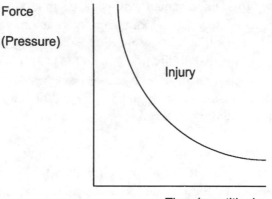

Fig. 2. Inverse relationship between force (pressure) and time (or repetition). As force (pressure) increases, the duration (time) or number (repetition) of force(s) required to cause tissue injury decreases. (Adapted from ref. *51*.)

strated that high rates of tissue deformation lead to cellular death, whereas comparable gradually applied loads do not *(52)*. It is therefore suggested that control of the velocity of the forefoot descending after heel strike by using ankle foot orthosis could possibly help in prevention of diabetic foot ulcers. The third mechanism of injury comes from repetitions of pressure, which in engineering terms would lead to an equivalent syndrome of mechanical fatigue. Mechanical fatigue is defined as failure of a structure or biologic tissue at a submaximal level to maintain integrity due to repeated bouts of loading. This type of injury seems to occur in the insensitive skin of the neuropathic foot.

The body will respond to repeated high pressures or microtrauma with callus formation in order to protect the skin from further damage. However, if callus formation becomes excessive, it will contribute to higher pressure, and calluses should therefore be removed at regular intervals *(28,29)*. Frequently ulcers are masked beneath callus, as high pressure builds up underneath the callus tissue. Not surprisingly, the presence of callus was found to be highly predictive of foot ulceration in a prospective study *(27)*.

Thus, it appears that peak pressure is not the only pressure parameter that is important in causing foot ulceration. There are several other factors to take into account, such as rate of increase of pressure, duration of these pressures, how frequently these pressures are applied to the skin of the foot, whether they are activity related, and so on. In addition, although foot pressures may be high during a barefoot pressure assessment, it is important to keep in mind that it is the combination of footwear, lifestyle factors, level of activity, tissue characteristics, and foot pressures that determines whether a person is going to develop foot ulcers.

Plantar Tissue Thickness in Relation to Foot Ulceration

An alternative to pressure measurement has been suggested in the form of assessment of plantar tissue thickness in the forefoot. Plantar tissue thickness has been strongly associated with plantar pressure, indicating a close relation between the amount of cushioning (soft tissue) available and the pressure distribution over the forefoot *(14,15)*. Furthermore, a strong relationship has been demonstrated between tissue thickness and history of ulceration in diabetic patients *(53,54)*. Loss of protective tissue in the plantar surface of the foot is thought to be caused by clawing of the toes, leading to a distal migration of the protective tissue from under the metatarsal heads, which leaves the remaining tissues susceptible to the resultant increased pressure levels under the metatarsal heads *(18,19)*. Atrophy of the intrinsic muscles of the foot in diabetic neuropathic patients has recently been confirmed using magnetic resonance imaging *(55)* and by demonstration of fatty infiltration in these muscles *(20)*. This suggests that the atrophic process leads to an imbalance between the short flexors and long extensors, contributing to the classic deformities of the neuropathic foot *(18,55)*. Furthermore, qualitative changes of the plantar fat pad were demonstrated in diabetic neuropathic patients. A nonspecific fibrotic process was observed beneath the metatarsal head, which will affect the intrinsic biomechanical properties of the plantar fat pad to act as a shock absorber and dissipate increased plantar pressures associated with neuropathy *(55)*.

Thus, plantar cushioning appears to be reduced in diabetic neuropathic patients, increasing the risk for developing prominent bones and high pressures and thereby increasing the risk for foot ulceration.

Foot Type and Foot Ulceration

Recent evidence suggests that feet with "abnormal" alignment of the forefoot or rearfoot exhibit a different loading pattern than normally aligned feet. Both nondiabetic and diabetic planus feet (everted rearfoot, inverted forefoot, and low arch) were reported to experience greater peak pressures than nondiabetic rectus feet (a neutral rearfoot and forefoot with normal arch morphology) *(56)*. These results confirmed some older data reported by Mueller and associates *(57)*, who demonstrated that certain foot types are associated with characteristic patterns of pressure distribution and callus formation on the feet. In this study a significant relationship between foot deformity and location of ulcer and callus was found in a group of diabetic patients with active ulceration. Foot deformity included typical fore- and rearfoot relationships, such as an uncompensated forefoot varus or forefoot valgus (in- or everted forefoot). Eighty-eight percent (15/17) of the subjects with one of these two deformities had ulcers located at the first or fifth metatarsal head. The results of this study confirm the theory of site of callus formation specific to certain foot types, as is widely used in podiatry practice; however, this is the first study to support this theory scientifically *(57)*. Similarly, a strong correlation between heel position during relaxed stance and metatarsal ulcer sites has been demonstrated *(58)*. Inverted heels were associated with lateral ulcers, whereas everted heels were associated with associated with medial ulcers ($r = 0.87$).

Thus, these studies indicate that the high pressures measured in these feet are not just caused by the effects of diabetes. However, it seems more reasonable to hypothesize that diabetic patients with foot type characteristics that differ from the norm are more likely to develop high foot pressures and ulceration than diabetic patients with normal foot morphology. In neuropathic patients with abnormal foot alignment, corrective insoles are contraindicated, as it is far more important to accommodate the foot and to reduce pressures at the high-pressure sites in order to prevent ulceration.

INTERVENTIONS TO REDUCE
FOOT PRESSURES AND FOOT ULCERATION

There are several ways to implement preventive measures to reduce the incidence of foot ulceration. Preventive care includes callus debridement as well as provision of pressure-reducing insoles and therapeutic footwear. Traditionally, callus is removed when it is excessively formed under the diabetic foot: however, only a few preliminary studies have addressed how callus buildup can be minimized. Colagiuri and colleagues *(59)* reported results of a small randomized placebo-controlled trial, investigating the efficacy of rigid orthotic in-shoe devices on plantar callus compared with conventional podiatric care. The results showed a reduction in callus grade in the orthotic group, with no change in the conventionally treated group. Foster and associates *(60)* investigated the efficacy of injecting collagen under callus in diabetic patients with previous neuropathic ulceration to improve subdermal cushioning and to spread weight-bearing forces. Patients were followed up for 8 months, and the active treatment group showed a 64% reduction of surface area of callus compared with 40% in the control group.

Appropriate management of callus is crucial in diabetic patients. Callus needs to be removed frequently, as it can build up quickly, with some patients needing debridement as often as every 3–4 weeks or sometimes even more frequently *(29)*.

The therapeutic use of liquid silicone injections in the foot has been suggested to improve cushioning at callus sites, corns, and localized painful areas *(61,62)*. Recently, a randomized placebo-controlled trial has shown the efficacy of injected liquid silicone to decrease peak plantar pressure and callus formation and increase plantar tissue thickness under silicone-treated areas *(63)*. This cushioning effect was still significant at 1 year following the injections. There were no side effects reported in this study, and in addition there is a large body of anecdotal evidence to support the safety of this procedure *(61)*. Anecdotal evidence also suggests that the bulk of the injected fluid remains for an indefinite period in the general area where it was originally injected. The results of the aforementioned randomized trial indicated that the magnitude of change after silicone injection was greater at injection sites with a lower baseline thickness and a higher baseline peak pressure (Fig. 3). A similar magnitude pressure-reducing effect was previously shown by Perry and colleagues *(64)*, who reported greatest pressure reduction (using cushioned running shoes) at sites with the highest initial pressure.

Thus, new exciting treatments to reduce the risk of foot ulceration have been developed. However, whether silicone injections can actually prevent foot ulceration needs to be confirmed in larger trials.

Surgical Interventions and Foot Ulceration

Different surgical methods have been suggested and used for reduction of foot pressures and prevention of ulceration. Surgical procedures include reconstructive and prophylactic measures. It is imperative to ensure that vascular supply is sufficient to ensure healing.

Surgical reconstruction when a gross foot deformity is present, such as in a Charcot foot, is mainly aimed at creating a foot shape that can be fitted in a shoe. Other interventions have a more specific aim of reducing foot pressures. For example, metatarsal

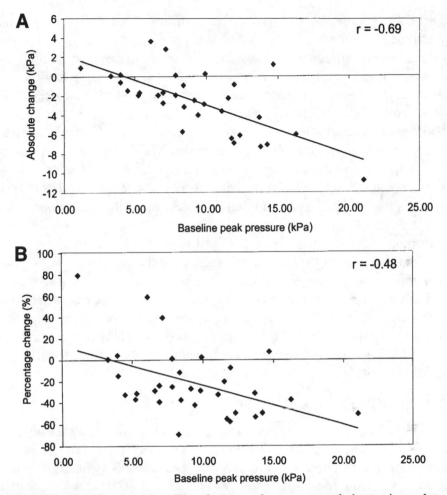

Fig. 3. Relationship between baseline plantar peak pressure and change in peak pressure after silicone injection treatment. Baseline plantar peak pressure was associated with absolute change (**A**) of pressure ($r = -0.69$) and percentage (**B**) change of pressure ($r = -0.48$).

head resection has been used to accelerate the healing of an open wound under a metatarsal head area, usually greatly exposed to high pressure. The hypothesis for improved healing rate and reduced ulcer recurrence rate using this procedure is that the pressure under the active or previous ulcer is greatly reduced, thereby allowing healing to occur or preventing recurrent foot ulceration. However, only limited evidence is available about the efficacy of this treatment. It is not known whether removal of one metatarsal head results in a transfer of peak pressure to other areas in the foot. The maximum follow-up with foot pressure measurements of patients who underwent this surgery in the literature is 6–8 weeks, at which time there may still be some swelling left, which could account for some of the plantar pressure reductions as measured in these patients *(65)*. However, no recurrent ulcers or transfer lesions were seen during a 6–20-month follow-up period. Another study reported favorable results of 34 metatarsal head resections for diabetic patients with chronic neuropathic ulceration, with no recurrence of ulcers during a 14 ± 11-month follow-up period *(66)*.

The efficacy of panmetatarsal head resection in neuropathic diabetic patients has been questioned, as the procedure does not appear to eliminate localized high-pressure areas (67). However, this report only included data on two patients (three feet), making generalization of results difficult. Previously reported success using this procedure is possibly related to improved footwear and care after surgery; unfortunately, foot pressure measurements were not included in this report (68).

Dorsiflexion metatarsal osteotomy has been suggested as an alternative to metatarsal head resection, as this procedure does not violate the MTPJ which may lead to transfer lesions to adjacent metatarsal heads (69). It elevates prominent metatarsal heads, thereby balancing the metatarsal heads and redistributing weight-bearing forces more evenly across the forefoot. Again, no pressure data are available to support this proposed mechanism of action.

Lengthening of the Achilles tendon has been suggested as a useful intervention for lowering foot pressures in the forefoot, by increasing the amount of dorsiflexion as a direct result of the procedure (70). It was shown in a small study that peak pressure in the forefoot was on average reduced by an amount of 27% at 8 weeks after the operation, compared with before the operation. In addition, dorsiflexion of the ankle joint had increased after the intervention. The suggested relationship between increase of dorsiflexion and reduced peak pressure is a confirmation of the earlier discussed limited joint mobility theory.

OFF-LOADING THE DIABETIC FOOT ULCER

Off-loading of the diabetic wound is a key factor in successful wound healing. Several devices have been described in the literature, most of them being effective in off-loading and healing of the wound. However, very little evidence is available on how effective different off-loading devices are with respect to healing time or reduction in plantar pressure and how these devices compare in their clinical effectiveness.

The total contact cast (TCC) is generally viewed as the gold standard for off-loading the diabetic wound; however, several useful alternatives exist (71). Although the TCC is probably the most effective in off-loading the wound, the problem with this method is that regular checking of the wound is difficult, as this means making a new cast after every check. In addition, casting is contraindicated in an acutely infected or ischemic foot. Other devices, such as the Scotchcast boot, removable casts, half shoes, and so on, are probably not as effective in off-loading; however, their main advantage is that regular inspection of the wound is possible. Obviously, this is at the same time also the main disadvantage, as the possibility of removing the device makes it very easy for patients not to comply with the off-loading treatment. Clearly, more studies are urgently needed in order to clarify which devices are successful in off-loading and how they compare in their clinical efficacy.

The Scotchcast boot is a well-padded plaster boot cut away by the ankle and made removable by cutting away the cast over the dorsum over the foot. Windows are cut under the ulcer, and the boot is worn with a cast sandal to increase patient mobility while the cast protects the ulcer from any pressure (72,73). Although the boot has been used very successfully for more than a decade in several UK clinics, to date there is no evidence available of comparison of healing rate of this type of cast with other casting modalities.

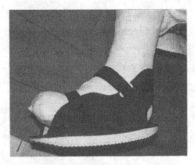

Fig. 4. Example of a total contact cast.

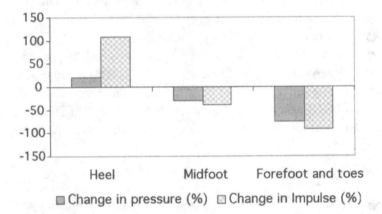

Fig. 5. Change in mean peak plantar pressure and impulse (pressure-time-integral) in the total contact cast compared with the shoe condition (cast shoe with a flat 0.5-inch PPT compliant insole). (Adapted from ref. *74*).

The TCC is a well-molded, minimally padded cast that maintains contact with the entire plantar aspect of the foot and lower leg (Fig. 4). It has been reported that a large proportion of the pressured reduction achieved in the forefoot of the TCC is transmitted along the cast wall or to the rearfoot *(74)* (Fig. 5). The advantage of the contact cast over other off-loading methods is that it is effective in reducing pressure, immobilizing tissues, and reducing edema; also, the patient cannot remove it. However, the cast can create secondary lesions, and the use of special dressings or topical agents is limited. Although the TCC is theoretically probably the most effective in ulcer healing, it requires a lot of expertise and time for application compared with other modalities. It is therefore not always a practical option in some clinics.

Removable cast walkers have shown to be effective in reducing peak pressure. The DH pressure relief walker and the prefabricated pneumatic walking brace (Air cast) were shown in two different studies to be as effective in reducing forefoot pressures as a TCC *(75,76)*. However, clinical data are still missing on the efficacy of healing foot ulcers of these casts.

Healing sandals have been shown to reduce pressures significantly, whereas postoperative shoes have not shown a significant effect on pressure *(77)*. Half-shoes have been shown to reduce peak pressure significantly at ulcer sites; however, they were less effective than TCC but more effective than felted foam and postoperative shoes *(78)*. Custom-made shoes come last of all off-loading treatment options. Therapeutic shoes and insoles are probably most optimally used as a preventive measure of ulcer development or recurrence and not for healing.

The ankle-foot orthosis has been suggested to be a useful alternative to casting techniques in order to off-load the diabetic foot during wound healing and to prevent ulceration *(79)*. It is proposed that an ankle-foot orthosis prevents high-velocity impact between the ground and the plantar surface of the foot, thereby controlling the rate of mechanical loading of the tissues. In fact, most casting techniques indirectly reduce rate of loading of the forefoot by immobilizing the ankle joint. There is only limited evidence on the efficacy of ankle-foot orthosis in ulcer healing and prevention; however, preliminary evidence indicates pressure reductions at ulcer sites ranging from 70 to 92% and significantly reduced loading rates *(79)*.

Thus, many off-loading modalities have been described to prevent (re)ulceration and to improve wound healing. Although several modalities have been shown to be successful in reducing foot pressures in the diabetic foot, not all have been shown to be clinically effective. Clearly, more clinical evidence is needed (i.e., randomized controlled trials) in order to improve clinical decision making in the prevention of diabetic foot ulcers.

REFERENCES

1. Nester CJ. Review of literature on the axis of rotation at the subtalar joint. *Foot* 1998;8: 111–118.
2. Sarrafian SK. Biomechanics of the subtalar joint complex. *Clin Orthop Res* 1993;290:17–26.
3. Wernick J, Volpe RG. Lower extremity function and normal mechanics, in *Clinical Biomechanics of the Lower Extremities* (Valmassy RL, ed.), Mosby Year Book, St Louis, 1996, pp. 2–57.
4. Hutton WC, Dhanendran M. The mechanics of normal and hallux valgus feet—a quantitative study. *Clin Orthop Res* 1981;157:7–13.
5. Root ML, Orien WP, Weed JH. *Clinical Biomechanics: Normal and Abnormal Function of the Foot*. Clinical Biomechanics, Los Angeles, 1977, p. 2.
6. Nack JD, Phillips RD. Shock absorption. *Clin Podiatr Med Surg* 1990;7:391–397.
7. Gibbs RC, Boxer MC. Abnormal biomechanics of feet and their cause of hyperkeratoses. *J Am Acad Dermatol* 1982;6:1061–1069.
8. Birke JA, Franks BD, Foto JG. First ray joint limitation, pressure, and ulceration of the first metatarsal head in diabetes mellitus. *Foot Ankle* 1995;16:277–284.
9. Boulton AJM. Late sequelae of diabetic neuropathy, in *Diabetic Neuropathy* (Boulton AJM, ed.), Marius Press, Carnforth, Lancashire, UK, 1997, pp. 63–76.
10. Mayfield JA, Reiber GE, Sanders LJ, Janisse D, Pogach LM. Preventive foot care in people with diabetes. *Diabetes Care* 1998;21:2161–2177.
11. Reiber GE, Vileikyte L, Boyko EJ, et al. Causal pathways for incident lower-extremity ulcers in patients with diabetes from two settings. *Diabetes Care* 1999;22:157–162.
12. Veves A, Murray HJ, Young MJ, Boulton AJM. The risk of foot ulceration in diabetic patients with high foot pressures; a prospective study. *Diabetologia* 1992;35:660–663.
13. Pham H, Armstrong DG, Harvey C, et al. Screening techniques to identify people at high risk for diabetic foot ulceration. A prospective multicenter trial. *Diabetes Care* 2000;23: 606–611.

14. Young MJ, Coffey J, Taylor PM, Boulton AJM. Weight bearing ultrasound in diabetic and rheumatoid arthritis patients. *Foot* 1995;5:76–79.

15. Abouaesha F, van Schie CHM, Boulton AJM. Predictive factors for foot ulceration (abstract). *Diabet Med* 2000;17(Suppl 1):22.

16. Ahroni JH, Boyko EJ, Forsberg RC. Clinical correlates of plantar pressure among diabetic veterans. *Diabetes Care* 1999;22:965–972.

17. Boyko EJ, Ahroni JH, Stensel V, et al. A prospective study of risk factors for diabetic foot ulcer. *Diabetes Care* 1999;22:1036–1042.

18. Boulton AJM, Betts RP, Franks CI, et al. Abnormalities of foot pressure in early diabetic neuropathy. *Diabet Med* 1987;4:225–228.

19. Myerson MS, Shereff MJ. The pathological anatomy of claw and hammer toes. *J Bone Joint Surg [Am]* 1989;71-A:45–49.

20. Suzuki E, Kashiwagi A, Hidaka H, et al. ^{1}H- and ^{31}P-magnetic resonance spectroscopy and imaging as a new diagnostic tool to evaluate neuropathic foot ulcers in type II diabetic patients. *Diabetologia* 2000;43:165–172.

21. Stokes IAF, Hutton WC, Stott JRR. Forces acting on the metatarsals during normal walking. *J Anat* 1979;129:579–590.

22. Hutton WC, Dhanendran M. A study of the distribution of load under the normal foot during walking. *Int Orthop (SICOT)* 1979;3:153–157.

23. Armstrong DG, Lavery LA. Elevated peak plantar pressures in patients who have Charcot arthropathy. *J Bone Joint Surg [Am]* 1998;80:365–369.

24. Garbalosa JC, Cavanagh PR, Wu G, et al. Foot function in diabetic patients after partial amputation. *Foot Ankle* 1996;17:43–48.

25. Lavery LA, Lavery DC, Quebedaux-Farnham TL. Increased foot pressures after great toe amputation in diabetes. *Diabetes Care* 1995;18:1460–1462.

26. Quebedeaux TL, Lavery LA, Lavery DC. The development of foot deformities and ulcers after great toe amputation in diabetes. *Diabetes Care* 1996;19:165–167.

27. Murray HJ, Young MJ, Hollis S, Boulton AJM. The association between callus formation, high pressures and neuropathy in diabetic foot ulceration. *Diabet Med* 1996;13:979–982.

28. Young MJ, Cavanagh PR, Thomas G, et al. The effect of callus removal on dynamic plantar foot pressures in diabetic patients. *Diabet Med* 1992;9:55–57.

29. Pitei DL, Foster A, Edmonds M. The effect of regular callus removal on foot pressures. *J Foot Ankle Surg* 1999;38:251–255.

30. Fernando DJS, Masson EA, Veves A, Boulton AJM. Relationship of limited joint mobility to abnormal foot pressures and diabetic foot ulceration. *Diabetes Care* 1991;14:8–11.

31. Veves A, Sarnow MR, Giurini JM, et al. Differences in joint mobility and foot pressure between black and white diabetic patients. *Diabet Med* 1995;12:585–589.

32. Frykberg RG, Lavery LA, Pham H, et al. Role of neuropathy and high foot pressures in dia-betic foot ulceration. *Diabetes Care* 1998;21:1714–1719.

33. Delbridge L, Perry P, Marr S, et al. Limited joint mobility in the diabetic foot: relationship to neuropathic ulceration. *Diabet Med* 1988;5:333–337.

34. Mueller MJ, Diamond JE, Delitto A, Sinacore DR. Insensitivity, limited joint mobility, and plantar ulcers in patients with diabetes mellitus. *Phys Ther* 1989;69:453–462.

35. Wordsworth P, Ogilvie D, Smith R, Sykes B. Joint mobility with particular reference to racial variation and inherited connective tissue disorders. *Br J Rheumatol* 1987;26:9–12.

36. Pountain G. Musculoskeletal pain in humans, and the relationship to joint mobility and body mass index. *Br J Rheumatol* 1992;31:81–85.

37. Vandervoort AA, Chesworth BM, Cunningham DA, et al. Age and sex effects on mobility on the human ankle. *J Gerontol* 1992;47:M17–M21.

38. Crisp AJ, Heathcote JG. Connective tissue abnormalities in diabetes mellitus. *J R Coll Phys* 1984;18:132–141.

39. Vlassara H, Brownlee M, Cerami A. Nonenzymatic glycosylation: role in the pathogenesis of diabetic complications. *Clin Chem* 1986;32:B37–B41.
40. Fitzcharles MA, Duby S, Waddell RW, Banks E, Karsh J. Limitation of joint mobility (cheiroarthropathy) in adult noninsulin-dependent diabetic patients. *Ann Rheum Dis* 1984; 43:251–257.
41. Pal B, Anderson J, Dick WC, Griffiths ID. Limitation of joint mobility and shoulder capsulitis in insulin- and non-insulin-dependent diabetes mellitus. *Br J Rheumatol* 1986;25:147–151.
42. Arkkila PET, Kantola IM, Viikari JSA, Ronnemaa T, Vohotalo MA. Limited joint mobility is associated with the presence but does not predict the development of microvascular complications in type 1 diabetes. *Diabet Med* 1996;13:828–833.
43. Mueller MJ, Minor SD, Sahrmann SA, Schaaf JA, Strube MJ. Differences in the gait characteristics of patients with diabetes and peripheral neuropathy compared to age-matched controls. *Phys Ther* 1994;74:299–313.
44. Andersen H, Mogensen PH. Disordered mobility of large joints in association with neuropathy in patients with long-standing insulin-dependent diabetes mellitus. *Diabet Med* 1996; 14:221–227.
45. Van Schie CHM, Boulton AJM. Joint mobility and foot pressure measurements in Asian and European diabetic patients: clues for difference in foot ulcer prevalence (abstract). *Diabetes* 2000;49(Suppl 1):A197.
46. Shaw JE, Boulton AJM. The pathogenesis of diabetic foot problems. An overview. *Diabetes* 1997;46(Suppl 2):S58–S61.
47. Boulton AJM, Kubrusly DB, Bowker JH, et al. Impaired vibratory perception and diabetic foot ulceration. *Diabet Med* 1986;3:335–337.
48. Bild DE, Selby JV, Sinnock P, et al. Lower-extremity amputation in people with diabetes. Epidemiology and prevention. *Diabetes Care* 1989;12:24–31.
49. McNeely MJ, Boyko EJ, Ahroni JH, et al. The independent contributions of diabetic neuropathy and vasculopathy in foot ulceration. How great are risks? *Diabetes Care* 1995;18:216–219.
50. Mueller MJ. Etiology, evaluation, and treatment of the neuropathic foot. *Crit Rev Phys Rehabil Med* 1992;3:289–309.
51. Kosiak M. Etiology and pathology of ischemic ulcers. *Arch Phys Med Rehabil* 1959;40:62–69.
52. Landsman AS, Meaney DF, Cargill II RS, Macarak EJ, Thibault LE. High strain tissue deformation. A theory on the mechanical etiology of diabetic foot ulcerations. *J Am Podiatr Assoc* 1995;85:519–527.
53. Brink T. Induration of the diabetic foot pad: another risk factor for recurrent neuropathic plantar ulcers. *Biomed Tech* 1995;40:205–209.
54. Gooding GA, Stess RM, Graf PM, et al. Sonography of the sole of the foot: evidence for loss of foot pad thickness in diabetes and its relationship to ulceration of the foot. *Invest Radiol* 1986;21:45–48.
55. Brash PD, J Foster, Vennart W, Anthony P, Tooke JE. Magnetic resonance imaging techniques demonstrate soft tissue damage in the diabetic foot. *Diabet Med* 1999;16:55–61.
56. Song J, Hillstrom HJ. Effects of foot type biomechanics and diabetic neuropathy on foot function, in *Proceedings of the XVIIth International Society of Biomechanics Congress*, Calgary, Alberta, Canada, 1999, p. 113.
57. Mueller MJ, Minor SD, Diamond JE, Blair VP. Relationship of foot deformity to ulcer location in patients with diabetes mellitus. *Phys Ther* 1990;70:356–362.
58. Bevans JS. Biomechanics and plantar ulcers in diabetes. *Foot* 1992;2:166–172.
59. Colagiuri S, Marsden LL, Naidu V, Taylor L. The use of orthotic devices to correct plantar callus in people with diabetes. *Diabetes Res Clin Prac* 1995;28:29–34.
60. Foster A, Eaton C, Dastoor N, et al. Prevention of neuropathic foot ulceration: a new approach using subdermal injection of collagen (abstract). *Diabet Med* 1988;5(Suppl 5):7.
61. Balkin SW, Kaplan L. Injectable silicone and the diabetic foot: a 25-year report. *Foot* 1991; 2:83–88.

62. Balkin SW. Fluid silicone implantation of the foot, in *Neale's Common Foot Disorders. Diagnosis and Management*, 5th ed (Lorimer D, ed.), Churchill Livingstone, Edinburgh, 1997, pp. 387–400.

63. Van Schie CHM, Whalley A, Vileikyte L, et al. Efficacy of injected liquid silicone in the diabetic foot to reduce risk factors for ulceration. A randomized double-blind placebo-controlled trial. *Diabetes Care* 2000;23:634–638.

64. Perry JE, Ulbrecht JS, Derr JA, Cavanagh PR. The use of running shoes to reduce plantar pressures in patients who have diabetes. *J Bone Joint Surg [Am]* 1995;77A:1819–1828.

65. Patel VG, Wieman TJ. Effect of metatarsal head resection for diabetic foot ulcers on the dynamic plantar pressure distribution. *Am J Surg* 1994;167:297–301.

66. Griffiths GD, Wieman TJ. Metatarsal head resection for diabetic foot ulcers. *Arch Surg* 1990;125:832–835.

67. Cavanagh PR. Elevated plantar pressure and ulceration in diabetic patients after panmetatarsal head resection: two case reports. *Foot Ankle Int* 1999;20:521–526.

68. Giurini JM, Basile P, Chrzan JS, Habershaw GM, Rosenblum BI. Pan metatarsal head resection: a viable alternative to the transmetatarsal amputation. *J Am Podiatr Med Assoc* 1993;83:101–107.

69. Fleischli JE, Anderson RB, Davis WH. Dorsiflexion metatarsal osteotomy for treatment of recalcitrant diabetic neuropathic ulcers. *Foot Ankle Int* 1999;20:80–85.

70. Armstrong DG, Stackpoole-Shea S, Nguyen H, Harkless L. Lengthening of the Achilles tendon in diabetic patients who are at high risk for ulceration of the foot. *J Bone Joint Surg [Am]* 1999;81A:535–538.

71. American Diabetes Association. Consensus Development on Diabetic Foot Wound Care. *Diabetes Care* 1999;22:1354–1360.

72. Jones GR. Walking casts: effective treatment for foot ulcers. *Practical Diabetes* 1991;8:131–132.

73. Knowles EA, Boulton AJM (1996). Use of the Scotchcast boot to heal diabetic foot ulcers, in *Proceedings of the 5th European Conference on Advanced Wound Care*. McMillan, London, 1996, pp. 199–201.

74. Shaw JE, His WL, Ulbrecht JS, et al. The mechanism of plantar unloading in total contact casts: implications for design and clinical use. *Foot Ankle Int* 1997;18:809–817.

75. Baumhauer JF, Wervey R, McWilliams J, Harris GF, Shereff MJ. A comparison study of plantar foot pressure in a standardized shoe, total contact cast, and prefabricated pneumatic walking brace. *Foot Ankle Int* 1997;18:26–33.

76. Lavery LA, Vela SA, Lavery DC, Quebedeaux TL. Reducing dynamic foot pressures in high-risk diabetic subjects with foot ulcerations. A comparison of treatments. *Diabetes Care* 1996;19:818–821.

77. Giacalone VF, Armstrong DG, Ashry HR, et al. A quantitative assessment of healing sandals and postoperative shoes in offloading the neuropathic diabetic foot. *J Foot Ankle Surg* 1997;36:28–30.

78. Fleischli JG, Lavery LA, Vela SA, Ashry H, Lavery DC. 1997 William J. Stickel Bronze Award. Comparison of strategies for reducing pressure at the site of neuropathic ulcers. *J Am Podiatr Med Assoc* 1997;87:466–472.

79. Landsman AS, Sage R. Off-loading neuropathic wounds associated with diabetes using an ankle-foot orthosis. *J Am Podiatr Med Assoc* 1997;87:349–357.

9

Clinical Examination of the Diabetic Foot and Identification of the At-Risk Patient

David G. Armstrong, DPM, Edward Jude, MD, Andrew J. M. Boulton, MD, and Lawrence B. Harkless, DPM

INTRODUCTION

The most common component in the pathway to amputation is the diabetic foot ulcer *(1,2)*. Although some progress has been made in increasing awareness of the problem of the etopathogenesis of diabetic foot ulceration, much work still needs to be done *(3,4)*. By the end of the first quarter of the present millennium, more than 300 million persons worldwide will have diabetes *(5)*. If we appreciate the fact that, at any one time, up to 7% of at-risk patients with diabetes have a diabetic wound *(6)* and that most ulcerations are entirely avoidable, the concept of prevention takes on a new urgency. In this chapter, we discuss the key evidence-based risk factors for ulceration, which may be broken down into three practical screening questions to identify patients at highest risk for skin breakdown. We then discuss seven essential questions to answer when both describing and classifying diabetic foot ulceration.

THREE KEY QUESTIONS FOR IDENTIFYING ULCER RISK

What are the factors that can be altered or for which we can accommodate? Clearly, all our patients with diabetes who present for care should be under the concomitant management of a primary care physician who should be monitoring and proactively controlling the patient's serum glucose. Working with that assumption, we must then evaluate the local (lower extremity) factors that the health care provider may address in his or her systematic examination of the diabetic foot.

1. Is There Loss of Protective Sensation?

Neuropathy is the major component of nearly all diabetic ulcerations *(8)*. Without loss of protective sensation, patients generally will not ulcerate. However, when such loss is present, patients may wear a hole in their foot much as a sensate patient might wear a hole in the stocking or shoe. Acceptable accuracy is represented by 4 or more absent sites (out of 10) using the Semmes-Weinstein 10-g monofilament wire or a vibration perception threshold (VPT) >25 V using a calibrated VPT meter *(9)*. These modalities,

From: *The Diabetic Foot: Medical and Surgical Management*
Edited by: A. Veves, J. M. Giurini, and F. W. LoGerfo © Humana Press Inc., Totowa, NJ

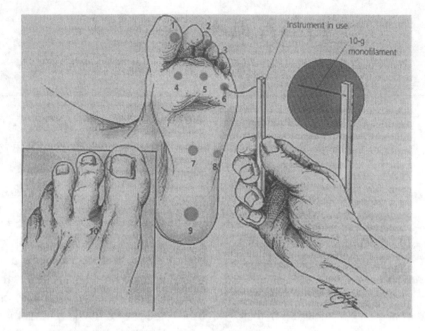

Fig. 1. Sites of testing for 10-g monofilament. Four or more imperceptible sites using a yes-no method of administration may be an optimal combination of sensitivity and specificity for identifying clinically significant loss of protective sensation. (From: *Am Fam Physician* 1998.)

when combined, yield a sensitivity of 100% and a 77% specificity. This has confirmed the previous work of numerous investigators who have described both devices as beneficial tools in assessing for neuropathy *(10–16)*.

Use of the Monofilament

The 10-g monofilament is a potentially valuable tool for identifying loss of protective sensation. However, one must use the device in a consistent manner to prevent over- or underreporting of clinically significant neuropathy. Testing may be carried out with a simple "yes-no" method of administration. The patient is placed supine in the examination chair with his or her eyes closed, and is instructed to say "yes" each time that he or she perceives the application of the monofilament. The device is applied until it bends and should be left in place for a minimum of 1 s. Measurements may be taken at each of 10 sites on the foot *(9–15)*. These include the first, third, and fifth digits plantarly, the first, third, and fifth metatarsal heads plantarly, the plantar midfoot medially and laterally, the plantar heel, and the midfoot dorsally (Fig. 1). In a clinical setting, it is best for the evaluator to have more than one monofilament available, as after numerous uses without a chance to "recover," the monofilament may buckle at a reduced amount of pressure, thus making it oversensitive and therefore less accurate. Furthermore, differences in materials used in manufacture and potential environmental factors may also change the characteristics of the monofilament *(17,18)*.

Use of a Vibration Perception Threshold Meter

A VPT meter is another useful adjunct to assist in clinical evaluation of nerve function. It is semiquantitative and potentially less prone to interoperator variation than the

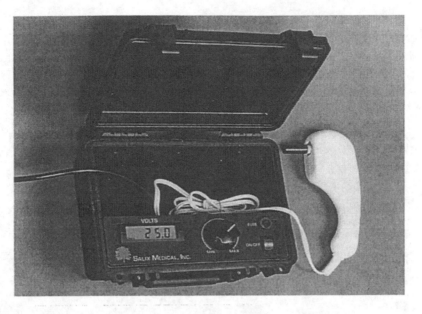

Fig. 2. The vibration perception threshold (VPT) meter. The vibrating tactor is placed at the distal pulp of the great toe. The amplitude (measured in volts) is increased on the base unit until the patient feels a vibration. This is termed VPT. A VPT >25 V may be an optimal combination of sensitivity and specificity for identifying clinically significant loss of protective sensation using this device.

10-g monofilament device. The VPT meter (Fig. 2; also known as a Biothesiometer or Neurothesiometer) is a hand-held device with a rubber tactor that vibrates at 100 Hz. The hand-held unit is connected by an electrical cord to a base unit. This unit contains a linear scale that displays the applied voltage, ranging from 0 to 50 V. The device is generally held with the tactor balanced vertically on the pulp of the toe. At this time, the amplitude is increased on the base unit until the patient can perceive a vibration. A mean of three readings (measured in volts) is generally used to determine the VPT for each foot.

Other tests exist to evaluate impaired neurologic status, and these may be performed in concert with one or more of the examinations above to give an even clearer picture of the patient's degree of sensory loss. These include deep tendon reflexes of patellar and Achilles tendons, sharp dull sensation, two-point discrimination, and sharp-dull sensation. Furthermore, a gross evaluation of a patient's feet may also provide valuable clues as to the patient's overall sensorimotor condition. Atrophy of the intrinsic muscles of the hands and feet is a late-stage condition frequently associated with polyneuropathy. This condition often leads to prominent digits and metatarsal heads, thus (in the face of sensory loss) causing a heightened risk for neuropathic ulceration. Similarly, bleeding into callus is a not uncommon condition associated with neuropathy. When present, the callused tissue (as with all callused tissue) should generally be debrided and inspected for the possible presence of underlying neuropathic ulceration or abscess. Failure to do this could lead to exacerbation of the condition by both covering up a potential fluid collection and further increasing plantar pressure *(8,19–24)* (Fig. 3).

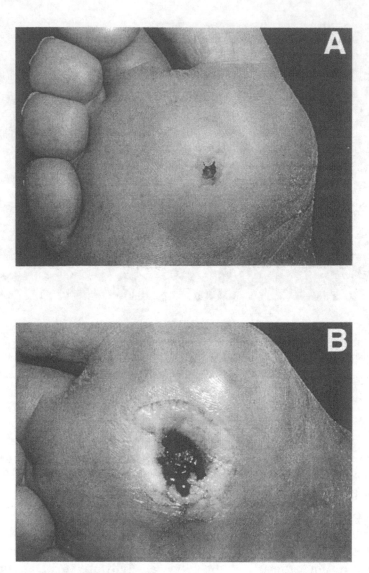

Fig. 3. Hemorrhage into callus (**A**) and subsequent underlying ulceration (**B**). Callus should generally be debrided beneath all pressure points. Not uncommonly, neuropathic patients may show bleeding into callus with an underlying ulceration.

2. Is There Deformity or Limited Joint Mobility?

Neuropathy and foot deformity, when combined with repetitive or constant stress, will ultimately lead to failure of the protective integument and ulceration. Characteristically, the highest plantar pressure is associated with the site of ulceration *(25–29)*. Deformity may be defined as any contracture or prominence that cannot be manually reduced. This is a simple, practical definition that can be used by all clinicians (regardless of specialty) to identify risk. Structural deformity is frequently accompanied by limited joint mobility. Nonenzymatic glycosylation of periarticular soft tissues may

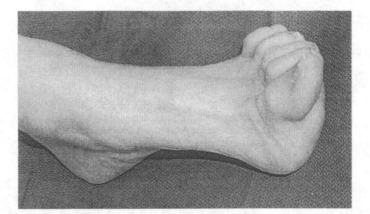

Fig. 4. Intrinsic muscular atrophy and foot deformity. Diabetic peripheral neuropathy also affects motor nerves, often causing atrophy of intrinsic musculature of the hand and foot. When this occurs, the extrinsic musculature works unopposed, thus causing hammering of the toes and retrograde buckling of the metatarsal heads. Thus, both the toes (dorsally) and the metatarsal heads (plantarly) are more prominent and therefore more prone to neuropathic ulceration.

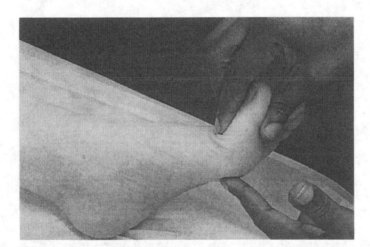

Fig. 5. Evaluation of first metatarsophalangeal joint dorsiflexion (limited joint mobility). Limited joint mobility is frequently encountered in patients with long-standing diabetes. This is most significant in the ankle joint (equinus) and in the forefoot. Less than 50 degrees of dorsiflexion at the first metatarsal phalangeal joint indicates clinically significant limited joint mobility.

limit joint motion in the person with diabetes, and neuropathy can lead to atrophy of the intrinsic musculature, which can cause hammering of digits *(30–32)* (Fig. 4). Limitation of motion reduces the foot's ability to accommodate for ambulatory ground reactive force and therefore increases plantar pressures *(33–37)*. We define limited joint mobility as simply <50 degrees of non-weight-bearing passive dorsiflexion of the hallux *(7,38)* (Fig. 5). Additionally, glycosylation may deleteriously affect the resiliency of the Achilles tendon, thereby pulling the foot into equinus and potentially further increasing the risk for both ulceration and Charcot arthropathy (Fig. 6).

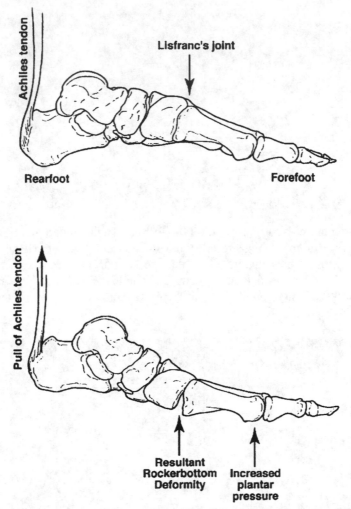

Fig. 6. Equinus and its relationship to elevated forefoot plantar pressure and Charcot arthropathy. Shortening or loss of natural extensibility of the Achilles tendon may lead to pulling of the foot into plantarflexion. This leads to increased forefoot pressure (increasing risk for plantar ulceration) and, in some patients, may be a component of midfoot collapse and Charcot arthropathy.

3. Is There a Previous History of Ulceration or Amputation?

A past history of previous ulceration or amputation heightens the risk for further ulceration, infection, and subsequent amputation *(1,7,39)*. This is generally caused by three key factors. First, following an ulceration, the skin plantar to that site may be less well fortified to accept repetitive stress and therefore more prone to subsequent breakdown. Second, persons with a partial foot amputation often develop local foot deformities secondary to biomechanical imbalances that may cause further foci of pressure *(40–42)* (Fig. 7). Certainly, those with a high-level amputation (below or above the knee) tend to be much more reliant on their remaining limb for transfer or ambulation and therefore may increase risk for tissue breakdown. Last, and perhaps most important, people with a history of ulceration or amputation have in general all the risk factors to reulcerate. This is evidenced by the fact that up to 6 in 10 persons with a history of ulceration will develop another one within 1 year of wound healing *(43,44)*.

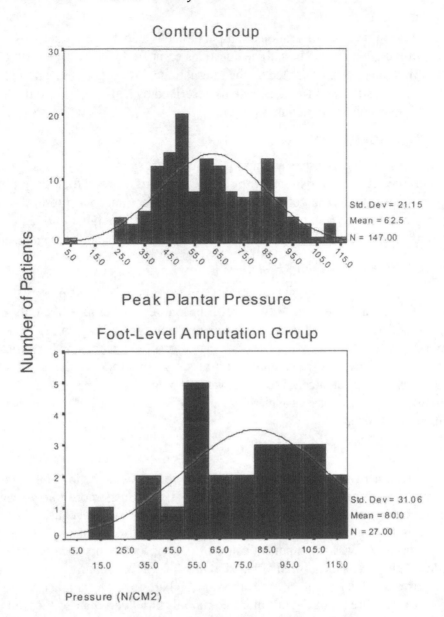

Fig. 7. Plantar pressures are higher following foot-level amputation. Partial foot amputation changes the architecture of the foot and therefore may affect its intrinsic stability. These histograms depict a generalized increase in peak plantar pressures in patients with diabetes who have undergone a foot-level amputation. (From: Armstrong DG, Lavery LA. Plantar pressures are higher in diabetic patients following partial foot amputation. *Ostomy Wound Manage* 1998; 44:30–32, 34, 36 passim.)

Cumulative Risk

When these three questions have been answered, one may then begin to assess degree of risk for ulceration. Lavery and co-workers *(7)* reported that the patient with neuropathy but no deformity or history of ulcer or amputation manifests a 1.7 times greater risk for ulceration compared with a patient without neuropathy. Neuropathy with concomitant deformity or limited joint mobility yields a 12.1 times greater risk. Lastly, the patient with a history of previous ulceration or amputation has a 36.4 times greater risk for presenting with another ulcer. These three questions compare to the first four categories in the classification system promoted by the International Working Group on the Diabetic Foot *(45)* and similar classification systems described by Rith-Najarian and coworkers *(46)* and Armstrong and colleagues *(47)*.

What About Vascular Disease?

Although vascular disease is an important factor that should be thoroughly assessed, it is generally not a strong risk factor for development of diabetic foot ulceration. It is, however, a powerful risk factor for *nonhealing of an ulcer* once it is present, and therefore it is a risk factor for amputation. This may be true for a number of other comorbid conditions once associated with ulcer development such as renal disease and smoking.

Assessment for Amputation Risk

Three key risk factors for lower extremity amputation include the presence of ulceration, infection, and ischemia. However, of these three, ischemia is the only one that can, in and of itself, precipitate a primary amputation. The other two factors rely on a host of concomitant or preceding factors to develop. For instance, most ulcers are preceded by neuropathy, deformity, and repetitive stress. In turn, most diabetic foot infections are preceded by an ulcer. Therefore, we will pragmatically discuss assessment for amputation risk in parts: assessment of vascular disease and assessment/classification of diabetic foot ulcers.

VASCULAR EVALUATION

Certainly, macrovascular disease is more common in the diabetic population. Commensurately, peripheral vascular disease (PVD) is five times more likely than in the nondiabetic population *(48)*. However, PVD is not the commonest cause of foot ulceration and is the underlying cause in only about one-fourth of all cases *(49,50)*. In a recent report, PVD was a component cause in 30% of foot ulcers seen in a two-center study *(8)*. The vessels most often affected in the diabetic are mainly in the calf including the posterior tibial, peroneal, and anterior tibial arteries. The smaller distal vessels (digital arteries) are probably not more commonly involved than in the nondiabetic population.

Claudication is the earliest symptom of peripheral vascular disease. It often later progresses to pain at rest. Often it may be difficult to make a distinction between painful neuropathy, necessitating a careful history and physical examination. Vascular assessment must include palpation of all lower extremity pulses. The femoral, popliteal, posterior tibial, and dorsalis pedis pulses may be examined. However, the presence of palpable pulses does not absolutely exclude peripheral vascular disease. Ankle brachial pressure index (ABPI) is a simple and easily reproducible method of diagnosing vascular insufficiency in the lower limbs. The ABPI is obtained by dividing the ankle by the brachial systolic pressures; the normal value is ≥ 0.95 *(51)*. The blood pressure at the ankle (dorsalis pedis or posterior tibial arteries) is measured using a Doppler ultrasound machine (Huntleigh Nesbit Evans Healthcare, UK). However, a normal ABPI may be deceiving, as medial arterial calcification of the foot vessels results in hardening of the arteries, which gives a falsely elevated ABPI. One can also assess the peripheral circulation by measuring the toe systolic pressure using either a strain-gauge sensor or a photoplethys-mograph, with a normal value considered one in excess of 4 kPa *(52,53)*. Trancutaneous oxygen tension (normal >40 mmHg) measurement has been used as a noninvasive measurement of limb perfusion *(54)*. Patients with occlusive disease have significantly reduced trancutaneous oxygen tension and this has been used to determine the possibility of ulcer and optimal amputation healing. Laboratory assessment of the peripheral circulation includes ultrasonic duplex scanning, color Doppler flow studies, and peripheral arteriograms. Peripheral angiogram is the gold standard for diagnosing vascular disease in the diabetic patient and also for planning vascular reconstruction. All these modalities, however, have significant limitations, not the least of which may be differences in technique and operator error. Therefore, a combination of modalities and detailed physical examination is always better than reliance on laboratory studies in isolation.

RISK FACTORS FOR AMPUTATION: ASSESSING AND CLASSIFYING THE WOUND

The importance of speaking a common language when communicating risk in the diabetic foot cannot be overstated. This tenet is most important when treating acute diabetic sequelae, such as the diabetic wound. A classification system, if it is to be clinically useful, should be easy to use, reproducible, and effective to communicate accurately the status of wounds in persons with diabetes mellitus. A variety of variables could be included in such a system, such as faulty wound healing, compliance issues, quality of wound granulation tissue, host immunity, nutritional status, and comorbidities. However, most of these variables are difficult to measure or categorize and can truly complicate a system. In contrast, three well-documented, relatively quantifiable factors associated with poor wound healing and amputation include depth of the wound *(55,56)*, presence of infection, and presence of concomitant ischemia *(57,58)*.

Although clearly important, a classification system has little value if the clinician using it does not approach each wound in a stepwise consistent, logical fashion. To that end, let us review such an approach.

Seven Essential Questions to Ask When Assessing a Diabetic Foot Wound

When using this approach, the first four questions are useful in terms of their descriptive value. The last three questions are most useful for their predictive qualities.

1. Where Is It Located?

Location of a wound and its etiology go hand in hand. Generally, wounds on the medial aspect of the foot are caused by constant low pressure (e.g., tight shoes), whereas wounds on the plantar aspect of the foot are caused by repetitive moderate pressure (e.g., repetitive stress on prominent metatarsal heads during ambulation).

2. How Large Is It?

Size of the wound plays a key role in determining duration to wound healing. To simplify wound diameter measurements, one may trace the wound on sterile acetate sheeting and tape this tracing into the chart (Fig. 8). The tracing can also be performed on the outer wrapping of an instrument sterilization pack (which would otherwise be

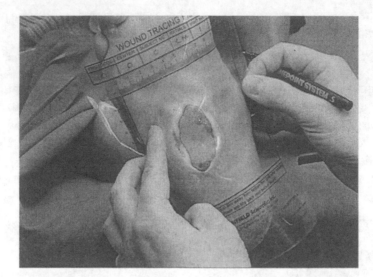

Fig. 8. Tracing the wound using a sterile acetate sheet. Wound tracing may yield far more reproducible results in measuring wound size than simply length by width measurement.

discarded). Recently, many centers have begun employing digital photography and computer-driven planimetric wound area calculations. This provides for potentially more consistent, accurate measurements and, ultimately, for comparison of wound healing rates with other centers regionally and beyond. In an evaluation of the reproducibility of wound measurement techniques, Wunderlich and co-workers *(59)* reported that wound tracing and digital planimetric assessment were by far more reliable than manual measurement of length and width.

3. What Does the Base Look Like?

When describing the base of a wound, one may use terms like granular, fibrotic, or necrotic. One may record the presence or absence of any drainage, which may be described as serous or purulent, with a further description of any odor or color, as necessary.

4. What Do the Margins Look Like?

The margins tell us a lot about the wound. If adequately debrided and off-loaded, they should adhere well to the surface of the underlying subcuticular structures, with a gentle slope toward normal epithelium. However, in the inadequately debrided, inadequately off-loaded wound, undermining of the leading edge normally predominates. This is caused by the *edge effect*, which dictates that an interruption in any matrix (in this case, skin), magnifies both vertical and shear stress on the edges of that interruption. This subsequently causes shearing from the underlying epithelium (making the wound larger by undermining) and increased vertical pressure (making the wound progressively deeper). If appropriately debrided and off-loaded, this effect will be mitigated. Nonetheless, the margins of the wound should be classified as undermining, adherent, macerated, and/or nonviable.

Subsequent to the first questions, which we term "descriptive," come the last three questions, which we term "classifiers." These classifiers can then be used to fit a patient into the University of Texas wound classification system (Table 1). This system has

Table 1
University of Texas Wound Classification System

Stage	Grade			
	0	1	2	3
A	Pre- or postulcerative lesion completely epithelialized	Superficial wound, not involving tendon, capsule, or bone	Wound penetrating to tendon or capsule	Wound penetrating to bone or joint
B	With infection	With infection	With infection	With infection
C	With ischemia	With ischemia	With ischemia	With ischemia
D	With infection and ischemia	With infection and ischemia	With infection and ischemia	With infection and ischemia

Table 2
Meggitt Wagner Wound Classification System

1. Superficial wound
2. Penetrates to tendon or bone
3. Deep with osteitis
4. Partial foot gangrene
5. Whole foot gangrene

evolved as a significant modification of the Wagner system (Table 2) to include concomitant depth, infection, and ischemia. Although both systems have been shown to be predictive of poor outcomes, the UT system has been shown to be significantly more predictive and complete *(60,61)*. Both, however, may be considered useful in a clinical scenario, depending on the preference of the clinician.

5. How Deep Is It? Are Underlying Structures Involved?

These two questions are closely related. Depth of the wound is the most commonly utilized descriptor in wound classification. Wounds are graded by depth. Grade 0 represents a pre- or postulcerative site. Grade 1 ulcers are superficial wounds through the epidermis or epidermis and dermis but do not penetrate tendon, capsule, or bone. Grade 2 wounds penetrate tendon or capsule. Grade 3 wounds penetrate bone or a joint. We have known for some time that wounds penetrating to bone are frequently osteomyelitic *(55)*. Additionally, we have observed that morbid outcomes are intimately associated with progressive wound depth.

Depth of the wound and involvement of underlying structures may best be appreciated through the use of a sterile blunt metallic probe (Fig. 9). The instrument is gently inserted into the wound and the dimensions of the wound explored. Additionally, bony involvement is typically readily appreciable thorough this method.

6. Is It Infected?

The definition of infection is not an easy one. Cultures, laboratory values, and subjective symptoms are all helpful. However, the diagnosis of an infection's genesis and resolution has and continues to be a clinical one. Although criteria for infection may be something less than clear-cut, there is little question that presence of infection is a

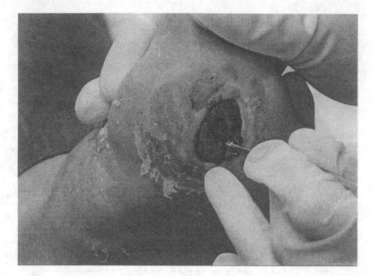

Fig. 9. Use of a sterile blunt instrument to probe wound. Probing the wound both for the sub-dermal dimensions and for involvement of underlying structures is an important part of wound assessment. Palpation of bone in a wound is strongly suggestive of osteomyelitis and should prompt further inspection.

prime cause of lower extremity morbidity and frequently evolves into wet gangrene and subsequent amputation. Therefore, in an effort to facilitate communication and effect consistent results, the foot care team should agree on criteria for this very important risk factor.

7. Is It Ischemic?

As discussed above, identification of ischemia is of utmost importance when evaluating a wound. If pulses are not palpable, or if a wound is slow to heal even in the face of appropriate off-loading and local wound care, noninvasive vascular studies are warranted, followed by a prompt vascular surgery consultation and possible intervention to improve perfusion and thereby effect healing.

SUMMARY

In conclusion, consistent, thoughtful assessment of the diabetic foot is of central importance in identifying risk for both ulceration and amputation (Fig. 10). Subsequent to the gathering of clinical data through sequential assessment, appropriate classification of the wound becomes paramount in our efforts to document and communicate the

Fig. 10. Flowchart for screening and treatment of the diabetic foot. This flowchart is adapted from the University of Texas Diabetic Foot Risk Classification and International Working Group on the Diabetic Foot Risk Classification systems. It is designed to assess comprehensively for risk of diabetic foot ulceration and amputation. The clinician begins by asking questions to assess for risk for amputation (ischemia, infection, and ulceration). Subsequently, the clinician may

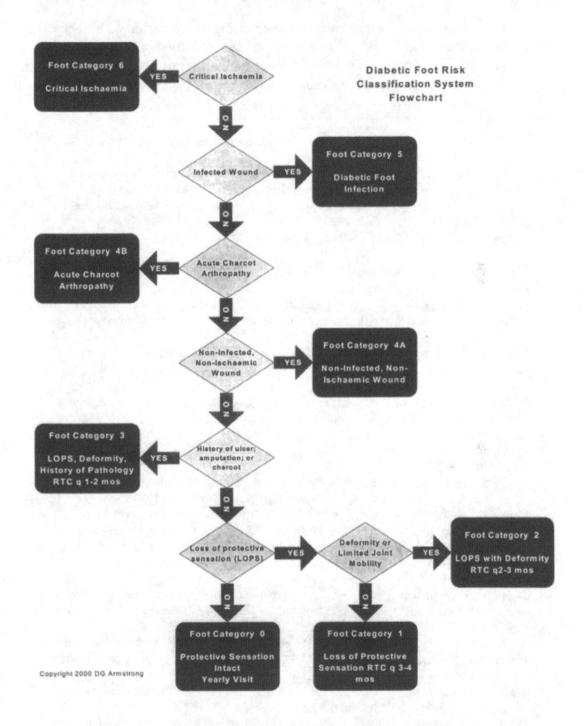

Diabetic Foot Risk Classification System Flowchart

Foot Category 6 — Critical Ischaemia

Critical Ischaemia — YES

Infected Wound — YES — Foot Category 5 — Diabetic Foot Infection

Acute Charcot Arthropathy — YES — Foot Category 4B — Acute Charcot Arthropathy

Non-Infected, Non-Ischaemic Wound — YES — Foot Category 4A — Non-Infected, Non-Ischaemic Wound

History of ulcer; amputation; or charcot — YES — Foot Category 3 — LOPS, Deformity, History of Pathology RTC q 1-2 mos

Loss of protective sensation (LOPS) — YES — Deformity or Limited Joint Mobility — YES — Foot Category 2 — LOPS with Deformity RTC q2-3 mos

Foot Category 0 — Protective Sensation Intact Yearly Visit

Foot Category 1 — Loss of Protective Sensation RTC q 3-4 mos

Copyright 2000 DG Armstrong

ask questions related to ulcer risk (neuropathy, deformity, history of previous ulcer or amputation). RTC, return to clinic for follow-up appointment. LOPS, loss of protective sensation (10-g monofilament). Patients with critical ischemia = prompt vascular surgery consultation. Patients with diabetic foot infection = consider infectious disease and/or surgical consultation. Patients with Charcot arthropathy = consider podiatric or orthopedic foot specialist evaluation. Patients with noninfected, nonischemic ulcers = consider frequent debridement, off-loading, and dressing of the wound by foot specialist. Patients in categories 0–3 should have regular preventative podiatric care.

level of risk to all members of the health care team caring for the person with diabetes. When this is accomplished, we believe that a significant reduction in lower extremity complications can indeed be realized locally. With dissemination of the tools and techniques for consistent examination, we believe that a global impact is well within reach.

REFERENCES

1. Pecoraro RE, Reiber GE, Burgess EM. Pathways to diabetic limb amputation: basis for prevention. *Diabetes Care* 1990;13:513–521.
2. Mayfield JA, Reiber GE, Sanders LJ, Janisse D, Pogach LM. Preventive foot care in people with diabetes [see comments]. *Diabetes Care* 1998;21:2161–2177.
3. Reiber GE. Diabetic foot care: financial implications and practice guidelines. *Diabetes Care* 1992;15(Suppl 1):29–31.
4. Reiber GE. Who is at risk of limb loss and what to do about it? *J Rehabil Res Dev* 1994;31: 357–362.
5. King H, Aubert RE, Herman WH. Global burden of diabetes, 1995–2025: prevalence, numerical estimates, and projections [see comments]. *Diabetes Care* 1998;21:1414–1431.
6. Abbott CA, Vileikyte L, Williamson S, Carrington AL, Boulton AJ. Multicenter study of the incidence of and predictive risk factors for diabetic neuropathic foot ulceration. *Diabetes Care* 1998;21:1071–1075.
7. Lavery LA, Armstrong DG, Vela SA, Quebedeaux TL, Fleischli JG. Practical criteria for screening patients at high risk for diabetic foot ulceration. *Arch Intern Med* 1998;158: 158–162.
8. Reiber GE, Vileikyte L, Boyko EJ, et al. Causal pathways for incident lower-extremity ulcers in patients with diabetes from two settings. *Diabetes Care* 1999;22:157–162.
9. Armstrong DG, Lavery LA, Vela SA, Quebedeaux TL, Fleischli JG. Choosing a practical screening instrument to identify patients at risk for diabetic foot ulceration. *Arch Intern Med* 1998;158:289–292.
10. Bloom S, Till S, Sönsken P, Smith S. Use of a biothesiometer to measure individual vibration thresholds and their variation in 519 non-diabetic subjects. *BMJ* 1984;288:1793–1795.
11. Young MJ, Breddy JL, Veves A, Boulton AJM. The prediction of diabetic neuropathic foot ulceration using vibration perception thresholds. *Diabetes Care* 1994;16:557–560.
12. Young MJ, Every N, Boulton AJ. A comparison of the neurothesiometer and biothesiometer for measuring vibration perception in diabetic patients. *Diabetes Res Clin Pract* 1993; 20:129–131.
13. Boulton AJ. Guidelines for diagnosis and outpatient management of diabetic peripheral neuropathy. European Association for the Study of Diabetes, EURODIAB. *Diabetes Metab* 1998;24(Suppl 3):55–65.
14. Kumar S, Fernando DJ, Veves A, et al. Semmes-Weinstein monofilaments: a simple, effective and inexpensive screening device for identifying diabetic patients at risk of foot ulceration. *Diabetes Res Clin Pract* 1991;13:63–67.
15. Mueller MJ. Identifying patients with diabetes who are at risk for lower extremity complications: use of Semmes-Weinstein monofilaments. *Phys Ther* 1996;76:68–71.
16. Olmos PR, Cataland S, O'Dorisio TM, et al. The Semmes-Weinstein monofilament as a potential predictor of foot ulceration in patients with non-insulin dependent diabetes. *Am J Med Sci* 1995;309:76–82.
17. Booth J, Young MJ. Differences in performance of commercially available 10-g monofilaments. *Diabetes Care* 2000;23:984–988.
18. Armstrong DG. The 10-g monofilament: the diagnostic divining rod for the diabetic foot? [editorial] [In Process Citation]. *Diabetes Care* 2000;23:887.
19. Murray HJ, Young MJ, Hollis S, Boulton AJ. The association between callus formation, high pressures and neuropathy in diabetic foot ulceration. *Diabet Med* 1996;13:979–982.

20. Young MJ, Cavanagh PR, Thomas G, et al. The effect of callus removal on dynamic plantar foot pressures in diabetic patients. *Diabet Med* 1992;9:55–57.

21. Pitei DL, Foster A, Edmonds M. The effect of regular callus removal on foot pressures. *J Foot Ankle Surg* 1999;38:251-255; discussion 306.

22. Collier JH, Brodbeck CA. Assessing the diabetic foot: plantar callus and pressure sensation. *Diabetes Educ* 1993;19:503–508.

23. Rosen RC, Davids MS, Bohanske LM, Lemont H. Hemorrhage into plantar callus and diabetes mellitus. *Cutis* 1985;35:339–341.

24. Ahroni JH, Boyko EJ, Forsberg RC. Clinical correlates of plantar pressure among diabetic veterans. *Diabetes Care* 1999;22:965–972.

25. Boulton AJ, Betts RP, Franks CI, Ward JD, Duckworth T. The natural history of foot pressure abnormalities in neuropathic diabetic subjects. *Diabetes Res* 1987;5:73.

26. Duckworth T, Betts RP, Franks CI, Burke J. The measurement of pressure under the foot. *Foot Ankle* 1982;3:130.

27. Armstrong DG, Lavery LA, Bushman TR. Peak foot pressures influence healing time of diabetic ulcers treated with total contact casting. *J Rehabil Res Dev* 1998;35:1–5.

28. Cavanagh PR, Ulbrecht JS, Caputo GM. Biomechanical aspects of diabetic foot disease: aetiology, treatment, and prevention. *Diabet Med* 1996;13(Suppl 1):S17–S22.

29. Birke JA, Novick ES, Hawkins ES, Patout C. A review of causes of foot ulceration in patients with diabetes mellitus. *J Prosthet Orthot* 1991;4:13–16.

30. Grant WP, Sullivan R, Soenshine DE, et al. Electron microscopic investigation of the effects of diabetes mellitus on the Achilles tendon. *J Foot Ankle Surg* 1997;36:272–278.

31. Rosenbloom AL, Silverstein JH, Lexotte DC. Limited joint mobility in childhood diabetics indicates increased risk for microvascular diseases. *N Engl J Med* 1982;305:191–194.

32. Rosenbloom AL. Skeletal and joint manifestations of childhood diabetes. *Pediatr Clin North Am* 1984;31:569–589.

33. Birke JA, Franks D, Foto JG. First ray joint limitation, pressure, and ulceration of the first metatarsal head in diabetes mellitus. *Foot Ankle* 1995;16:277–284.

34. Lavery LA, Lavery DC, Quebedeax-Farnham TL. Increased foot pressures after great toe amputation in diabetes. *Diabetes Care* 1995;18:1460–462.

35. Frykberg RG, Lavery LA, Pham H, et al. Role of neuropathy and high foot pressures in diabetic foot ulceration [In Process Citation]. *Diabetes Care* 1998;21:1714–1719.

36. Fernando DJS, Masson EA, Veves A, Boulton AJM. Relationship of limited joint mobility to abnormal foot pressures and diabetic foot ulceration. *Diabetes Care* 1991;14:8–11.

37. Armstrong DG, Stacpoole-Shea S, Nguyen HC, Harkless LB. Lengthening of the Achilles tendon in diabetic patients who are at high risk for ulceration of the foot. *J Bone Joint Surg [Am]* 1999;81A:535–538.

38. Birke J, Cornwall MA, Jackson M. Relationship between hallux limitus and ulceration of the great toe. *Sports Phys Ther J Orthop* 1988;10:172–176.

39. Goldner MG. The fate of the second leg in the diabetic amputee. *Diabetes* 1960;9:100–103.

40. Armstrong DG, Lavery LA. Plantar pressures are higher in diabetic patients following partial foot amputation. *Ostomy Wound Manage* 1998;44:30–32, 34, 36 passim.

41. Quebedeaux TL, Lavery LA, Lavery DC. The development of foot deformities and ulcers after great toe amputation in diabetes. *Diabetes Care* 1996;19:165–167.

42. Murdoch DP, Armstrong DG, Dacus JB, et al. The natural history of great toe amputations. *J Foot Ankle Surg* 1997;36:204–208.

43. Uccioli L, Faglia E, Monticone G, et al. Manufactured shoes in the prevention of diabetic foot ulcers. *Diabetes Care* 1995;18:1376–378.

44. Helm PA, Walker SC, Pulliam GF. Recurrence of neuropathic ulcerations following healing in a total contact cast. *Arch Phys Med Rehabil* 1991;72:967–970.

45. International Working Group on the Diabetic Foot. *International Consensus on the Diabetic Foot*. EASD, Amsterdam, 1999.

46. Rith-Najarian SJ, Stolusky T, Gohdes DM. Identifying diabetic patients at risk for lower extremity amputation in a primary health care setting. *Diabetes Care* 1992;15:1386–1389.
47. Armstrong DG, Lavery LA, Harkless LB. Who's at risk for diabetic foot ulceration? *Clin Podiatr Med Surg* 1998;15:11–19.
48. Steiner G. Diabetes and atherosclerosis; epidemiology and intervention trials, in *Atherosclerosis X* (Woodford FP, Davingnon J, Sniderman A, eds.), Elsevier, Amsterdam, 1995, pp. 13–93.
49. Edmonds ME. Experience in a multidisciplinary diabetic foot clinic, in *The Foot in Diabetes* (Connor H, Boulton AJM, Ward JD, eds.), John Wiley & Sons, New York, 1987, pp. 121–131.
50. Thompson FJ, Veves A, Ashe H, et al. A team approach to diabetic foot care—the Manchester experience. *Foot* 1991;1:75–82.
51. Weitz JI, Byrne J, Clagett GP, et al. Diagnosis and treatment of chronic arterial insufficiency of the lower extremities: a critical review. *Circulation* 1996;94:3026–3049.
52. Holstein P, Lassen NA. Healing of ulcers on the feet correlated with distal blood pressure measurements in occlusive arterial disease. *Acta Orthop Scand* 1980;51:995–1006.
53. Orchard TJ, Strandness DE. Assessment of peripheral vascular disease in diabetes: report and recommendation of an international workshop. *Diabetes Care* 1993;83:685–695.
54. Franzeck UK, Talke P, Bernstein EF, Golbranson FL, Fronek A. Transcutaneous PO_2 measurements in health and peripheral arterial occlusive disease. *Surgery* 1982;91:156–163.
55. Grayson ML, Balaugh K, Levin E, Karchmer AW. Probing to bone in infected pedal ulcers. A clinical sign of underlying osteomyelitis in diabetic patients. *JAMA* 1995;273:721–723.
56. Birke JA, Novick A, Patout CA, Coleman WC. Healing rates of plantar ulcers in leprosy and diabetes. *Lepr Rev* 1992;63:365–374.
57. Reiber GE, Pecoraro RE, Koepsell TD. Risk factors for amputation in patients with diabetes mellitus: a case control study. *Ann Intern Med* 1992;117:97–105.
58. Mayfield JA, Reiber GE, Nelson RG, Greene T. A foot risk classification system to predict diabetic amputation in pima indians. *Diabetes Care* 1996;19:704–709.
59. Wunderlich RP, Peters EJ, Armstrong DG, Lavery LA. Reliability of digital videometry and acetate tracing in measuring the surface area of cutaneous wounds. *Diabetes Res Clin Pract* 2000;49:87–92.
60. Armstrong DG, Lavery LA, Harkless LB. Validation of a diabetic wound classification system: the contribution of depth, infection, and vascular disease to the risk of amputation. *Diabetes Care* 1998;21:855–859.
61. Oyibo SO, Jude EB, Tarawneh I, et al. A comparison of two diabetic foot ulcer classification systems. *Diabetes* 2000;49(Suppl 1):A33.
62. Armstrong DG, Lavery LA. Diabetic foot ulcers: prevention, diagnosis and classification. *Am Fam Physician* 1988;57:1325–1332, 1337–1338.

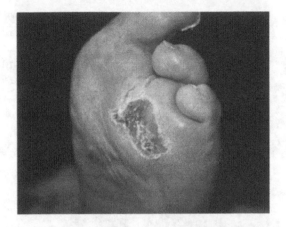

Color Plate 1. Diabetic foot with plantar callus. (*Fig. 1, Chapter 13; see* discussion on pp. 252–253.)

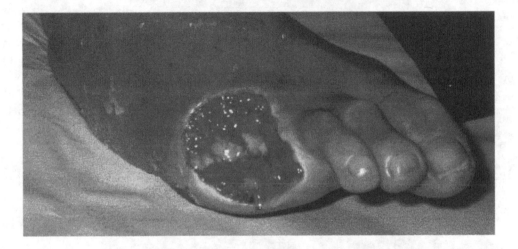

Color Plate 2. Diabetic foot post surgical debridement. (*Fig. 3, Chapter 13; see discussion* on pp. 254–255.)

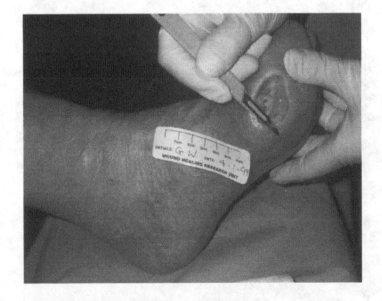

Color Plate 3. Sharp debridement of diabetic foot ulcer. (*Fig. 4, Chapter 13; see* discussion on pp. 254–255.)

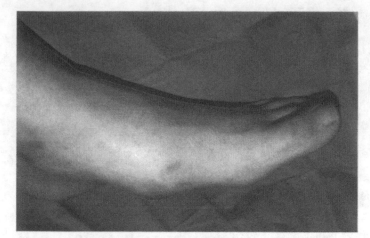

Color Plate 4. A grade 0 foot with callous formation is indicative of high foot pressures, requiring treatment and accommodation with orthotic devices. (*Fig. 2, Chapter 14*; *see* discussion on pp. 280–281.)

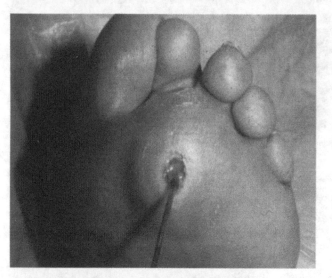

Color Plate 5. The presence of synovial drainage from an ulceration is indicative of joint involvement and requires resection of that joint. (*Fig. 3, Chapter 15; see* discussion on p. 297).

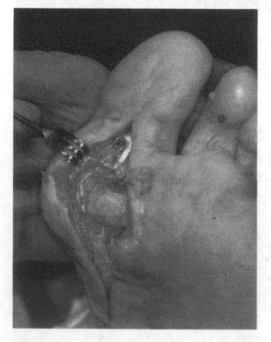

Color Plate 6. Osteomyelitis of the first metatarsophalangeal joint is best addressed by elliptical excision of the ulcer with resection of the joint. Adequate resection of the first metatarsal should be performed to assure complete eradication of the infected bone. (*Fig. 4, Chapter 15; see* discussion on pp. 297–299.)

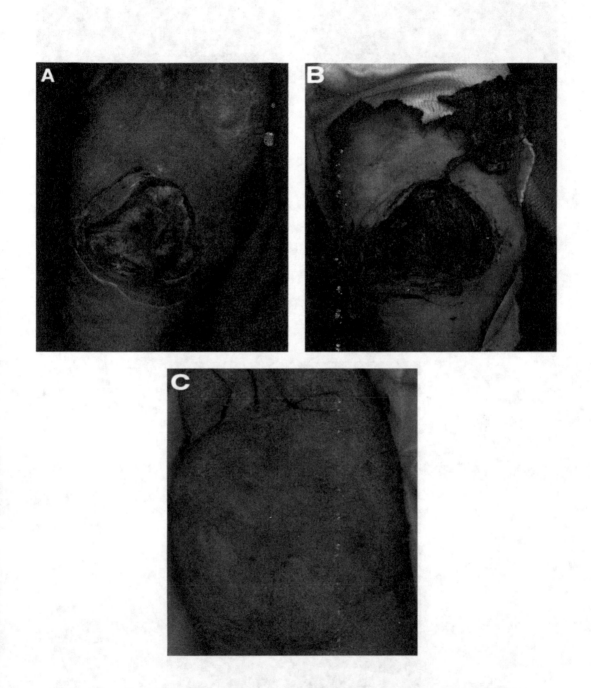

Color Plate 7. (**A**) Infection of midfoot with full-thickness necrosis of skin, subcutaneous tissue, and plantar aponeurosis. (**B**) Intraoperative view showing excised plantar fascia and intact flexor digitorum brevis muscle. (**C**) Skin grafted directly to muscle provided stable coverage. (*Fig. 11, Chapter 17; see* discussion on p. 361.)

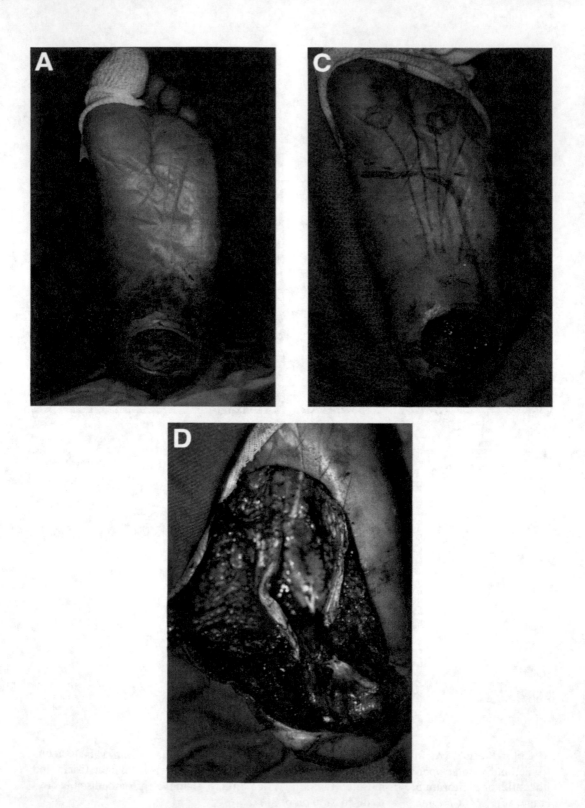

Color Plate 8. (**A**) Example of frequently encountered neuropathic ulcer, involving most of weight-bearing heel. (**C**) After debridement of bone and soft tissue, a thin skin flap was designed for rotation; the distal incision is at least 3 cm posterior to metatarsal heads. (**D**) Skin flap elevated, and flexor brevis muscle transposed into ulcer. (*Fig. 16, Chapter 17; see discussion on p. 366.*)

10

Radiographic Changes of the Diabetic Foot

Yvonne Cheung, MD, Mary Hochman, MD,
and David P. Brophy, MD, FFRRCSI, FRCR, MSCVIR

INTRODUCTION

Foot infections are among the most common causes of hospitalization in the diabetic population, accounting for 20% of all diabetes-related admissions. Complicated foot infections may require treatment by amputation—as many as 6–10% of all diabetic patients will undergo amputation for treatment of infection *(1–3)*, accounting for 57% of nontraumatic lower extremity amputations *(4–6)*. The scope of the problem is compelling. Infections and complicated vascular diabetic foot problems result in 50,000 amputations a year in the United States *(7)*. The Centers for Disease Control and Prevention (CDC) estimated the annual treatment cost of amputees within this group at $1.2 billion for the year 1997. However, this figure does not include the cost of rehabilitation, prosthetic devices, or lost income *(8)*. These treatment costs are likely to escalate, as the prevalence of diabetes is on the rise. The latest epidemiology study shows an increase of the overall prevalence of diabetes from 4.9% in 1990 to 6.5% in 1998 *(9)*.

Information derived from imaging studies can play an important role in management of complicated foot problems in the diabetic patient. Soft tissue abnormalities such as abscesses and cellulitis can be identified, osteomyelitis may be detected, the extent of abnormal marrow can be depicted, neuroarthropathic changes can be diagnosed and followed over time, distribution of atherosclerotic lesions can be noninvasively mapped, and the effectiveness of revascularizaton procedures can be evaluated. A variety of studies are currently available for imaging the diabetic foot. To use these imaging studies effectively, it is important to understand the unique strengths and weaknesses of each modality, as they apply to the particular clinical problem in question. The goal of this chapter is to review the modalities available for imaging of the diabetic foot infection and to highlight their relative utilities in clinical problem solving.

INFECTION IN THE DIABETIC FOOT

Risk Factors

Many factors contribute to infection in the diabetic foot including peripheral neuropathy *(10)* and vascular insufficiency *(11)*. Repetitive minor trauma to an insensitive neuropathic foot, exacerbated by abnormal biomechanics or ill-fitting shoes, causes

From: *The Diabetic Foot: Medical and Surgical Management*
Edited by: A. Veves, J. M. Giurini, and F. W. LoGerfo © Humana Press Inc., Totowa, NJ

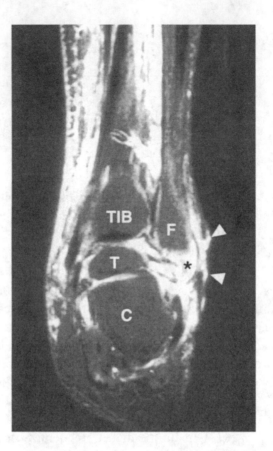

Fig. 1. Osteomyelitis deep to ulcer on MRI. Coronal STIR image of the left foot of a diabetic patient shows an area of marrow edema (*) at the tip of the fibula (F). Overlying this focus of abnormal marrow is an ulcer surrounded by diffuse soft tissue swelling (arrowheads). These findings represent osteomyelitis. C, calcaneus; TIB, tibia; T, talus.

areas of increased plantar pressure to develop calluses that predispose to ulcer development. Deep to the callus and clinically occult, an ulcer forms insidiously *(12,13)*. Direct extension of infected ulcers or soft tissue infection leads to osteomyelitis *(14)* (Fig. 1). These infections are usually polymicrobial and involve both anaerobic and aerobic pathogens.

Soft Tissue Abnormalities

Soft tissue abnormalities associated with the diabetic foot include soft tissue edema, cellulitis, abscess, ulcers, sinus tracts, tenosynovitis, joint effusions, and arthritis *(15–17)*. The importance of differentiating these conditions lies in their differing management: abscess necessitates prompt surgical drainage, septic arthritis requires surgical debridement, and cellulitis generally entails antibiotic therapy.

Soft tissue edema and swelling are common findings in the diabetic patient. Soft tissue swelling can occur in the absence of infection, owing to vascular insufficiency or peripheral neuropathy *(17)* (Fig. 2). However, soft tissue swelling can also reflect the presence of cellulitis, that is, soft tissue infection of the superficial soft tissues. Cellulitis

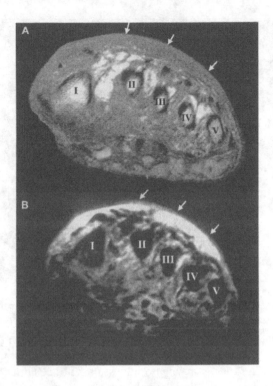

Fig. 2. Dorsal soft tissue swelling in a diabetic patient. Coronal MR (**A**) T1-weighted and (**B**) STIR images acquired at the level of the midmetatarsal shafts show diffuse dorsal soft tissue swelling (small arrows). The swelling or edema is dark on T1 (**A**) and bright on STIR (**B**). I–V, first to fifth metatarsals.

along the dorsum of the foot usually occurs secondary to surface infections in the nails, toes, or web spaces. Simple cellulitis is generally diagnosed clinically, without the need for imaging. The major indication for imaging of patients with cellulitis is suspected underlying deep infection, such as soft tissue abscess, osteomyelitis, or septic arthritis.

Osteomyelitis

Osteomyelitis of the foot occurs up to 15% of diabetic patients *(16)*. Bone infection results from local extension of soft tissue infection (Fig. 1). Callus and ulcers serve as the conduit for infection to spread to deep soft tissue compartments, bones, and joints. The most common sites of soft tissue infection and secondary osteomyelitis are foci of increased plantar pressure, such as the metatarsal heads and the calcaneus (Fig. 3). Evaluation of foot ulcers is important because >90% of osteomyelitis cases result from contiguous spread of infection from soft tissue to bone *(7)*. Newman et al. further demonstrate a clear relationship between ulcer depth and osteomyelitis: 100% of the ulcers that expose bone and 82% of the moderately deep-seated ulcers have osteomyelitis on bone biopsy *(2)* (Fig. 1).

Recognition of osteomyelitis in the diabetic foot is difficult both clinically and radiographically. Ability to probe a pedal ulcer through to bone (Fig. 4) has been reported as a useful index of underlying osteomyelitis in a diabetic patient *(18)* and is commonly used to guide decisions regarding treatment. Nonetheless, clinical judgment was shown

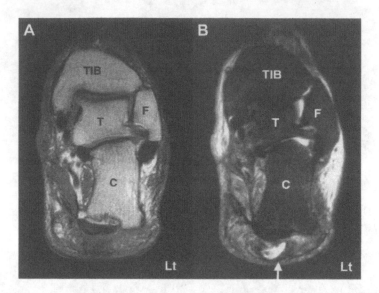

Fig. 3. Deep ulcer and inflammation beneath a focus of high plantar pressure on MRI. A diabetic patient presented with soft tissue swelling and inflammation of the left foot. Coronal T1-weighted (**A**) and STIR (**B**) images of the left ankle show a fluid collection surrounded by an area of inflammation (arrow) in the plantar fat pad. Both the inflammation and fluid collection are dark on T1-weighted (**A**) and of varying brightness on STIR (**B**) images. The overlying skin appears intact. Normal marrow signal in the calcaneus excludes osteomyelitis. F, fibula; TIB, tibia; T, talus.

to be a poor indicator of infection. The technique of probe to bone, only 68% sensitive, may underestimate the incidence of bone involvement, according to Newman et al. *(2)*. In the same study, 18 of 19 pedal ulcers did not expose bone nor display inflammation yet contained osteomyelitis. Other clinical parameters such as fever and leukocytosis are unreliable in the diabetic patient. Only 18% of patients with clinically severe osteomyelitis were febrile *(14)*. Neither fever nor leukocytosis predicts the necessity for surgical exploration *(19)*.

IMAGING MODALITIES

Accurate diagnosis in the diabetic patient translates to differentiation between bone and soft tissue infection, characterization of soft tissue abnormalities, and mapping of atherosclerotic disease for surgical intervention. The imaging modalities that are useful in the evaluation of the diabetic foot infections include radiography, computed tomography (CT), ultrasound (US), skeletal scintigraphy, and magnetic resonance imaging (MRI) and angiography (MRA). Imaging techniques vary in their sensitivity for detection of osteomyelitis, with specificity limited in the presence of cellulitis, peripheral ischemia, and diabetic neuroarthropathy (Table 1). In the appropriate setting, however, noninvasive imaging can aid in diagnosis and treatment planning.

Radiography

Radiography remains the first screening examination in any patient with suspected infection. Calcification in the interdigital arteries identifies an unsuspected diabetic

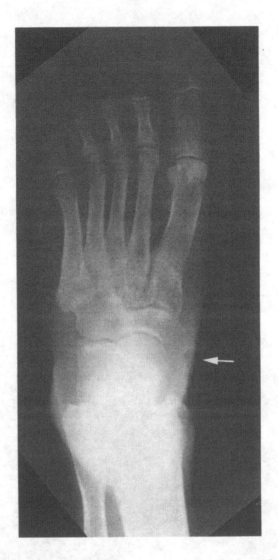

Fig. 4. Osteomyelitis of the navicular on radiography. AP view of the right foot shows a deep ulcer (arrow) surrounding the navicular. The medial cortex of the navicular is destroyed, representing osteomyelitis. On clinical exam, exposed bone was evident at the ulcer.

patient because these vessels rarely calcify in a nondiabetic patient. Gas is readily detected on radiographs (Fig. 5). Denser foreign bodies, such as metal and lead-containing glass, are radioopaque and generally are visible on x-ray. Detection of nonmetallic foreign bodies and subtle soft tissue calcifications may entail radiographs acquired with a soft tissue technique (i.e., using low kV).

Both soft tissue edema and cellulitis display increase density and thickening of the subcutaneous fat. Infection may result in blurring of the usually visible fat planes. Focal fluid and callus will both demonstrate local increased density in the soft tissues. Ulcers may or may not be visible depending on their size and orientation. In general, all these soft tissue abnormalities are more clearly evident at physical exam.

The presence of soft tissue swelling, periosteal new bone formation, cortical bone destruction, focal osteopenia, and permeative radiolucency are diagnostic for osteomy-

Table 1
Compilation of Sensitivity and Specificity
of Various Imaging Modalities in the Diagnosis of Osteomyelitis

	Range of sensitivity (%)	Range of specificity (%)	Compiled sensitivity/ specificity (%/%)	References
Radiography	52–93	33–92	61/72	*(2,20–28)*
Three-phase bone scan in patients without bone complications			94/95	Review of 20 published reports *(29)*
Three-phase bone scan in patients with bone complications			95/33	*(29)*
In-111-labeled WBC	75–100	69–100	93/80	*(8,23,24,30-33)*
Combined gallium and bone scan			81/69	*(29)*
MR imaging	29–100	67–95	96/87	*(8,25,27, 28,34,35)*

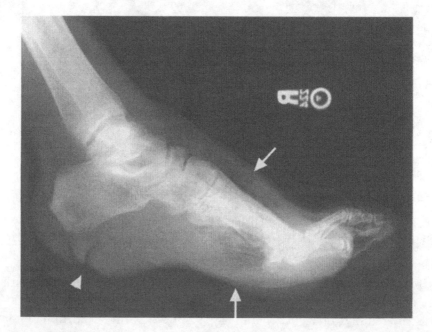

Fig. 5. Soft tissue air and deep ulcers on radiography. The lateral view of the right foot from a diabetic patient shows subcutaneous air (arrows) in both dorsal and plantar soft tissues surrounding the metatarsals. A deep ulcer dissects the heel fat pad (arrowhead).

elitis (Table 2 and Fig. 4). These osseous changes only become evident after osteomyelitis has been present for 10–14 days and require up to a 50% bone loss before becoming image evident *(36)*. Thus, radiography is less sensitive compared with other imaging modalities. Most studies report a sensitivity of 52–93% and a specificity of 33–92% for detection of osteomyelitis (Table 1).

Table 2
Radiographic Findings of Acute Osteomyelitis

Cortical bone destruction

Permeative radiolucency

Focal osteopenia or focal osteolytic lesion

Periosteal new bone formation

Soft tissue swelling

Not restricted to documentation of osteomyelitis, soft tissue abnormalities, and subcutaneous air (Fig. 5), radiographs can demonstrate changes associated with neuroarthropathy. Correlative radiographs, when used as roadmaps for subsequent imaging exams, may clarify postsurgical changes, fractures, foreign bodies, gas, foot deformities, and bony variants. All of these may cause unnecessary confusion on MR or nuclear medicine imaging.

Nuclear Medicine Studies

The three most commonly employed nuclear medicine tests are bone, gallium, and labeled leukocyte studies. All are considered highly sensitive to the presence of both soft tissue infection and osteomyelitis (Table 1). When prior bone changes (i.e., neuroarthropathy, trauma, degenerative changes) are present, indium-labeled leukocyte scan provides the best overall sensitivity and specificity (Table 1).

Three-Phase Technetium Bone Scan

Traditionally, triple-phase bone scan (TPBS) has been the test used for the workup of suspected osteomyelitis in patients with negative radiographs. TPBS involves intravenous injection of radioactive technetium-99m methylene diphosphonate, followed by imaging with a gamma camera at three distinct time points. Images acquired every 2–5 s immediately following injection provide a radionuclide angiogram (the flow phase) and may demonstrate asymmetrically increased blood flow to the region of interest. The second (blood pool phase) is obtained within 10 min and reveals soft tissue inflammation. A delayed phase is acquired 2–4 h after the injection. This third phase demonstrates areas of active bone turnover, which have incorporated the radionuclide tracer and are seen as focal hot spots of increased tracer activity. The tracer is taken up by bone in an amount dependent on the degree of osteoblastic activity.

Osteomyelitis results in increased uptake in all three phases, whereas simple cellulitis demonstrates increased uptake in the first two phases (Fig. 6). However, there are many causes of positive bone scans. In general, a positive delay scan is seen when there is an underlying process that promotes bone remodeling, e.g., healing fracture, neuropathic osteoarthropathy, recent surgery. False negatives may occur when the radiotracer fails to reach the foot because of diminished vascular flow. This is of particular concern in the diabetic with atherosclerotic disease.

Schauwecker's *(29)* literature review of 20 published reports shows a compiled mean sensitivity and specificity of 94% and 95%. Unfortunately, these data apply only to patients without previous bone deformities. In the diabetic patient with complicated bone conditions, a more common clinical presentation, the sensitivity remains at 95%, but the

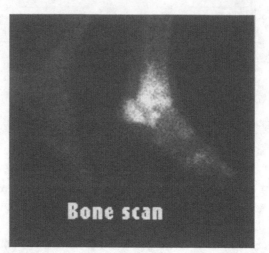

Fig. 6. Osteomyelitis of left tibia. Delayed phase of a three-phase bone scan. This lateral view shows diffuse tracer activity about the ankle joint of a febrile diabetic patient. A similar increase in tracer activity is noted on both the first and second phase (not shown) of the three-phase bone scan. Findings represent osteomyelitis.

specificity declines to 33%. Thus the American College of Radiology (ACR)-sponsored appropriateness criteria for detection of osteomyelitis recommends a TPBS only when there is absence of radiographic findings of bone complications *(37)*. When the bone scan is normal, there is little chance of osteomyelitis, and the investigation can stop at this point. If the bone scan shows a focal abnormality, a subsequent labeled leukocyte study or MRI is necessary. Gallium scan is a good alternative if labeled leukocyte scan or MRI is not available.

Gallium Scan

Gallium-67 citrate localizes in areas of infection. If the gallium scan is normal, osteomyelitis can be excluded. By itself, gallium is not very specific for the diagnosis of osteomyelitis because gallium accumulates not only at sites of infection but also at sites of increased bone remodeling, as seen in trauma *(38)*. Gallium scan images frequently lack spatial resolution, which preclude separation of bone from soft tissue uptake *(28)* (Fig. 7). If the gallium scan is positive, assessment of osteomyelitis requires a supplementary bone scan to improve specificity *(39)*, the rationale of a combined bone/gallium exam being that the uptake on bone scan can be used to account for the bony remodeling portion of the gallium uptake. The criteria for diagnosis of osteomyelitis in a combined bone and gallium exam are summarized in Table 3.

Schauwecker *(29)* showed the sensitivity and specificity of this technique to be 81% and 69%, respectively. However, he also observed that more than half of the combined bone and gallium exams were equivocal. This technique, therefore, is only helpful when the study reads positive or negative. Although the relative high number of equivocal exams makes this modality less advantageous, gallium scan remains a useful alternative if labeled leukocyte scan or MRI is not available.

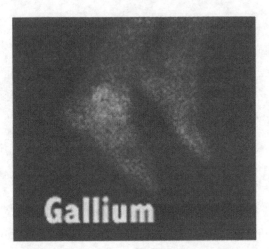

Fig. 7. Osteomyelitis of left tibia: gallium scan. The increase in gallium activity in the distal tibia of a diabetic patient suggests osteomyelitis. However, the lack of resolution of the image precludes separation of bone and soft tissue inflammation.

Table 3
Criteria for a Combined Bone
and Gallium Exam for Diagnosis of Osteomyelitis

Gallium uptake exceeds bone scan uptake

Gallium and bone scan uptake are spatially incongruent

Labeled Leukocyte Scan

Labeled leukocyte scans, also known as labeled white blood cell scans, are performed by extracting patient's blood, fractionating the leukocytes from the blood, incubating the white blood cells with the either indium 111-oxine or technetium-hexamethylpropylene amine oxime (Tc-HMPAO) in order to label them, and then reinjecting the labeled white blood cells into the same patient. Imaging is performed 16–24 h later, using a standard gamma camera. Theoretically, labeled white blood cells only accumulate at sites of infection and not at sites of increased osteoblastic activity and should be extremely useful in the diagnosis of complicated osteomyelitis (Fig. 8).

Indium-labeled leukocyte scan offers the best sensitivity and specificity among the three readily available scintigraphic techniques (Table 1). A compilation of sensitivities and specificities from seven studies reports 93% and 89%, respectively *(8,23,24, 30–33)*. In addition, Newman *(8)* suggested that indium-labeled leukocyte imaging could be used to monitor response to therapy, with images reverting to normal in 2–8 weeks after commencement of antibiotic therapy.

Despite their potential advantages and reported high sensitivity and specificity, indium-labeled leukocyte scans have not completely displaced other imaging modalities. Recent data show uptake of indium-labeled leukocytes in as many as 31% of noninfected neuropathic joints *(40)*. These false-positive exams stem from the inability to determine

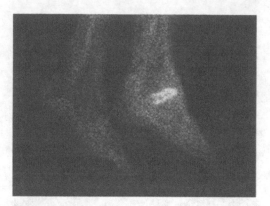

Fig. 8. Osteomyelitis: indium-labeled leukocyte scan. Increase in indium accumulation about the ankle represents the focus of osteomyelitis in a patient with swelling and fever. *Staphylococcus aureus* grew from the marrow aspiration.

whether labeled leukocytes located outside the typical marrow distribution represent infection or merely an atypical site of hematopoietic activity *(41)*. Atypical patterns of marrow distribution may accompany fractures, orthopedic hardware, infarctions, and tumors. False-negative examinations may occur when the procedure for labeling the leukocytes is inadequate *(42)*. Rarely a problem in the forefoot *(2)*, where the osseous structures are equidistant from both dorsal and plantar skin surfaces, detection of osteomyelitis in the mid- and hind foot is compromised by the anatomic complexity associated with the latter structures *(40,41)*. Interpreting labeled leukocyte study in conjunction with bone scan can make some improvement in the accuracy.

Tc-HMPAO-labeled leukocyte scans are reported to be as accurate as indium-labeled leukocyte studies in the diagnosis of osteomyelitis. This technique of labeling has the advantage of providing the results on the same day and depositing a much lower radiation dose. Its major drawback is that it does not permit simultaneous acquisition of combined bone and labeled leukocyte data.

Other disadvantages intrinsic to any labeled leukocyte studies include complexity of the labeling process, high cost, and the general availability of the test, not to mention the risks related to handling of blood products.

Newer Radiopharmaceuticals

Newer radioactive agents for imaging osteomyelitis are undergoing trials with favorable results. These include 18F fluorodeoxyglucose (FDG) imaging using a positron emission tomography (PET) coincidence camera technique *(43)*, antigranulocyte antibodies labeled with technetium or polyclonal immunoglobulins labeled with indium, and radiolabeled peptides *(44–46)*. With a high degree of accuracy and improved resolution on the few preliminary studies, these new modalities hold promise for detection of osteomyelitis in the diabetic patients.

Computed Tomography

CT scan is useful for detection of radiographically occult foreign bodies, even those that are not traditionally considered radiopaque (e.g., wood). It is superior to radiog-

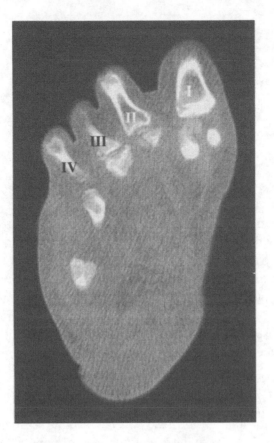

Fig. 9. Metatarsal osteonecrosis on CT. The second and third metatarsal heads are flattened. The radiolucencies beneath the deformed metatarsal heads represent subchondral fractures. CT exquisitely demonstrates these cortical abnormalities.

raphy in detection of cortical destruction (Fig. 9), periostitis, and soft tissue or intraosseous gas. These findings of acute osteomyelitis during the early stages of infection may be difficult to detect on radiography but can frequently be documented on CT. The sequestrum (a focus of necrotic bone insulated from living bone by granulation tissue), which is related to chronic osteomyelitis, is exquisitely displayed on CT images. This necrotic focus carries a characteristic CT finding of a dense bone spicule in the medullary cavity surrounded by soft tissue density *(7,47)*. While CT scans performed with iodinated intravenous contrast may detect abscess, MRI and ultrasound, possessing superior soft tissue contrast resolution, are better suited to imaging of fluid collections. Neither generally requires contrast enhancement. Thus, employment of CT for this purpose should be weighed against the risk of contrast-induced complications.

The data on sensitivity or specificity of CT for diagnosis of diabetic pedal osteomyelitis, however, are scant. There appears to be little enthusiasm for CT as a diagnostic test for osteomyelitis probably because of the potential risk arising from ionizing radiation exposure and contrast reaction.

Ultrasound

Ultrasound is well suited to evaluation of superficial soft tissues and to guide aspiration of fluid collection. Imaging of superficial soft tissues requires use of a high-frequency

Table 4
Indications for MRI in Detection of Infection

Characterize soft tissue abnormalities

Exclude osteomyelitis

Preoperative assessment

transducer, often in conjunction with a stand-off pad. Abscesses are seen as hypoechoic collections with increased through-transmission (that is, tissue deep to the abscess appears more echogenic than expected because the sound waves are attenuated less by fluid in the abscess than by the soft tissue surrounding the abscess). However, an abscess may become isoechoic to surrounding tissues or display lack of posterior enhancement when its contents become proteinaceous, thus evading detection. Joint effusions are often visible as hypoechoic on ultrasound but may be less evident when their contents are complex. Despite its ability to detect fluid collections, sonography cannot determine the presence or absence of infection within the fluid, nor can sonography offer any information on osteomyelitis. Thus, ultrasound is best employed for purpose of guiding aspiration.

Magnetic Resonance Imaging

MRI is notable for its high intrinsic soft tissue contrast, that is, it depicts the full spectrum of soft tissues without the use of intravenous contrast. It readily delineates an infection's extent, guides surgery, characterizes soft tissue abnormalities, and excludes osteomyelitis *(48)* (Table 4). Its advantages over scintigraphy are precise anatomic definition and improved lesion characterization *(49,50)*. The range of magnetic resonance (MR) techniques available is expansive. A brief review of pulse sequences, MR contrast, imaging planes, and optimization of techniques will be presented.

Pulse Sequences

The sequences frequently employed in MRI for detection of bone and soft tissue abnormalities include T1, T2, short tau inversion recovery (STIR), and T1 with fat saturation.

T1 SEQUENCE (SHORT TE/SHORT TR)

This sequence depicts pathology in detailed anatomy. The normal fatty marrow that is bright or hyperintense on T1 images clearly highlights abnormal marrow that is dark or hypointense (Fig. 10).

STIR SEQUENCE

Normal marrow is dark or of low signal on STIR images. Pathology and fluid collections become bright or of high signal (Fig. 10). Thus, it is a highly sensitive sequence to screen for lesions and fluid collections. Its disadvantage is that the anatomic detail depicted on this pulse sequence is inferior to that of the T1 sequence.

T1 WITH FAT SATURATION (FAT SAT) SEQUENCE

This sequence best documents enhancement following injection of gadolinium (Fig. 11). When fat signal is suppressed, both normal fatty marrow and pathology are gener-

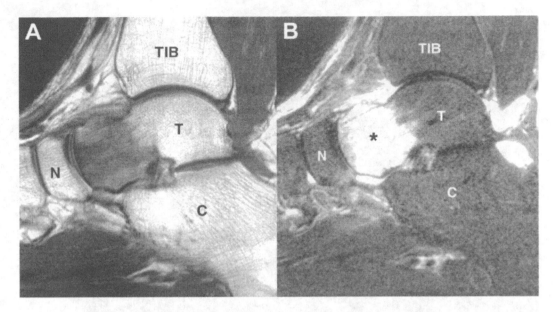

Fig. 10. Bone bruise and marrow edema on MRI. Sagittal images of the ankle show marrow edema or bone bruise (*), which is dark on T1-weighted image (**A**) and bright on STIR (**B**) image. This patient sustained trauma to the anterior talus. This marrow edema pattern is non-specific and is similar to the marrow changes in osteomyelitis. Specificity and accuracy can be improved by administration of gadolinium, as osteomyelitis frequently shows marrow enhancement. C, calcaneus; N, navicula; T, talus; TIB, tibia.

ally dark or low in signal. Any bright or high signal represents a focus of enhancement. The drawback of this sequence is inhomogeneous fat suppression, which generates signal abnormalities that lead to erroneous diagnosis. This is a common problem in the foot where uniform fat suppression is difficult. Comparing the postcontrast images with an additional set of precontrast fat-suppressed images or STIR images can minimize this problem.

T2 SEQUENCE (LONG TE/LONG TR)

A commonly employed sequence that is less sensitive than the STIR sequence in detection of marrow abnormality. Abnormal marrow, fluid collection and cellulitis are bright or hyperintense on this sequence.

Gadolinium

Intravenous injection of a gadolinium-containing contrast agent improves the sensitivity of the diagnosis of osteomyelitis (Fig. 11). Gadolinium concentrates in areas of infectious or noninfectious inflammation and produces hyperintense signal on T1 images. As fat is also hyperintense on a T1 sequence, images are acquired using a fat suppression technique. Normal marrow in the foot is predominantly composed of fat and is hypointense on the fat-suppressed images. This overall dark background allows inflamed tissue to be displayed conspicuously. The accuracy for diagnosis of osteomyelitis is higher in the contrast-enhanced studies (89%) than in non-contrast-enhanced studies (78%) *(51)*. The nephrotoxicity of gadolinium is significantly less than that of the iodinated compounds and is generally safe when used in diabetic patients with elevated renal functions.

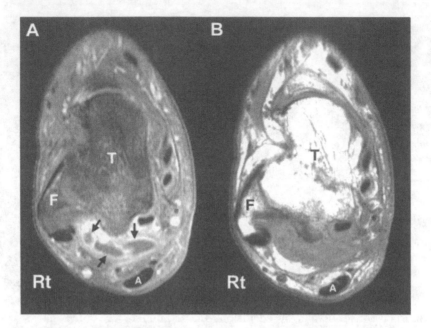

Fig. 11. Soft tissue abscess on MRI. Axial images of the ankle in a diabetic patient who presented with a posterior abscess. The T1-weighted image with fat suppression and gadolinium (**A**) is more specific than the T1 image without contrast or fat suppression (**B**) in detection of the abscess. Administration of contrast shows rim enhancement (black arrows, **A**) of the abscess, which is dark on the T1-weighted (**B**) image. The suppression of surrounding fat signal further highlights the contrast enhancement (**A**). A, Achilles tendon; F, fibula; T, talus.

Marrow enhancement, which accompanies osteomyelitis, however, is nonspecific and can be seen in osteonecrosis and fracture.

Imaging Planes

All three planes, (sagittal, coronal, and axial) of the foot are necessary. To minimize confusion in orientation, the axial plane of the foot refers to the short axis of the metatarsals, and the coronal plane denotes their long-axis image. The presence of foot deformities mandates imaging in oblique planes. Careful attention to imaging planes minimizes volume-averaging artifacts and improves diagnostic accuracy.

Optimization of Technique

Acquisition of high-resolution images requires meticulous technique (Table 5). MR-sensitive markers denote the area of interest and ulceration. The smallest field of view encompassing the entire lesion produces higher resolution images. Employment of a surface coil, commonly the knee coil, improves image resolution. Imaging both feet in the head coil, utilizing a large field of view, significantly degrades image quality and is not recommended.

MRI is contraindicated in patients who have pacemakers and other electronic implants, ferromagnetic cranial aneurysm clips, and intraocular metal. Most claustrophobic patients can be imaged with sedation or the use of an open architecture magnet. Weight limitations for obese patients currently range from 300 to 450 pounds, depending on the mag-

Table 5
Optimization of MR Techniques

MR markers denoting ulcers and inflammation
Small surface coil
Small field of view
Oblique imaging planes

net. Although patients with orthopedic hardware can usually be imaged, assessment of the area immediately surrounding the hardware is frequently limited by distortion of the local magnetic field.

Imaging Features

Cellulitis manifests as an ill-defined area in the subcutaneous fat that is of low signal on T1 and high signal on STIR *(16)* (Fig. 2). This signal pattern is nonspecific and is common to both cellulitis and noninfected edema. Gadolinium administration may identify uncomplicated cellulitis, which typically shows uniform enhancement of the subcutaneous edema *(15)*.

Abscess presents as a focal low T1 signal and high STIR and T2 signal lesion. Only the wall of the abscess enhances following administration of gadolinium on fat-suppressed T1 images (Fig. 11). Without the use of intravenous gadolinium, abscess may not be clearly evident *(51)* (Fig. 11). The enhancing rim was believed to correspond to the granulation tissue in the pseudocapsule *(52)*. The presence of rim enhancement and mass effect differentiates abscess collection from phlegmonous change or cellulitis *(15)* (Fig. 11). The latter typically shows diffuse enhancement (Fig. 2). Ring enhancement, however, is a sensitive but nonspecific sign for abscess and has been described in necrotic tumors, seromas, ruptured popliteal cysts, and hematomas *(51)*.

The center of the abscess, composed of pus, may present with variable signal intensity depending on its proteinaceous contents. T1 shortening by the proteinaceous material may produce intermediate to hyperintense T1 signal, thus comparison to a precontrast fat-suppressed image becomes essential.

The diagnosis of septic arthritis is generally made clinically and confirmed by percutaneous joint aspiration or surgery *(15)*. The MR appearance of septic arthritis consists of joint effusions and intraarticular debris. Following administration of intravenous gadolinium, there is intense synovial enhancement. Periarticular reactive marrow edema, occasionally seen in the bone marrow surrounding an infected joint, may demonstrate gadolinium enhancement without the presence of osteomyelitis *(15)*. This constellation of findings is suggestive but not specific for infection and can also be seen in inflammatory conditions such as rheumatoid arthritis and seronegative arthropathies.

The primary MRI finding in osteomyelitis is abnormal marrow signal that enhances. The abnormal marrow is low (dark) on T1 images and high (bright) on STIR images. Following intravenous administration of gadolinium contrast, the abnormal marrow enhances, seen as a bright focus on the fat suppressed T1 images. Secondary signs of osteomyelitis include cortical interruption, periostitis (seen as enhancement at the margins

Table 6
MRI Findings of Osteomyelitis

Primary signs
  Hyperintense (bright) STIR signal sequence and
  Hypointense (dark) T1 signal sequence
  Enhancing marrow following Gd on T1 (fat sat) sequence

Secondary MR signs
  Periosteal reaction
  Subperiosteal abscess
  Periostitis, manifested by periosteal enhancement
  Cortical destruction
  Ulcer
  Sinus tract

of the periosteum; *16,53*), and cutaneous ulcer or sinus tract in contiguity with the abnormal marrow. A negative MRI successfully excludes osteomyelitis and predicts nonoperrative management *(48)* (Fig. 3).

The sensitivity and specificity compiled from seven MRI studies are 96% and 87% respectively *(8,25,27,28,34,35)*.

Another important use of MRI is in surgical planning. As foot-sparing surgical procedures are increasingly performed in the ambulatory patient, accurate depiction of the extent of marrow involvement becomes paramount *(51)* (Fig. 10). Marrow involvement is best depicted on either T1 or STIR images.

Despite all the attributes of MRI, it has several limitations. MRI of the infected diabetic foot yields a significant number of false-positive diagnoses. Abnormal marrow signal can also be seen with neuroarthropathy, fractures (Fig. 12), and occasionally osteonecrosis. The hyperemic phase of neuroarthropathy may similarly display enhancing marrow edema indistinguishable from osteomyelitis. Use of MR imaging for following the infection's therapeutic response to treatment is limited and remains to be defined.

Angiography

Angiography is indicated in the diabetic patients with nonhealing ulcers or osteomyelitis requiring endovascular and surgical planning. Almost without exception, these patients with nonhealing foot ulcers will have severe stenoocclusive disease involving all three runoff vessels of the calf (anterior tibial, posterior tibial, and peroneal arteries) (Fig. 13). In this patient population, 20% of peripheral bypass grafts will have to extend to a pedal artery. The distal anastomosis is either to the dorsalis pedis artery or the proximal common plantar artery trunk *(54)*. Thus detailed mapping of arterial disease from the abdominal aorta to the pedal vessels is necessary.

Traditionally, vascular imaging has been performed using conventional angiography. Conventional angiography is an invasive procedure performed in the angiographic suite under fluoroscopic (real-time x-ray imaging) guidance. A thin, flexible catheter is inserted into the aorta or arteries, usually via a femoral artery approach. A relatively large bolus

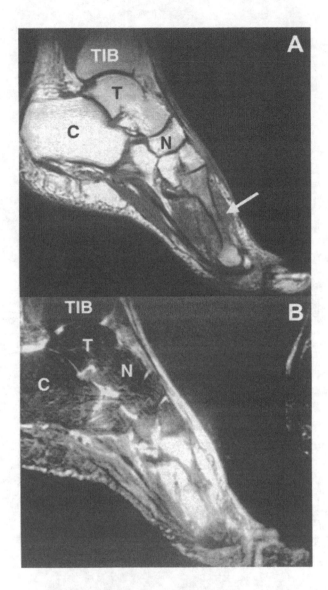

Fig. 12. Stress fracture on MRI. Sagittal T1-weighted (**A**) and STIR (**B**) MR images of the foot demonstrate cortical irregularity of the mid-third metatarsal shaft. The marrow beneath the cortical irregularity shows low T1 signal (**A**) of marrow edema. On the STIR image (**B**), the marrow of the entire metatarsal shaft becomes bright or hyperintense. The fracture line remains dark and is highlighted by bright edematous marrow. Marked soft tissue swelling is also better seen on the STIR images (**B**). C, calcaneus; N, navicular; TIB, tibia; T, talus.

of iodinated contrast is injected into the intraluminal catheter, and rapid sequence radiographs are exposed. Although examination of the abdominal aorta and iliac vessels can readily be performed with a multi-sidehole catheter in the abdominal aorta, examination of the femoral, popliteal, tibioperoneal, and pedal arteries entails placement of an ipsilateral external iliac artery catheter. Selective catheter placement can also limit contrast burden in a patient group predisposed to renal insufficiency.

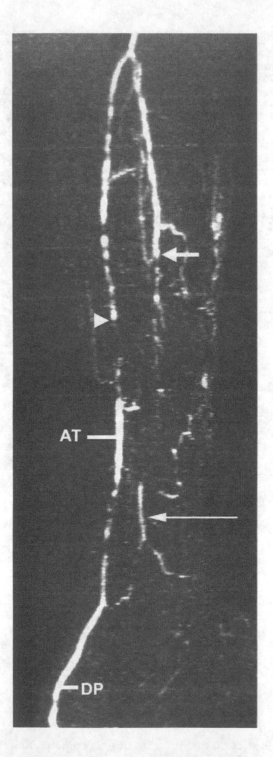

Fig. 13. Time of flight MR angiogram of the leg and foot from beneath the knee to the foot in a diabetic with ischemic foot ulcer demonstrates occlusion of the peroneal and both anterior (arrowhead) and posterior tibial (arrow) arteries. There is reconstitution of a small distal peroneal artery (long arrow) and the anterior tibial, which, although severely diseased distally, continues as a good-caliber dorsalis pedis (DP) artery. Bypass to the dorsalis pedis artery with vein graft allowed ulcer healing and ultimately resumption of normal weight bearing. AT, anterior tibial artery.

The risks of the procedure include radiation exposure, potential for bleeding, injury to the vessel wall with or without dislodgment of embolic material, and risk of renal failure or allergic reaction from the iodinated contrast. Not infrequently, vascular disease and slow flow can disrupt the timing of the exam, with resultant failure to demonstrate the distal vessels. This is especially problematic when demonstration of distal vessels is the key to planning a bypass graft procedure. The major advantage of conventional angiography is that it provides access to perform not only diagnostic but also therapeutic vascular procedures, including angioplasty, atherectomy, stenting, and thrombolysis.

Magnetic Resonance Angiography

More recently, MRI has come to play a role in the imaging of arterial disease, in the form of MR angiography or MRA. MRA has the benefit of providing detailed anatomy of the arterial disease yet bypassing arterial catheter placement with its complications and the need for nephrotoxic contrast material administration. Time-of-flight (TOF) and gadolinium-enhanced MRA are the preferred techniques for MRA of the lower extremity *(55,56)*.

The TOF MRA technique relies on a non-contrast-enhanced, flow-sensitive MR sequence. Computer postprocessing of the MR data generate coronal, sagittal, or oblique reconstructions that mimic the appearance of conventional angiograms. TOF MRA can be particularly time consuming, lasting 1–2 h, in order to cover the distance from the aortic bifurcation to the distal lower extremity. Cardiac gating, employed during image acquisition, improves image quality but significantly lengthens exam time, especially when the patient has cardiac arrhythmia or in on β-blocker medication. TOF MRA images exaggerate the degree of stenoocclusive disease and are more prone to motion and susceptibility artifact.

Gadolinium-enhanced MRA relies on intravenous injection of a small volume of gadolinium contrast and fast imaging that is timed to follow the passage of the contrast bolus optimally through the arteries. This technique has the advantage of short scan time, reduced motion, and susceptibility artifacts. It is more accurate than TOF MRA exam in depiction of the grade of stenoocclusive disease. It uses a much smaller volume of contrast than conventional angiography and therefore generates a smaller osmotic load and subsequently a lower incidence of nephrotoxicity. However, visualization of the arteries may be limited by venous enhancement (Fig. 14) or suboptimal arterial filling related to inaccurate timing of data acquisition.

OSTEOMYELITIS VERSUS NEUROARTHROPATHY

Differentiation between osteomyelitis and neuroarthropathy is often difficult. Certain neuroarthropathic changes resemble osteomyelitis. To better understand their differences, the imaging characteristics of neuroarthropathy will be presented here. Frykberg provides an extensive discussion of Charcot changes in Chapter 12 of this book.

Loss of both pain and proprioceptive sensation is believed to cause repetitive trauma leading to diabetic neuroarthropathy *(16)*. Although devastating, the incidence of neuropathic joints in the diabetic is surprisingly low, at 0.1–0.5%.

The joints of the forefoot and midfoot are commonly involved. The distribution of neuroarthropathy in diabetic patients is 24% in the intertarsal region, 30% in the

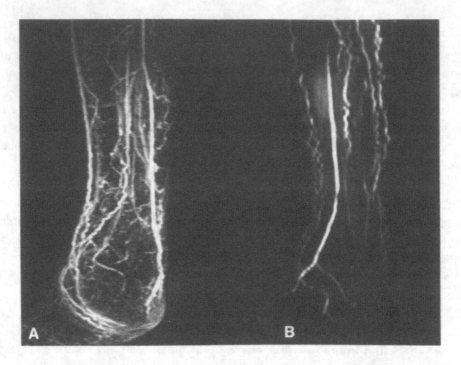

Fig. 14. MRA. (**A**) Gadolinium-enhanced MRA shows inaccurate timing of data acquisition with both arterial and venous enhancement limiting identification of arterial disease, a pitfall of gadolinium-enhanced MR angiogram. (**B**) MRA of the same patient selectively depicts the arterial flow and demonstrates typical severe occlusive disease of all three tibioperoneal arteries with reconstitution of a distally mildly diseased anterior tibial continuing as a good-caliber dorsalis pedis artery.

tarsometatarsal joint (Fig. 15), and 30% in the metatarsophalangeal joints. Abnormalities of the ankle (11%) and interphalangeal (4%) joints are less frequent *(57)*.

Two classical forms of neuroarthropathy, the atrophic and hypertrophic have been described *(58)*. The atrophic form, representing the acute resorptive or hyperemic phase, is characterized by osteopenia (Fig. 15) and osseous resorption. This form frequently appears in the forefoot and the metatarsophalangeal joints, leading to partial or complete disappearance of the metatarsal heads and proximal phalanges. Osteolytic changes produce tapering or " pencil-pointing" of phalangeal and metatarsal shafts. Marrow changes in the atrophic or hyperemic form show hyperintense STIR and hypointense T1 signal and mimic those of osteomyelitis.

The hypertrophic form, representing the healing or reparative phase, is characterized by sclerosis, osteophytosis, and a radiographic appearance of extreme degenerative change (Fig. 16). In its early phase, the hypertrophic form of neuroarthropathy may be confused with osteoarthritis. Concurrent osseous fragmentation, subluxation, or dislocation predominate in the intertarsal and tarsometatarsal joints. Ruptured ligaments in the mid- and forefoot cause dorsal lateral displacement of the metatarsals in relation to the tarsal bones. This classic finding resembles an acute Lisfranc's fracture-dislocation. Disruption of the talonavicular and calcaneocuboid joints causes collapse of the longi-

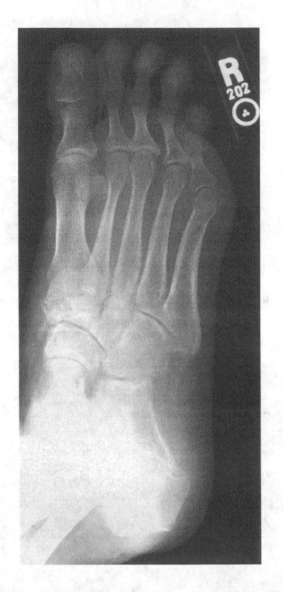

Fig. 15. Neuroarthropathy of the midfoot on radiography. Oblique image of the foot demonstrates diffuse osteopenia of the forefoot. The first and second cuneiforms are fragmented and are surrounded by osseous debris.

tudinal arch with subsequent plantar displacement of the talus (Fig. 17). These changes produce the classic "rocker-bottom" deformity *(59)*. Recognition of this deformity is important because it creates new pressure points that may lead to callus formation and finally ulcerations (Fig. 18). Attempts to classify neuropathic joints into these two classical forms may be difficult as a mixed pattern, composed of both forms, occurs in 40% of neuropathic joints *(60)*.

Other than the characteristic findings of diffuse dark marrow signal on T1, STIR, and T2 images associated with hypertrophic neuroarthropathy, there is no easy method of distinguishing between osteomyelitis and neuroarthropathy. Secondary findings such as involvement of the midfoot and multiple joints, absence of cortical destruction, presence

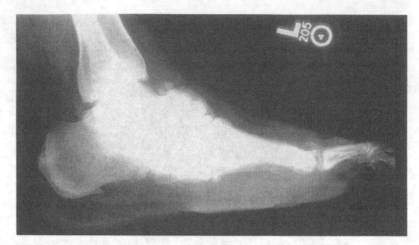

Fig. 16. Hypertrophic phase of neuroarthropathy on radiography. Lateral image of the foot shows the hypertrophic form of neuroarthropathy, characterized by sclerosis, osteophytosis, and radiographic appearance of extreme degenerative change. In its early phase, it may be confused with osteoarthritis.

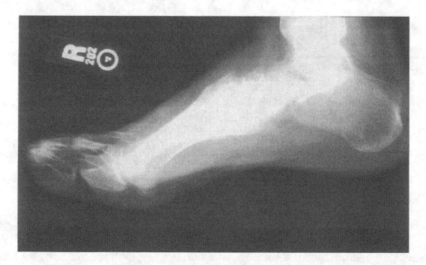

Fig. 17. Midfoot deformity related to neuroarthropathy on radiography. Lateral radiograph demonstrates dorsal dislocation of the tarsometatarsal joints leading to reversal of the normal arch of the foot. The metatarsal bases are superiorly subluxed. Progression of the subluxation will finally result in rocker bottom deformity.

of small cyst-like lesions, and some distance between soft tissue infection and bone changes favor a diagnosis of neuroarthropathy *(16)* (Table 7). In contrast, osteomyelitis prefers the toes or metatarsal heads, focal cortical lesions, and close proximity to the ulcer.

Approaches to Diagnosis of Pedal Osteomyelitis in the Diabetic Patient

Figure 19 suggests an algorithm for imaging pedal osteomyelitis in the diabetic patient.

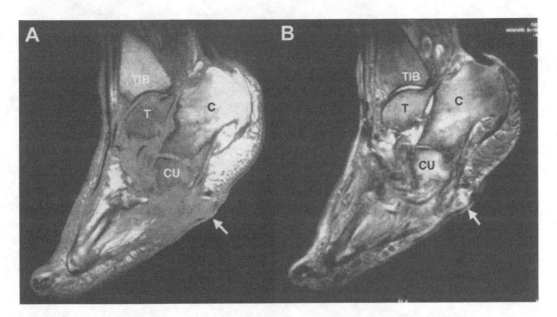

Fig. 18. Rocker bottom deformity and ulceration at focus of high plantar pressure on MRI. (**A**) Sagittal T1-weighted and (**B**) STIR images show disruption of the talonavicular joint causing collapse of the longitudinal arch. These changes produce the classic rocker bottom deformity (49). Recognition of this deformity is important because it creates new pressure points that lead to callus and ulcer formation (arrow). The diffuse marrow edema, associated with neuroarthropathy of the tarsal bones, mimics osteomyelitis. T, talus; CU, cuboid; C, calcaneus; TIB, tibia.

Table 7
Osteomyelitis vs. Neuroarthropathy

	Favors osteomyelitis	Favors neuroarthropathy
Radiography		
Location	Forefoot, metatarsal heads, and toes	Midfoot
Cortical destruction	Absent	Discrete cortical lesion
Soft tissue ulcer	Some distance from soft tissue infection or ulcer	Beneath or close to the ulcer or soft tissue infection
Magnetic resonance		
Signal characteristics of the abnormal marrow	Hyperintense STIR or T2 marrow signal. This signal pattern overlaps the hyperemic phase of neuroarthropathy and acute fracture	Hypointense marrow signal on all T1, T2, and STIR sequences. This signal pattern corresponds to the hypertrophic phase of neuroarthropathy
Cysts	Cysts are not common in osteomyelitis	Well-marginated cysts like lesions, hypointense on T1 and hyperintense on T2

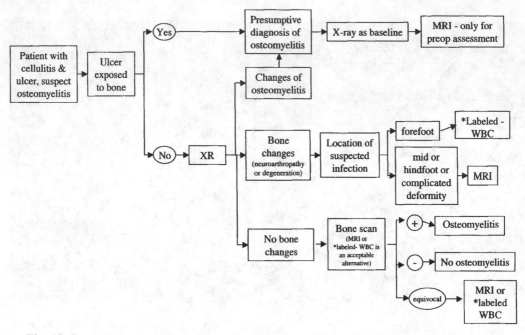

Fig. 19. Suggested approach to diagnosis of osteomyelitis in diabetic foot infection. *, labeled-WBC, labeled leukocyte scan. If labeled leukocyte scan is unavailable, may replace with gallium scan.

Soft Tissue Ulceration Exposing Bone

When the soft tissue ulcer exposes bone, no imaging is needed to confirm the diagnosis of osteomyelitis. Radiography is appropriate to provide a baseline and to document bone complications.

Soft Tissue Inflammation (Ulcers and or Cellulitis) with no Exposed Bone

Radiography further separates the patients into two groups. If the radiographs are normal and the clinical suspicion for osteomyelitis is high, a three-phase bone scan can efficiently exclude or detect osteomyelitis. MRI or labeled leukocyte study is an acceptable alternative (37). A gallium scan may replace labeled leukocyte study if the latter is not available (61). Unlike plain radiographs, these modalities become positive in the first few days of infection. In light of their high sensitivity, these studies provide a high negative predictive value for osteomyelitis. If the bone scan is equivocal, supplementary imaging with either MRI or labeled leukocyte scans is required.

When the radiographs are abnormal, showing neuroarthropathic, degenerative or traumatic changes, either labeled leukocyte scan or MRI is acceptable. Their choice depends on the location of the suspected osteomyelitis. If the inflammation is in the forefoot, an indium leukocyte study efficiently identifies osteomyelitis. When the infection is in the mid- or hindfoot, MRI adequately separates bone from soft tissue inflammation.

SUMMARY

Imaging plays an important role in the assessment of the diabetic patient with foot problems. Nuclear medicine and MRI techniques generally detect osteomyelitis, characterize various soft tissue abnormalities, and depict the extent of bone involvement. MR angiographic studies assess foot vessel runoff when conventional angiography fails to detect additional vascular lesions that are distal to a focus of obstruction. Nevertheless, distinguishing osteomyelitis from concurrent neuropathic change remains a challenge. Only with an understanding of the unique strengths and weaknesses of each modality, as they apply to the particular clinical problem in question, can these wide variety of imaging studies be utilized in an effective and efficienct manner.

ACKNOWLEDGMENTS

Special thanks to Dr. Anthony Parker, for his guidance and editorial assistance in this manuscript.

REFERENCES

1. Scher KS, Steele FJ. The septic foot in patients with diabetes. *Surgery* 1988;104:661–666.
2. Newman LG, Waller J, Palestro CJ, et al. Unsuspected osteomyelitis in diabetic foot ulcers. Diagnosis and monitoring by leukocyte scanning with indium in 111 oxyquinoline [see comments]. *JAMA* 1991;266:1246–1251.
3. Kaufman M, Bowsher, JE. Preventing diabetic foot ulcers. *Medsurg Nurs* 1994;3:204.
4. Bild DE, Selby JV, Sinnock P, et al. Lower-extremity amputation in people with diabetes. Epidemiology and prevention. *Diabetes Care* 1989;12:24–31.
5. Ecker ML, Jacobs BS. Lower extremity amputation in diabetic patients. *Diabetes* 1970;19: 189–195.
6. Penn I. Infections in the diabetic foot, in *The Foot in Diabetes* (Sammarco GJ, ed.), Lea & Febiger, Philadelphia, 1991, pp. 106–123.
7. Gold RH, Tong DJ, Crim JR, Seeger LL. Imaging the diabetic foot. *Skeletal Radiol* 1995; 24:563–571.
8. Newman LG. Imaging techniques in the diabetic foot. *Clin Podiatr Med Surg* 1995;12:75–86.
9. Mokdad A, Ford E, Bowman B, et al. Diabetes trends in the US: 1990–1998. *Diabetes Care* 2000;23:1278–1283.
10. Horowitz SH. Diabetic neuropathy. *Clin Orthop* 1993;296:78–85.
11. Edmonds ME, Roberts VC, Watkins PJ. Blood flow in the diabetic neuropathic foot. *Diabetologia* 1982;22:9–15.
12. Murray HJ, Young MJ, Hollis S, Boulton AJ. The association between callus formation, high pressures and neuropathy in diabetic foot ulceration. *Diabet Med* 1996;13:979–982.
13. Gooding GA, Stess RM, Graf PM, et al. Sonography of the sole of the foot. Evidence for loss of foot pad thickness in diabetes and its relationship to ulceration of the foot. *Invest Radiol* 1986;21:45–48.
14. Bamberger DM, Daus GP, Gerding DN. Osteomyelitis in the feet of diabetic patients. Long-term results, prognostic factors, and the role of antimicrobial and surgical therapy. *Am J Med* 1987;83:653–660.
15. Linklater J, Potter HG. Emergent musculoskeletal magnetic resonance imaging. *Top Magn Reson Imaging* 1998;9:238–260.
16. Marcus CD, Ladam-Marcus VJ, Leone J, et al. MR imaging of osteomyelitis and neuropathic osteoarthropathy in the feet of diabetics. *Radiographics* 1996;16:1337–1348.
17. Moore TE, Yuh WT, Kathol MH, el-Khoury GY, Corson JD. Abnormalities of the foot in patients with diabetes mellitus: findings on MR imaging. *AJR* 1991;157:813–816.
18. Grayson ML, Gibbons GW, Balogh K, Levin E, Karchmer AW. Probing to bone in infected pedal ulcers. A clinical sign of underlying osteomyelitis in diabetic patients [see comments]. *JAMA* 1995;273:721–723.

19. Cook TA, Rahim N, Simpson HC, Galland RB. Magnetic resonance imaging in the management of diabetic foot infection. *Br J Surg* 1996;83:245–248.
20. Park HM, Wheat LJ, Siddiqui AR, et al. Scintigraphic evaluation of diabetic osteomyelitis: concise communication. *J Nucl Med* 1982;23:569–573.
21. Segall GM, Nino-Murcia M, Jacobs T, Chang K. The role of bone scan and radiography in the diagnostic evaluation of suspected pedal osteomyelitis. *Clin Nucl Med* 1989;14:255–260.
22. Seldin DW, Heiken JP, Feldman F, Alderson PO. Effect of soft-tissue pathology on detection of pedal osteomyelitis in diabetics. *J Nucl Med* 1985;26:988–993.
23. Keenan AM, Tindel NL, Alavi A. Diagnosis of pedal osteomyelitis in diabetic patients using current scintigraphic techniques. *Arch Intern Med* 1989;149:2262–2266.
24. Larcos G, Brown ML, Sutton RT. Diagnosis of osteomyelitis of the foot in diabetic patients: value of ^{111}In-leukocyte scintigraphy. *AJR* 1991;157:527–531.
25. Nigro ND, Bartynski WS, Grossman SJ, Kruljac S. Clinical impact of magnetic resonance imaging in foot osteomyelitis [published erratum appears in J Am Podiatr Med Assoc 1993; 83:86]. *J Am Podiatr Med Assoc* 1992;82:603–615.
26. Oyen WJ, Netten PM, Lemmens JA, et al. Evaluation of infectious diabetic foot complications with indium-111-labeled human nonspecific immunoglobulin G. *J Nucl Med* 1992; 33:1330–1336.
27. Weinstein D, Wang A, Chambers R, Stewart CA, Motz HA. Evaluation of magnetic resonance imaging in the diagnosis of osteomyelitis in diabetic foot infections. *Foot Ankle* 1993; 14:18–22.
28. Yuh WT, Barloon TJ, Sickels WJ, Kramolowsky EV, Williams RD. Magnetic resonance imaging in the diagnosis and followup of idiopathic retroperitoneal fibrosis. *J Urol* 1989; 141:602–605.
29. Schauwecker DS. The scintigraphic diagnosis of osteomyelitis. *AJR* 1992;158:9–18.
30. McCarthy K, Velchik MG, Alavi A, et al. Indium-111-labeled white blood cells in the detection of osteomyelitis complicated by a pre-existing condition. *J Nucl Med* 1988;29:1015–1021.
31. Maurer A, Millmond S, Knight L, et al. Infection in diabetic osteoarthropathy: use of indium-labeled leukocytes for diagnosis. *Radiology* 1986;161:221–225.
32. Splittgerber GF, Spiegelhoff DR, Buggy BP. Combined leukocyte and bone imaging used to evaluate diabetic osteoarthropathy and osteomyelitis. *Clin Nucl Med* 1989;14:156–160.
33. Schauwecker DS, Park HM, Burt RW, Mock BH, Wellman HN. Combined bone scintigraphy and indium-111 leukocyte scans in neuropathic foot disease. *J Nucl Med* 1988;29:1651–1655.
34. Wang A, Weinstein D, Greenfield L, et al. MRI and diabetic foot infections. *Magn Reson Imaging* 1990;8:805–809.
35. Beltran J, Campanini DS, Knight C, McCalla M. The diabetic foot: magnetic resonance imaging evaluation. *Skeletal Radiol* 1990;19:37–41.
36. Bonakdar-Pour A, Gaines VD. The radiology of osteomyelitis. *Orthop Clin North Am* 1983; 14:21–37.
37. Alazraki N, Dalinka M, Berquist T, et al. Imaging diagnosis of osteomyelitis in patients with diabetes mellitus, in *American College of Radiology ACR Appropriateness Criteria*. American College of Radiology, Reston, VA, 2000, pp. 303–310.
38. Losbona R, Rosenthall L. Observations on the sequential use of 99mTc-phosphate complex and 67Ga imaging in osteomyelitis, cellulitis, and septic arthritis. *Radiology* 1977;123:123–129.
39. Seabold JE, Flickinger FW, Kao SC, et al. Indium-111-leukocyte/technetium-99m-MDP bone and magnetic resonance imaging: difficulty of diagnosing osteomyelitis in patients with neuropathic osteoarthropathy. *J Nucl Med* 1990;31:549–556.
40. Palestro CJ, Torres MA. Radionuclide imaging in orthopedic infections. *Semin Nucl Med* 1997;27:334–345.

41. Abreu SH. Skeletal uptake of indium 111-labeled white blood cells. *Semin Nucl Med* 1989; 19:152–155.
42. Zhuang H, Duarte PS, Pourdehand M, Shnier D, Alavi A. Exclusion of chronic osteomyelitis with F-18 fluorodeoxyglucose positron emission tomographic imaging. *Clin Nucl Med* 2000;25:281–284.
43. Babich JW, Graham W, Barrow SA, Fischman AJ. Comparison of the infection imaging properties of a 99mTc labeled chemotactic peptide with 111In IgG. *Nucl Med Biol* 1995;22: 643–648.
44. Fischman AJ, Babich JW, Barrow SA, et al. Detection of acute bacterial infection within soft tissue injuries using a 99mTc-labeled chemotactic peptide. *J Trauma* 1995;38:223–227.
45. Rubin RH, Fischman AJ. The use of radiolabeled nonspecific immunoglobulin in the detection of focal inflammation. *Semin Nucl Med* 1994;24:169–179.
46. Magid D, Fishman EK. Musculoskeletal infections in patients with AIDS: CT findings. *AJR* 1992;158:603–607.
47. Horowitz JD, Durham JR, Nease DB, et al. Prospective evaluation of magnetic resonance imaging in the management of acute diabetic foot infections. *Ann Vasc Surg* 1993;7:44–50.
48. Chandnani VP, Beltran J, Morris CS, et al. Acute experimental osteomyelitis and abscesses: detection with MR imaging versus CT [see comments]. *Radiology* 1990;174:233–236.
49. Beltran J, McGhee RB, Shaffer PB, et al. Experimental infections of the musculoskeletal system: evaluation with MR imaging and Tc-99m MDP and Ga-67 scintigraphy. *Radiology* 1988;167:167–172.
50. Morrison WB, Schweitzer ME, Wapner KL, et al. Osteomyelitis in feet of diabetics: clinical accuracy, surgical utility, and cost-effectiveness of MR imaging. *Radiology* 1995;196:557–564.
51. Beltran J. MR imaging of soft-tissue infection. *Magn Reson Imaging Clin North Am* 1995; 3:743–751.
52. Morrison WB, Schweitzer ME, Batte WG, Radack DP, Russel KM. Osteomyelitis of the foot: relative importance of primary and secondary MR imaging signs. *Radiology* 1998; 207:625–632.
53. Pomposelli FB Jr, Marcaccio EJ, Gibbons GW, et al. Dorsalis pedis arterial bypass: durable limb salvage for foot ischemia in patients with diabetes mellitus. *J Vasc Surg* 1995;21: 375–384.
54. Cotroneo AR, Manfredi R, Settecasi C, Prudenzano R, Di Stasi C. Angiography and MR-angiography in the diagnosis of peripheral arterial occlusive disease in diabetic patients. *Rays* 1997;22:579–590.
55. Kreitner KF, Kalden P, Neufang A, et al. Diabetes and peripheral arterial occlusive disease: prospective comparison of contrast-enhanced three-dimensional MR angiography with conventional digital subtraction angiography. *AJR* 2000;174:171–179.
56. Holmes GB Jr, Hill N. Fractures and dislocations of the foot and ankle in diabetics associated with Charcot joint changes. *Foot Ankle Int* 1994;15:182–185.
57. Sequeira W. The neuropathic joint. *Clin Exp Rheumatol* 1994;12:325–337.
58. Zlatkin MB, Pathria M, Sartoris DJ, Resnick D. The diabetic foot. *Radiol Clin North Am* 1987;25:1095–1105.
59. Brower A, Allman R. Pathogenesis of the neuropathic joint: neurotraumatic versus neurovascular. *Radiology* 1981;139:349–354.
60. Donohoe KJ. Selected topics in orthopedic nuclear medicine. *Orthop Clin North Am* 1998; 29:85–101.

11

Microbiology and Treatment of Diabetic Foot Infections

Adolf W. Karchmer, MD

INTRODUCTION

The foot of patients with diabetes mellitus is affected by several processes that not only contribute to the development and progression of infection but on occasion alter the appearance of the foot in ways that may obscure the clinical features of local infection. Neuropathy involving the motor fibers supplying muscles of the foot causes asymmetric muscle weakness, atrophy, and paresis, which in turn result in foot deformities and maldistribution of weight (or pressure) on the foot surface. Dysfunction of the sensory fibers supplying the skin and deeper structural elements of the foot allows minor and major injury to these tissues to proceed without appreciation by the patient. As a result of neuropathy, the foot may be dramatically deformed, ulcerate in areas of unperceived trauma (mal perforans), and on occasion be warm and hyperemic in response to deep structural injury (acute Charcot's disease). This warmth and hyperemia may be misinterpreted as cellulitis, and an ulceration (although a major portal of entry for infection) may be uninfected. In the patient with diabetes, peripheral neuropathy may develop in isolation or commonly in parallel with atherosclerotic peripheral vascular disease. The latter involves major inflow vessels to the lower extremity but is commonly associated with occlusive lesions of the tibial and peroneal arteries between the knee and ankle. The resulting arterial insufficiency can alter the appearance of the foot and obscure infection. Rubor may reflect vascular insufficiency rather than inflammation, and conversely pallor may mute the erythema of acute infection. Gangrene and necrosis may be primarily ischemic or may reflect accelerated ischemia in the setting of infection. In sum, the diagnosis of infection involving the foot in patients with diabetes requires a careful detailed examination of the lower extremity and its blood supply.

DIAGNOSIS

Infection involving the foot is diagnosed clinically. Finding purulent drainage (pus) or two or more signs or symptoms of inflammation (erythema, induration, pain, tenderness, or warmth) is indicative of infection. Clinical signs on occasion belie the significance and severity of infection. A minimally inflamed but deep ulceration may be associated with underlying osteomyelitis (1). Serious limb-threatening infection may not result in

From: *The Diabetic Foot: Medical and Surgical Management*
Edited by: A. Veves, J. M. Giurini, and F. W. LoGerfo © Humana Press Inc., Totowa, NJ

Table 1
Classification of Severity of Foot Infection in Patients with Diabetes Mellitus

	Features[a]			
Classification	Superficial ulcer or cellulitis	Deep soft tissue or bone involved	Tissue necrosis or gangrene	Systemic toxicity or metabolic instability
Mild	+	−	−	−
Moderate	+	± (no gas/fasciitis)	± (minimal)	−
Severe	+	±	±	+

[a]+, present; −, not present; ±, may or may not be present.
From: Lipsky BA. Problems of the foot in diabetic patients, in *The Diabetic Foot* (Bowker JH, Pfeifer MA, eds.), 2001.

systemic toxicity. For example, among patients hospitalized for limb-threatening infection only 12–35% have significant fever *(2–4)*. In fact, fever in excess of 102°F suggests infection involving deeper spaces in the foot with tissue necrosis and undrained pus, extensive cellulitis, or bacteremia with hematogenous seeding of remote sites. Open skin wounds and ulcerations are often contaminated or colonized by commensal organisms that on occasion become pathogens. As a consequence, cultures, although essential in the assessment of the microbiology of foot infections, do not in isolation establish the presence of infection. Unless the cultured material is obtained from deep tissue planes by percutaneous aspiration, the results of cultures must be interpreted in the clinical context.

SEVERITY

Multiple classification schemes have been designed to define the severity of foot wounds or infection. The Wagner system has been used commonly, but only one of six grades includes infection *(5)*. The University of Texas classification of foot wounds uses four grades, each of which can be modified by the presence of ischemia, infection, or both *(6)*. Grade 0 is a previously ulcerated lesion that is completely epithelialized; grade 1 is a superficial wound not involving the tendon or joint capsule; grade 2 wounds penetrate to the tendon or joint capsule; and grade 3 wounds penetrate to the bone or joint. Increasing depth of the wounds and complications of ischemia or infection in this classification have been associated with increased likelihood of amputation *(6)*. Lipsky *(7)* has proposed a classification that utilizes depth of a wound, presence of ischemia, presence of infection, and systemic toxicity to designate severity of wound infection (Table 1).

A simple practical classification of foot infection into limb threatening or non-limb threatening has also been described *(8)*. In this scheme, infection is categorized primarily based on depth of the tissues involved, this being largely a function of depth of a predisposing ulceration and the presence or absence of significant ischemia. Patients with non-limb-threatening infection have superficial infection involving the skin, lack major systemic toxicity, and do not have significant ischemia. What might have been a non-limb-threatening infection becomes limb threatening in the face of severe ischemia. If an ulceration is present in a non-limb-threatening infection, it does not penetrate fully through skin. Limb-threatening infection, which is not categorized as such based on severe ischemia, involves deeper tissue planes, with the portal of entry being an ulcer that has penetrated subcutaneous tissue or potentially tendon, joint, or bone. Although limb-threatening infections may be dramatic, with extensive tissue necrosis, purulent drainage, edema, and erythema, they may be cryptic as well. Thus, an infected deep ulcer with a rim of cellulitis that is ≥2 cm in width is considered limb threatening. Note that hyperglycemia occurs almost universally in patients with non-limb-threatening and limb-threatening infection. In contrast, significant fever occurs in only 12–35% of patients with limb-threatening infection *(2–4)*. Fever is found primarily in patients with extensive cellulitis and lymphangitis, infection (abscesses) loculated in the deep spaces of the foot, bacteremia, or hematogenously seeded remote sites of infection.

This simplified scheme accommodates the more complex University of Texas wound classification and that proposed by Lipsky. Unless the foot is compromised by severe ischemia, patients with foot infections categorized as University of Texas grade 0 (or mild infection by Lipsky) would be considered to have non-limb-threatening infection. Those with infection categorized as University of Texas grade 1–3 (or by Lipsky's scheme as moderate to severe) would have limb-threatening infection. In contrast to the University of Texas scheme, the classification of foot infection into non-limb-threatening and limb-threatening groups has not been demonstrated to correlate with the risk of amputation *(6)*. Nevertheless, this simple classification, when adjusted for prior medical therapy and antibiotic exposure, allows one to anticipate the organisms causing wound infections and thus is an excellent point of departure from which to plan empiric antimicrobial therapy.

MICROBIOLOGY

Cultures of open foot ulcers cannot be used to establish the presence of infection. Foot ulcers, whether infected or not, will contain multiple comensal or colonizing bacteria, some of which have the potential to become invasive pathogens. As a foot ulcer transitions from uninfected to infected, organisms isolated from the ulcer cavity include both colonizing flora and invasive pathogens. Assigning specific significance to organisms isolated from ulcers may be difficult and has resulted in some investigators calling cultures from specimens obtained through the ulcer unreliable. In contrast, reliable specimens are those obtained aseptically at surgery, by aspiration of pus, or by biopsy of the infected tissue across intact skin. Although the organisms recovered from reliable specimens are likely to be invasive pathogens, it is unlikely that cultures of reliable specimens yield all the pathogens present, and obtaining these specimens is often impractical. Sapico and colleagues demonstrated that the organism cultured from specimens obtained by aspiration or by curettage of the cleansed ulcer base were most concordant with those isolated from necrotic infected tissue excised from an area adjacent to the ulcer base *(9,10)*. Cultures of aspirated material failed to yield pathogens recovered from curettage or excised tissue in 20% of patients. Wheat et al. *(11)* found poor concordance between organisms isolated from specimens obtained through an ulceration and those recovered from specimens obtained without traversing the ulceration. Cultures obtained through the ulcers were more likely to yield comensals and antibiotic-resistant gram-negative bacilli than were the more reliable specimens.

As a consequence of the variable specimens examined as well as the microbiologic techniques used to culture specimens, i.e., inconsistent and incomplete efforts to recover anaerobic bacteria, the precise microbiology of foot infections is not established. Although the microbiology from clinical reports, in which most specimens are obtained through the ulceration, requires interpretation to adjust for the inclusion of organisms of known low invasive potential and likely to be comensals or colonizers, it is possible to sense the major pathogens causing non-limb-threatening and limb-threatening foot infections. Similarly, when surgical or aspiration specimens are not readily available for culture, antibiotic therapy can be designed with reasonable confidence based on the culture results from specimens obtained by curettage of the ulcer base. The exception to the utility of ulcer cultures is in the design of antimicrobial therapy for osteomyelitis when the infected bone is to be debrided piecemeal, as opposed to resected en bloc. In this situation, more precise biopsy-based culture information is highly desirable.

In non-limb-threatening infections, particularly those occurring in patients who have not previously received antimicrobial therapy, *Staphylococcus aureus* and streptococci, particularly group B streptococci, are the predominant pathogens *(12–14)*. *S. aureus* has been isolated from >50% of these patients, and in more than 30% *S. aureus* is the only bacterium isolated *(12)*.

Limb-threatening foot infections are generally polymicrobial. Cultures from these infections yield on average 4.1–5.8 bacterial species per culture. Both gram-positive cocci and gram-negative rods are commonly isolated from a single lesion, and in 40% of infections both aerobic and anaerobic organisms are recovered *(2,9–11,13,15)* (Table 2). Individual cultures have yielded on average 2.9–3.5 aerobes and 1.2–2.6 anaerobes *(16)*. *S. aureus*, streptococci, and facultative gram-negative bacilli (*Proteus* species, *Enterobacter* species, *Escherichia coli*, and *Klebsiella* species) are the predominant aerobic pathogens in these infections. Among the anaerobes, *Peptostreptococcus* species, *Prevotella* species, and *Bacteroides* species, including those of the *B. fragilis* group, are recovered frequently *(16,17)*. *Clostridium* species are recovered infrequently. Although anaerobes are recovered from 41–53% of limb-threatening infections, in clinical trials with optimal methods these organisms can be recovered from 74–95% of these infections *(16)*. The frequency of isolating anaerobic bacteria is greatest in those patients with the most severe infections, particularly those in whom infection involves necrotic gangrenous tissue and amputation is often required. Nevertheless, the clinical features of foot infections, beyond those that allow categorization as non-limb threatening or limb threatening, are not sufficiently sensitive clues to the microbiology of these infections. Fetid infections suggest infection with anaerobes; however, anaerobes including *B. fragilis* may be recovered from infections that are not particularly foul smelling. Hence, clinical clues beyond the major categorization of infections are not sufficient to predict the microbiology of foot infections.

The spectrum of bacterial species recovered from foot infections, especially those that are limb threatening, can be dramatically altered by prior failed antimicrobial therapy. Whereas *Pseudomonas aeruginosa*, *Acinetobacter* species, and other antibiotic-resistant facultative gram-negative bacilli are uncommon in previously untreated infections, these organisms are not infrequent isolates from infected chronic ulcers *(2)*. Similarly,

Table 2
Microbiology of Limb-Threatening Infections in Patients with Diabetes[a]

Organisms	% of Patients					
	Gibbons et al. (42)[b]	Wheat et al. (54)	Hughes et al. (50)	Bamberger et al. (51)	Scher et al. (65)	Grayson et al. (96)
Aerobic						
S. aureus	22	20	25	22	23	54
S. epidermidis	12	17	14	19	18	12
Enterococcus spp.	16	15	17			28
Streptococcus spp.	13	23	20	41	54	55
Corynebacterium spp.	7	11		8		
E. coli	7	5	3	1	19	6
Klebsiella spp.	4	6	7	4	10	5
Proteus mirabilis	11	9	11	5	36	9
Enterobacter spp.	3	4	7	7		9
Other						
Enterobacteriaceae	2	15	5	7	50	17
P. aeruginosa	3	4	0	5	15	8
Acinetobacter spp.	1	0	0	0		7
Anaerobic						
Gram-positive cocci	21	30	40	14	52	12
Bacteroides fragilis		2	5	4		
Bacteroides melaninogenicus		3	11			
Other						
Bacteroides spp.	6	12	2	5	55	30
Clostridium spp.	2	3	1	3	23	
Other anaerobes			13	2	20	14
Number isolates/infection	2.76	3.31	3.62	2.88	5.76	2.77

[a]Specimens obtained by various routes, including deep ulcer swabs, curettage of the ulcer base, aspiration or tissue biopsy, except Wheat et al., who excluded specimens obtained through the ulcer cavity.
Data from refs. 2, 11, 15, 31, 35, and 38.
[b]Number in parentheses.

211

methicillin-resistant *S. aureus* may be encountered commonly in patients with chronically infected foot ulcers that have persisted in spite of multiple prior courses of antimicrobial therapy. These resistant bacteria are probably acquired nosocomially or alternatively emerge from endogenous flora during the repetitive hospitalization and antibiotic treatment of patients with nonhealing foot ulcers. Accordingly, when selecting an antimicrobial regimen to treat a foot infection in a patient who has had multiple hospitalizations and prior courses of antibiotics, physicians should anticipate the presence of antibiotic-resistant pathogens.

The role of relatively avirulent bacteria, many of which are part of skin flora that are often isolated from cultures of specimens obtained through an ulcer, is uncertain. *Staphylococcus epidermidis* has been recovered, usually in conjunction with other bacteria, from 15–35% of these infections and may not reflect ulcer colonization. On the other hand, *S. epidermidis* has been isolated from reliable foot specimens with similar frequency to *S. aureus*, suggesting that these organisms may be pathogens in some patients *(11)*. Enterococci, viridans streptococci, and *Corynebacterium* species, organisms that are often considered contaminants and not pathogens when isolated from skin and soft tissue infections, are among the isolates recovered frequently from polymicrobial limb-threatening foot infections. When recovered from specimens in conjunction with typical pathogens, these organisms are often disregarded as contaminants. Often, foot infections respond to therapy with antimicrobials that are active in vitro against the pathogens but not against these presumed contaminants *(16,18)*. Although these observations support the designation of these organisms as contaminants, they could also indicate that with the eradication of major pathogens, host defenses and surgical debridement can control these less virulent organisms. On occasion enterococci, viridans streptococci, or *Corynebacterium* species are isolated from uncontaminated specimens and may even be the sole bacterial isolate from an infection *(12,19)*. Thus, these organisms should not be routinely disregarded but rather interpreted in the clinical context.

MICROBIOLOGIC ASSESSMENT

Clinically uninfected ulcers should not be cultured. When infection is present, a microbiologic diagnosis will usually facilitate subsequent therapy, particularly in the setting of limb-threatening infection or failure of prior antimicrobial therapy *(3,8,14)*. Although cultures of tissue obtained aseptically at surgery or purulent specimens aspirated percutaneously are more likely to contain only true pathogens, obtaining these specimens before initiating therapy is often either impractical or not feasible (no abscess present). Accordingly, after cleansing the skin and debriding any overlying eschar, specimens for culture should be obtained before initiating therapy by curettage of the necrotic base of the ulcer. Specimens should be handled and processed as both routine wound cultures and primary anaerobic cultures. If patients are febrile, blood cultures should also be obtained before initiating antimicrobial therapy. During the initial days of therapy and with debridement, specimens from necrotic purulent tissue or exposed bone should be recultured. Concurrent antimicrobial therapy may preclude isolation of susceptible organisms during effective therapy; however, resistant organisms missed on the initial cultures can be recovered from these specimens. Osteomyelytic bone in the forefoot (visible or detectable on probing) that will be totally resected does not require specific cultures. Infected bone in the midfoot or posterior foot that can be probed should be biopsied, ideally approaching the bone for culture through a route other than the ulcer. Here, where debridement is likely to be piecemeal, rather than en bloc resection of all involved bone, precise microbiologic data from bone are required so that optimal antimicrobial therapy can be selected. Bone that remains unexposed after debridement and wherein osteomyelitis is suspected based on radiologic findings is not routinely biopsied. Careful clinical and radiologic follow-up of this bone will often resolve the question of osteomyelitis without the potential hazards of an invasive procedure.

TREATMENT

Debridement and Surgery

With the exception of cellulitis or lymphangitis arising from an unrecognized (or microscopic) portal of entry, infected foot lesions generally require debridement. Debridement should be done surgically rather than by chemical or enzymatic agents *(20)*. For apparent non-limb-threatening infections, debridement may be limited but nevertheless allows full evaluation of the portal of entry and prepares the site for culture. Occasionally, what appeared to be a non-limb-threatening infection is discovered on debridement to actually be limb threatening, with extension of infection to deep tissue planes. Limb-threatening infection by virtue of extension to deep tissue planes requires surgical debridement *(3,8)*. Early surgical intervention can reduce the duration of hospitalization and the need for major amputations *(21)*. Failure to debride necrotic tissue and drain purulent collections increases the risk of amputation *(3,8,21)*. Percutaneously placed drains or aspiration drainage is inadequate, rather, devitalized tissue must be resected and purulent collections drained by incision. Uncertainty about the patient's arterial circulation status should not delay initial debridement. Effective debridement may require multiple procedures as the extent of tissue destruction becomes progressively more apparent. If the infection has destroyed the function of the foot or if it threatens the patient's life, a guillotine amputation to allow prompt control of the infection with a subsequent definitive closure is advised *(22)*.

Antibiotic Therapy

Antimicrobial treatment of foot infections in patients with diabetes is begun empirically and thereafter revised based on the results of cultures, which were obtained prior to therapy and on occasion during therapy, and the clinical response of the infection. Knowledge of the spectrum of bacteria that cause non-limb-threatening infection and limb-threatening infection, as well as the changes in these organisms that might have been induced by selected circumstances, e.g., prior antimicrobial treatment, serves as the basis for selecting effective empiric therapy. The potential toxicity of various antibiotics for individual patients and the unique vulnerability of patients with diabetes as a group must be considered. Thus, for this population with an increased frequency of renal disease, the availability of nonnephrotoxic antimicrobials with potent activity against gram-negative bacilli renders the aminoglycosides relatively undesirable and unnecessary. Antibiotic therapy is administered intravenously when patients are systemically ill, have severe local infection, are unable to tolerate oral therapy, or are infected by bacteria that are not susceptible to available oral antimicrobials. Some antimicrobials are fully bioavailable after oral administration, e.g., selected fluoroquinolones (levofloxacin), clindamycin, and metronidazole, and, when appropriate microbiologically, could often be used in lieu of parenteral therapy initially. After control of infection, continued therapy can commonly be effected with oral agents. For patients who require prolonged courses of parenteral therapy, e.g., for osteomyelitis, generally treatment can be provided in an outpatient setting *(23)*.

Topical antimicrobials, including silver sulfadiazine, polymixin, gentamicin, and mupirocin, have been used to treat selected soft tissue infections; however, this approach has not been studied in foot infections. In randomized trials, a cationic peptide antimicrobial, pexiganin acetate (not yet approved by the Food and Drug Administration), used as a 1% cream applied topically, was nearly as effective (85–90%) as oral ofloxacin in treating mildly infected foot ulcers *(24)*. Although antimicrobials have been applied topically to foot infections, it seems unlikely that the topical route would result in effective tissue concentrations of the antimicrobial. Accordingly, topical therapy should only be used to supplement effective systemic therapy and then with the realization that its efficacy is not established.

The potential therapeutic or prophylactic benefits of systemic antibiotic therapy in patients with uninfected neuropathic ulcers is a subject of debate. One controlled trial showed no benefit from antibiotic therapy *(25)*. In view of the potential adverse consequences, including colonization with resistant bacteria, antibiotic therapy is not recommended for clinically uninfected neuropathic ulcer *(20)*. Similarly, continuation of antibiotics beyond a limited course that was sufficient to eradicate infection has not been required to accomplish healing ulcers that remain open *(12,26)*.

Empiric therapy for patients with non-limb-threatening infection, many of whom can be treated as outpatients, is directed primarily at staphylococci and streptococci *(20)* (Table 3). Lipsky et al. *(12)* demonstrated that oral therapy with clindamycin or cephalexin for 2 weeks in patients with previously untreated non-limb-threatening foot infection resulted in satisfactory clinical outcome in 96 and 86%, respectively *(12)*. Caputo et al. *(14)*, in a retrospective study, reported that 54 of 55 patients with non-limb-threatening infections were improved or cured with oral therapy, primarily first-generation cephalosporins or dicloxacillin, directed at staphylococci and streptococci *(14)*. If patients with superficial ulcers present with more extensive cellulitis that warrants hospitalization and parenteral antimicrobial treatment, cefazolin should be effective. However, if prior microbiologic data or antimicrobial therapy suggests that infection might be caused by methicillin-resistant *S. aureus*, therapy should be initiated with vancomycin. Quinupristin/dalfopristin and linezolid, which can be administered intravenously or orally, have provided effective treatment of skin soft tissue infection caused by methicillin-resistant *S. aureus* and could be considered alternatives to vancomycin *(27–29)*. The duration of treatment, which in the final analysis is determined by the time course of the clinical response, is usually 1–2 weeks.

Multiple antibiotics have been demonstrated to be effective therapy in prospective treatment trials of complicated skin and soft tissue infections, many of which were foot infections. Additionally, some of these antimicrobials have been proved effective in prospective studies of foot infections, many of which have been limb threatening: amoxicillin-clavulanate, ampicillin-sulbactam, piperacillin-tazobactam, ticarcillin-clavulanate, cefoxitin, ceftizoxime, ciprofloxacin, ofloxacin, trovafloxacin, and imipenem/cilastatin

Table 3
Selected Antibiotic Regimens for Initial Empiric Therapy
of Foot Infections in Patients with Diabetes Mellitus

Infection	Antimicrobial regimen[a]
Non-limb threatening	Cephalexin 500 mg p.o. q6h
	Clindamycin 300 mg p.o. q8h
	Amoxicillin-clavulanate (875/125 mg) one q12h
	Dicloxacillin 500 mg p.o. q6h
	Levofloxacin 500–750 mg p.o. qd
Limb threatening	Ceftriaxone 1 g IV daily plus clindamycin 450–600 mg IV q8h[b]
	Ciprofloxacin 400 mg IV q12h plus clindamycin 450–600 mg IV q8h
	Ampicillin/sulbactam 3 g IV q6h
	Ticarcillin/clavulanate 3.1 g IV q4–6h
	Piperacillin/tazobactam 3.375 g IV q4h or 4.5 g IV q6h
	Fluoroquinolone[c] IV plus metronidazole 500 mg IV q6h
Life threatening	Imipenem cilastatin 500 mg IV q6h
	Piperacillin/tazobactam 4.5 g IV q6h plus gentamicin[d] 1.5 mg/kg IV q8h
	Vancomycin 1 g IV q12h plus gentamicin plus metronidazole

[a]Doses for patients with normal renal function.
[b]An alternative is cefotaxime 2 g IV q8h.
[c]Fluoroquinolone with increased activity against gram-positive cocci, e.g., levofloxacin 500–750 mg IV qd.
[d]Can be given as single daily dose 5.1–7.0 mg/kg/d.

(2,18,30–32). In comparative prospective (sometimes blinded) trials of treatment for limb-threatening foot infections, the clinical and microbiologic response rates for the studied agents have been similar, and no single agent has been proved superior to all others.

In selecting empiric therapy for limb-threatening foot infections, reasonable principles emerge from clinical trials and other published studies *(3,8,20)*. The choice of agents used empirically should be based on the known polymicrobial nature of these infections with modifications, where appropriate, to address anticipated highly resistant pathogens that might have been selected in the process of prior hospitalizations and treatment. Although empiric therapy should be effective against an array of Enterobacteriaceae and anaerobes, including *B. fragilis*, especially in the more severe infection where there is tissue necrosis and gangrene, therapy should always be effective against *S. aureus* and group B streptococci. Drug selection should attempt to minimize toxicity and be cost effective. Glucose metabolism (control of blood sugar) should be pursued aggressively. In limb-threatening infection (but not in life-threatening infection), the initial empiric therapy does not have to be effective in vitro for all potential pathogens. Broad-spectrum therapy that is active against many, but not necessarily all, gram-negative bacilli, and against anaerobes, *S. aureus*, and streptococci when combined with good wound care is as effective as even broader spectrum antimicrobial therapy. Thus, in a randomized blinded trial, ampicillin-sulbactam therapy was not only as effective as imipenem-cilastatin at the end of treatment, but on initial evaluation of responses on day 5 the two regimens also performed comparably *(2)*. Thus, in infections in which initial cultures yielded organisms resistant to ampicillin-sulbactam but susceptible to imipenem-cilastatin, patients with limb-threatening infections treated with ampicillin-sul-bactam responded as well as those treated with imipenem-cilastatin. Adequate debride-ment not only shortens required duration of therapy but is required for effective therapy.

Empiric antimicrobial treatment should be reassessed between days 3 and 5 of treat-ment in the light of culture results and clinical response. When therapy is unnecessarily broad spectrum (effective therapy for the bacteria isolated could be achieved by less broad-spectrum antimicrobials with possible cost savings, avoidance of toxicity, or a reduction in selective pressure for emergence of antimicrobial resistance) and patients have responded clinically, treatment regimens should be simplified based on culture data. If a bacteria resistant to the current therapy has been recovered and yet the clinical response is satisfactory, treatment need not be expanded. Alternatively, if in the face of an isolate resistant to treatment the response to therapy is unsatisfactory, the wound should be examined for necrotic tissue that has not been debrided, the adequacy of arterial circulation must be assessed, and because the resistant organism might be a pathogen (rather than colonizing flora), antimicrobial therapy should be expanded to treat this isolate as well as others.

A number of regimens have been recommended as reasonable initial empiric therapy of limb-threatening infections *(8,20)* (Table 3). Some antimicrobials that have been used to treat these infections in the past are, because of gaps in their spectrum of activ-ity versus the typically anticipated pathogens, no longer considered ideal when used alone: cefuroxime, cefamandole, cefoxitin, cefotetan, ceftazidime, and ciprofloxacin. Trovafloxacin, which possesses an appropriate spectrum of activity for this infection and was effective in early trials, is not advocated for routine therapy because of potential hepatotoxicity, but it remains available for severe infections in hospitalized patients *(33)*. It is likely that new fluoroquinolones with a spectrum of activity similar to trovaflox-acin will be studied as single agents for treatment of these infections. If patients with limb-threatening infections have had extensive prior antimicrobial therapy and hospital-izations, highly antibiotic-resistant pathogens should be anticipated and empiric therapy must be expanded, perhaps using regimens similar to those advocated for life-threaten-ing foot infections.

Patients with life-threatening infections, e.g., those with hypotension or severe keto-acidosis, should be treated with maximal regimens (Table 3). If highly resistant gram-negative bacilli are anticipated, gentamicin or another aminoglycoside is advocated. Similarly, if infection with methicillin-resistant *S. aureus* is suspected, vancomycin should be utilized.

The duration of antimicrobial therapy for severe soft tissue foot infection is based on the temporal response to wound care and antimicrobial therapy. Two weeks of therapy is often effective; however, some recalcitrant infections will require longer courses of treat-ment *(2)*. After acute infection has been controlled, antimicrobial therapy that was begun parenterally should be changed to oral therapy with comparable orally bioavail-able antibiotics. Even if the ulcer has not fully healed, antibiotics can in general be discontinued when evidence of infection has resolved. Persistent ulcers must be man-aged with wound care, including avoidance of weight bearing, so that healing can be achieved and the ulcer eliminated as a portal for later infection. The occurrence of bacte-remia, especially if remote sites are seeded, may require extended therapy. Note that *S.*

aureus bacteremia entails a distinct risk for secondary endocarditis *(34)*. These patients should be evaluated carefully including an assessment for endocarditis with a transesophageal echocardiogram.

The antibiotic therapy of osteomyelitis must be coordinated with the surgical debridement of the involved bone. Several reports have suggested that osteomyelitis of bones in the foot can be cured or at least arrested for extended periods with minimal debridement and prolonged courses of antimicrobial therapy *(4,32,35)*. Others have suggested that cure rates for osteomyelitis (where bone destruction is evident or bone is visible or detectable by probing) will be enhanced by aggressive debridement, and even excision of all infected bone when feasible in the forefoot *(3,8,36)*. If all infected bone is resected en bloc, e.g., amputation of a phalanges or phalanges and the related distal metatarsal, the infection has in essence been converted to a soft tissue process and can be treated accordingly. The bacteriology defined by wound cultures can be used to guide therapy, and antibiotic treatment can often be abbreviated, i.e., 2–3 weeks *(2,3,8,37)*. In contrast, if osteomyelitis involves bones that cannot be resected en bloc without disruption of the functional integrity of the foot, debridement must be done in a piece-meal fashion. As a result, the adequacy of the debridement cannot be ensured, and the management strategy must be altered. In this setting, bone cultures to allow precise targeting of antimicrobial therapy are necessary, antimicrobial therapy must be administered in a manner that results in adequate serum concentration (intravenously or orally) for a prolonged period (at least 6 weeks), and adequate blood supply to infected tissues must be ensured *(3,37)*.

OUTCOME

The effective treatment of foot infection is far more than the administration of antibiotics that are active in vitro against the implicated pathogens. Optimal therapy involves the integration of wound care, control of glucose metabolism, antibiotic therapy, debridement and possibly reconstructive foot surgery, and (when ischemia is a limiting factor) vascular reconstruction *(20)*. The knowledge and skills to achieve an optimal outcome often require the collaboration of multiple care providers, including diabetologists, infectious disease specialists, podiatrists, and vascular surgeons. With appropriate care a satisfactory clinical response can be anticipated in 90% of patients with non-limb-threatening infection and at least 60% of those with limb-threatening infection. Limb-threatening infections may require foot-sparing amputations, but salvage of a weight-bearing foot is usually achievable. Vascular reconstruction, especially bypass grafts to pedal arteries that restore pulsable flow to the foot, decrease major amputations and allow foot-sparing/foot-salvage surgery.

REFERENCES

1. Newman LG, Waller J, Palestro CJ, et al. Unsuspected osteomyelitis in diabetic foot ulcers: diagnosis and monitoring by leukocyte scanning with indium and 111 oxyquinoline. *JAMA* 1991;266:1246–1251.
2. Grayson ML, Gibbons GW, Habershaw GM, et al. Use of ampicillin/sulbactam versus imipenem/cilastatin in the treatment of limb-threatening foot infections in diabetic patients. *Clin Infect Dis* 1994;18:683–693.

3. Karchmer AW, Gibbons GW. Foot infections in diabetes: evaluation and management, in *Current Clinical Topics in Infectious Diseases* (Remington JS, Swartz MN, eds.), Blackwell Scientific Publications, Boston, 1994, pp. 1–22.

4. Pittet D, Wyssa B, Herter-Clavel C, et al. Outcome of diabetic foot infections treated conservatively. *Arch Intern Med* 1999;159:851–856.

5. Wagner FW Jr. The diabetic foot and amputation of the foot, in *Surgery of the Foot* (Mann RA, ed.), Mosby, St. Louis, 1986, pp. 421–455.

6. Armstrong DG, Lavery LA, Harkless LB. Validation of a diabetic wound classification system. The contribution of depth, infection, and ischemia to risk of amputation. *Diabetes Care* 1998;21:855–859.

7. Lipsky BA. Problems of the foot in diabetic patients, in *The Diabetic Foot* (Bowker JH, Pfeifer MA, eds.), Mosby, St. Louis, MO, 2001, pp. 467–480.

8. Caputo GM, Cavanagh PR, Ulbrecht JS, Gibbons GW, Karchmer AW. Assessment and management of foot disease in patients with diabetes. *N Engl J Med* 1994;331:854–860.

9. Anonymous. The infected foot of the diabetic patient: quantitative microbiology and analysis of clinical features. *Rev Infect Dis* 1984;6:S171–S176.

10. Sapico FL, Canawah HN, Witte JL, et al. Quantitative aerobic and anaerobic bacteriology of infected feet. *J Clin Microbiol* 1980;12:413–413.

11. Wheat LJ, Allen SD, Henry M, et al. Diabetic foot infections: bacteriologic analysis. *Arch Intern Med* 1986;146:1935–1940.

12. Lipsky BA, Pecoraro RE, Larson SA, Hanley ME, Ahroni JH. Outpatient management of uncomplicated lower-extremity infections in diabetic patients. *Arch Intern Med* 1990;150: 790–797.

13. Lipsky BA, Pecoraro RE, Wheat LJ. The diabetic foot: soft tissue and bone infection. *Infect Dis Clin North Am* 1990;4:409–432.

14. Caputo GM, Ulbrecht JS, Cavanagh PR, Juliano PJ. The role of cultures in mild diabetic foot cellulitis. *Infect Dis Clin Pract* 2000;9:241–243.

15. Scher KS, Steele FJ. The septic foot in patients with diabetes. *Surgery* 1988;104:661–666.

16. Gerding DN. Foot infections in diabetic patients: the role of anaerobes. *Clin Infect Dis* 1995; 20(Suppl 2):S283–S288.

17. Johnson S, Lebahn F, Peterson LP, Gerding DN. Use of an anaerobic collection and transport swab device to recover anaerobic bacteria from infected foot ulcers in diabetics. *Clin Infect Dis* 1995;20(Suppl 2):S289–S290.

18. Lipsky BA, Baker PD, Landon GC, Fernau R. Antibiotic therapy for diabetic foot infections: comparison of two parenteral-to-oral regimens. *Clin Infect Dis* 1997;24:643–648.

19. Watanakunakorn C, Burkert T. Infective endocarditis at a large community teaching hospital, 1980–1990: a review of 210 episodes. *Medicine* 1993;72:90–102.

20. American Diabetes Association: consensus development conference on diabetic foot wound care, April 7–8, 1999, Boston, Massachusetts. *Diabetes Care* 1999;22:1354–1360.

21. Tan JS, Friedman NM, Hazelton-Miller C, Flanagan JP, File TM Jr. Can aggressive treatment of diabetic foot infections reduce the need for above-ankle amputation? *Clin Infect Dis* 1996;23:286–291.

22. McIntyre KE Jr, Bailey SA, Malone JM, Goldstone J. Guillotine amputation in the treatment of non-salvageable lower extremity infections. *Arch Surg* 1984;119:450–453.

23. Fox HR, Karchmer AW. Management of diabetic foot infections, including the use of home intravenous antibiotic therapy. *Clin Podiatr Med Surg* 1996;13:671–682.

24. Lipsky BA, McDonald D, Litka PA. Treatment of infected diabetic foot ulcers: topical MSI-78 vs. oral ofloxacin. *Diabetologia* 1997;40(Suppl 1):482–482.

25. Chantelan E, Tanudjaja T, Altenhofer F, et al. Antibiotic treatment for uncomplicated neuropathic forefoot ulcers in diabetes: a controlled trial. *Diabet Med* 1996;13:156–155.

26. Jones EW, Edwards R, Finch R, Jaffcoate WJ. A microbiologic study of diabetic foot lesions. *Diabet Med* 1984;2:213–215.

27. Drew RH, Perfect JR, Srinath L, et al. Treatment of methicillin-resistant *Staphylococcus aureus* infections with quinupristin-dalfopristin in patients intolerant of or failing prior therapy. *J Antimicrob Chemother* 2000;46:775–784.

28. Leach TS, Schaser RJ, Todd WM, Hafkin B, Kaja RW. Clinical efficacy of linezolid for complicated skin and soft tissue infections caused by MRSA, in *Abstracts of the 38th Annual Meeting of the Infectious Diseases Society of America* 2000;Sept 7–10:abstract 60.

29. Nichols RL, Graham DR, Barriere SL, et al. Treatment of hospitalized patients with complicated gram-positive skin and skin structure infections: two randomized, multicentre studies of quinupristin/dalfopristin versus cefazolin, oxacillin or vancomycin. *J Antimicrob Chemother* 1999;44:263–273.

30. Beam TR Jr, Gutierrez I, Powell S, et al. Prospective study of the efficacy and safety of oral and intravenous ciprofloxacin in the treatment of diabetic foot infections. *Rev Infect Dis* 1989;11(Suppl 5):S1163–S1163.

31. Hughes CE, Johnson CC, Bamberger DM, et al. Treatment and long-term follow-up of foot infections in patients with diabetes or ischemia: a randomized, prospective, double-blind comparison of cefoxitin and ceftizoxime. *Clin Thera* 1987;10(Suppl A):36–49.

32. Peterson LR, Lissack LM, Canter K, et al. Therapy of lower extremity infections with ciprofloxacin in patients with diabetes mellitus, peripheral vascular disease, or both. *Am J Med* 1989;86:801–808.

33. Anonymous. Unpublished data. *Pfizer, Inc.*, 2001.

34. Cooper G, Platt R. *Staphylococcus aureus* bacteremia in diabetic patients: endocarditis and mortality. *Am J Med* 1982;73:658–662.

35. Bamberger DM, Daus GP, Gerding DN. Osteomyelitis in the feet of diabetic patients: long-term results, prognostic factors and the role of antimicrobial and surgical therapy. *Am J Med* 1987;83:653–660.

36. Van GH, Siney H, Danan JP, Sachon C, Grimaldi A. Treatment of osteomyelitis in the diabetic foot. *Diabet Care* 1996;19:1257–1260.

37. Lipsky BA. Osteomyelitis of the foot in diabetic patients. *Clin Infect Dis* 1997;25:1318–1326.

38. Gibbons GW, Eliopoulos GM. Infections of the diabetic foot, in *Management of Diabetic Foot Problems* (Kozak GP, Hoar CS Jr, Rowbotham RL, eds.), WB Saunders, Philadelphia, 1984, pp. 97–102.

12

Charcot Changes in the Diabetic Foot

Robert G. Frykberg, DPM, MPH

INTRODUCTION

J.-M. Charcot's classic work on the "arthropathies of locomotor ataxia" was first published in 1868 while he was the Chief Physician at the Salpetrière in Paris *(1,2)*. In describing the joint affections of patients with tabes dorsalis, he noted severe deformities, crepitations, and instability, with gradual degrees of healing over time. Of primary importance, he believed these changes to be secondary to the underlying disease, in which there was an associated *nutritive* deficiency in the spinal cord. Although lesions in this structure are far less frequently involved in the pathogenesis of neuroarthropathy than peripheral nerve lesions, Charcot was certainly intuitive in this regard. In his own words,

> How often have not I seen persons, not yet familiar with this arthropathy, misunderstand its real nature, and, wholly preoccupied with the local affection, even absolutely forget that behind the disease of the joint there was a disease far more important in character, and which in reality dominated the situation... *(1)*.

Although W. Musgrave in 1703 and later J.K. Mitchell in 1831 ostensibly described osteoarthropathy associated with venereal disease and spinal cord lesions, respectively, Charcot's name remains synonymous with neuropathic arthropathies of multiple etiologies *(2–5)*.

W.R. Jordan in 1936 *(6)* was the first to fully recognize and report on the association of neuropathic arthropathy with diabetes mellitus. In his comprehensive review of the neuritic manifestations of diabetes, he described a 56-year-old woman with diabetes of approximately 14 years who presented with "a rather typical, painless Charcot joint of the ankle." His description typifies the classic presentation we now commonly recognize in patients with long-standing diabetes and neuropathy. Subsequently, Bailey and Root *(7)* in their 1947 series noted that 1 in 1100 patients with diabetes mellitus developed neurogenic osteoarthropathy.

In the classic 1972 Joslin Clinic review of 68,000 patients by Sinha et al. *(8)*, 101 patients were encountered with diabetic Charcot feet. This ratio of 1 case in 680 patients with diabetes brought greater attention to this disorder and characterized the affected patients' clinical and radiographic presentations. In the subsequent 30 years there has been a significant increase in the number of reports on diabetic osteoarthropathy, its

From: *The Diabetic Foot: Medical and Surgical Management*
Edited by: A. Veves, J. M. Giurini, and F. W. LoGerfo © Humana Press Inc., Totowa, NJ

complications, and management *(6–10)*. The prevalence of this condition is highly variable, ranging from 0.15% of all diabetic patients to as high as 29% in a population of only neuropathic diabetic subjects *(2,8,10,11)*. The data concerning the true frequency of osteoarthropathy in diabetes, however, is limited by the small number of prospective or population-based studies currently available. Much of the data we rely on are based on retrospective studies of small single-center cohorts. Nonetheless, the incidence of Charcot cases reported is very likely an underestimation since many cases go undetected, especially in the early states *(2,11,12)*. The frequency of diagnosis of the diabetic Charcot foot appears to be increasing as a result of increased awareness of its signs and symptoms *(13)*. Although the original descriptions of neuropathic osteoarthropathy were attributed to patients with tertiary syphilis, diabetes mellitus has now become the disease most often associated with this severe foot disorder.

ETIOLOGY

Charcot foot (neuropathic osteoarthropathy) can be defined as a noninfectious and progressive condition of single or multiple joints characterized by joint dislocation, pathologic fractures, and severe destruction of the pedal architecture that is closely associated with peripheral neuropathy *(2,9,14)*. Almost uniformly, trauma of some degree when superimposed on the neuropathic extremity precipitates the cascade of events leading to the joint destruction. Osteoarthropathy, therefore, may result in debilitating deformity or even amputation *(4,12,15)*. Neuroarthropathy can result from various disorders that have the potential to cause a peripheral neuropathy. With the decline in numbers of patients with tertiary syphilis since Charcot's time and the concomitant rise in the prevalence of diabetes mellitus, the latter disease has now become the primary condition associated with Charcot joints. Table 1 lists the various neuropathic disorders that can compromise joint mechanisms including their predilection for sites of involvement *(2,8,9,13)*.

Several conditions can produce radiographic changes similar to those of Charcot joints. These include acute arthritides, psoriatic arthritis, osteoarthritis, osteomyelitis, osseous tumors, and gout. These joint affectations in the presence of neuropathy make the correct diagnosis even more difficult to ascertain *(8)*. Nonetheless, the characteristics of the joint changes, site for predilection, and even age of the patient assist in determining the true underlying diagnosis.

The primary risk factors for this potentially limb-threatening deformity are the presence of dense peripheral sensory neuropathy, normal circulation, and a history of preceding trauma, often minor in nature *(4,12,16)*. There is no apparent predilection for either sex *(2)*. Trauma is not limited to injuries such as sprains or contusions. Foot deformities, prior amputations, joint infections, or surgical trauma may result in stress sufficient to lead to Charcot joint disease *(10)*. Other factors possibly implicated in the etiology of osteoarthropathy are metabolic abnormalities, renal transplantation, immunosuppressive/steroid therapy, impaired cartilage growth, and nonenzymatic glycosylation *(2)*.

Although the exact pathogenesis may vary from patient to patient, it is undoubtedly multifactorial in nature *(2,10,13,16)*. The *neurotraumatic* (German) theory has traditionally been proposed as the primary etiology of osteoarthropathy, in which neuropathy and repeated trauma produce eventual joint destruction. The loss or diminution of pro-

Table 1
Diseases Causing Neuropathic Osteoarthropathy

Disorder	Predilection site
Diabetes mellitus	Foot and ankle, knee, spine
Tabes dorsalis	Knee, shoulder, hip, ankle, spine
Syringomyelia	Shoulder, elbow, cervical spine
Leprosy	Foot, ankle, hand
Spina bifida	Hip and knee
Meningomyelocele	Foot and ankle
Congenital insensitivity to pain	Ankle and foot
Chronic alcoholism	Foot
Peripheral nerve injury	Ankle and knee
Sciatic nerve severance	Ankle and knee
Spinal cord injury	Varies
Hysterical insensitivity to pain	
Myelodysplasia	
Multiple sclerosis	
Poliomyelitis	
Riley-Day syndrome	
Intraarticular injections	
Paraplegia	

tective sensation allows repetitive micro- or macrotrauma, producing intracapsular effusions, ligamentous laxity, and joint instability. With continued use of the injured extremity, further degeneration ensues, which eventually results in a Charcot joint. Underlying sensory neuropathy resulting from any disorder is therefore a prerequisite under this theory of pathogenesis. However, the neurotraumatic theory does not explain all accounts of Charcot arthropathy, especially its occurrence in bedridden patients (2,4,9–12).

The *neurovascular reflex* (French) theory, in contrast, proposes that increased peripheral blood flow owing to autonomic neuropathy leads to hyperemic bone resorption (17). This theory might indeed correspond to Charcot's original hypothesis of a central "nutritional" defect, although we now recognize this process as a peripheral nerve disorder. Autonomic neuropathy results in an impairment of vascular smooth muscle tone and consequently produces a vasodilatory condition in the small arteries of the distal extremities. In concert with associated arteriovenous shunting, there is a demonstrable increase in bone blood flow in the neuropathic limb. The resultant osteolysis, demineralization, and weakening of bone can predispose to the development of neuroosteoarthropathy (2,16–19). A recent study demonstrates an imbalance between the normally linked bone resorption and production in patients with osteoarthropathy (20). Specifically, greater osteoclastic than osteoblastic activity was noted in acute neuroarthropathy, suggesting an explanation for the excessive bone resorption during the acute stage.

The actual pathogenesis of Charcot arthropathy is probably a combined effect of both the neurovascular and neurotraumatic theories (13,16,18). It is generally accepted that trauma superimposed on a well-perfused but severely neuropathic extremity can

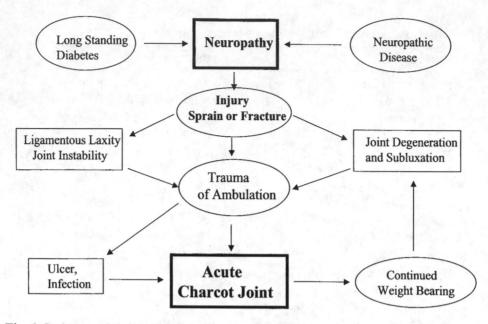

Fig. 1. Pathogenesis of diabetic neuropathic osteoarthropathy. (From: Frykberg RG. Charcot foot: an update on pathogenesis and management, in *The Foot in Diabetes*, 3rd ed. (Boulton et al., eds.), John Wiley, Chichester, UK, 2000, pp. 235–260.

precipitate the development of an acute Charcot foot. The presence of sensory neuropathy renders the patient unaware of the initial precipitating trauma and often profound osseous destruction taking place during ambulation. The concomitant autonomic neuropathy with its associated osteopenia and relative weakness of the bone predisposes it to fracture *(21)*. A vicious cycle then ensues whereby the insensate patient continues to walk on the injured foot, thereby allowing further damage to occur *(9,12,13)*. With added trauma and fractures in the face of an abundant hyperemic response to injury, massive swelling soon follows. Capsular and ligamentous distention or rupture is also a part of this process, leading to the typical joint subluxations and loss of normal pedal architecture and culminating in the classic rocker bottom Charcot foot. The amount of joint destruction and deformity that results is highly dependent on the time at which the proper diagnosis is made and when non-weight-bearing immobilization is begun *(9)*. A simplified cycle of the pathogenesis of Charcot joints is illustrated in (Fig. 1).

Often it is a fracture, either intra- or extraarticular, that initiates the destructive process. This had not been fully appreciated until Johnson *(22)* presented a series of cases in which diabetic patients developed typical Charcot joints after sustaining neuropathic fractures. Additionally, amputation of the great toe or first ray, often a consequence of infection or gangrene in the diabetic patient, may lead to neuropathic joint changes in the lesser metatarsophalangeal (MTP) joints (Fig. 2). Presumably, this is a stress-related factor secondary to an acquired biomechanical imbalance. Intraarticular infection can also be implicated as an inciting event leading to this end point. In effect, almost any inflammatory or destructive process introduced to a neuropathic joint has the potential for creating a Charcot joint.

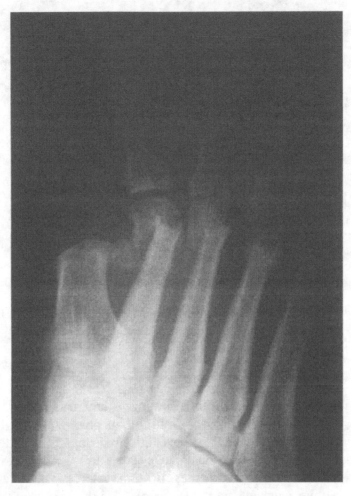

Fig. 2. Neuropathic changes (fractures) in the lesser metatarsal heads after a first ray amputation. Biomechanical imbalances and increased stress presumably lead to these changes.

CLASSIFICATION OF CHARCOT ARTHROPATHY

The most common classification system of Charcot arthropathy is based on radiographic appearance as well as physiologic stages. The *Eichenholtz classification* divides osteoarthropathy into developmental, coalescence, and reconstructive stages *(23)*. The *developmental* stage is characterized by fractures, debris formation, and fragmentation of cartilage and subchondral bone. This is followed by capsular distention, ligamentous laxity, and varying degrees of subluxation and marked soft tissue swelling. Synovial biopsy at this time will show osseous and cartilaginous debris embedded in a thickened synovium, which is pathognomonic for the disease *(23)*. The *coalescence* stage is marked by the absorption of much of the fine debris, a reduction in soft tissue swelling, bone callus proliferation, and consolidation of fractures. Finally, the *reconstructive* stage is denoted by bony ankylosis and hypertrophic proliferation with some restoration of stability when this stage is reached. In certain cases, however, severe osseous disintegration occurs owing to prolonged activity. In these situations the condition may be

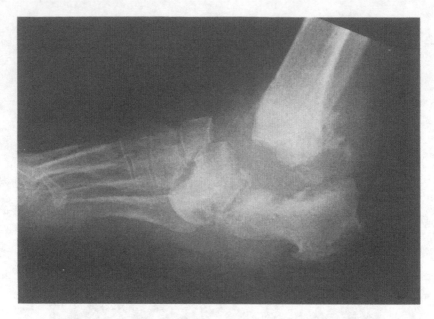

Fig. 3. Osteolysis of the talus and disintegration of the ankle and subtalar joints.

referred to as chronically active, and little healing, if any, takes place. Although the system is radiologically very descriptive and useful, its practical clinical applicability is less so. In clinical practice, the initial developmental stage is considered *active* or *acute*, whereas the coalescent and reconstructive stages are considered to be the *quiescent* or reparative stages. A more recent classification system has been described based on anatomic sites of involvement, but it does not describe the activity of the disease *(2)*.

RADIOGRAPHIC FINDINGS

Radiographically, osteoarthropathy takes on the appearance of a severely destructive form of degenerative arthritis. Serial x-rays will customarily demonstrate multiple changes occurring throughout the process and can assist in monitoring disease activity *(10)*. Rarely will nucleotide scanning, computed tomography (CT), or magnetic resonance imaging (MRI) be necessary to establish the diagnosis. The acute or developmental stage is marked by an abundance of soft tissue edema, osteopenia, multiple fractures, loose bodies, dislocations, or subluxations. These radiographic findings are fairly typical of noninfective bone changes associated with diabetes and have been described well by Newman *(24)*. In addition to alterations in the normal pedal architecture, the metatarsal heads and phalanges will frequently demonstrate atrophic changes, often called diabetic *osteolysis (12)*. Synonyms for this phenomenon include a "sucked candy" appearance, "pencil pointing," or "hourglass" deformities of the phalanges, or mortar and pestle deformity of the MTP joints. Massive osteolysis can also occur in the rearfoot during the acute stage, especially in the ankle and subtalar joints (Fig. 3). These changes will often coexist with the obvious ankle fractures that initiated the destruc-

Table 2
Radiographic Changes in Osteoarthropathy

Stage	Atrophic Changes	Hypertrophic Changes	Miscellaneous
Acute	Osteolysis— resorption of bone Metatarsal heads, phalangeal diaphyses, MTP, subtalar, ankle osteopenia	Periosteal new bone, intraarticular debris, joint mice, fragments, osteophytes, architectural collapse, deformity	Joint effusions, subluxations, fractures, soft tissue edema, medial arterial calcification, ulceration
Quiescent	Distal metatarsal and rearfoot osteolysis, bone loss	Periosteal new bone, marginal osteophytes, fracture, bone callus, rocker bottom, midfoot or ankle deformity, ankylosis	Resorption of debris, diminished edema, sclerosis, ulceration

tive process. Medial arterial calcification is another associated but unrelated finding frequently observed in these patients.

Chronic reparative or quiescent radiographic changes include hypertrophic changes such as periosteal new bone formation, coalescence of fractures and bony fragments, sclerosis, remineralization, and a reduction in soft tissue edema (22,24,25). Rocker bottom deformities, calcaneal equinus, dropped cuboid, or other deformities not previously appreciated may also become visible, especially when taking weight-bearing images. Table 2 summarizes the varieties of radiographic changes found in osteoarthropathy.

Sanders and Frykberg (2,10) describe typical neuropathic osteoarthropathy patterns of joint involvement based on joint location in diabetic patients. These patterns may exist independently or in combination with each other as determined through clinical and radiographic findings. They are illustrated in Fig. 4 and are described as follows: pattern I, forefoot—MTP joints; pattern II, tarsometatarsal (Lisfranc's) joint; pattern III, midtarsal and navicular-cuneiform joints; pattern IV, ankle and subtalar joints; and pattern V, calcaneus (calcaneal insufficiency avulsion fracture).

Pattern I: Forefoot

Pattern I encompasses atrophic changes or osteolysis of the MTP and interphalangeal joints with the characteristic sucked candy appearance of the distal metatarsals (24) (Fig. 5). Frequently, atrophic bone resorption of the distal metatarsals and phalanges accompanies other changes found in the midfoot and rearfoot. An infectious etiology has been proposed for these findings, although osteolysis can occur without any prior history of joint sepsis. Ten to 30% of the neuropathic osteoarthropathies have been categorized in various reports as pattern I (2,8).

Pattern II: Tarsometatarsal (Lisfranc's) Joint

Pattern II involves Lisfranc's joint, typically with the earliest clue being a very subtle lateral deviation of the base of the second metatarsal at the cuneiform joint. Once the stability of this "keystone" is lost, the Lisfranc joint complex will often subluxate dorso-

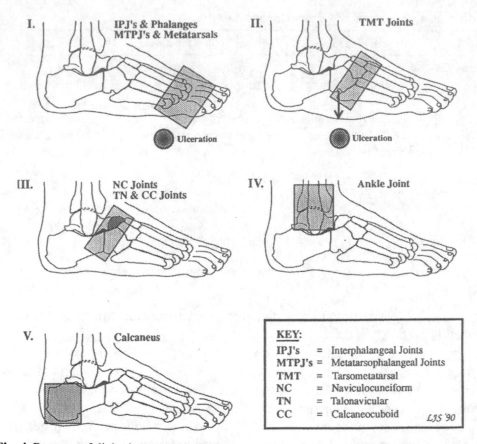

Fig. 4. Patterns of diabetic osteoarthropathy based on anatomic sites of involvement. (From: Sanders LJ, Frykberg RG. Diabetic neuropathic osteoarthropathy: the Charcot foot, in *The High Risk Foot in Diabetes Mellitus* (Frykberg RG, ed.), Churchill Livingstone, New York, 1991, pp. 297–338. Used with permission.)

laterally. Fracture of the second metatarsal base allows for greater mobility in which subluxation of the other metatarsal bases will occur. The rupture of intermetatarsal and tarsometatarsal ligaments plantarly will also allow a collapse of the arch during normal weight bearing, leading to the classic rocker bottom deformity. Compensatory contracture of the gastrocnemius muscle will frequently follow and create a further plantarflexory moment to accentuate the inverted arch. This pattern is also commonly associated with plantar ulcerations at the apex of the collapse, which typically involves the cuboid or cuneiforms (2,16,19). This was the most frequent pattern of presentation for diabetic Charcot feet in the Sinha series and represents the most common presentation in clinical practice (8) (Fig. 6).

Pattern III: Midtarsal and Naviculocuneiform Joints

Pattern III incorporates changes within the midtarsal (Chopart's) joint with the frequent addition of the naviculocuneiform joint. As described by Newman (26) and Lesko and Maurer (27), spontaneous dislocation of the talonavicular joint with or without fragmentation characterize this pattern. Newman further suggests that isolated talona-

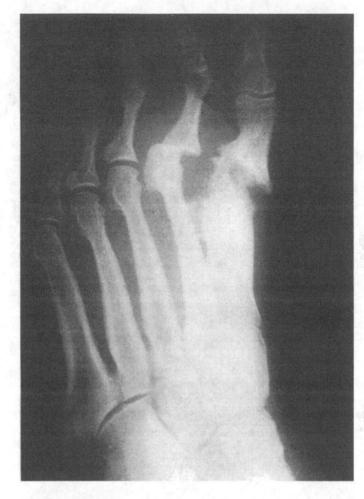

Fig. 5. Pattern I: Osteolytic changes involving the first metatarsals and phalanx are evident without any current infection documented.

vicular joint subluxation might even be considered as an entity separate from osteoarthropathy, although still an important element of noninfective neuropathic bone disease *(24,26)*. Lisfranc's joint changes (pattern II) are often seen in combination with pattern III deformities of the lesser tarsus (Fig. 7).

Pattern IV: Ankle and Subtalar Joint

Pattern IV involves the ankle joint, including the subtalar joint and body of the talus (Fig. 8). Disintegration of the talar body is equivalent to the central tarsal disintegration of Harris and Brand *(28)*. The destructive forces are created by joint incongruity and continued mechanical stress, which eventually erodes the talus. Massive osteolysis is frequently observed in this pattern with attendant ankle or subtalar subluxation and angular deformity. As noted, tibial or fibular malleolar fractures are frequently seen in association with osteoarthropathy in this location and most likely precipitated the development of the joint dissolution. Pattern IV Charcot is found in approximately 10% of reported cases *(2,8,10,29)*.

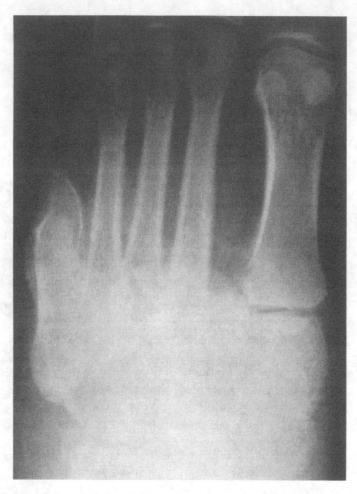

Fig. 6. Pattern II: Lisfranc's joint dislocation with associated fractures are evident in this common presentation of the Charcot foot.

Pattern V: Calcaneus (Calcaneal Insufficiency Avulsion Fracture)

Pattern V, the least common presentation (approx 2%), is characterized by extraarticular fractures of the calcaneus (posterior pillar). This osteopathy is usually included in the neuropathic osteoarthropathy classification; however, there is no joint involvement (Fig. 9). This is more appropriately considered a neuropathic fracture of the body or, more commonly, the posterior tuberosity of the calcaneus. El-Khoury and Kathol and colleagues *(30,31)* have termed this entity the "calcaneal insufficiency avulsion fracture".

CLINICAL PRESENTATION

The classic presentation for acute osteoarthropathy includes several characteristic clinical findings (Table 3). Typically, the patient with a Charcot foot will have had a long duration of diabetes, usually in excess of 12 years. Although all age groups can be affected, a review of the literature in this regard indicates that most of patients are in

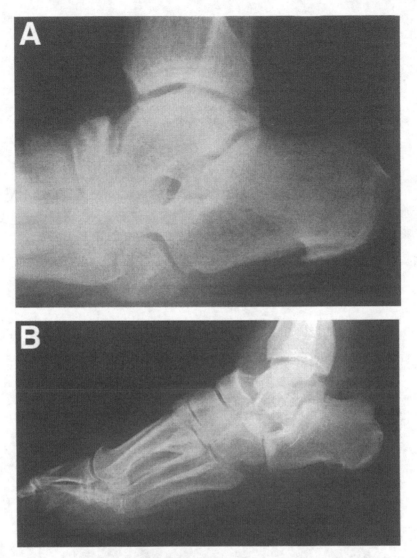

Fig. 7. Pattern III: (**A**) Talonavicular dislocation with "dropped cuboid" and plantarflexed calcaneus. (**B**) Talonavicular dislocation with early subtalar and calcaneal-cuboid subluxation. Note absence of fractures or osteochondral defects.

their sixth decade (midfifties) *(2)*. There does not appear to be a predilection for either sex. Although unilateral involvement is the most frequent presentation, bilateral Charcot feet can be found in 9–18% of patients *(4,8)*.

The initial presentation for acute Charcot arthropathy is usually quite distinct in that a diabetic patient will seek attention for a profoundly swollen foot that is difficult to fit into a shoe (Fig. 10). Although classically described as painless, 75% of these patients will complain of pain or aching in an otherwise insensate foot *(4)*. Almost uniformly, an antecedent history of some type of injury can be elicited from the patient. When no such history is available, the precipitating event might simply have gone unrecognized in the neuropathic limb.

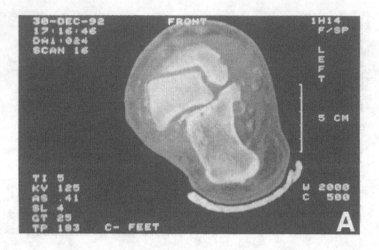

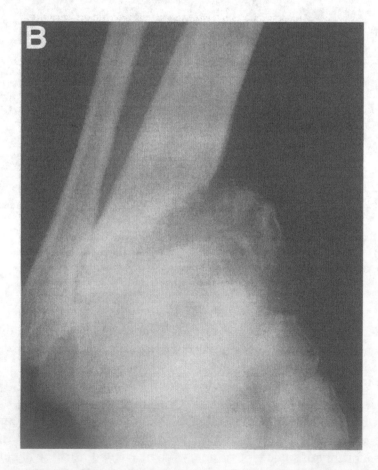

Fig. 8. Pattern IV: (**A**) Subtalar joint dislocation diagnosed on CT scan. (**B**) Acute ankle Charcot arthropathy with medial malleolar fracture and medial displacement of foot.

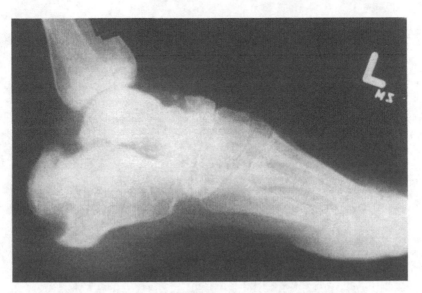

Fig. 9. Pattern V: Calcaneal insufficiency avulsion fracture of the calcaneus.

Table 3
Clinical Features of Acute Charcot Joint

Vascular	Neuropathic	Skeletal	Cutaneous
Bounding pedal pulse	Absent or diminished:	Rocker bottom deformity	Neuropathic ulcer
Erythema	Pain	Medial tarsal subluxation	Hyperkeratoses
Swelling	Proprioception	Digital subluxation	Infection
Warmth	Deep tendon reflex	Rearfoot equinovarus	
	Anhidrosis	Rearfoot subluxation	
		Hypermobility	

On examination, the pulses will be characteristically bounding even through the grossly edematous foot *(12,16)*. Occasionally, however, the swelling will obscure one or both pedal pulses. In concert with the hyperemic response to injury, the foot will also be somewhat erythematous and warm. The skin temperature elevation can be ascertained by dermal infrared thermometry and will contrast with the unaffected side by 3–8°C *(2, 4,29)*. There is always some degree of sensory neuropathy in which reflexes, vibratory sense, proprioception, light touch, and/or pain (pinprick) are either diminished or absent *(9)*. As mentioned, the patients will usually relate some localized pain, although this is often mild in comparison with the deformity present *(11,12)*. Motor neuropathy can present as a foot drop deformity or with intrinsic muscle atrophy. Triceps surae equinus can sometimes be ascertained initially but cannot at this time be considered a precipitating or causal factor for osteoarthropathy. Autonomic neuropathy, which coexists with somatosensory neuropathy, can be clinically appreciated by the presence of anhidrosis with very dry skin and/or thick callus. Another fairly frequent cutaneous finding is a plantar neuropathic ulceration, especially in chronic or chronically active Charcot feet.

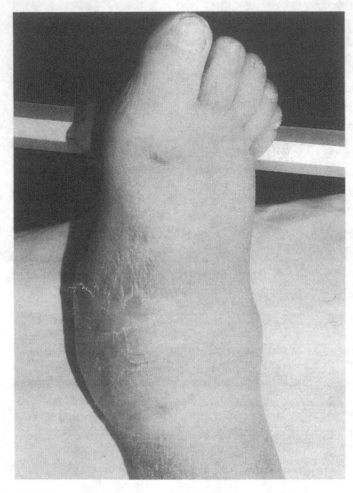

Fig. 10. Acute Charcot ankle with profound foot and leg edema.

A concomitant ulceration will therefore raise questions of potential contiguous osteo-myelitis *(10,19)*.

The skeletal changes frequently manifest as obvious deformity of the medial midfoot with collapse of the arch and/or rocker bottom deformity (Fig. 11). Associated find-ings might often include hypermobility with crepitus, significant instability, and ankle deformity.

CLINICAL DIAGNOSIS OF ACUTE CHARCOT ARTHROPATHY

Plain radiographs are invaluable for ascertaining the presence of osteoarthropathy in a warm, swollen, insensate foot *(16,32)*. In most cases, no further imaging studies will be required to make the correct diagnosis. With a concomitant wound, it may initially be difficult to differentiate between acute Charcot arthropathy and osteomyelitis solely based on plain radiographs *(10,15)*. Additional laboratory studies may prove useful in determining the appropriate diagnosis. Leukocytosis can often suggest acute osteomye-litis; however, this normal response to infection can be blunted in persons with dia-

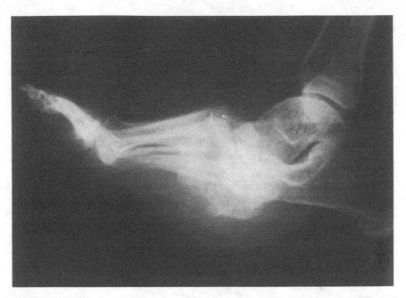

Fig. 11. Radiograph of rocker bottom Charcot foot with collapse of the midfoot.

betes *(33)*. Although the erythrocyte sedimentation rate (ESR) may also be elevated in the case of acute infection, it often responds similarly to any inflammatory process and is therefore nonspecific. When the ulcer probes to bone, a bone biopsy is indicated and should be considered the most specific method of distinguishing between osteomyelitis and osteoarthropathy in these circumstances *(16)*. A biopsy consisting of multiple shards of bone and soft tissue embedded in the deep layers of synovium is pathognomonic for neuropathic osteoarthropathy *(23)*.

Technetium (Tc) bone scans are relatively expensive and generally nonspecific in assisting in the differentiation between osteomyelitis and acute Charcot arthropathy *(34)*. Indium scanning, although still expensive, has been shown to be more specific *(35)*. Additional studies helpful in differentiating Charcot arthropathy from osteomyelitis include Tc-hexamethyl-propyleneamine-oxime (Tc-HMPAO)-labeled white blood cell scans and MRI *(36,37)*. However, no study is 100% accurate in distinguishing these entities. Clinical judgment, therefore, remains of paramount importance in properly assessing and managing these patients.

CONSERVATIVE MANAGEMENT

Immobilization and reduction of stress are considered the mainstays of treatment for acute Charcot arthropathy *(4,10,12–16,29)*. Non-weight bearing on the affected limb for 8–12 weeks removes the continual trauma and should promote conversion of the active Charcot joint to the quiescent phase. This author advocates complete non-weight bearing through the use of crutches, wheelchair, or other assistive modalities during the initial acute period. Although it is an accepted form of treatment, three-point crutch gait may in fact increase pressure to the contralateral limb, thereby predisposing it to repetitive stress and ulceration or neuroarthropathy *(27)*. A short leg plaster or fiberglass non-weight-bearing cast can additionally be used for acute Charcot joint without ulceration or occasionally with superficial noninfected ulcerations *(2,4,9)*. A

Table 4
Off-Loading/Immobilizing Devices
Used in the Management of Charcot Feet

Wheelchair
Crutches
Walker
Elastic bandage or Jones dressing
Unna's boot
Total contact cast
Bivalved cast
Posterior splint
Fixed ankle walking brace
Patellar tendon-bearing brace
Charcot restraint orthotic walker (CROW)
Surgical shoe with custom inlay

soft compressive dressing or Unna's boot is most frequently used in this regard, however. Following a relatively brief period of complete off-loading, a rapid reduction in edema and pain will occur. Although there is no uniform consensus, some centers advocate the initial use of a weight-bearing total contact cast in the management of acute osteoarthropathy *(4,32,38,39)*. Such casts need to be changed at least weekly to adjust to the changes in limb volume as the edema decreases. When deeper or infected ulcerations are present, frequent debridements and careful observation are required. These patients will therefore benefit from removable immobilization devices or bivalved casts.

Off-loading with or without immobilization should be anticipated for approximately 3–6 months, depending on the severity of joint destruction *(4,10,16,29)*. Conversion to the reparative phase is indicated by a reduction in pedal temperature toward that of the unaffected side and a sustained reduction in edema *(2,4,10,14,16,29)*. This should be corroborated with serial radiographs indicating consolidation of osseous debris, union of fractures, and a reduction in soft tissue edema *(12)*.

When the patient enters the quiescent phase, management is directed at a gradual resumption of weight bearing with prolonged or permanent bracing *(4,13,16,38,39)*. Care must be taken to wean the patient gradually from non-weight bearing to partial to full weight bearing with the use of assistive devices (i.e., crutches, cane, or walker). Progression to *protected* weight bearing is permitted, usually with the aid of some type of ambulatory immobilizing device. Through the use of appropriately applied total contact casts or other immobilizing ambulatory modalities (i.e., fixed ankle walker, bivalved casts, total contact prosthetic walkers, patellar tendon-bearing braces, and so on), most patients may safely ambulate while bony consolidation of fractures progresses *(10,16,32,40–42)* (Table 4). Charcot restraint orthotic walkers (CROW) or other similar total contact prosthetic walkers have gained acceptance as useful protective modalities for the initial period of weight bearing *(40–43)*. These custom-made braces usually incorporate some degree of patellar tendon bearing as well as a custom foot bed with a rocker sole (Fig. 12).

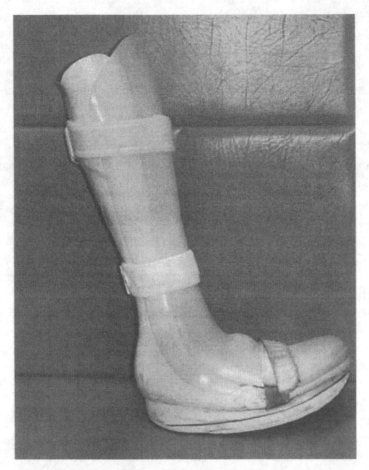

Fig. 12. Total contact custom orthosis with rocker sole.

The mean time of rest and immobilization (casting followed by removable cast walker) prior to return to permanent footwear is approximately 4–6 months *(2,4,12,13, 15,29)*. Feet must be closely monitored during the time of transition to permanent footwear to ensure that the acute inflammatory process does not recur. Forefoot and midfoot deformities (patterns I–III) often do well with custom full-length inserts and comfort or extra depth shoes once bracing is no longer required *(16)*. Healing sandals made from full-length custom inserts placed into a surgical shoe often serve as interim footwear prior to wearing permanent footwear *(12)*. Severe midfoot deformities will often require the fabrication of custom shoes to accommodate the misshapen foot. Rearfoot osteoarthropathy with minimal deformity may require only a deep, well-cushioned shoe with a full-length orthotic device. For mildly unstable ankles without severe deformity or joint dissolution, high-top custom shoes can sometimes provide adequate stability against transverse plane rotational forces. The moderately unstable ankle will benefit from an ankle foot orthosis (AFO) and a high-top therapeutic shoe. The severely unstable or maligned rearfoot will require a patellar tendon-bearing (PTB) brace incorporated into a custom shoe *(32,44,45)*. The PTB brace has reportedly decreased the rearfoot mean peak forces by at least 32% *(45)*.

In the setting of altered bone mineral density (BMD) in patients with diabetes and neuropathy, there has been recent interest in the adjunctive use of bisphosphonate therapy in acute Charcot arthropathy (21,46,47). These pyrophosphate analogs are potent inhibitors of osteoclastic bone resorption and are widely used in the treatment of osteoporosis and Paget's disease. Although one uncontrolled study of six patients found significant reductions in foot temperature and alkaline phosphatase levels compared with baseline, it is hard to draw meaningful conclusions because of the small size and lack of a control group (46). A subsequent randomized trial from this same group was performed using a single intravenous infusion of pamidronate compared with saline infusion (47). The treatment group had significant falls in temperature and markers of bone turnover in subsequent weeks, in contrast to the control subjects. However, no differences in clinical or radiographic outcomes were reported. Until definitive controlled outcome studies are performed that concurrently measure serum markers of osteoclastic activity and attempt to control for treatment effects from simple off-loading, bisphosphonate use can only be considered an unproved ancillary treatment for active osteoarthropathy.

Another modality that has been applied to the management of acute neuroarthropathy is electrical bone stimulation (48–50). In one study of 31 subjects randomized to either casting alone or cast with combined magnetic field (CMF) electrical bone stimulation, there was a significant reduction in time to consolidation of the Charcot joints in the study group (11 vs. 24 weeks) (49). Although this is a promising modality, larger well-controlled studies are necessary.

SURGICAL THERAPY

Neuropathic arthropathy should not be considered primarily a surgical disorder. On the contrary, there is an abundance of support in the literature confirming the need for initial attempts at conservative therapy to arrest the destructive process by converting the active Charcot joint to its quiescent, reparative stage (2,4,10,15,16,29,32). As indicated by Johnson in 1967 (22), the three keys to treatment of this disorder should be prevention first, followed by early recognition, and after diagnosis, protection from further injury until all signs of "reaction" have subsided. Surgery should be contemplated only when attempts at conservative care (as previously outlined) have failed to provide a stable, plantigrade foot. Additionally, when uncontrollable shearing forces result in recurrent plantar ulcerations or in those unusual cases that demonstrate continued destruction despite non-weight bearing, procedures such as simple bone resections, osteotomies, midfoot or major tarsal reconstruction, and ankle arthrodeses might become necessary (15,16,22,38–40,51–53).

Surgery on the Charcot foot has recently gained more acceptance in clinical practice, but it is not a new concept. In 1931, Steindler (54) first reviewed his series of operative results in tabetic patients including one subtalar arthrodesis. He, like Samilson et al. (55), Harris and Brand (28), and Johnson (22) many years later, recommended early recognition of the arthropathy, immediate protection from external deforming forces, and early operative stabilization when significant malalignment and instability precluded further conservative treatment. Samilson et al. in 1959 (55) and Heiple and Cammarn in 1966 (56) were early to recognize the necessity for compressive internal fixation and prolonged immobilization in effectuating a solid bony fusion.

In 1966, Harris and Brand *(28)* provided insight into this disorder associated with leprosy and described their five patterns of "disintegration of the tarsus". Full immobilization was always deemed imperative as an initial treatment; however, when progression continued or an unsatisfactory result was obtained, early surgical fusion was advocated. A year later Johnson *(22)* published his large series, which established the need for early recognition and protection to allow the acute inflammatory response to subside prior to surgical intervention. As he stated, "Appropriate surgery on neuropathic joints, performed according to these principles, should be undertaken with great respect for the magnitude of the problem but not with dread." Johnson clearly favored osteotomy or arthrodesis in selected patients with quiescent Charcot joints and deformity in order to restore more normal alignment. Since the trauma of surgery could result in further absorption of bone during the acute stage, great emphasis was placed on resting the part until there was clinical and radiographic evidence of repair. Only then could surgery be attempted with a favorable chance for success.

Indications and Criteria

Instability, gross deformity, and progressive destruction despite immobilization are the primary indications for surgical intervention in neuroarthropathy *(2,10,16,52)*. Additionally, recurrent ulceration overlying resultant bony prominences of the collapsed rear-, mid-, and forefoot may require partial ostectomy to effect final healing when performed in conjunction with appropriate footwear therapy *(38,57)*. Pain or varying degrees of discomfort will frequently accompany the deformity and may be refractory to conservative care in some patients. Attributable to chronic instability, this can be effectively eliminated by limited arthrodeses at the primary focus of the neuroarthropathy (Fig. 13).

Lesko and Maurer *(27)* and Newman *(24,26)*, in their considerations of spontaneous peritalar dislocations, advocate primary arthrodesis for those acute cases in which there is a reducible luxation in the absence of significant osseous destruction. Since these luxations may be the initial event in the sequence leading to typical osteoarthropathy, early intervention following a period of non-weight bearing has been recommended to counteract forces that would most likely lead to further progression of the deformity.

Age and overall medical status should also weigh heavily in the decision regarding suitability for surgery. With the recognition that arthrodeses and major reconstructions will require cast immobilization and non-weight bearing for up to 6 months, selection of the appropriate patient is critical to a successful outcome *(4,52,53)*. Since most patients with osteoarthropathy are in their sixth to seventh decades and may likely have coexistent cardiovascular or renal disease *(2,10)*, careful consideration must be given to the risk versus benefit of lengthy operative procedures and the attendant prolonged recuperation. As mentioned, a simple bone resection or limited arthrodesis might suffice in an older patient with a rocker bottom deformity prone to ulceration, as opposed to a complete reconstruction of the midfoot *(19,57)*. The former procedures can be done under local anesthesia relatively quickly, require a shorter convalescence, are prone to fewer complications, and can provide a stable, ulcer-free foot when maintained in protective footwear. Nevertheless, major foot reconstructions and arthrodeses are certainly indicated in those healthier patients with severe deformity, instability, or recurrent ulcerations who have not satisfactorily responded to conservative efforts *(16,22,51–53)*. In

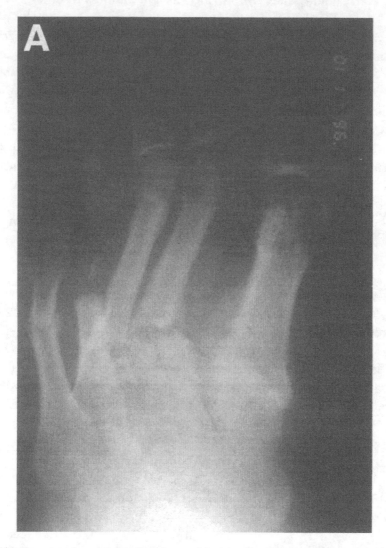

Fig. 13. (A) Preoperative x-ray of patient with dorsally dislocated first metatarsal-cuneiform joint and several metatarsal fractures.

all cases, however, the patient must be well educated as to the necessity for strict compliance with postoperative immobilization and non-weight bearing for as long as 6–12 months.

An acute deformity, either a spontaneous dislocation or the more advanced fracture-dislocation paradigmatic of osteoarthropathy, must always be rested and immobilized prior to any attempted surgery. Surgery during the active stage will usually compound and exacerbate the bone atrophy indicative of this inflammatory stage of destruction. Hence, it is often counterproductive as well as detrimental to operate on these feet until they have been converted to the quiescent, reparative stage. One recent report, however, indicates successful arthrodeses rates with preserved foot function in patients with acute arthropathy of the midfoot *(60)*. Nevertheless, this small retrospective study

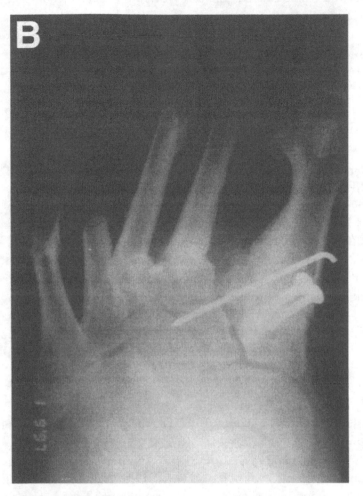

Fig. 13. (B) Stability, resolution of symptoms, and complete healing was achieved with a limited arthrodesis of the first ray.

needs confirmation through larger trials prior to adopting this approach in routine management of the acute Charcot foot.

Ostectomy of plantar prominences in the face of recalcitrant or recurrent neuropathic ulceration is perhaps the most frequent procedure performed on Charcot feet *(2,15,38, 39,57–59)*. Such operations are fairly easy to perform and do not generally require lengthy periods of immobilization beyond attaining wound closure. Surgical approaches are varied, with direct excision of ulcers by ellipse or rotational local flaps predominating *(57–59)*. Alternative incisions are performed adjacent to ulcers or prominences, through either a medial or lateral approach. One recent report suggests that excisions of medial plantar prominences fare better and present fewer complications than those under the lateral midfoot *(58)*. However, an earlier study reviewing experience with only lateral column ulcers reported an 89% overall healing rate *(59)*. A flexible approach to both incision and soft tissue coverage, including tissue transfer, is therefore required for optimal outcomes in cases of midfoot plantar ulceration *(58,59)*.

Arthrodesis of unstable Charcot joints of the midfoot and rearfoot frequently becomes necessary to provide a useful, plantigrade foot when bracing or footwear therapy have been unsuccessful *(16,22,38,39,52,53)*. Major foot reconstruction is also an attractive alternative to amputation in patients with chronic or recurrent ulceration. Thompson and Clohisy *(61)* recommend reconstructive surgery for Charcot deformities unable to function with load-sharing orthoses. Commonly a tendo-Achilles lengthening precedes the fusion to ultimately diminish the plantarflexory forces contributing to pedal destruction *(16,39)*. The preferred method for arthrodesis remains open reduction with solid internal fixation for noninfected Charcot joints, whereas external fixation is utilized when there is suspected infection of the joint fusion site *(16,22,51,62)*. The operative fusion technique requires meticulous excision of the synovium, open manipulation, and precise osteotomies prior to rigid fixation *(22)*. The cannulated screw system is useful since temporary fixation is achieved while recreating "normal" pedal architecture. After copious lavage, a surgical drain is placed before primary wound closure.

Postoperatively, the patient immediately undergoes immobilization of the foot with a posterior splint or bivalve cast. The patient must adhere to strict bed rest and prevent lower extremity dependency for several days until the soft tissue swelling subsides and serial below-knee casting begins. The patient will remain non-weight bearing for a minimum of 2–3 months prior to considering partial weight bearing *(4,51)*. Advancement to a weight-bearing cast, total contact cast, or walking brace will follow after evidence of consolidation.

Complications

Traditionally, surgery on neuropathic joints had been met with a good deal of failure including high rates of nonunion, pseudoarthrosis, and infection *(2)*. Most such occurrences can now be attributed to a failure of appreciation of the natural history of osteoarthropathy and lack of attention to the necessary criteria and the basic tenets of surgery on Charcot joints, as previously discussed. Even with this knowledge, however, complications can ensue in these high-risk feet during the immediate postoperative period and beyond.

Infection can be a major sequel of surgery and of course can threaten the success of an attempted arthrodesis site as well as the limb itself. Most longitudinal studies and reports of surgery on Charcot joints indicate a certain percentage of patients in whom osteomyelitis or severe infection developed that necessitated major amputation *(22,29, 39,51)*. Therefore, caution must constantly be exercised in these patients to ensure that infection or osteomyelitis is controlled and eradicated prior to reconstructive surgery. Perioperative antibiotic therapy is certainly indicated in these compromised patients, and, once present, infection must be aggressively treated.

Pseudoarthrosis and nonunion are very troublesome complications in nonneuropathic patients undergoing arthrodesis or osteotomy. However, this is not always the case in neuropathic patients undergoing the same type of reconstructive procedures. As long as stability and satisfactory alignment are achieved, a failure of complete arthrodesis or union is not necessarily considered a failure of surgery *(22)*. Just as they will not sense the discomfort of posttraumatic arthritis in unreduced fracture-dislocations, these patients will have no symptoms from a stable, well-aligned nonunion. Nonetheless, the surgical prin-

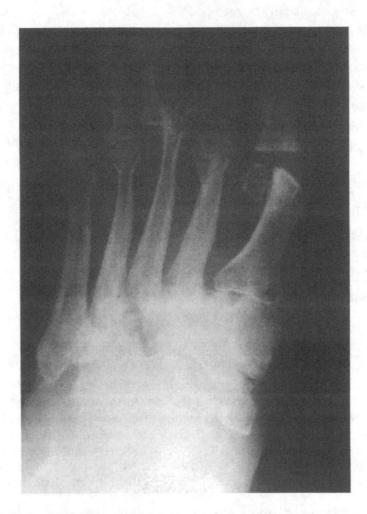

Fig. 14. Resection of the first MTP joint in this neuropathic patient eventually led to the development of pattern I, II, and III changes, presumably because of biomechanical alterations.

ciples for achieving solid union, as previously discussed, must always be followed when operating on these patients.

Since the trauma of surgery in itself can potentially incite an acute reaction in a chronic neuropathic joint, one must always treat the newly operated foot as an active Charcot joint. Furthermore, Clohisy and Thompson *(63)* make a strong argument for prophylactic immobilization of the contralateral extremity to prevent the development of an acute deformity on the supporting foot. Ablative or corrective procedures of the forefoot can also have detrimental effects on adjacent structures as well as on the midfoot and rearfoot *(2)*. Biomechanical alterations will result in increased areas of vertical and shear stress in new sites, which will then be predisposed to ulceration and osteoarthropathy (Fig. 14). Therefore, surgery of any kind on the neuropathic foot must be performed with discretion and with attention to proper postoperative care to obviate the occurrence of these potentially destructive sequelae.

Amputation should usually be regarded as a procedure of last resort in neuropathic patients and not as a normal consequence of osteoarthropathy. Although this outcome can sometimes represent a failure in early recognition and management, amputation usually results from overwhelming postoperative infection or late-stage ulcerations. Unfortunately, amputation will always be a necessary consideration in this complicated group of patients. In certain situations, amputation might be the *best* alternative to a difficult reconstruction in an unstable patient or in those patients who do not wish to engage in the lengthy recuperative period that follows major arthrodeses. However, it must be reserved for those extremities beyond salvage after all other attempts at conservative and reconstructive care have failed.

REFERENCES

1. Charcot JM. Sur quelques arthropathies qui paraissent dépendre d'une lesion du cerveau ou de la moelle epinière. *Arch Physiol Norm Pathol* 1868;1:161.
2. Sanders LJ, Frykberg RG. Diabetic neuropathic osteoarthropathy: Charcot foot, in *The High Risk Foot in Diabetes Mellitus* (Frykberg RG, ed.), Churchill Livingstone, New York, 1991, pp. 297–338.
3. Kelly M. John Kearsley Mitchell and the neurogenic theory of arthritis. *J Hist Med* 1965; 20:151–157.
4. Armstrong DG, Todd WF, Lavery LA, Harkless LB, Bushman TR. The natural history of acute Charcot's arthropathy in a diabetic foot specialty clinic. *Diabet Med* 1997;14:357–363.
5. Mitchell JK. On a new practice in acute and chronic rheumatism. *Am J Med Sci* 1831;8:55.
6. Jordan WR. Neuritic manifestations in diabetes mellitus. *Arch Intern Med* 1936;57:307.
7. Bailey CC, Root HF. Neuropathic foot lesions in diabetes mellitus. *N Engl J Med* 1947;236: 397.
8. Sinha S, Munichoodappa G, Kozak GP. Neuroarthropathy (Charcot joints) in diabetes mellitus. Clinical study of 101 cases. *Medicine* 1972;52:191.
9. Frykberg RG, Kozak GP. Neuropathic arthropathy in the diabetic foot. *Am Fam Physician* 1978;17:105.
10. Sanders LJ, Frykberg RG. Charcot neuroarthropathy of the foot, in *Levin and O'Neals the Diabetic Foot,* 6th ed. (Bowker JH, Pfeiffer MA, eds.), Mosby, St. Louis, 2001, p. 439.
11. Cofield RH, Morrison MJ, Beabout JW. Diabetic neuroarthropathy in the foot: patient characteristics and patterns of radiographic change. *Foot Ankle* 1983;4:15.
12. Frykberg RG, Kozak GP. The diabetic Charcot foot, in *Management of Diabetic Foot Problems,* 2nd ed. (Kozak GP, Campbell DR, Frykberg RG, Habershaw GM, eds.), WB Saunders, Philadelphia, 1995, pp. 88–97.
13. Frykberg RG. Charcot foot: an update on pathogenesis and management, in *The Foot in Diabetes,* 3rd ed (Boulton AJM, Connor H, Cavanagh PR, eds.), John Wiley & Sons, Chichester, UK, 2000, pp. 235–260.
14. International Working Group on the Diabetic Foot. *International Consensus on the Diabetic Foot.* Amsterdam, The Netherlands, 1999.
15. Banks AS. A clinical guide to the Charcot foot, in *Medical and Surgical Management of the Diabetic Foot* (Kominsky SJ, ed.), Mosby Yearbook, St. Louis, 1994, pp. 115–143.
16. Frykberg RG, Armstrong DG, Giurini J, et al. Diabetic foot disorders: a clinical practice guideline. *J Foot Ankle Surg* 2000;39(Suppl 1):2–60.
17. Brower AC, Allman RM. Pathogenesis of the neuropathic joint: neurotraumatic vs neurovascular. *Radiology* 1981;139:349.
18. Edelman SV, Kosofsky EM, Paul RA, et al. Neuro-osteoarthropathy (Charcot's joint) in diabetes mellitus following revascularization surgery. *Arch Intern Med* 1987;147:1504.

19. Banks AS, McGlamry ED. Charcot foot. *J Am Podiatr Med Assoc* 1989;79:213.
20. Gough A, Abraha H, Li F, et al. Measurement of markers of osteoclast and osteoblast activity in patients with acute and chronic diabetic Charcot neuroarthropathy. *Diabet Med* 1997;14:527–531.
21. Young MJ, Marshall A, Adams JE, Selby PL, Boulton AJM. Osteopenia, neurological dysfunction, and the development of Charcot neuroarthropathy. *Diabetes Care* 1995;18:34–38.
22. Johnson JTH. Neuropathic fractures of joint injuries. Pathogenesis and rationale of prevention and treatment. *J Bone Joint Surg [Am]* 1967;49A:1.
23. Eichenholtz SN. *Charcot Joints*. Charles C Thomas, Springfield, IL, 1966.
24. Newman JH. Non-infective disease of the diabetic foot. *J Bone Joint Surg [Br]* 1981;63B:593.
25. Clouse ME, Gramm HF, Legg M, et al. Diabetic osteoarthropathy. Clinical and roentgenographic observations in 90 cases. *AJR* 1974;121:22.
26. Newman JH. Spontaneus dislocation in diabetic neuropathy: a report of six cases. *J Bone Joint Surg [Br]* 1979;61B:484.
27. Lesko P, Maurer RC. Talonavicular dislocations and midfoot arthropathy in neuropathic diabetic feet:natural course and principles of treatment. *Clin Orthop* 1989;240:226.
28. Harris JR, Brand PW. Patterns of disintegration of the tarsus in the anaesthetic foot. *J Bone Joint Surg [Br]* 1966;48B:4.
29. Fabrin J, Larsen K, Holstein PE. Long-term follow-up in diabetic Charcot feet with spontaneous onset. *Diabetes Care* 2000;23:796–800.
30. El-Khoury GY, Kathol MH. Neuropathic fractures in patients with diabetes mellitus. *Radiology* 1980;134:313.
31. Kathol MH, El-Khoury GY, Moore TE, et al. Calcaneal insufficiency avulsion fractures in patients with diabetes mellitus. *Radiology* 1991;180:725.
32. Caputo GM, Ulbrecht J, Cavanagh PR, Juliano P. The Charcot foot in diabetes: six key points. *Am Fam Physician* 1998;57:2705–2710.
33. Armstrong DG, Lavery LA, Sariaya M, Ashry H. Leukocytosis is a poor indicator of acute osteomyelitis of the foot in diabetes mellitus. *J Foot Ankle Surg* 1996;35:280–283.
34. Keenan AM, Tindel NL, Alavi A. Diagnosis of pedal osteomyelitis in diabetic patients using current scintigraphic techniques. *Arch Intern Med* 1989;149:2262–2266.
35. Schauwecker DS, Park HM, Burt RW, Mock BH, Wellman HN. Combined bone scintigraphy and indium-111 leukocyte scans in neuropathic foot disease. *J Nucl Med* 1988;29:1651–1655.
36. Blume PA, Dey HM, Daley LJ, et al. Diagnosis of pedal osteomyelitis with Tc-99m HMPAO labeled leukocytes. *J Foot Ankle Surg* 1997;36:120–126.
37. Croll SD, Nicholas GG, Osborne MA, Wasser TE, Jones S. Role of magnetic resonance imaging in the diagnosis of osteomyelitis in diabetic foot infection. *J Vasc Surg* 1996;24:266–270.
38. Pinzur MS, Sage R, Stuck R, Kaminsky S, Zmuda A. A treatment algorithm for neuropathic (Charcot) midfoot deformity. *Foot Ankle* 1993;14:189–197.
39. Myerson MS, Henderson MR, Saxby T, Short KW. Management of midfoot diabetic neuroarthropathy. *Foot Ankle Int* 1994;15:233–241.
40. Sella EJ, Barrette C. Staging of Charcot neuroarthropathy along the medial column of the foot in the diabetic patient. *J Foot Ankle Surg* 1999;38:34–40.
41. Giurini JM. Applications and use of in-shoe orthoses in the conservative management of Charcot foot deformity. *Clin Podiatr Med* 1994;11:271.
42. Morgan JM, Biehl WC, Wagner FW. Management of neuropathic neuropathy with the Charcot restraint orthotic walker. *Clin Orthop* 1993;296:58.
43. Mehta JA, Brown C, Sargeant N. Charcot restraint orthotic walker. *Foot Ankle Int* 1998;19:619–623.

44. Guse ST, Alvine FG. Treatment of diabetic foot ulcers and Charcot neuroarthropathy using the patellar tendon-bearing brace. *Foot Ankle* 1997;18:675.
45. Saltzman CL, Johnson KA, Goldstein RH, Donnelly RE. The patellar tendon-bearing brace as treatment for neuropathic arthropathy: a dynamic force monitoring study. *Foot Ankle* 1992;13:14.
46. Selby PL, Young MJ, Boulton AJM. Bisphosphonates: a new treatment for diabetic Charcot neuroarthropathy? *Diabet Med* 1994;11:28.
47. Jude EB, Page S, Donohue M, et al. Pamidronate in diabetic Charcot neuroarthropathy: a randomized placebo controlled trial (Abstract). *Diabetologia* 2000;43(Suppl 1):A62.
48. Beir RR, Estersohn HS. A new treatment for Charcot joint in the diabetic foot. *J Am Podiatr Med Assoc* 1987;77:63.
49. Hanft JR, Goggin JP, Landsman A, et al. The role of combined magnetic field bone growth stimulation as an adjunct in the treatment of neuroarthropathy/Charcot joint: an expanded pilot study. *J Foot Ankle Surg* 1998;37:510–515.
50. Grady JF, O'Connor KJ, Axe T, et al. Use of electrostimulation in the treatment of diabetic neuroarthropathy. *J Am Podiatr Med Assoc* 2000;90:287–294.
51. Papa J, Myerson M, Girard P. Salvage, with arthrodesis, in intractable diabetic neuropathic arthropathy of the foot and ankle. *J Bone Joint Surg [Am]* 1993;75A:1056.
52. Pinzur MS. Benchmark analysis of diabetic patients with neuropathic (Charcot) foot deformity. *Foot Ankle Int* 1999;20:564–567.
53. Myerson MS, Alvarez RG, Lam PW. Tibiocalcaneal arthrodesis for the management of severe ankle and hindfoot deformities. *Foot Ankle Int* 2000;21:643–650.
54. Steindler A. The tabetic arthropathies. *JAMA* 1931;96:250.
55. Samilson RL, Sankaran B, Bersani FA, Smith AD. Orthopedic management of neuropathic joints. *Arch Surg* 1959;78:115.
56. Heiple KG, Cammarn MR. Diabetic neuroarthropathy with spontaneous peritalar fracture-dislocation. *J Bone Joint Surg [Am]* 1966;48A:1177.
57. Leventen EO. Charcot foot—a technique for treatment of chronic plantar ulcer by saucerization and primary closure. *Foot Ankle* 1986;6:295.
58. Catanzariti AR, Mendocino R, Haverstock B. Ostectomy for diabetic neuroarthropathy involving the midfoot. *J Foot Ankle Surg* 2000;39:291–300.
59. Rosenblum BI, Giuini JM, Miller LB, Chrzan JS, Habershaw GM. Neuropathic ulcerations plantar to the lateral column in patients with Charcot foot deformity: a flexible approach to limb salvage. *J Foot Ankle Surg* 1997;36:360–363.
60. Simon SR, Tejwani SG, Wilson DL, Santner TJ, Denniston NL. Arthrodesis as an early alternative to nonoperative management of Charcot arthropathy of the diabetic foot. *J Bone Joint Surg [Am]* 2000;82-A:939–950.
61. Thompson RC, Clohisy DR. Deformity following fracture in diabetic neuropathic osteoarthropathy: operative management of adults who have type-I diabetes. *J Bone Joint Surg [Am]* 1993;75A:1765.
62. Schon LC, Marks RM. The management of neuroarthropathic fracture-dislocations in the diabetic patient. *Orthop Clin North Am* 1995;26:375–392.
63. Clohisy DR, Thompson RC. Fractures associated with neuropathic arthropathy in adults who have juvenile-onset diabetes. *J Bone Joint Surg [Am]* 1988;70A:1192.

13

Principles of Treatment of the Chronic Wound

Joseph E. Grey, MB BCh, PhD, MRCP,
Vanessa Jones, MSc, RGN, NDN, RCNT, PGCE,
and Keith G. Harding, MB ChB, MRCGP, FRCS

"I dressed the wound and God healed it"

Ambroïse Paré

INTRODUCTION

The effective use of dressings is essential to ensure the optimal management of diabetic foot ulcers. Although there is a wealth of literature on the subject of diabetic foot ulceration, much of this literature signally fails to mention the use of dressings in the treatment of diabetic foot ulcers. The reasons are manifold; in the main this may be due to a lack of evidence to support an effect on increasing the rate of healing in diabetic foot ulcers, although there may be other benefits to the patient. The appropriate choice of dressing is an important and integral part of the treatment of the diabetic foot ulcer. This choice should, where possible, be made as part of a interdisciplinary approach to the assessment and treatment of the person with a diabetic foot ulcer.

THE INTERDISCIPLINARY APPROACH

Diabetic foot ulceration is the cause of a great deal of morbidity and is the most common reason for hospital admission in diabetic patients. Annually 2–3% of diabetics will develop a foot ulcer *(1–5)*. Although most of these heal, up to 15% of diabetics will develop a chronic ulcer during their lifetime *(6,7)*. In those diabetics who require lower limb amputation, 70–90% will be preceded by foot ulceration *(8)*.

The etiology of diabetic foot ulceration is multifactorial, and care should reflect this fact. The advent of the interdisciplinary diabetic foot clinic has seen a dramatic improvement in care, leading to increased healing rates of diabetic foot ulcers. Furthermore, it has also contributed to a reduction in the previously very high rates of amputation so characteristic of diabetic foot ulceration. Indeed, the incidence of amputations in patients treated in dedicated multidisciplinary diabetic foot clinics has dropped by between 50 and 70% *(9–11)*. The interdisciplinary team should comprise or have access to a diabetologist, specialist wound healing nurses, orthotist, podiatrist/chiropodist, occupational therapist, physiotherapist, orthopedic surgeon, vascular surgeon, and pharmacist. In such circumstances most diabetic foot ulcers will heal with appropriate care and intervention.

From: *The Diabetic Foot: Medical and Surgical Management*
Edited by: A. Veves, J. M. Giurini, and F. W. LoGerfo © Humana Press Inc., Totowa, NJ

Table 1
Assessment of Diabetic Foot Ulcers

General medical and diabetic history

Blood tests—glucose, Hb_{A1C}, U+E, protein

Wound swab

Examination of feet
  Ulcer classification/staging, e.g., Wagner classification
  Ulcer attributes: necrosis/slough
    Gangrene
    Infection
    Exudate
    Wound shape and depth
    Cavity/sinus/tracks
  Skin surrounding ulcer
  Callus
  Foot deformity, Charcot joint
  Radiologic investigation as indicated

Neurologic investigation
  Tendon reflexes
  128-Hz tuning fork
  Semmes-Weinstein monofilament
  Biothesiometer
  Pain

Peripheral vasculature
  Dorsalis pedis/posterior tibial pulses
  Ankle-brachial pressure index
  Duplex lower limbs
  Transcutaneous oxygen saturation
  Hallux blood pressure

Infection
  Superficial
  Deep
  Osteomyelitis

Diabetic foot ulcers arise through a complex interplay of three major factors: neuropathy and ischemia are the primary causes, with superadded infection completing the triad, often leading to a downward spiral in the condition of the ulcer. It will be obvious that before deciding on an appropriate dressing a thorough assessment of the diabetic foot and ulcer should be undertaken and the effects of neuropathy, ischemia and infection addressed (Table 1).

The choice of dressing is less critical than other treatment modalities in achieving healing, although modern dressings may well confer significant benefits to the patient and clinician in the overall management of the ulcer. These modalities include pressure off-loading, debridement of callus, treatment of infection, arterial reconstruction, and tight glycemic control. A detailed assessment of the foot is required to take into account the neurologic, vascular, and infection status of the foot. A detailed description of all parts of the investigation and management of the diabetic foot is beyond the scope of this chapter but is addressed in other chapters.

WOUND DRESSINGS

Throughout history a variety of materials have been used as wound dressings in order to arrest bleeding, absorb exudate, ease pain, and protect the wound. These materials have included cobwebs, dung, leaves, animal fat, and honey *(12)*. A composite dressing of animal fat, honey, and lint said to have been used in 2000 BC may have been the first example of a complex interactive dressing that would have been nonadherent, osmotically and enzymatically active, antibacterial, and an exudate absorber *(13)*.

It was not until the mid-20th century that the possible beneficial effects of dressings that occluded the wound and created a moist wound environment began to be understood and studied. Up until this time, the practice had been to keep the wound dry in an attempt to prevent bacterial infection. However, initial work by Odland *(14)* in the 1950s demonstrated that if a blister was left intact it healed faster than if it was deroofed.

The seminal work on the beneficial effects of occlusive dressings was a small study carried out by Winter in 1962 *(15)*. Working on the domestic pig, he showed that reepithelialization of acute wounds occurred twice as fast if they were occluded and kept moist, compared with wounds left exposed or those treated with conventional (for the time) dressings. These findings were reproduced by Hinman and Maibach *(16)* in work on the effects on moist wound healing in humans with acute wounds and have since been confirmed by many other investigators.

The results of these investigations led to the concept of moist wound healing, the dressing providing a moist environment at the wound-dressing interface. Much work has been undertaken in an attempt to elucidate the reason for faster healing in occluded wounds. Occlusive dressings may modify the biology of the wound environment *(17)*. The dressings may maintain the viability of cells, thus enabling them to modulate, produce, and release growth factors *(18)*. Such work has, however, highlighted a difference in the environment created by moist healing of acute and chronic wounds.

When acute wounds are occluded, there is increased release of proteolytic enzymes including collagenase. This facilitates autolytic debridement through degradation of collagen, cells, and bacteria and subsequent keratinocyte migration from the wound edge, leading to faster reepithelialization of the wound *(19)*. These processes are often diminished or absent in diabetics *(20)*. The acute wound fluid that accumulates under occlusive dressings has been shown to stimulate in vitro growth of fibroblasts and endothelial cells *(21)*. Platelet-derived growth factor (PDGF), transforming growth factor-β (TGF-β), and epidermal growth factor (EGF) have been found in acute wound fluid *(22,23)*. These growth factors are known to be involved in the chemotaxis, migration, stimulation, and proliferation of cells and matrix materials necessary for wound healing to occur.

In contrast, the mechanism of action of moist healing in chronic wounds under occlusive dressings is less well understood, possibly in part because of the lack of a good animal model *(24,25)*. Fluid from occluded chronic wounds differs from that from acute wounds and has been found to be inhibitory to the proliferation of a variety of cells necessary for wounds to heal *(26–28)*.

The major anxiety in the use of occlusive dressings on chronic wounds has been the fear of increased infection. This has proved unfounded. Although bacterial colonization increases under occlusive dressings, the rate of infection is lower than in wounds without occlusive dressings *(29–31)*. Indeed, infection rates of 7.1% with conventional dressings compared with only 2.6% under occlusive dressings were reported in a review by Field and Kerstein *(18)*.

Selection of Dressing

The now accepted tenet of moist wound healing has brought with it a vast and bewildering array of dressings from which to chose. However, there is a paucity of adequate trials and reliable data on the efficacy of many of these dressings in the healing of chronic wounds. What is needed is investigation of the strength of the evidence for treatment of diabetic foot ulcers similar to that carried out by the Agency for Health Care Policy and Research (AHCPR) on the evidence for treatment of pressure ulcers. These guidelines have confirmed a beneficial effect of moist wound healing in the treatment of chronic pressure ulcers *(32)*. Such evidence on the treatment of diabetic foot ulcers is to a large extent lacking. Not until the relatively recent introduction of technologies such as tissue engineering do we see any large randomized controlled studies and meaningful data.

This lack of conclusive data coupled with the lack of guidelines for the use of suitable dressings to treat diabetic foot ulcers is a potential source of confusion. Indeed, choice of dressing is often dictated by local tradition and personal experience. This practice has been highlighted in results of a questionnaire sent to diabetic specialist nurses and state-registered chiropodists in the United Kingdom and Ireland: Fisken and Digby *(33)* asked which dressings these specialists would use on various categories of ulcer in a person with diabetes. They found that up to eight dressing types were chosen for the same type of ulcer, the most popular being hydrocolloids, hydrogels, alginates, and low/nonadherent dressings. It was not clear whether this seemingly almost random choice of dressing arose as a result of lack of information or whether it did not matter which dressing was used as long as there was one! In consequence, some clinicians do not use these modern products even though they may be more convenient and cost effective.

The absence of a systematic framework for dressing choice will create the potential to delay wound healing if inappropriate dressings are used. Clearly, inappropriate dressings will have added financial implications. This said, however, although occlusive dressings can be expensive, used appropriately they may be cost effective since fewer dressings are required. In consequence, overheads, particularly staff time (perhaps the most expensive component of wound management) will be reduced.

Properties of the Ideal Dressing

Modern dressings are designed to promote and maintain a moist wound environment in the different phases of wound healing. The properties of the (elusive) ideal dressing are summarized in Table 2. Perhaps not unsurprisingly, no single dressing meets all the criteria. It should be borne in mind that conventional dressings are not designed to

Table 2
Properties of the Ideal Dressing

Creates and maintains a moist wound environment
Promotes wound healing
Provides thermal insulation
Provides mechanical protection
Requires infrequent changing
Safe to use, nontoxic, nonsensitizing, hypoallergenic
Free from particulate contaminants
Does not adhere to the wound
Allows removal without pain or trauma
Capable of absorbing excess exudate
Allows wound monitoring
Allows gaseous exchange
Conformable
Impermeable to microorganisms
Acceptable to the patient
Easy to use
Cost effective

withstand the high and repetitive forces exerted on the sole of the foot *(34)*, and their properties may therefore be altered. Furthermore, foot ulcer dressings may have an impact on the fit of footwear. In consequence, the ideal properties of a dressing for people with diabetic footwear have been simplified as follows *(35)*:

- Does not take up too much space in the shoe
- Does not increase the risk of infection
- Absorbs exudate
- Can be changed frequently.

Types of Dressing

Wound dressings may be described as passive, active, or interactive *(36)*. Although passive dressings simply have a protective function, both active and interactive dressings create a moist environment at the wound-dressing interface. Furthermore, interactive dressings are also believed to modify the biology of the wound environment, in particular modulating and stimulating cell proliferation via growth factor release *(18)*. Interactive dressings include the alginates, foams, hydrocolloids, hydrogels, semipermeable films, cadexomer iodine, hydrofibers, and, although technically not dressings, living skin equivalents (e.g., Dermagraft, Apligraf). These dressings also promote debridement and may enhance granulation and reepithelialization.

Traditional dressings such as gauze, absorbent cellulose, and wet-to-dry saline dressings have several disadvantages compared with newer products. When dry, these dressings adhere to the wound bed and often cause bleeding when removed *(37)*. Moreover, there is a risk of damaging the new epithelium. These dressings are prone to bacterial contamination, especially if *strike-through* (leakage of exudate) occurs *(38)*. Any exudate buildup may lead to maceration of the skin, with the potential for further skin erosion or ulceration *(39)*. Removal of dry dressings may also be painful to the patient.

Table 3
Criteria for Determining Choice of Dressing

Wound attributes	Type of dressing	Rationale for use
Necrosis/slough	Surgical or mechanical debridement	Promote autolysis and healing
	Enzymatic debrider; hydrogel	Decrease risk of infection
Gangrenous	Dry; low/nonadherent	Prevent formation of wet gangrene
Infection	No adhesive dressing	Daily dressing change
	Alginates; low/nonadherent; foams	
Exudate		
Low	Low/nonadherent foam; film; hydrocolloid	Maintain moist environment
High	Alginates; foam	Prevent strike-through/maceration
Wound shape and depth		
Flat		
Low exudate	Low/nonadherent film; hydrocolloid	Maintain moist environment
High exudate	Foams	Prevent maceration
Cavity		
No sinus	Hydrogel; hydrocolloid paste; alginate rope	Maintain moist environment
	Foam cavity dressings	
Sinus tracks	Alginate rope; hydrogel	Fill the cavity

To maintain a moist wound environment, frequent changes of traditional dressings are necessary. In contrast, the newer active and interactive dressings are designed to be left in place for several days. This leads to reduced risk of contamination, causes minimum disruption to the delicate wound tissue and may reduce cost *(40)*. This is, however a contentious area. Whereas it may be appropriate to dress clean, nonnecrotic ulcers twice or three times a week, frequent dressing changes have been advocated, especially for infected diabetic foot ulcers, in order to allow daily inspection of the wound *(41–43)*.

Clearly, no one dressing will be suitable for all types of wounds or all stages of wound healing. Data on the use of modern dressings in the treatment of the diabetic foot ulcer are scant, and the rationale for the use of certain dressings is derived from their use in the treatment of other wound types. The appropriate choice of dressings will depend on the characteristics of the ulcer, based on parameters such as the presence of necrosis, infection, slough, granulation, reepithelialization, exudate, wound shape, presence of sinuses, and so on. Suggestions for appropriate dressings dependent on these characteristics are given in Table 3.

Regular assessment of both wound and dressing should be undertaken. Studies on the efficacy of dressings in the treatment of chronic wounds (venous leg ulcers) have suggested that unless a significant reduction in wound size occurs within 2–4 weeks of commencement of therapy, that therapy is likely to fail *(44)*.

Predressing Wound Preparation

Integral to the good care of the diabetic foot ulcer before application of a dressing is debridement of the wound. Debridement involves removal of necrotic and devitalized tissue and callus (Fig. 1; *see* Color Plate 1, following p. 178) associated with the chronic

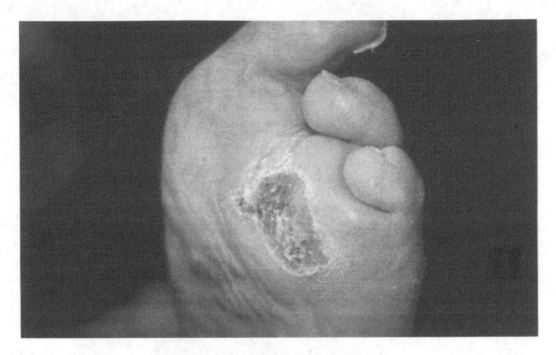

Fig. 1. Diabetic foot with plantar callus.

wound. The presence of such material prevents accurate assessment of the wound and may lead to underestimation of the extent of the diabetic foot ulcer. Debridement also allows for a reduction in the pressure on the capillary bed and wound edge, as well as drainage of any exudate and pus, and may increase antibiotic penetration to the infected wound *(45)*.

The causes of necrosis are multifactorial. They include poor blood flow, hyperkeratosis (callus), abnormal pressure, thermal injury, or surgical complications, all of which may involve both dermis and epidermis and subcutaneous tissues. Moreover, the diabetic's impaired inflammatory response coupled with cellular hypoxia reduces the phagocytic capacity of neutrophils, leading to accumulation of bacteria and dead cells and subsequent slough formation.

The necrotic material ranges in color and consistency from hard, black, leathery eschar to soft, almost liquid yellow slough (Fig. 2). Chronic wound eschar consists of collagen, chondroitin sulfate, fibronectin, and elastin, although this varies between individuals *(46)*. Eschar is inelastic and may prevent wound contraction, thereby delaying wound healing *(47)*. Slough is composed of leukocytes, fibrin, cell debris, and bacteria *(12)*. The presence of necrotic and devitalized tissue may prevent or delay wound healing *(48,49)*. One possible reason for this may be that devitalized tissue becomes a nidus for, and enhances the growth of, pathogenic microorganisms *(50)*. The removal of the necrotic material may therefore reduce the risk of infection and facilitate wound healing *(51,52)*.

Techniques of Debridement

A variety of debridement techniques are employed today. The choice of technique should be dictated by systemic and local factors, availability of materials and resources, and the experience of the practitioner. It should be noted that it is not always appropriate

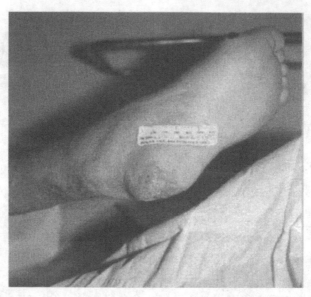

Fig. 2. Sloughy diabetic heel ulcer. Note also presence of eschar over medial aspect of first metatarsopharlyngeal joint.

to debride necrotic tissue. Any suspicion of vascular disease causing necrosis should prompt the involvement of a vascular surgeon. A gangrenous toe, for example, should not be debrided or dressed with occlusive dressings. If vascular intervention is not possible, then it may be more appropriate to leave the toe to undergo autoamputation *(53)*.

Autolytic Debridement

Autolysis promotes the use of the body's own enzymes to break down devitalized tissue and separate it from healthy tissue. The central cell responsible for this process is the macrophage, which releases proteolytic enzymes to degrade the devitalized tissue *(54)*. Autolysis is facilitated by a moist environment and forms the basis for using occlusive dressings such as hydrogels and hydrocolloids, which maintain such an environment. However, the use of hydrocolloids in the treatment of diabetic foot ulcers is controversial, and they tend not to be the first choice for debridement in such circumstances. Cadexomer iodine, which has antibacterial properties, may also be used to promote autolytic debridement *(55)*. Autolytic debridement may be a slow process, which may therefore have devastating consequences for the diabetic foot ulcer. It may also lead to maceration of the periwound skin if the wound exudate is not adequately controlled or the surrounding skin protected.

Sharp and Surgical Debridement

Both sharp and surgical methods of debridement are the most rapid methods of removing devitalized tissue *(56,57)*. Although the two terms are often used interchangeably, they are not synonymous. Surgical debridement (Fig. 3; *see* Color Plate 2, following p. 178) involves excision of dead tissue and may also include opening of sinuses and wound pockets, thus allowing drainage of wound exudate or pus *(58)*. It should be carried out by a skilled clinician. If the debridement is to be extensive, it should be performed in the operating theater while the patient is anesthetized. This should not be

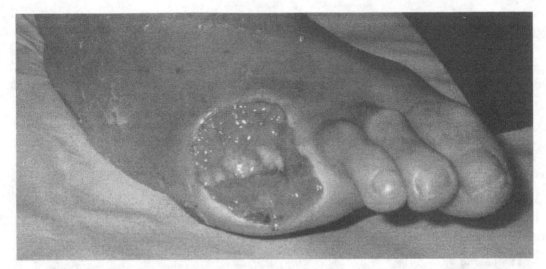

Fig. 3. Diabetic foot post surgical debridement.

undertaken lightly, rather, it should be done expeditiously and judiciously to prevent the risk of infection spreading.

Sharp, or conservative, debridement (Fig. 4; *see* Color Plate 3, following p. 178) plays an important part in the management of the diabetic foot and diabetic foot ulceration. This involves removal of slough and loose, hanging, avascular and necrotic tissue. Equally importantly, it is the method of choice to remove the callus surrounding diabetic foot ulceration. Experienced personnel associated with diabetic foot clinics such as podiatrists, physicians, surgeons, and specialist nurses should carry out sharp debridement.

Sharp debridement may be painful in the sensate foot and may require the use of topical anesthetic (e.g., EMLA [lidocaine/prilocaine]) *(59)*. Pain is a protective mechanism, and special care should be taken in the sharp debridement of the insensate foot, as the patient may not be able to alert the practitioner that he/she is debriding vital tissue! Other potential hazards of sharp debridement include bleeding that is difficult to control and sepsis. Special care should be taken when debriding an infected ulcer.

Chemical Debridement

Many chemicals have been used to deslough wounds. There is evidence that substances such as hypochlorite and hydrogen peroxide may damage healthy tissue *(12, 60)*. In view of their potentially toxic effects, such chemicals are now rarely used. However, applications of short duration (5–7 days) are sometimes used by some with the healthy tissue protected *(53)*.

Enzymatic Debridement

A variety of enzymatic agents have been developed to debride necrotic and sloughy wounds without damaging healthy tissue surrounding the wound. These include crab-derived collagenase *(61)*, collagenase from krill *(62)*, sutilans, and papain. A combination of streptokinase and streptodornase (Varidase) has been used to debride diabetic foot ulcers *(63)*.

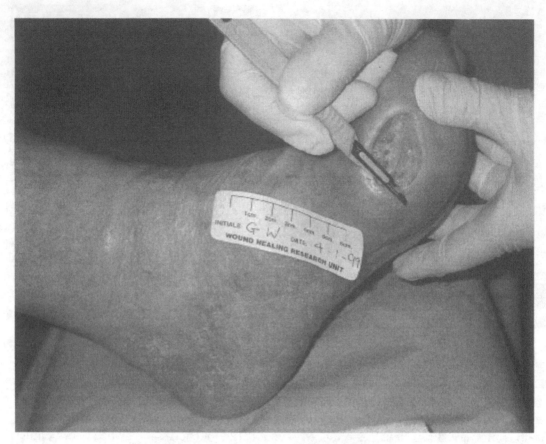

Fig. 4. Sharp debridement of diabetic foot ulcer.

The products may be applied directly to the wound bed or injected into or under the devitalized tissue. If the necrotic material is very hard, then the eschar should be incised prior to application. Many of the enzymatic preparations are, however, used with occlusive dressings, prompting the question of whether it is the enzyme or the moist wound environment created by the dressing that is responsible for the debridement.

Enzymatic debridement is expensive and requires a certain amount of skill to apply; as yet there is little scientific support for its use *(53)*. It should also be remembered that these products are potentially allergenic *(64)*, and appropriate safeguards should be taken.

Mechanical Debridement

Wet-to-dry debridement represents a simple form of mechanical debridement. Moistened saline gauze is applied to the wound, allowed to dry and harden, and then removed with the attached devitalized tissue. Unfortunately, this method also has the potential to disrupt the wound bed, remove viable and nonviable tissue, and cause pain to the patient when sensation is intact *(65)*.

More hi-tech approaches to mechanical debridement involve the use of high-pressure irrigation, whirlpool hydrotherapy, and ultrasound. These treatments loosen and soften the devitalized tissue between dressing changes. These newer methods, along with the traditional wet-to-dry method, are not recommended for use with diabetic foot ulcers.

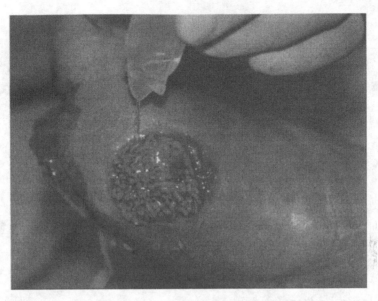

Fig. 5. Removing maggots of *Lucilia sericata* from a diabetic foot ulcer following a period of debridement. (Courtesy of Dr. Steven Thomas, Bridgend, UK.)

Biosurgical Debridement

The beneficial effects of maggot (fly larvae) have been recognized for many centuries. However, more recently there has been a resurgence in their use as debriding agents, and they have been used on a wide range of sloughy and necrotic wounds including diabetic foot ulcers (Fig. 5). The most commonly used larvae are those of the green bottle fly (*Lucilia sericata*). They have a voracious appetite for devitalized tissue while avoiding healthy tissue *(66)*, externally and internally digesting it along with a variety of microorganisms. They may also be effective against methicillin-resistant *Staphylococcus aureus (67)*.

The larvae are applied to the wound surface and covered with a hydrocolloid dressing to avoid damage to healthy tissue from the proteases, which they secrete. Care should be exercised when using them on plantar diabetic foot ulcers as they may get squashed! Larval therapy is suitable for debriding dry gangrenous areas, thus avoiding the potential for maceration that may accompany autolytic debridement *(68)*. As with many therapies used in wound healing, much of the data for maggot therapy comes from case histories using small numbers of patients *(69)*.

SPECIFIC WOUND DRESSINGS

Hydrocolloid Dressings

One of the first interactive dressings to be developed was the hydrocolloid dressing (Fig. 6). Most hydrocolloids are occlusive dressings designed to create and maintain a moist wound environment, although semiocclusive hydrocolloids also exist. Numerous hydrocolloids are on the market, generally based on the gelling agent sodium carboxymethylcellulose combined with absorbent polymers and an adhesive.

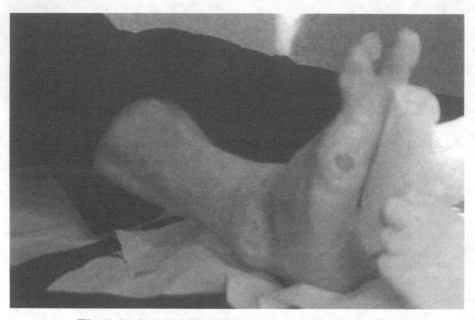

Fig. 6. Hydrocolloid being applied to diabetic foot ulcer.

Hydrocolloids are able to absorb a moderate amount of wound exudate, causing a gel to be formed on the wound surface, which maintains a moist wound environment. The volume of exudate absorbed by hydrocolloids (and, indeed, other dressings) is partly dependent on the moisture vapor transmission rate (MVTR) of the backing layer, which controls the loss of water vapor from the dressing. A low MVTR makes the hydrocolloids almost impermeable to water vapor, thus facilitating a moist wound environment. This attribute promotes rehydration and autolytic debridement, making hydrocolloids particularly useful in treating wounds covered with eschar *(70,71)*. It has been demonstrated that clothing, dressings, bedclothes, and footwear affect the MVTR of hydrocolloids *(20,72)*. This has obvious implications for the volume of exudate that the hydrocolloid can handle.

It has been observed by Thomas and coworkers *(73)* that hydrocolloids may reduce the volume of exudate by up to 50%: the authors postulate that exudate accumulated under the intact hydrocolloid causes increased pressure, which prevents further fluid loss from the capillaries. However, when the hydrocolloid dressing becomes saturated, the liquefied yellow-brown gel, which may be malodorous, may leak out. This may lead to maceration of the surrounding skin in heavily exuding wounds (Fig. 7). It has been suggested, therefore, that hydrocolloids are best avoided on plantar and heel diabetic foot ulcers as the periwound skin is susceptible to maceration *(74,75)*. Other authorities opine that hydrocolloids may be used on diabetic foot ulcers with light to moderate exudate, i.e., Wagner stage I or II *(76,77)*.

Hydrocolloids probably do not simply facilitate autolytic debridement through a moist wound environment. They have been shown to retain growth factors under the dressing *(78)* and also to promote granulation and epithelialization *(36)*.

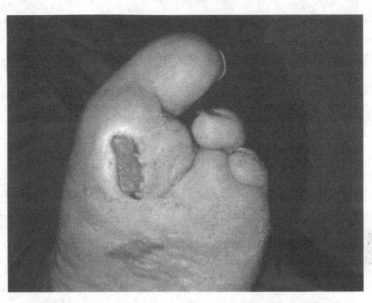

Fig. 7. Diabetic foot ulcer with surrounding maceration.

Infection and Hydrocolloids

Infection of diabetic foot ulcers is the cause of considerable morbidity and mortality. The role of hydrocolloids with respect to diabetic foot ulcers and infection is somewhat controversial.

Initial fears that occlusive dressings and a moist wound environment would lead to an increase in infection appear to be unfounded. A review of controlled trials revealed an infection rate of 7.1% under conventional dressings compared with only 2.6% under occlusive dressings (*18*). Bacterial overgrowth is reported to be inhibited, as hydrocolloids provide a physical barrier and also lower the subdressing pH (*12,29,79*). The growth of *Pseudomonas* has been reported to be inhibited by hydrocolloids (*80*) possibly because of the low pH and hypoxic environment (*81*). It has also been demonstrated that polymorphonuclear lymphocytes infiltrate occluded wounds more effectively than dry-dressed wounds (*82*). Moreover, hydrocolloids have been shown to minimize airborne dispersal of pathogens during dressing changes (*83*). This has obvious implications for infection control and may decrease the risk of cross-infection.

Despite the evidence that the microenvironment created by hydrocolloids appears to optimize the conditions necessary for control of potential pathogens (*81*), there has been concern that the use of hydrocolloids may lead to a deterioration of diabetic foot ulcers. A retrospective review of diabetic foot ulcers dressed with hydrocolloids has not revealed an increase in infection rates compared with other dressings (*31*).

Two cases of deterioration of infected ulcers following 3- and 7-day treatment with hydrocolloids have been reported (*84*), although the duration of treatment indicates inappropriate use of the dressing. A further report of eight cases of deterioration of diabetic foot ulcers dressed with hydrocolloids has been reported by Foster and coworkers

(41). In each of these cases, however, the hydrocolloids were applied for between 5 and 7 days. Furthermore, some of the ulcers were infected prior to application of the hydrocolloid. In such cases one would question both the choice of dressing and the excessive length of treatment.

Infection should be treated as a serious issue in the diabetic foot ulcer. Diabetics have a poor response to infection, and a limb- or life-threatening infection can develop startlingly rapidly. Clearly, more work is needed in this area. Randomized, controlled trials are under way and should shed light on this contentious issue.

Frequency of Change of Hydrocolloids

The frequency of dressing change is a further area of debate. Hydrocolloids are designed to be left on the wound for several days. Many authorities are of the opinion that hydrocolloids may be used on appropriate (noninfected) wounds for more than 1 day *(75,76, 85–90)*. Others dissent, recommending daily dressing changes to allow regular inspection of the ulcer *(43,91,92)*. Patients with infected diabetic foot ulcers have the potential for serious deterioration, and thus frequent dressing change combined with appropriate antibiotic therapy is necessary *(42,93)*. McInnes *(90)*, however, opines that ischemic or infected wounds may be inspected at least every 3 days.

There is a dearth of meaningful studies investigating the frequency of hydrocolloid changes in the treatment of diabetic foot ulcers. We are, therefore, left to try and extrapolate from several descriptive and comparative trials. Apelqvist and co-workers *(94)* reported that hydrocolloids used on clean, nonnecrotic diabetic foot ulcers were changed an average of two to three times a week. Dennison *(95)* examined patients with diabetic foot ulcers weekly for 12 weeks and reported that Granuflex (a hydrocolloid) and Intrasite (a hydrogel) were the main dressings used to treat necrotic sloughy wounds. However, it was not clear whether any of these lesions were infected.

In a comparative trial of Cutinova Hydro (a hydrocolloid) versus Allevyn, dressings were changed on average every 2–3 days *(96)*. Although 75% of the patients were receiving concurrent antibiotics, there was no indication that these patients' dressings were changed more frequently. Laing *(86)* noted that hydrocolloids had been left in place for 1 week in association with total contact casts without infection developing in the diabetic foot ulcer. *Pseudomonas* was cultured from some of the wounds without any obvious signs of clinical infection. This is a noteworthy finding, which is at odds with a previous study showing that hydrocolloids inhibited growth of *Pseudomonas (80)*.

Hydrocolloids are favored by many nurses to treat diabetic foot ulcers as they do not require a secondary dressing. In one study hydrocolloids were shown to be the second most popular dressing used by chiropodists and diabetic specialist nurses to dress diabetic foot ulcers *(97)*. Hydrocolloids take up less space than conventional dressings, making them less likely to affect shoe-fit *(93,98)*. Care should be exercised when using hydrocolloids to dress plantar lesions, as rucking of the dressings may occur and lead to development of high pressure in such areas. They have been shown not to stick to wounds when removed and to cause minimal trauma to the healing wound *(77,88)*. The reduced frequency of dressing change has an impact on cost (although this must be of secondary consideration in the at-risk diabetic foot), especially in treating patients in the community, where the bulk of the cost is associated with transport and staff time *(94,99)*.

Alginate Dressings

Alginates are naturally occurring polysaccharides composed of the sugars *mannuronic* and *guluronic* acids. They are found primarily as the sodium salt in members of one the main divisions of algae, the brown algae (Phaeophyceae). Alginates have found widespread uses since they were first purified in the late 19th century. Alginates are considered to be nontoxic and nonallergenic. They are used in a variety of textiles, foodstuffs, and drinks as thickeners and stabilizing agents and are extensively used by the pharmaceutical industry, not exclusively for the manufacture of alginate wound dressings. Indeed, although there is not firm proof, seaweed itself is purported to have been used to heal wounds under the guise of various names including the "mariner's cure". Alginates were initially used on wounds to achieve hemostasis in the middle of the 20th century. It was not until the 1980s that they began to be used again on any great scale in wound healing and on a variety of wounds.

Structure

Alginates are composed of distinct sequences of mannuronic and guluronic acids and regions of mixed sequences of both. It is the relative proportions and arrangements of these sequences that confer the physical and chemical attributes of the alginates and their subsequent use as a dressing *(100)*.

Alginate dressings are composed either of 100% calcium alginate or a combination of calcium and sodium alginate, usually in a 4:1 ratio. When the calcium-rich alginate interacts with the sodium-rich wound exudate, ion exchange occurs, leading to the formation of a hydrophilic gel on the wound surface and providing the conditions necessary for a moist wound healing environment.

Calcium alginates rich in guluronic acid tend to have a stable structure when in contact with wound fluid. They are strong but brittle, and the gel formed on contact with wound fluid tends to be hard. Calcium alginates rich in mannuronic acid, on the other hand, absorb fluid to a greater extent owing to the ion exchange between calcium and the sodium-rich wound exudate. This results in increased fluid uptake and faster gel formation than guluronic acid-rich alginates. Alginates rich in mannuronic acid, therefore, form softer gels and are more absorbent than those rich in guluronic acid *(100)*. The replacement of a proportion of calcium by sodium ions in the calcium/sodium alginates leads to a dressing in which the production of the hydrophilic gel on contact with wound fluid is accelerated *(101)*. Depending on the ratio of mannuronic to guluronic acids, alginates can absorb between 15 and 20 times their own weight of fluids *(102)*.

The absorptive capacity of alginates makes them eminently suited to the treatment of heavily exuding wounds. Diabetic foot ulcers are at risk of maceration owing to the pooling of exudate and are, providing appropriate safeguards are observed, suitable to be dressed with alginates. However, diabetic foot ulcers that are initially exuding should be examined frequently so that wounds with diminishing volumes of exudate do not cause the alginate to remain dry and hard, which in turn could lead to obstruction of drainage or to areas of increased pressure.

Attributes

Alginates rich in mannuronic acid (e.g., Sorbsan) form soft hydrophilic gels on exposure to wound exudate and can thus generally be removed from the wound by irrigation

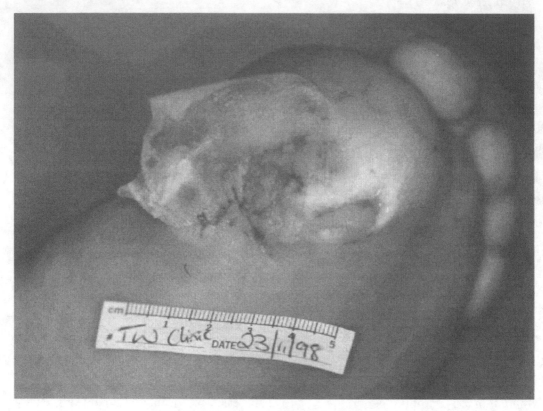

Fig. 8. Alginate on wet diabetic foot ulcer.

with normal saline (Figs. 8 and 9). Those alginates rich in guluronic acid (e.g., Kaltostat) often appear relatively intact, even after sometimes prolonged exposure to wound fluid. They may not wash off the wound and may be removed intact with a gloved hand or pair of forceps. Although ease of removal is a major attribute of alginates, one should not be misled into believing that alginates are nonadherent. Indeed, several studies have reported problems removing alginates from wounds. For example, in one study almost 20% of alginate dressings adhered to the wound *(35)*.

In common with other modern wound dressings, alginates are costly. However, they are reportedly cost effective since they potentially decrease the number of dressing changes required, thus reducing nursing time and allowing the patient to be discharged earlier from hospital *(103,104)*. Studies have also shown that alginates are easy to use and acceptable to the patient *(105–107)*. There is, however, no conclusive evidence for reduction of healing time in diabetic foot ulcers dressed with alginates.

A variety of composite alginate dressings are currently on the market, e.g., alginate/ hydrocolloid, alginate/hydrogel, alginate/collagen. Again, few reliable trials have been carried out on these products, and it is difficult to ascertain whether these composites have any advantage over the traditional calcium or calcium/sodium alginates. For example, Fibracol (an alginate/collagen dressing) has been compared with saline-moistened dressings in the treatment of diabetic foot ulcers *(107)*. This type of composite alginate is theoretically a potentially attractive development, especially given the difficulties

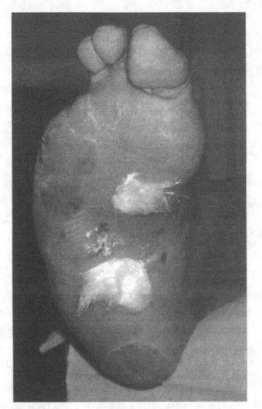

Fig. 9. Alginate on dry diabetic foot ulcers.

diabetics have with collagen formation in wounds, although evidence for such an effect is still required. The patients were reviewed weekly for up to 8 weeks or until wound healing. Although the mean reduction in wound area and incidence of wound healing were higher in the Fibracol treatment group, these failed to reach statistical significance. Seemingly paradoxically, the mean time (not statistically significant) to healing was longer in the Fibracol-treated group.

Biodegradability

Assumptions that fibers of retained alginates are enzymatically degraded by the host have, in the past, given rise to the claim that these dressings are biodegradable. However, reports from both animal and human studies indicate that this may not be the case. Subcutaneous implants of Kaltostat in rats showed no significant degradation over a 12-week study period *(108)*. There was an initial foreign body reaction, which subsided, followed by development of fibrous sheaths around the Kaltostat. It was concluded that the Kaltostat did not pose a toxic risk, nor was its use contraindicated for hemostasis in surgery.

Similar results have been recorded in humans. Remnants of alginate have been found in a tooth socket 12 weeks after a tooth extraction *(109)*. A subsequent account of the use of Kaltostat following tooth extraction reported the development of a florid foreign body giant cell reaction 7 months after extraction *(110)*. Giant cell foreign body reactions have also been reported following the use of Kaltostat in clean surgical cavity wounds *(106,111)*. Such reports are few and have occurred in small and tortuous cavities, not unlike the conditions found with diabetic foot ulcers, with small openings and sinuses. It is advisable, therefore, that alginates be removed as carefully and meticulously as any other dressing used on diabetic foot ulcers. It should be noted, however, that there have been reports that the retained alginate fibers disappear as the wound matures *(112)*.

There are many anecdotal reports that alginates enhance the wound healing process. This may not be solely owing to the promotion of a moist wound environment. Alginates have been shown to stimulate human fibroblasts while inhibiting the proliferation of human keratinocytes and endothelial cells *(113)*. They have also been shown to induce proinflammatory growth factor production by human monocytes *(114)*. This latter study demonstrated that alginates rich in mannuronic acid stimulated growth factor production 10-fold more than those rich in guluronic acid, leading to the hypothesis that mannuronic acid residues were responsible for the effect. A similar conclusion was reached in other studies *(115)*.

In contrast, it has been reported that certain alginates rich in guluronic acid also stimulate the production of tumor necrosis factor-α (TNF-α, a proinflammatory growth factor) from human macrophages *(116)*. This study reported that Kaltostat (guluronic-rich), Sorbsan (mannuronic-rich), Seasorb (guluronic-rich), and Tegagen HG (mannuronicrich) all stimulated production of TNF-α to varying degrees. However, polymixin-B (an inhibitor of lipopolysaccharide) abolished the response in all but Kaltostat-treated macrophages, in which the level was only reduced. It was postulated, therefore, that the growth factor stimulation in macrophages is a function of an activity associated with the insoluble alginate fibers related not only to the relative proportions of guluronic to mannuronic acids but also to the their polymeric arrangement. Indeed, lipopolysaccharide and polymannuronic acid alginates share a common binding site on the macrophage *(117)*.

The role of TNF-α in wound healing is controversial. In chronic, nonhealing, noninfected wounds there is a selective deficit of TNF-α, whereas other proinflammatory growth factors (e.g., interleukin-1, interleukin-8) are present at high levels *(118)*. Large numbers of macrophages are present in the chronic, noninfected granulation tissue but produce only low levels of TNF-α *(119,120)*. It is possible, therefore, that TNF-α induction by alginates, and indeed, other bioactive dressings, may recruit fresh leukocytes, thus restarting the wound healing cascade necessary for healing to occur.

Alginates and Infection

The specter of infection is ever present in patients with diabetic foot ulcers, and, once again, the use of alginates in the treatment of infected diabetic foot ulcers is controversial. The potential risks of treating diabetic foot ulcers with alginates arise from the fact that the ulcers often have small openings with a larger interior wound cavity. This makes dressing and, more importantly, its removal, difficult. There have been some reports of infected plantar diabetic foot ulcers treated with alginates *(35,121)*. In these cases the infection was caused by a not unforeseeable problem with alginates: The alginate dried and hardened, preventing free drainage of exudate, with subsequent deterioration of the ulcer. In addition, the number of cases reported were small, and the results should therefore be viewed within the context of care.

Such problems may be minimized by ensuring that the alginate is used on appropriate wounds, does not dry out, and is not left on the wound for inappropriately long periods. Dry alginate may be mistaken for callus and inadvertently left on the wound, leading to problems such as infection and abnormal pressure. To obviate these potential problems, alginates should be loosely laid into sinuses and the number of sheets or ropes used recorded. Alginate ribbons such as Sorbsan may be more easily irrigated from the diabetic foot ulcer cavity.

Studies have shown that alginates may be used in wounds such as diabetic foot ulcers without causing serious infection. A comparison of Sorbsan with gauze in the treatment of diabetic foot ulcers found no incidence of serious infection and no apparent risk of exacerbating infection *(122)*. In vitro work with Sorbsan has demonstrated a significant inhibition of *Staphylococcus aureus* with no increase in growth of *Pseudomonas*, *Streptococcus*, or *Bacteroides fragilis (123)*.

Results of a survey of the management of fungating wounds and radiation-damaged skin indicated that Sorbsan was superior to Kaltostat in the treatment of infected, necrotic, and malodorous wounds *(124)*. It is known that alginates can stimulate the production of TNF-α, and it is possible that the alginates, via their action on macrophages, also have a role in the control of infection of the wound.

Alginates are eminently suited to treat moderately to highly exuding wounds. They may also be useful in infected diabetic foot ulcers provided they are removed thoroughly and changed daily. Caution should be exercised in wounds that have only a low level of exudate. A potential drawback to the use of alginates, especially in the treatment of diabetic foot ulcers, is the need for secondary dressings to keep them in place.

Hydrogel Dressings

Hydrogels are composed of insoluble polymers, which contain hydrophilic sites allowing interaction with aqueous solutions, absorbing and retaining significant volumes of water *(12)* (Fig. 10). Indeed, the hydrogel matrix may contain up to 96% water. They are able to transmit oxygen and water vapor, with fluid permeability dependent on the secondary dressing necessary to keep the hydrogel in place *(24)*. They are absorbent and semitransparent. Hydrogels facilitate autolysis and therefore promote debridement, by rehydrating the wound. The process of debridement is often impaired in diabetics, in part owing to defective leukocyte activity *(125)*.

Hydrogel dressings are available in two basic forms: (1) the flexible sheet form, which has a stable structure although it may swell and increase in volume as fluid is absorbed; and (2) the amorphous form, which does not have a fixed structure and becomes more fluid and less viscous as fluid is absorbed. The amorphous hydrogels have been used in a wide range of wound types and conditions to achieve debridement *(126)*. A variety of hydrogel dressings are commercially available. Their formulations and consequently their absorptive and hydrative capacities vary considerably *(127)*. This will obviously impact on the wound.

Many case reports and clinical trials have investigated the use of hydrogels as a debriding agent *(64,128–130)*, and many of these were carried out in patients with venous leg ulcers or pressure ulcers. However, there are few data on the use of hydrogels in the treatment of diabetic foot ulcers. There is often good reason for excluding diabetic foot ulcers from clinical trials. The presence of slough or necrotic tissue, for example, often

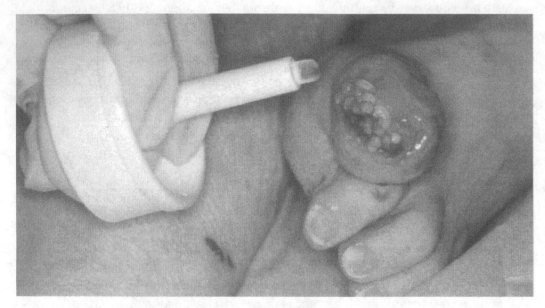

Fig. 10. Hydrogel being applied to diabetic ulcer.

heralds underlying peripheral vascular disease, thus requiring other intervention. Assessment of the vascular supply to the area is thus essential before deciding on treatment. Use of moist dressings such as hydrogels is generally not appropriate for the management of patients with peripheral vascular disease and associated ischemic and often gangrenous tissue. Intrasite, a hydrogel, has, however, been used successfully as a pretreatment on dry gangrene prior to the application of larvae *(68)*. Where dry gangrene occurs adjacent to slough and necrosis, sharp debridement is a more appropriate intervention *(131)*.

A variety of newer hydrogels (e.g., Sterigel, Nu-Gel, GranuGel, Purilon, Aquaform) have been trialled and have shown good clinical results *(132–135)*. They are able to deal with a mildly exuding wound, a feature that was not associated with the earlier products, leading to fewer dressing changes and thus to a reduction in cost. Composite hydrogels have also been developed comprising, for example, hydrogel and hydrocolloid (Granugel) or hydrogel and alginate (Purilon, Nu-Gel). These formulations may offer advantages in the management of diabetic foot wounds when there is a large amount of tissue loss following debridement. They should be changed on a daily basis.

Although the use of hydrogels in the treatment of neuropathic diabetic foot ulcers is perhaps controversial, they may have a role in the treatment of large amounts of tissue loss complicated by thick eschar when surgical debridement is not an option.

Hydrogels and Infection

The data on the effect of hydrogels on infection in diabetic foot ulcers are not extensive. In vitro work with Intrasite has shown that bacterial growth is not supported due to its bacteriostatic activity *(136)*. Application of Intrasite to neuropathic diabetic foot ulcers was not associated with bacterial growth at times 0, 24, 48, and 72 hours after application *(137)*.

Hydrogels may be considered appropriate for the treatment of diabetic foot ulcers as long as the wound is properly assessed and the practitioner realizes that frequent dressing changes are required and that any infection requires treatment with systemic antibiotics.

Iodine Dressings

The use of antisepsis in the treatment of ulceration is controversial, as antiseptics have been found to be harmful to healing wounds, especially in animal models. However, although no clinical studies have demonstrated harm from their use, none has shown any benefits.

Iodine is an antiseptic that, at high concentrations, can be toxic to human cells. It is also toxic to bacteria and fungi *(138,139)*. Bacteria are more sensitive to its effects than fibroblasts, leading to the hypothesis that iodine may be used for antisepsis without impairing wound healing *(140)*. Furthermore, penetration through wound tissue leads to a concentration gradient of iodine, further reducing its toxicity *(141)*. Development of bacterial resistance to iodine is reportedly low *(142)*. The antimicrobial effects of iodine are rapidly impaired in the presence of organic substances such as exudate and proteins on the wound surface *(143)*.

Elemental iodine is almost insoluble in water, may lead to skin irritation and hypersensitivity, and may be absorbed systemically *(142)*. Compounds of iodine linked to a nonionic surfactant called *iodophores* have been developed to overcome the potential problems of molecular iodine *(143)*. Currently two types of iodophore are commercially available. These include povidone-iodine and cadexomer-iodine, which differ in their characteristics and mechanism of release of iodine *(144)*. Both iodophores are used for their cleansing and debridement properties and may have an impact on the prevention of wound infection.

Povidone-Iodine

At high concentrations povidone-iodine has been shown to be toxic to fibroblasts in vitro, to inhibit wound contraction, and to have a deleterious effect on wound healing in animals *(60,145,146)*. However, it is bactericidal at low dilutions, with a maximum activity in the range of 0.1–1.0% *(147)*. The carrier molecule, polyvinyl-pyrrolidine, is able to deliver the iodine directly to the cell surface. Povidone-iodine has been shown to provide effective antibacterial prophylaxis in patients with burns *(148)*. There is lack of evidence of its efficacy in other wound types, and it should not be substituted for systemic antimicrobial therapy, especially in patients with diabetic foot ulcers.

Inadine (Fig. 11) is a commonly used povidone-iodine dressing. It appears to have minimal systemic effects *(131)*. There is, however, a potential effect on the thyroid gland, especially in those patients taking sulphonamides or sulphonylureas, which may inhibit thyroid hormone synthesis *(149)*. Thyroid function tests should be monitored before and during any treatment with iodine-containing dressings. It has also been suggested that serum iodide concentrations be measured in patients with renal impairment, which occurs frequently in diabetics *(150)*.

Cadexomer-Iodine

Cadexomer-iodine consists of microspheres formed from a three-dimensional lattice of cross-linked starch chains *(cadexomers)*. The hydrophilic beads so formed contain 0.9% (w/w) iodine. Upon contact with wound fluid, the beads swell, slowly releasing

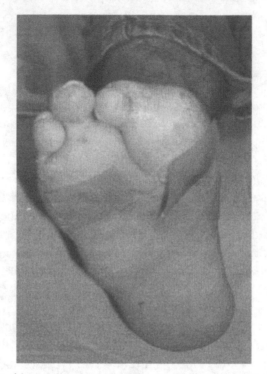

Fig. 11. Application of Inadine to diabetic foot ulcer.

the iodine at low concentrations and resulting in a concentration gradient with the lowest levels of iodine at the wound surface. This method of delivery allows for prolonged delivery of iodine. Two formulations of cadexomer-iodine are currently in use: Iodosorb, formulated as an ointment, and Iodoflex, formulated as a paste.

Cadexomer-iodine dressings have the ability to remove debris and bacteria from the wound *(12,151)*. Unlike povidone-iodine, cadexomer-iodine has good fluid absorption properties; 1 g of cadexomer-iodine is able to absorb up to 7 mL of fluid *(152)*.

Cadexomer-iodine may also have bioactive properties. An in vitro study demonstrated that cadexomer-iodine was able to stimulate macrophages to produce the proinflammatory growth factor TNF-α, which has been found to be at low levels in chronic wounds *(153)*. Cadexomer-iodine is sensitive to hydrolysis by enzymes found in most body fluids and is thus biodegradable *(12)*.

Various studies have confirmed the place of cadexomer-iodine in the management of sloughy and infected wounds. A multicenter trial investigating the effects of cadexomer-iodine compared with older standard treatment on leg ulcers reported that cadexomer-iodine promoted pain reduction, removal of exudate and debris, stimulation of granulation tissue, and infection reduction *(154)*. Cadexomer-iodine has been reported to be effective in the treatment of dirty, malodorous venous leg ulcers *(155)*.

Cadexomer-iodine also compares favorably with other dressings in the treatment of chronic wounds including the diabetic foot ulcers *(152)*. Trials of Iodosorb on diabetic foot ulcers have reported it to be useful in the treatment of exudate, leading to a favorable healing rate *(156,157)*.

Cadexomer-iodine may be used throughout the wound healing process, although its major indication is in debriding sloughy and infected ulcers. The dressing should be changed when it is saturated with fluid and its color changes from brown to gray, indicating that all the iodine has been released *(157)*. Prolonged use of cadexomer-iodine may lead to significant systemic absorption of iodine. Iodosorb may cause local stinging on application.

It should be clear from the foregoing account that the range of dressings is enormous and that there is no ideal dressing. Other classes of dressings exist, such as the hydrofibers and foams. These have not been discussed owing to lack of meaningful data for their use on diabetic foot ulcers. Indeed, the evidence for all dressings in relation to the treatment of diabetic foot ulcers is limited, and case histories, local traditions, and personal experience are often employed when choosing a dressing. Randomized controlled trials of the dressings are needed to assess their use on diabetic foot ulcers, although this is not always possible because of the often parlous state of diabetic foot ulcers, their potential for infection, and their rapid deterioration. The advent of the newer types of treatment for chronic ulcers such as growth factor therapy and bioengineered living skin equivalents has been accompanied by such trials, though these products are still at an early stage clinically.

GROWTH FACTORS AND BIOENGINEERING

An in-depth account of growth factors and bioengineered skin substitutes is beyond the scope of this chapter, and these are discussed elsewhere. Although they are not dressings, they are becoming as easy to apply as conventional dressings, and many are currently used in specialist wound care services. In the future they will be even more widely used (within certain defined circumstances) and thus a brief introduction to each is included here. It should be noted though, that (as with conventional dressings) their use is not without controversy.

Growth Factors

Growth factors are secreted regulatory proteins that control survival, growth, differentiation, and effector functions of tissue cells. They may act in a paracrine, autocrine, and sometimes endocrine fashion. There is a potential for confusion in the terminology used to describe these chemical messengers. In the context of wound healing, the term growth factor encompasses, among others, the terms cytokine, interleukin, colony-stimulating factor peptide inflammatory mediator, interferon, tumor necrosis factor, and so on. Thus a *growth factor* may belong to the *interleukin* family, initiate *colony stimulation*, and be released from the cell as a *cytokine*. Furthermore, growth factors were named according to their first documented behavior, cell of origin, or target cell, and the name belies their subsequently discovered multiple functions. Thus basic fibroblast growth factor may be secreted by a macrophage and stimulate angiogenesis as well as influencing fibroblasts! Falanga *(158)* has, therefore, proposed the term *multifunctional peptide* to reflect their multiple activities and to clear up some of this confusion.

Growth factors may have inhibitory or stimulatory actions depending on the local wound environment and their interaction with each other at any given time in the wound healing process *(159)*. The ability to produce pure human growth factors through recombinant DNA technology has allowed their study in both scientific and clinical contexts.

Of the growth factors studied to date, PDGF has been extensively used in clinical trials on diabetic foot ulcers. Macrophages, vascular endothelium, fibroblasts, and platelets are known to secrete PDGF *(160)*. It is thought to exert a pivotal effect on the initiation of wound healing as it is among the first growth factors to be released by the platelets on wounding and sets in train the cascade of events leading to wound healing.

Levels of PDGF have been reported to be lower in chronic wounds than in healing wounds, or they may be inappropriately low for the stage of wound healing *(161)*. PDGF has also been shown to stimulate the formation of granulation tissue and thus promote wound healing *(162)*. Unsurprisingly, therefore, PDGF has received much attention in an attempt to restart stalled chronic wounds including diabetic foot ulcers *(163–168)*.

Diabetics have impaired immunity and are at risk of developing foot infections that cause considerable morbidity and mortality. Granulocyte colony-stimulating factor (G-CSF) is known to stimulate differentiation, release, and function of neutrophils, and its concentration rises during bacterial sepsis *(169,170)*. Studies of G-CSF in the treatment of diabetes with foot infections have yielded promising results.

Vascular endothelial growth factor (VEGF) has been used in gene transfer studies in an attempt to stimulate angiogenesis in ischemic limbs *(171)*. Studies are at an early stage, but results indicate that this form of therapy has exciting potential.

One conclusion that may be drawn from many of the studies on growth factors is that application of single growth factors may not be sufficient to accelerate wound healing in the diabetic patient. Wound healing is a complex process, and it is not surprising that application of single growth factors to chronic wounds may not provide the stimulus necessary to restart it. Results of studies investigating the efficacy of, for example, G-CSF and VEGF illustrate the benefit of growth factor monotherapy when specific defects are identified. At every step of the (non-)healing process, we are tempted by the potential of growth factor therapy. If it were possible to identify growth factors that are deficient, overexpressed, present in abnormal ratios, or being broken down, then the use of single or multiple growth factors may become a realistic option in the treatment of the chronic wound.

Bioengineering

The development of bioengineered skin substitutes has proceeded apace since the first in vitro cultivation of keratinocyte sheets in the mid-1970s *(172)*. Furthermore, over the past decade there has been an active search for a biologic substance capable of reproducing the structure and function of skin. As a result, a number of bioengineered skin substitutes have been licensed and are in clinical use. These skin substitutes may be classified according to their structure as follows:

- Fibroblast-derived *dermal* substitutes, e.g., Dermagraft
- Keratinocyte-derived *epidermal* substitutes, e.g., Vivoderm
- Composite substitutes composed of dermal and epidermal components, e.g., Apligraf.

Most skin substitutes are allogeneic, being produced from neonatal fibroblasts and keratinocytes. They are, therefore, within defined limits, available off the shelf. Autologous epidermal substitutes derived from the patient's own keratinocytes are also commercially available.

The exact mechanism of action of skin substitutes is still a matter of conjecture and much research. The type of substitute used will influence the mechanism of action. Initially it was thought that skin substitutes would provide permanent skin cover. It is now believed that they act as a temporary wound covering, eventually being replaced by host cells *(173)*. However, it has been suggested that some substitutes become vascularized remodeling with time and leading to graft integration analogous to autologous skin grafting *(174)*.

Both fibroblasts and keratinocytes secrete growth factors in physiologic amounts, which may stimulate wound healing by, for example, controlling cell proliferation, inducing angiogenesis, and modifying the inflammatory response. In addition, the extracellular matrix of the skin substitute may act as a smart matrix, recruiting cells necessary for healing to occur into the wound *(175)*. Clearly this is not a simple process and probably involves a complex interplay of many processes.

Rejection of the skin substitute or development of immune sensitization does not appear to be a problem. It is thought that this may be due to the lack of antigen-presenting cells and the fact that neonatal fibroblasts lack the HLA-DR surface antigens, which are responsible for generating allograft rejection *(176–178)*.

The development of bioengineered skin equivalents represents an exciting innovation in the treatment of diabetic foot ulcers. They should not as yet be used as first-line therapy, rather, they should be kept for use on difficult to heal ulcers in a specialist wound care center. One of the potential drawbacks to all skin equivalents is their expense. This said, however, it has been estimated that when Dermagraft is used to treat diabetic foot ulcers not only are more ulcers healed at a faster rate, but its use results, in the United Kingdom, in a saving of almost £1000 over conventional therapy *(179)*. Nevertheless, the cost of new therapies is a real issue with implications for health care resources in both public and private health care systems. This includes not only the direct costs of the therapy but also, for example, the preparation and application of some of these new therapies, which can be labor and time intensive.

The preceding account illustrates that a wide variety of topical treatments for diabetic foot ulcers exist. Much of their use, however, lacks a truly evidence-based approach. More studies are needed to validate individual treatments, and comparative trials of (especially) the newer therapies are also required. In addition, the practitioner needs a fundamental understanding of basic and applied knowledge relating to conventional and newer therapies. Moreover, until all the processes of wound healing are elucidated and understood, treatment of diabetic foot ulcers will continue to pose a major challenge.

REFERENCES

1. Palumbo PJ, Melton LJ. *Peripheral Vascular Disease and Diabetes. Diabetes in America.* US Government Printing Office, Washington, DC, 1985.
2. Reiber GE. The epidemiology of diabetic foot problems. *Diabet Med* 1996;13:S6–S11.
3. Walters DP, Gatling W, Mullee MA, Hill RD. The distribution and severity of diabetic foot disease: a community study with comparison to a non-diabetic group. *Diabet Med* 1992;9:354–358.
4. Borssen B, Bergenheim T, Lithner F. The epidemiology of foot lesions in diabetic patients aged 15–50 years. *Diabet Med* 1990;7:438–444.

5. Moss SE, Klein R, Klein BEK. The prevalence and incidence of lower extremity amputation in a diabetic population. *Arch Intern Med* 1992;152:610–616.
6. Reiber GE, Boyko EJ, Smith G. Lower extremity foot ulcers and amputation in diabetes, in *National Diabetes Data Group. Diabetes in America*. National Institutes of Health, Bethesda, MD, 1995, pp. 409–428.
7. Moss SE, Klein R, Klein BEK. The prevalence and incidence of lower extremity amputation in a diabetic population. *Arch Intern Med* 1992;152:610–616.
8. Grunfeld C. Diabetic foot ulcers: etiology, treatment and prevention. *Adv Intern Med* 1991; 37:103–132.
9. Edmonds ME, Blundell MP, Morris H, et al. Improved survival of the diabetic foot—the role of a specialised foot clinic. *Q J Med* 1986;60:763–771.
10. Larsson J, Apelqvist J, Agardh CD, et al. Decreasing incidence of major amputation in diabetic patients: a consequence of a multidisciplinary foot care approach? *Diabet Med* 1995;12:770–776.
11. McCabe CJ, Stevenson RC, Dolan AM. Evaluation of a diabetic foot screening and protection programme. *Diabet Med* 1998;15:80–84.
12. Thomas S. *Wound Management and Dressings*. The Pharmaceutical Press, London. 1990.
13. Ladin DA. Understanding dressings. *Clin Plast Surg* 1998;25:433–441.
14. Odland G. The fine structure of the inter-relationship of cells in the human epidermis. *J Biophys Biochem Cytol* 1958;4:529–535.
15. Winter G. Formation of the scab and the rate of epithelialisation of superficial wounds in the skin of the young domestic pig. *Nature* 1962;193:293–294.
16. Hinman CD, Maibach H. Effect of air exposure and occlusion on experimental human skin wounds. *Nature* 1963;200:377–378.
17. Chen WYJ, Rogers AA, Lydon MI. Characteriztion of biologic properties of wound fluid collected during early stages of wound healing. *J Invest Dermatol* 1992;99:559–564.
18. Field CF, Kerstein MD. Overview of wound healing in a moist environment. *Am J Surg* 1994;1A:2S–6S.
19. Rovee DT, Kurowsky CA, Labun J, et al. Effect of local wound environment on epidermal healing, in *Epidermal Wound Healing* (Maibach HI, Rovee DT, eds.), Yearbook Medical Publishers, Chicago, 1972, pp. 159–181.
20. Jones V, Gill D. Hydrocolloid dressings and diabetic foot lesions. *Diabet Foot* 1998;1: 127–134.
21. Katz MH, Alvarez AF, Kirsner RS, et al. Human wound fluid from acute wounds stimulates fibroblasts and endothelial cell growth. *J Am Acad Dermatol* 1991;25:1054–1058.
22. Deuel TF, Kawahara RS, Mustoe TE, Pierce AF. Growth factors and wound healing: platelet-derived growth factor as a model cytokine. *Annu Rev Med* 1991;42:567–584.
23. King LE, Carpenter GF. Epidermal growth factor, in *Biochemistry and Physiology of the Skin* (Goldsmith LA, ed.), OUP, New York, NY, 1983, pp. 269–281.
24. Choucair M, Phillips T. A review of wound healing and dressing materials. *Wounds* 1996; 8:165–172.
25. Phillips TJ, Dover JS. Leg ulcers. *J Am Acad Dermatol* 1991;25:965–987.
26. Bucalo B, Eaglstein WH, Falanga V. The effect of chronic wound fluid on cell proliferation in-vitro. *J Invest Dermatol* 1989;92:408.
27. Grinnell F, Ho CH, Wysocki A. Degradation of fibronectin and vitronectin in chronic wound fluid: analysis by cell blotting, immunoblotting and cell adhesion assays. *J Invest Dermatol* 1992;98:410–416.
28. Bucalo B, Eaglstein WH, Falanga V. Inhibition of cell proliferation by chronic wound fluid. *Wound Rep Regen* 1993;1:181–186.
29. Mertz PM, Marshall DA, Eaglstein WH. Occlusive wound dressings to prevent bacterial invasion and wound infection. *J Am Acad Dermatol* 1985;12:662–668.

30. Helfman T, Ovington L, Falanga L. Occlusive dressings and wound healing. *Clin Dermatol* 1994;12:121–127.

31. Knowles EA, Westwood B, Young MJ, et al. A retrospective study of the use of Granuflex and other dressings in the treatment of diabetic foot ulcers, in *Proceedings of the 3rd European Conference on Advances in Wound Management*. Macmillan, London, 1993, pp. 117–120.

32. van Rijswijk L. Clinical practice guidelines: moving into the 21st century. *Ostomy Wound Manage* 1999;45(Suppl 1A):47S–53S.

33. Fisken RA, Digby M. Which dressing for diabetic foot ulcers? *Pract Diabetes Int* 1996; 13:107–109.

34. Baker NR. Foot ulcer management. *J Wound Care* 1997;6: Resource file supplement.

35. Foster AVM, Greenhill MT, Edmonds ME. Comparing two dressings in the treatment of diabetic foot ulcers. *J Wound Care* 1994;3:224–228.

36. Hansson, C. Interactive wound dressings. A practical guide to their use in older patients. *Drugs Aging* 1997;11:271–284.

37. Wijetunge DB. Management of acute and traumatic wounds: main aspects of care in adults and children. *Am J Surg* 1994;167(Suppl):56s–60s.

38. Lawrence C. Dressings and wound infection. *Am J Surg* 1994;167(Suppl):21s–24s.

39. Eaglstein WH. Occlusive dressings. *J Dermatol Surg Oncol* 1993;19:716–720.

40. Jones V, Harding K. Choosing wound dressings for the community patient. *Prescriber* 1995;19 December:25–32.

41. Foster AVM, Spencer M, Edmonds ME. Deterioration of diabetic foot lesions under hydrocolloid dressings. *Pract Diabetes Int* 1997;14:62–64.

42. Boulton AJM, Knowles A, Jackson N. Use of alginate and hydrocolloid dressings in diabetic foot lesions. *Pract Diabetes Int* 1997;14:148.

43. Vowden K. Diabetic foot complications. *J Wound Care* 1997;6:4–8.

44. Arnold T, Stanley J, Fellows E. Prospective multicenter study for managing lower extremity venous ulcers. *Ann Vasc Surg* 1994;8:356–362.

45. Jones V. Selecting a dressing for the diabetic foot: factors to consider. *Diabet Foot* 1998; 1:48–52.

46. Thomas AML, Harding, KG, Moore K. The structure and composition of chronic wound eschar. *J Wound Care* 1999;8:285–287.

47. Constantine B, Bolton LA. A wound model for ischemic ulcers in the guinea pig. *Arch Dermatol Res* 1986;278:429–431.

48. Bergstrom, N, Bennett MA, Carlston, CE, et al. *Treatment of Pressure Ulcers. Clinical Practice Guideline 15*. Publication no. 95–0652. Public Health Service Agency for Health Care Policy and Research, Washington, DC, 1994.

49. Goode PS. Consensus on wound debridement. A United States perspective. *Eur Tissue Rep Soc* 1995;2:104.

50. Mulder GD. Cost-effective management care. Gel vs. wet-to-dry debridement. *Ostomy Wound Manage* 1995;41:896–900.

51. Razor B, Martin L. Validating sharp wound debridement. *J Enterost Nurs* 1991;18:105–110.

52. Harding KG, Dunkley P, Wood RAB, et al. *The Wound Programme*. Centre for Medical Education, University of Dundee, Dundee, Scotland, 1992.

53. Bale S. A guide to wound debridement. *J Wound Care* 1997;6:179–182.

54. Clark RAF. Mechanisms of cutaneous wound repair, in *Haematology in General Medicine* (Fitzpatrick TB, et al., eds.), McGraw-Hill, New York, 1993.

55. Mertz P, Davis S, Brewer L, et al. Can antimicrobials be effective without impairing wound healing? The evaluation of cadexomer iodine ointment. *Wounds* 1994;6:184–193.

56. Fowler E, van Rijswijk L. Using wound debridement to help achieve goals of care. *Ostomy Wound Manage* 1995;41(Suppl)235–265.

57. Bale S, Jones V. Assessment and planning of individualised care, in *Wound Care Nursing: A Patient Centred Approach.* Balliere Tindall, London, 1997.

58. Vowden KR, Vowden P. Wound debridement, part 2: sharp techniques. *J Wound Care* 1999;8:291–294.

59. Hansson C, Holm J, Lillieborg S, et al. Repeated treatment with lidocaine/prilocaine cream (EMLA) as a topical anesthetic for the cleansing of venous leg ulcers: a controlled study. *Acta Derm Venereol* 1993;73:231–233.

60. Brennan SS, Leaper DJ. The effects of antiseptics on the healing wound: a study using the rabbit ear chamber. *Br J Surg* 1985;82:780–782.

61. Glyvanstev SP, Adamyan AA, Sakharov I. Crab collagenase in wound debridement. *J Wound Care* 1997;6:13–16.

62. Mekkes JR, Le Poole IC, Das PK, Bos JD, Westerhof W. Efficient debridement of necrotic wounds using proteolytic enzymes derived from Antarctic krill: a double blind placebo-controlled study in a standardised animal wound model. *Wound Rep Regen* 1998; 6:50–57.

63. Levin ME. The diabetic foot: pathophysiology, evaluation and treatment, in *The Diabetic Foot* (Levin ME, O'Neall LW, eds.), Mosby, St. Louis, MO, 1988.

64. Colin D, Kurring PA, Yvon C. Managing sloughy pressure sores. *J Wound Care* 1996;5: 444–446.

65. Baxter CR, Rodehaver GT. Interventions, in *New Directions in Wound Healing.* ER Squibb, New York, 1990.

66. Sherman RA, Wyte F, Vulpe M. Maggot therapy for treating pressure ulcers in spinal cord injury patients. *Spinal Cord Med* 1995;18:71–74.

67. Courtney M. The use of larval therapy in wound management in the UK. *J Wound Care* 1999;8:177–179.

68. Rayman A, Stansfield G, Woollard T, et al. Use of larvae in the treatment of the diabetic necrotic foot. *Diabet Foot* 1998;1:7–13.

69. Thomas S, Jones M, Shutler S, Jones S. Using larvae in modern wound management. *J Wound Care* 1996;5:60–69.

70. Thomas S. Hydrocolloids update. *J Wound Care* 1992;1:27–30.

71. Thomas S. *A Prescribers Guide to Dressings and Wound Management Materials.* Value for Money Unit, Cymru, Wales, 1996.

72. Lawrence JC. Moist wound healing: critique 1. *J Wound Care* 1995;4:368–370.

73. Thomas S, Fear M, Humphreys J, et al. The effects of dressings on the production of exudate from venous leg ulcers. *Wounds* 1996;8:145–150.

74. Tovey F. Diabetic foot ulceration. *Wound Manage* 1993;3:12–14.

75. Conroy M. The diabetic foot, in *Proceedings of the Fourth European Conference on Advances in Wound Management.* Macmillan, London, 1994, pp. 115–116.

76. Barnett A. Prevention and treatment of the diabetic foot ulcer. *Br J Nurs* 1992;2:7–10.

77. Jeffcoate W, Macfarlane R. The Diabetic Foot. Chapman and Hall, London, 1995.

78. Ono I, Gunji H, Zhang JZ, Maruyama K, Kaneko F. Studies on cytokines related to wound healing in donor site wound fluid. *J Dermatol Sci* 1995;10:241–245.

79. Varghese MC, Balin AK, Carter M Caldwell D. Local environment of chronic wounds under synthetic dressings. *Arch Dermatol* 1986;122:52–57.

80. Gilchrist B, Reed C. The bacteriology of chronic venous ulcers treated with occlusive hydrocolloid dressings. *Br J Dermatol* 1989;121:337–344.

81. Bowler PG. The role of occlusive dressings in infection control. *Wound Manage* 1996;1: 5–6.

82. Saymen DG, Holder NP. Control of surface wound infection: skin versus synthetic grafts. *Appl Microbiol* 1973;25:921–934.

83. Bowler PG, Jones SA, Davies BJ Coyle E. Infection control properties of some wound dressings. *J Wound Care* 1999;8:499–502.

84. Lithner F. Adverse effects on diabetic foot ulcers of highly adhesive hydrocolloid occlusive dressing. *Diabetes Care* 1990;13:814–815.

85. Pizzey M. Which dressing for diabetic leg ulcers? *Diabetes Rev* 1993;2:8–10.

86. Laing P. Diabetic foot ulcers. *Am J Surg* 1994;1A(Suppl):31s–36s.

87. Young M, Young C. Footwork. *Nurs Times* 1994;90:66–71.

88. Knowles A. Diabetic foot ulceration. *Nurs Times* 1996;92:65–68.

89. Booth J, McInnes A, Birch I. A pressure measurement tool for plantar wound management. *J Wound Care* 1997;6:458–460.

90. McInnes A. Diabetic foot ulceration. *Nurs Times* July 9, 1997.

91. Foster AVM. Chiropody care for diabetic feet. *Pract Diabetes* 1993;10:44–45.

93. Knowles EA, Jackson NJ. Care of the diabetic foot. *J Wound Care* 1997;6:227–230.

94. Apelqvist J, Ragnarson-Tenvall G, Larsson J. Topical treatment of diabetic foot ulcers: an economic analysis of treatment alternatives and strategies. *Diabet Med* 1994;12:123–128.

95. Dennison D. Diabetic foot wounds. *J Tissue Viab* 1993;3:58–60.

96. Clever H, Dreyer M. Comparing two wound dressings for the treatment of neuropathic diabetic foot ulcers, in *Proceedings of the Fifth European Conference on Advances in Wound Management.* Macmillan, London, 1995, pp. 201–202.

97. Fisken RA, Digby M. Which dressing for diabetic foot ulcers? *J Br Podiatr Med* 1997;52: 20–22.

98. Morgan D. *Formulary of Wound Management Products*, 7th ed. Euromed Communications, Haselmere, 1997.

99. Bale S, Banks V, Harding KG. Problems and pitfalls of doing cost-effectiveness studies, in *Proceedings of the Fourth European Conference on Advances in Wound Management.* Macmillan, London, 1992, pp. 45–47.

100. Thomas S. Alginate dressings in surgery and wound management—part 1. *J Wound Care* 2000;9:56–60.

101. Qin Y, Gilding DK. Alginate fibres and wound dressings. *Med Dev Tech* November, 1996, pp. 32–41.

102. Jones V. Alginate dressings and diabetic foot lesions. *Diabet Foot* 1999;2:8–14.

103. Thomas S, Tucker CA. Sorbsan in the management of leg ulcers. *Pharm J* 1989;243:706–709.

104. Fannucci D, Seese J. Multifaceted use of calcium alginates: a painless, cost-effective alternative for wound care management. *Ostomy Wound Manage* 1991;37:16–22.

105. Chaloner D, Fletcher M. Clinical trials: comparing dressings. *Nurs Stand* 1992;7:9–11.

106. Berry DP, Bale S, Harding KG. Dressings for cavity wounds. *J Wound Care* 1996;5:10–13.

107. Donaghue VM, Chrzan JS, Rosenblum BI. Evaluation of a collagen alginate wound dressing in the management of diabetic foot ulcers. *Adv Wound Care* 1998;11:114–119.

108. Lansdown AB, Payne MJ. An evaluation of the local reaction and biodegradation of calcium sodium alginate (Kaltostat) following subcutaneous implantation in the rat. *J R Coll Surg Edinb* 1994;39:284–288.

109. Matthew LR, Browne JW, et al. Tissue response to a haemostatic alginate wound dressing in tooth extraction sockets. *Br J Oral Maxillofac Surg* 1993;31:163–169.

110. Odell EW, Oades P, Lombardi T. Symptomatic foreign body alginate. *Br J Oral Maxillofac Surg* 1994;32:178–179.

111. Schmidt RJ, Turner TD. Calcium alginate dressings [letter]. *Pharm J* 1986;236:578.

112. Blair SD, Backhouse CM, Harper R Matthews J McCollum CM. Comparison of absorbable materials for surgical haemostasis. *Br J Surg* 1988;75:969–971.

113. Doyle JW, Roth TP, Smith RM Li YQ Dunn RM. Effects of calcium alginate on cellular wound healing processes modelled in vitro. *J Biomed Mater Res* 1996;32:561–568.

114. Otterlei MA, Sundan A, Skjak-Braek G, et al. Similar mechanisms of action of defined polysaccharides. Lipopolysaccharides: characterization of binding and tumor necrosis factor alpha induction. *Infect Immun* 1993;61:1917–1925.

115. Kulseng B, Skjak-Braek G, Folling I, et al. TNF production from peripheral blood mononuclear cells in diabetic patients after stimulation with alginate and lipopolysaccharide. *Scand J Immunol* 1996;43:335–340.

116. Thomas S. Alginate dressings in surgery and wound management: part 3. *J Wound Care* 2000;9:163–166.

117. Skjak-Braek G, Espevik T. Application of alginate gels in biotechnology and biomedicine. *Carbohydrates Eur* 1996;14:19–25.

118. Thomas A, Harding, KG, Moore K. Alginates from wound dressings activate human macrophages to secrete tumour necrosis factor-α. *Biomaterials* 2000;21:1797–1802.

119. Moore K, Ruge F, Harding KG. T-lymphocytes and the lack of activated macrophages in wound margin biopsies from chronic leg ulcers. *Br J Dermatol* 1997;137:188–194.

120. Moore K, Thomas A, Ruge F, Harding KG. A human tissue explant culture system for the study of wound biology, in *Proceedings of the Sixth European Conference on Advances in Wound Management.* Macmillan, New York, 1997, pp. 19–22.

121. Lawrence IG, Lear JT, Burden AC. Alginate dressings and the diabetic foot ulcer. *Pract Diabetes Int* 1997;14:61–62.

122. Pecoraro RE, Ahroni JH. Evaluation of Sorbsan in the treatment of diabetic foot and lower extremity ulcers, presentation at the Fifth Annual Symposium on Advanced Wound Care, New Orleans, LA, 1992.

123. Cazzaniga AL, Marshall DA, Mertz PM. The effect of calcium alginate dressing on the multiplication of bacterial pathogens in vitro, presentation at the Fifth Annual Symposium on Advanced Wound Care, New Orleans, LA, 1992.

124. Thomas S. Current practices in the management of fungating lesions and radiation damaged skin. SMTL, Bridgend, 1992.

125. Elkeles RS, Wolfe JHN. The diabetic foot: ABC of vascular disease. *BMJ* 1991;303:1053–1055.

126. Dealey C. *The Care of Wounds.* Blackwell Science, London, 1994.

127. Thomas S, Hay NP. Assessing the hydroaffinity of hydrogel dressings. *J Wound Care* 1995; 3:89–91.

128. Stewart AJ, Leaper DJ. Treatment of chronic leg ulcers in the community: a comparative trial of Sterisorb and Iodosorb. *Phlebology* 1987;2:115–121.

129. Thomas S, Fear M. Comparing two dressings for wound debridement. *J Wound Care* 1993; 2:272–274.

130. Flanagan M. The efficacy of a hydrogel in the treatment of wounds with non-viable tissue. *J Wound Care* 1995;4:264–267.

131. Jones V. Use of hydrogels and iodine in diabetic foot ulcers. *Diabet Foot* 1999;2:47–54.

132. Gibson B, Hofman D, Nelson A, et al. A clinical investigation of two hydrocolloid gels for the treatment of chronic wounds. Poster presentation, in *Proceedings of Symposium on Advanced Wound Care.* Health Management Publications, Philadelphia, PA, 1995.

133. Thomas S, Hay NP. In-vitro investigation of a new hydrogel dressing. *J Wound Care* 1996; 5:130–132.

134. Young T, Williams C, Benbow M, et al. A study of two hydrogels used in the management of pressure sores, in *Proceedings of the Sixth European Conference on Advances in Wound Management.* Macmillan, London, 1997, pp. 103–106.

135. Bale S, Banks V, Hagelstein S. A comparison of the amorphous hydrogels in the debridement of pressure sores. *J Wound Care* 1998;7:65–68.

136. McCulloch D. An investigation into the effects of Intrasite gel on the in-vitro proliferation of aerobic and anaerobic bacteria (poster), in *Proceedings of the Second European Conference on Advances in Wound Management.* MacMillan, London, 1993, p. 207.

137. Schipani E, Romanelli M, Piaggesi A, et al. Long-term application of hydrocolloid gel in neuropathic diabetic foot ulcers: evaluation of sterility, in *Proceedings of the Sixth European Conference on Advances in Wound Management.* MacMillan. London, 1997, p. 256.

138. Zamora JL. Chemical and microbiologic characteristics and toxicity of povidone-iodine solutions. *Am J Surg* 1986;151:400–406.
139. Lacey RW, Catto A. Action of povidone-iodine against methicillin-sensitive and -resistant cultures of *Staphylococcus aureus*. *Postgrad Med J* 1993;69:S78–S83.
140. Lineweaver W, Howard R, Soucy D, et al. Topical antimicrobial toxicity. *Arch Surg* 1985; 120:267–270.
141. Moore DJ. The use of antiseptics in wound care: critique 3. *J Wound Care* 1996;5:46–47.
142. Dela Cruz F, Brown DH, Leikin JB Franklin C Hryhorczuk DO. Iodine absorption after topical administration. *West J Med* 1987;146:43–45.
143. Lawrence JC. The use of iodine as an antiseptic agent. *J Wound Care* 1998;7:421–425.
144. Gilchrist B.. Should iodine be reconsidered? *Nurs Times* 1997;43:6–7.
145. Geronemus RG, Mertz PM, Eaglstein WH. Wound healing: the effects of topical agents. *Arch Dermatol* 1979;115:1311–1313.
146. Kashyap A, Beezhold D, Wiseman J, et al. Effect of povidone-iodine ointment on wound healing. *Am Surg* 1995;61:486–491.
147. Gordon J. Clinical significance of MRSA in UK hospitals and the relevance of povidone-iodine in their control. *Postgrad Med* 1993;69(Suppl 3):S106–S116.
148. Lawrence JC. Burn bacteriology during the last 50 years. *Burns* 1992;18(Suppl):S23–S29.
149. Johnson & Johnson. *Inadine: Your Questions Answered.* J&J Medical, Ascot, UK, 1997.
150. Aronoff GR, Friedman SJ, Doedens DJ, Lavelle KJ. Increased serum iodide concentrations from iodine absorption through wounds treated topically with povidone iodine *Am J Med Sci* 1980;279:173–176.
151. Moberg S, Hoffman L, Grennet ML Holst A. A randomised trial of cadexomer iodine in decubitus ulcers. *J Am Geriatr Soc* 1983;31:462–465.
152. Sundberg J, Meller L. A retrospective review of the use of cadexomer iodine in the treatment of chronic wounds. *Wounds* 1997;9:68–86.
153. Moore K, Thomas A, Harding KG. Iodine released from the wound dressing Iodosorb modulates the secretion of cytokines by human macrophages. *Int J Biochem Cell Biol* 1997; 29:163–171.
154. Skog E, Arnesjo B, Troeng T, et al. A randomised trial comparing cadexomer iodine and standard treatment in the out-patient management of chronic venous ulcers. *Br J Dermatol* 1983;109:73–83.
155. Steele K, Irwin G, Dowds N. Cadexomer iodine in the management of venous ulcers in general practice. *Practitioner* 1986;230:63–68.
156. Apelqvist J, Larsson J, Stenstrom A. Cadexomer iodine gel in the treatment of deep diabetic foot ulcers, in *Proceedings of the First European Conference on Advances in Wound Management*. Macmillan, London, 1992, pp. 91–92.
157. Apelqvist J, Ragnarson-Tenvall G. Cavity foot ulcers in diabetic patients: a comparative study of cadexomer iodine ointment and standard treatment. *Acta Derm Venereol* 1996; 76:231–235.
158. Falanga V. Growth factors and wound repair. *J Tissue Viab* 1992;2:101–104.
159. Cox DA. Growth factors in wound healing. *J Wound Care* 1993;6:339–342.
160. Lynch SE, Nixon JC. Role of platelet-derived growth factor in wound healing: synergistic effects with growth factors. *Proc Natl Acad Sci USA* 1987;84:7696–7697.
161. Cooper DM, Yu EZ, Hennesey P Ko F Robson MC. Determination of endogenous cytokines in chronic wounds. *Ann Surg* 1994;219:688–692.
162. Ross R. Platelet-derived growth factor. *Lancet* 1989;331:1179–1182.
163. Steed DL. Clinical evaluation of recombinant human platelet-derived growth factor for the treatment of lower extremity diabetic ulcers. *J Vasc Surg* 1995;21:71–81.
164. d'Hemecourt PA, Smiell JM, Karim MR. Sodium carboxymethylcellulose aqueous-based gel vs. becaplermin gel in patients with non-healing lower extremity diabetic ulcers. *Wounds* 1998;10:69–75.

165. Wieman TJ. Clinical efficacy of becaplermin (rhPDGF-BB) gel. *Am J Surg* 1998;176(Suppl 2A):74S–79S.

166. Wieman TJ, Smiell JM, Su Y. Efficacy and safety of a topical gel formulation of recombinant human platelet-derived growth factor-BB (becaplermin) in patients with chronic neuropathic diabetic ulcers: a phase III, randomized, placebo-controlled, double-blind study. *Diabetes Care* 1998;21:822–827.

167. Young M. Becaplermin and its role in healing neuropathic diabetic foot ulcers. *Diabet Foot* 1999;2:105–107.

168. Smiell JM. Clinical safety of becaplermin (rhPDGF-BB) gel. *Am J Surg* 1988;176(Suppl 2A):68S–73S.

169. Dale DC, Liles WC, Summer WR, Nelson S. Granulocyte colony stimulating factor (G-CSF): role and relationships in infectious diseases. *J Infect Dis* 1995;172:1061–1075.

170. Gough A, Clapperton M, Rolando N, et al. Randomised placebo-controlled trial of granulocyte-colony stimulating factor in diabetic foot infection. *Lancet* 1997;350:855–859.

171. Isner JM, Pieczek A, Schainfeld R, et al. Clinical evidence of angiogenesis after arterial gene transfer of phVEGF$_{165}$ in patient with ischaemic limb. *Lancet* 1996;348:370–373.

172. Rheinwald JG, Green H. Serial cultivation of strains of human epidermal keratinocytes: the formation of keratinizing colonies from single cells. *Cell* 1975;6:331–344.

173. Phillips T. Cultured epidermal allografts: a temporary or permanent solution? *Transplantation* 1991;51:937–941.

174. Sabolinski ML, Alvarez O, Auletta M Mulder G Parentau NL. Cultured skin as a smart material for healing wounds: experience in venous ulcers. *Biomaterials* 1996;17:311–320.

175. Phillips TJ. New skin for old. *Arch Dermatol* 1998;134:344–349.

176. Cuono CB, Langdon R, Birchall N, Barttelbort S, McGuire J. Composite autologous-allogeneic skin replacement development and clinical application. *Plast Reconstr Surg* 1987;80:626–627.

177. Eaglstein WH, Irionodo M, Laszio K. A composite skin substitute (Graftskin) for surgical wounds. *Dermatol Surg* 1995;21:839–843.

178. Falanga V, Margolis D, Alvarez O, et al. Healing of venous ulcers and lack of clinical rejection with an allogeneic cultured human skin equivalent. *Arch Dermatol* 1998;134:293–300.

179. McColgan M, Foster A, Edmonds M. Dermagraft in the treatment of diabetic foot ulcers. *Diabet Foot* 1998;1:75–78.

14

Local Care of the Diabetic Foot

Philip Basile, DPM and Barry I. Rosenblum, DPM

INTRODUCTION

Diabetic foot ulcers continue to pose a serious threat to patients with diabetes. The presence of an ulcer significantly increases the risk of amputation. Although treatment of an ulcer depends on the combination of medical and surgical management, many ulcers will heal with conservative care. Local care of the diabetic foot requires that the practitioner have the ability not only to treat ulcerations but also to recognize these problems early on so as to prevent their worsening. This knowledge is paramount for healing diabetic ulcers and preventing infection and subsequent amputation. The goal of healing the diabetic foot in the outpatient setting focuses on maintaining an intact skin envelope. If this fails, infection may develop and amputation may ensue. It is the goal of the practitioner to recognize the at-risk diabetic foot as well as address those problems that may give rise to infection and amputation (1,2).

As stated in previous chapters, the at-risk diabetic foot may present with sensory changes consistent with neuropathy, leading to skin breakdown unrecognized by the patient. This may or may not be complicated by arterial insufficiency that will contribute to nonhealing. In addition, the presence of infection may also decrease the ability to heal a neuropathic foot lesion.

CLASSIFICATION OF DIABETIC FOOT ULCERS

Many classification systems have been described in the literature pertaining to the diabetic foot. Perhaps the most commonly referred to system has been that proposed by Wagner (3). His classification system is a useful tool in categorizing the neuropathic foot complicated by ischemia. In addition, others have described systems that attempt to include infection and ischemia, in order to predict healing and outcomes. Most recently, classification systems described by Brodsky and Lavery have been developed in order to be more inclusive of all types of neuropathic foot lesions and to have the ability to better predict outcomes and response to therapy (4). The ideal system should allow the practitioner to communicate the appearance of the ulcer with as few as descriptive terms as possible.

From: *The Diabetic Foot: Medical and Surgical Management*
Edited by: A. Veves, J. M. Giurini, and F. W. LoGerfo © Humana Press Inc., Totowa, NJ

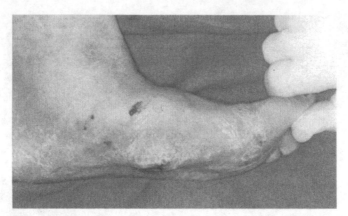

Fig. 1. Wasting of intrinsic musculature resulting in prominence of the metatarsal heads makes the grade 0 foot susceptible to ulcerations.

ULCER ASSESSMENT

Prior to embarking on a treatment plan for a foot ulcer, the wound needs to be assessed. Many parameters need to be addressed, including the extent of neuropathy, the vascular status, and the presence of infection. A detailed history needs to be taken and a com-plete evaluation of the foot performed. This examination should include an evaluation of the sensory system and the perfusion to the foot. Absence of peripheral pulses requires further diagnostic workup of the circulation, with likely referral to the vascular surgeon. Infection needs to be assessed, including the relative depth of the ulcer, as obtained with a sterile probe, in addition to the possible presence of other signs of infection, such as erythema, edema, warmth, or drainage from the wound.

Grade 0 Foot

A grade 0 foot, as defined by the Wagner system *(3)*, is the at-risk foot without ulceration. By definition, this foot has sensory neuropathy. The foot may present with a preulcerative or postulcerative lesion. The grade 0 foot is characterized by the presence of one or more risk factors. Clinically significant sensory neuropathy may be detected by screening tools such as the Semmes-Weinstein 5.07 monofilament wire or tuning fork *(5)*. Areas of sensory neuropathy should be carefully mapped out so as to identify the at-risk areas of the foot. Other risk factors may coexist such as motor neuropathy or high foot pressures. The foot should be closely inspected for corns or calluses, as they will identify potentially vulnerable areas and are indicative of high foot pressures (Figs. 1 and 2; *see* Color Plate 4, following p. 178).

The management of grade 0 feet is primarily accomplished through a program of education and prevention. Patients should be educated as to the risks associated with the neuropathic foot and the early signs of inflammation, irritation, and infection. They should also be educated about the early treatment of these conditions. Early treatment involves identifying the cause for these conditions.

Prevention is the hallmark of management of these feet and should include daily inspection by the patient or family member. Shoegear modification should be discussed

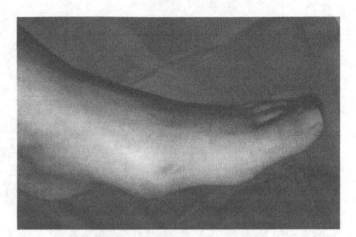

Fig. 2. A grade 0 foot with callous formation is indicative of high foot pressures, requiring treatment and accommodation with orthotic devices.

with the patient when necessary to accommodate bony deformities. High plantar foot pressures can be accommodated with orthoses and padded hosiery (6,7).

An additional technique used to modify pressure points is the habit of changing one's shoes every 4 hours. This has several advantages in preventing ulcerations. Since each shoe has a slightly different pressure point, rotating shoes also rotates pressure points. This prevents the accumulation of pressure over any one area of the foot for extended periods. Additionally, the outer soles and leather uppers of shoes fatigue with time; the longer one wears a shoe, the less shock absorption and support the shoe will provide. Changing shoes regularly also affords patients the opportunity to inspect their feet frequently, allowing for the detection of lesions before they become significant problems.

Regular visits to the foot specialist should be part of the patient's routine. The foot should be inspected at every visit. Pulses should be palpated and any lesion should be noted. Any callous should be debrided, as these alone can lead to high foot pressures (8). The patient should be instructed on the proper care of the nails and skin. Moisturizing creams should be prescribed for dry, scaly skin so as to avoid fissures. The interdigital spaces should also be inspected for cracking or evidence of tinea pedis.

Grade 1 Foot

Grade one ulcerations are those that have penetrated beyond the epidermis (4) (Fig. 3). These ulcerations are indicative of two or more risk factors: peripheral sensory neuropathy and at least one other risk factor. Ulcerations should be evaluated for size, depth, and location. Careful attention should be paid to the structures involved as well as to the presence of infection. The presence of drainage, as well as the type of drainage, should be noted. Cultures are of limited usefulness at this stage, as the ulceration will most assuredly be colonized with multiple organisms representing primarily skin flora (9). Typically, grade 1 ulcerations have not progressed beyond the dermis. The underlying cause should be identified.

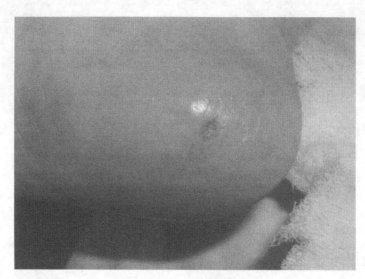

Fig. 3. The grade 1 foot is characterized by superficial tissue breakdown involving the epidermis and no deeper structures. Abnormal foot architecture such as that occurring in Charcot joint disease is a risk of foot ulceration.

Ulcers should be debrided to remove any hyperkeratotic tissue surrounding the ulcer and any nonviable tissue at the base of the ulceration *(10)*. Debridement by any method allows for better visualization of the ulcer field, as well as a better ability to assess the overall depth of the defect. In addition, there is some evidence that debridement allows for an increase in local growth factors, important to allow the healing cycle to begin.

There are four types of debridement: enzymatic, autolytic, mechanical, and surgical. Enzymatic debridement is the utilization of topical agents that have the ability to degrade proteins, thus destroying necrotic tissue. The use of this type of debridement is limited *(11)*. Patients with large eschars or decubitus lesions may benefit from this type of debridement, allowing for a slow eradication of the necrotic area. Autolytic debridement is simply the process by which tissues will remove debris once the proper environment has been established for the wound, i.e., adequate arterial perfusion and optimal moisture. An occlusive dressing will contribute to this type of debridement. Mechanical debridement includes the use of wet to dry dressings whereby the proper type of gauze sponge will slightly adhere to the tissues and gently remove nonviable materials. This method is widely used as an adjunct to sharp debridement.

Surgical debridement has been shown to be the best method for creating the proper environment for wound healing *(11–13)*. The authors concur with the work of Steed et al. *12–13)* and believe that an overall aggressive approach to debridement needs to be taken when dealing with wounds of any grade. Sharp debridement may be done with a scalpel and should be carried down through any necrotic or nonviable tissue until a bleeding ulcer bed is created. The debridement should also be carried to the wound margins, with care taken to uncover any undermining of the wound edges. This type of debridement may be done in the office setting in the face of dense neuropathy; however, if there is any possibility of the patient being sensate enough to feel pain during the procedure, then it should be done in the operating room where anesthesia may be provided.

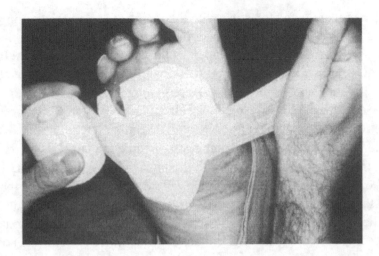

Fig. 4. The felted foam dressing is an effective modality to off-load a grade 1 ulceration.

Following debridement, which is a mainstay of therapy, the foot, and specifically the wound, must be off-loaded to eliminate all pressure from the site of ulceration *(14)*. Historically, the gold standard for eliminating pressure is total non-weight-bearing, either with crutches or a walker. However, most patients are unlikely to comply with this regimen entirely. Therefore, several methods of compromise for off-loading the foot have been devised. Total contact casting, commercially available removable boots, and half-shoes have been described as ways of off-loading the foot and reducing pressures *(15–18)*. The authors' preferred method of off-loading ulcerations is the felted foam dressing *(19)* (Fig. 4).

Compliance with non-weight-bearing is often a problem when dealing with the diabetic patient who presents with a foot ulceration. Recommendations may be made to remain non-weight-bearing via the use of crutches or a walker, but quite frequently these instructions are not followed. As a practical, cost-effective alternative to the total contact cast, the authors have described the felted foam dressing for the conservative treatment of ulcerations that may be classified as Wagner grade 1 or grade 2 *(19)*.

The felted foam dressing is a simple approach toward offloading the insensate foot with a plantar ulcer. Its ease of use, cost effectiveness, and reproducibility make it an important adjunct to the physician's ability to heal neuropathic ulcers. Application of the felted foam dressing requires the following: ¼-inch felted foam, which is essentially a ¼-inch piece of foam laminated to a thin layer of felt, rubber cement, a self-adhering gauze, and tape. The practitioner's choice of dressing(s) may be applied to the wound.

Prior to application of the felted foam, the wound needs to be measured. With a template, the appropriate aperture may be cut into the dressing, specifically the felted foam. Recently, the authors have been utilizing a double thickness of the felted foam, resulting in a ½-inch accommodative pad beneath the sole of the foot. Once the appropriate size aperture, or window, has been cut, care must be taken to skive the edges of the dressing with a scissor. This is done on the edges of the dressing, as well as along the aperture closest to the actual ulcer. This step is performed so as to not to leave an "edge effect" *(20)*.

Once this has been completed, the foot is painted with the rubber cement, along with both sides of each piece of the felted foam. Once this has dried, the two ¼-inch pieces of felted foam are laminated together, with the foam always on the bottom and the felt on top. Once this has been accomplished, the felt top layer is attached directly to the skin. The self-adherent gauze is then wrapped around the foot to secure the dressing. An important point here is the method by which the self-adherent gauze is applied to the foot. This should never be done in a continuous, circumferential manner around the foot. The disadvantage of this method is the possibility of a local tourniquet effect, with the likelihood of inducing a focal area of ischemia *(20)*, rather, the self-adherent gauze should be wrapped in an "over and back" technique that relies on the self-adhering properties of the bandage, along with the underlying skin adherent. This may be carried to the dorsum of the foot, ending just short of the midline, and then reversing direction to the sole of the foot. Once this has been accomplished, then a window may be cut into the plantar surface of the dressing, allowing not only application of whatever dressing is recommended by the practitioner but also direct visualization of the lesion. A surgical healing shoe is then dispensed to the patient, to be worn whenever ambulating. In fact, these pads are often left in place for approximately 10–14 days, at which time they are removed, the wound is assessed, and reapplication done if necessary.

The benefits of this type of therapy are multiple. Clearly it is an easy dressing to apply. The dressing changes to be done by the patient only require the removal of a small gauze square, similar to the ones used in hospital settings. Any topical dressing may be applied with this technique and secured to the foot/felted foam dressing with adhesive tape. The wound may be inspected on a more frequent basis, something not seen with the total contact cast. The disadvantages are few. Primarily, the patient is required to keep the foot dry while the bandage is in place. This includes showers and baths, unless the patient is successful at keeping the foot dry during this activity. In addition, care must be taken to ensure that there is an adequate fit of the dressing. On occasion, if the patient is extremely active, then the dressing will start to shrivel and eventually fall off. It must be stressed to the patient with a grade 1, and sometimes grade 2, foot that limited ambulation is absolutely recommended. The surgical shoe often serves as a reminder of this point.

The ulceration is dressed daily to provide a moist environment conducive to wound healing. Harsh undiluted chemicals should be avoided, as they can be toxic to granulation tissue *(21,22)*. Topical antibiotics have limited usefulness in this setting. When an infection is suspected, it is best treated with systemic antibiotics, which are only recommended when clinical signs of infection are present (i.e., erythema, purulent drainage). Overzealous use of antibiotics may lead to superinfection or development of resistant strains. Exceptions to this rule include patients with severe peripheral vascular disease or patients on immunosuppressive medications, such as renal transplant patients, in whom even the most superficial ulcer may be limb threatening.

Ulcerations that recur may warrant surgical correction of an underlying structural deformity. Digital arthroplasties, metatarsal osteotomies, metatarsal head resections, midfoot and hindfoot ostectomies, joint arthrodeses, and Achilles tendon lengthenings have all proved useful in the prevention of recurrent ulcerations *(23–28)*.

Grade 2 Foot

Continued weight bearing on grade 1 lesions will cause ulcerations to become deeper *(4)* (Fig. 5). These will go beyond the dermis and can involve deeper structures such as

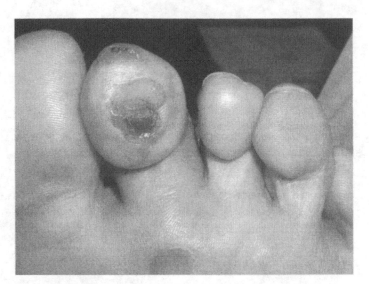

Fig. 5. A rigidly contracted digit can be irritated by the toebox of a shoe, creating a grade 2 ulceration.

tendons, ligaments, joint capsules, or neurovascular structures. At this point the lesion is considered grade 2 *(3)*. Radiographs should be taken in all grade 2 ulcerations to evaluate for osteomyelitis *(29,30)*. To be considered a grade 2 lesion, films should be negative for osteomyelitis and bone cannot be probed. Management of these ulcerations is dependent on accurate assessment of ulcer depth. The ulcer base and periphery should be gently probed with a stainless steel blunt probe to determine undermining or the presence of any penetrating sinus tracts and involvement of deeper structures. This simple technique has an 80% specificity and 89% positive predictive value for diagnosing osteomyelitis. This helps avoid invasive, more expensive diagnostic tests such as bone or leukocyte scans and magnetic resonance imaging (MRI) *(31)*. Radionuclide scans, MRIs, and bone biopsies are often recommended for diagnosing osteomyelitis *(32–34)*. However, false positives and negatives occur with any of these modalities. Grayson et al. *(31)* have shown that the ability to probe bone with a blunt sterile probe is reliable and cost effective in diagnosing osteomyelitis.

The involvement of any of the above deeper structures should alert the clinician to the possible need for hospitalization, complete bed rest, and empiric use of broad-spectrum antibiotics *(35)*. Once the patient is hospitalized, the foot should be drained dependently and packed open. This can often be performed at the bedside in severely neuropathic patients. However, if the infection appears to be undermining adjacent tissues, the patient should be brought to the operating room, where a thorough incision, drainage, and debridement can be performed *(35)*. Generally for an ulcer to be considered grade 2, deep abscesses are not present. Any sinus tract should be explored and drained, and all nonviable tissue should be excised. This should be done thoroughly and aggressively, even if a complete tenectomy is necessary. Deeper cultures should be taken at this time. Preferably tissue should be sent instead of a swab *(36)*. Intravenous antibiotics can then be adjusted to cover the exact organisms *(36)*.

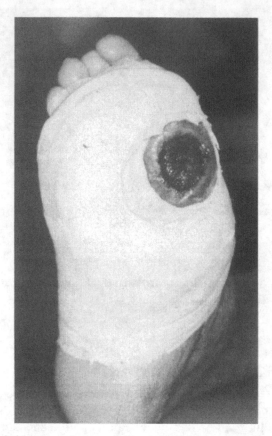

Fig. 6. Adequate debridement of ulceration requires removal of all exuberant callous tissue and necrotic tissue, revealing a clean granular base.

An aggressive incision and drainage or debridement of a foot with underlying ische-mia should not be delayed (Fig. 6). Adequate drainage of the infected foot is impera-tive. Delaying surgery may lead to further tissue loss and potential limb loss, even with a grade 2 lesion *(37)*. Consultation with a vascular surgeon as well as arterial studies should be initiated immediately. If these studies could not be scheduled before the incision and drainage, surgery should not be delayed. A more expedient scheduling of arteriography and lower extremity revascularization is likely if the vascular surgeon is consulted early *(38)*. Dressing changes and wound packing should be done at least twice a day. Subsequent bedside debridements while waiting to perform definitive closure is often necessary *(35)*.

Once the tissues appear to be granulating, and following adequate control of infec-tion, thought can be given to a definitive treatment of the ulceration and any underlying bony deformity. Delayed primary closure of the wound will allow for primary wound healing and earlier ambulation. Some clinicians prefer to wait for secondary wound healing to take place. The myriad of topical agents available today may hasten the heal-ing process. This is covered in greater detail in other chapters. However, while this is perfectly appropriate, it often requires prolonged periods of non-weight-bearing, and the resultant area of scar tissue may not be suited for weight bearing. For these reasons the authors' tendency is to close wounds primarily whenever possible.

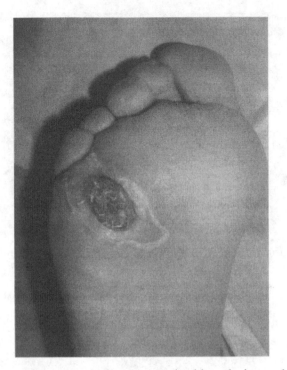

Fig. 7. Grade 3 ulcerations are typically characterized by a lesion underlying a metatarsal head involving deep structures such as tendon, joint, capsule, or bone.

Not all grade 2 ulcerations require hospitalization *(10)*. Although rare, ulcerations over exposed tendon and capsule have the ability to granulate. Outpatient treatment of these lesions must follow the same principles of treating grade 1 ulcerations, namely, strict adherence to non-weight-bearing and weekly debridement. The same strategies to off-load grade 1 ulcerations (i.e., felted foam dressings, total contact casts, and so on) should be applied to grade 2 ulcerations. Because there tends to be more drainage with these ulcerations, dressings should be changed more regularly, often twice a day. It is often prudent to have these performed by a health care professional such as a visiting nurse, who is trained in recognition of the early signs of infection. Oral antibiotics, although often not necessary in grade 1 ulcerations, are more commonly prescribed in grade 2 ulcerations because of the depth of the lesion, the vital structures involved, and the presence of drainage, creating an ideal environment for bacterial growth.

Grade 3 Foot

Deep infection that results in abscess formation and bone involvement is characteristic of the grade 3 foot *(35)* (Figs. 7 and 8). These may result from unresponsive grade 2 ulcerations, aggressive bacterial infections, or, not uncommonly, puncture wounds resulting in direct inoculation of bone. Because of the depth of these ulcerations, the presence of abscess, and the possibility of bone infection, hospitalization and surgical intervention are required.

As with deeply infected grade 2 ulcerations, adequate drainage of infection is key in managing grade 3 lesions *(35)*. Once again, the sinus tract must be explored, and any

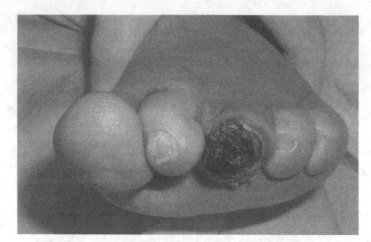

Fig. 8. A sock stuffed into the end of a shoe resulted in minor trauma and focal gangrenous changes.

undrained abscess or devitalized tissue must be thoroughly debrided. In cases of severe infection, open ray amputations become necessary to control the spread of infection.

Once the infection has cleared and healthy granulation tissue appears, thought can be given to surgical reconstruction of the wound and the foot. This may involve simple delayed primary closure or more complicated reconstructive surgery, including additional bone resections, tissue flaps, or skin grafts *(39)*. No one technique can be applied to all wounds. A flexible approach to wound closure will maximize limb salvage. These lesions often require maximum use of all members of the diabetic foot team *(38,40)*.

The long-term management of the grade 3 foot emphasizes prevention of transfer ulcerations. Because ablative surgery is common in the grade 3 foot, transfer of pressure to adjacent areas of the foot is expected. Prevention of chronically recurrent ulcerations requires the use of appropriate orthoses, prescription footwear, and regular podiatry visits. At each visit orthoses and shoes should be inspected for signs of early wear and breakdown. These should be replaced immediately when found to be worn down. The goal of long-term care is to distribute plantar foot pressures more evenly along the entire plantar aspect of the foot, thus avoiding concentration of pressure over any one focal area.

Grade 4 Foot

Grade 4 lesions are particularly challenging. Such patients often present with a variety of underlying risk factors, making overall management difficult. Peripheral vascular disease, osteomyelitis, sepsis, and extensive tissue loss necessitates the cooperation of all members of the limb salvage team. Consultations with vascular surgeons, podiatrists, plastic surgeons, and orthopedic surgeons are often required. The primary goal in the management of these lesions is to limit tissue loss.

Minor trauma in the face of severe arterial insufficiency can result in gangrenous changes of the skin *(41)*. This most commonly occurs at the distal end of extremities since this is where end-arteries are typically found. Lack of adequate perfusion and oxygenation will initially cause focal necrosis that may cause increasing amounts of tissue loss. These changes are most commonly referred to as dry gangrene.

Overwhelming infection may also result in gangrenous changes either from marked edema of local tissue or from infective vasculitis, both of which result in occlusion of digital arterial branches *(42)*. Infective vasculitis will typically lead to wet gangrene.

Initial therapy of these lesions is dependent on identifying the underlying cause. Gangrene resulting from arterial insufficiency should be treated with immediate vascular assessment and lower extremity revascularization (when possible) to minimize tissue loss *(37,43)*.

Grade 5 Foot

Extensive necrosis of the foot characterizes the grade 5 foot. The direct cause is arterial occlusion and failure of arterial inflow. Primary amputation is the only treatment for extensive gangrene. However, these patients should undergo vascular assessment and revascularization whenever possible to reduce tissue loss and to allow for amputation at the most distal level that will support healing. In many instances, the outcome of therapy for the grade 5 foot is similar to that seen with the grade 4 foot.

REFERENCES

1. Thomson FJ, Veves A, Ashe H, et al. A team approach to diabetic foot care—the Manchester experience. *Foot* 1991;1:75–82.
2. Edmonds ME, Blundell MP, Morris HE, et al. Improved survival of the diabetic foot: the role of the specialist foot clinic. *Q J Med* 1986;232:763–771.
3. Wagner FW. The dysvascular foot: a system for diagnosis and treatment. *Foot Ankle* 1981; 2:64.
4. Lavery LA, Armstrong DG, Harkless LB. Classification of diabetic foot wounds. *J Foot Ankle Surg* 1996;35:528–531.
5. Olmos PR, Cataland S, O'Dorisio TM, et al. The Semmes-Weinstein monofilament as a potential predictor of foot ulceration in patients with noninsulin-dependent diabetes. *Am J Med Sci* 1995;309:76–82.
6. Veves A, Masson EA, Fernando DJS, Boulton AIM. Use of experimental padded hosiery to reduce foot pressures in diabetic neuropathy. *Diabetes Care* 1989;12:653–655.
7. Veves A, Masson EA, Fernando DJS, Boulton AIM. Studies of experimental hosiery in diabetic neuropathic patients with high foot pressures. *Diabet Med* 1990;7:324–326.
8. Young MJ, Cavanagh PR, Thomas G, et al. The effect of callus removal on dynamic plantar pressures in diabetic patients. *Diabet Med* 1992;9:55–57.
9. Joseph WS, Axler DA. Microbiology and antimicrobial therapy of diabetic foot infections. *Clin Podiatr Med Surg* 1990;7:467–481.
10. Caputo OM, Cavanagh PR, Ulbrecht JS, Gibbons OW, Karchmer AW. Assessment and management of foot disease in patients with diabetes. *N Engl J Med* 1994;331:854–860.
11. Eaglestein W, Falanga V. Chronic wounds. *Surg Clin North Am* 1997;77:689–700.
12. Steed DL, Diabetic Ulcer Study Group. Clinical evaluation of recombinant human platelet-derived growth factor for the treatment of lower extremity diabetic ulcers. *J Vasc Surg* 1995;21:71–81.
13. Steed DL, Donohoe D, Webster MW, Lindsley L. Diabetic Ulcer Study Group. Effect of extensive debridement and treatment on the healing of diabetic foot ulcers. *J Am Coll Surg* 1996;183:61–64.
14. Young MJ, Veves A, Boulton AJM. The diabetic foot: aetiopathogenesis and management. *Diabetes Metab Rev* 1993;9:109–127.
15. Pollard JP, LeQuesne LP. Methods of healing diabetic forefoot ulcers. *BMJ* 1983;286: 436–437.

16. Burden AC, Jones OR, Jones R, Blandford RL. Use of the Scotchcast boot in treating diabetic foot ulcers. *BMJ* 1983;286:1555–1557.
17. Coleman WC, Brand PW, Birke JA. The total contact cast: a therapy for plantar ulcerations on insensitive feet. *J Am Podiatr Assoc* 1984;74:548–552.
18. Mueller MJ, Diamond JE, Sinacore DR. Total contact casting in treatment of diabetic plantar ulcers. *Diabetes Care* 1989;12:384–388.
19. Ritz G, Kushner D, Friedman S. A successful technique for the treatment of diabetic neurotrophic ulcers. *J Am Podiatr Med Assoc* 1992;82:479–481.
20. Giurini J. Diabetic ulcers. *J Am Podiatr Med Assoc* 1992;82:594.
21. Kucan JO, Robson MC, Heggers JP, Ko F. Comparison of silver sulfadiazine, povidone-iodine and physiologic saline in the treatment of chronic pressure ulcers. *J Am Geriatr Soc* 1981;29:232–235.
22. Lineweaver W, Howard R, Soucy D, et al. Topical antimicrobial activity. *Arch Surg* 1985; 120:267–270.
23. Gudas CJ. Prophylactic surgery in the diabetic foot. *Clin Podiatr Med Surg* 1987;4:445–458.
24. Tillo TH, Oiurini JM, Habershaw OM, Chrzan JS, Rowbotham JL. Review of metatarsal osteotomies for the treatment of neuropathic ulcerations. *J Am Podiatr Med Assoc* 1990;80: 211–217.
25. Jacobs RL. Hoffman procedure in the ulcerated diabetic neuropathic foot. *Foot Ankle* 1982; 3:142–149.
26. Giurini JM, Basile P, Chrzan JS, Habershaw GM, Rosenblum BI. Panmetatarsal head resection: a viable alternative to the transmetatarsal amputation. *J Am Podiatr Med Assoc* 1993; 83:101–107.
27. Giurini JM, Rosenblum HI. The role of foot surgery in patients with diabetes. *Clin Podiatr Med Surg* 1995;12:119–127.
28. Rosenblum BI, Giurini JM, Chrzan JS, Habershaw GM. Preventing loss of the great toe with the hallux interphalangeal joint arthroplasty. *J Foot Ankle Surg* 1994;33:557–560.
29. Newman LG, Waller J, Palestro CJ, et al. Unsuspected osteomyelitis in diabetic foot ulcers: diagnosis and monitoring by leukocyte scanning with indium in 111 oxyquinoline. *JAMA* 1991;266:1246–1251.
30. Keenan AM, Tindel NL, Alavi A. Diagnosis of pedal osteomyelitis in diabetic patients using current scintigraphic techniques. *Arch Intern Med* 1989;149:2262–2266.
31. Grayson ML, Gibbons GW, Halogh K, Levin E, Karchmer AW. Probing to bone in infected pedal ulcers: a clinical sign of underlying osteomyelitis in diabetic patients. *JAMA* 1995; 273:721–723.
32. Hetherington VJ. Technetium and combined gallium and technetium scans in the neurotrophic foot. *J Am Podiatr Assoc* 1982;72:458–463.
33. Morrison WB, Schweitzer ME, Wapner KL, et al. Osteomyelitis in feet of diabetics: clinical accuracy, surgical utility, and cost-effectiveness of MR imaging. *Radiology* 1995;196: 557–564.
34. Yuh WTC, Corson ILL, Baraniewski HM, et al. Osteomyelitis of the foot in diabetic patients: evaluation with plain film, Tc-MDP bone scintigraphy, and MR imaging. *AJR* 1989;152: 795–800.
35. Gibbons GW. The diabetic foot: amputations and drainage of infection. *J Vasc Surg* 1987;5: 791–793.
36. Wheat LJ, Allen SD, Henry M, et al. Diabetic foot infections: bacteriologic analysis. *Arch Intern Med* 1986;146:1935–1940.
37. Taylor LM, Porter JM. The clinical course of diabetic patients who require emergent foot surgery because of infection or ischemia. *J Vasc Surg* 1987;6:454–459.
38. LoGerfo FW, Gibbons GW, Pomposelli FH Jr, et al. Trends in the care of the diabetic foot: Expanded role of arterial reconstruction. *Arch Surg* 1992;127:617–621.

39. Attinger CE. Use of soft tissue techniques for the salvage of the diabetic foot, in *Medical and Surgical Management of the Diabetic Foot* (Kominsky SJ, ed.), Mosby-Year Book, Boston, 1994.
40. Gibbons OW, Marcaccio EJ Jr, Burgess AM, et al. Improved quality of diabetic foot care, 1984 vs 1990: reduced length of stay and costs, insufficient reimbursement. *Arch Surg* 1993; 128:576–581.
41. Pecoraro RE, Reiber GE, Burgess EM. Pathways to diabetic limb amputation: basis for prevention. *N Engl J Med* 1994;331:854–860.
42. Edmonds M, Foster A, Oreenhill M, et al. Acute septic vasculitis not diabetic micro angiopathy leads to digital necrosis in the neuropathic foot. *Diabet Med* 1992;9(Suppl):P85.
43. Klamer TW, Towne JB, Bandyk DF, Bonner MJ. The influence of sepsis and ischemia on the natural history of the diabetic foot. *Am Surg* 1987;53:490–494

15

Surgical Treatment of the Ulcerated Foot

John M. Giurini, DPM

INTRODUCTION

Foot ulceration with infection is one of the leading causes of hospitalization for patients with diabetes mellitus. Although solid data on the true incidence and prevalence of diabetic foot ulcerations does not exist, it is believed that approximately 15% of patients with diabetes will develop a foot or leg ulceration in their lifetime (1). The rate of recidivism is also staggering in this population, with 50% of ulcerations recurring within 18 months. The number of lower extremity amputations among diabetic patients has been well documented for years. Diabetic patients are 15 times more likely to undergo a major lower extremity amputation than nondiabetic patients, with the total number of major limb amputations being over 50,000 (2).

When one considers there are 16 million people in the United States with diagnosed or undiagnosed diabetes mellitus, this places not only a significant sociologic impact on the health care system but an enormous economic impact as well (3). It is estimated that in 1992 in the United States, the direct and indirect cost for care of the diabetic patient was $91.8 billion. In comparison, $20.4 billion was spent in 1987. Treatment of diabetic foot infections cost $300 million/year and lower extremity amputations $600 million/year (1,3). These numbers are so staggering that the Department of Health and Human Services has set as a goal of Healthy People 2000 a 40% reduction in diabetic amputations by the year 2000 (4).

The ability to achieve this goal requires a thorough understanding of the risk factors for ulcerations and amputations. Current algorithms take advantage of recent advances in antimicrobial therapy, wound healing strategies including topical growth factors, and surgical intervention. One of the key components in establishing successful outcomes is identifying a dedicated team of health care professionals to manage these complex problems (5–8).

GOALS OF SURGERY

There was a time not too long ago when surgery on the diabetic patient was to be avoided at any cost. In the past 5 years, however, surgical intervention has been more readily accepted as a form of treatment and prevention of chronic ulcerations.

From: *The Diabetic Foot: Medical and Surgical Management*
Edited by: A. Veves, J. M. Giurini, and F. W. LoGerfo © Humana Press Inc., Totowa, NJ

Table 1
Surgical Goals in the Insensate Patient

Reduce risk for ulceration/amputation

Reduce foot deformity

Provide stable foot for ambulation

Reduce pain

Improve appearance of foot

As with any surgery, the goals of the procedure must be clearly delineated. This is no different in patients with diabetes. What is different are the goals of surgery in patients with neuropathy as opposed to patients with normal sensation. The primary reason for surgical intervention in patients with normal sensation is to reduce a painful condition by correcting an underlying deformity. In the absence of pain as in the neuropathic foot, the primary goal of surgery is to reduce the risk of lower extremity amputation by eliminating a focus of osteomyelitis or correcting those structural factors or deformities leading to ulcerations (Table 1).

PREOPERATIVE EVALUATION

A detailed present and past medical history, past surgical history, list of current medications, and identification of risk factors such as smoking and nephropathy is critical to proper perioperative risk assessment. Patients with long-standing diabetes mellitus will often present with cardiac and renal complications, which must be managed to reduce the morbidity and mortality of the local foot procedure *(9)*. The surgeon would be well advised to obtain consultations with cardiology, nephrology, endocrinology, and vascular surgery when appropriate.

A detailed social history has become increasingly important over the years as more of the burden for a patient's aftercare is placed on the family. Because most patients will require daily dressing changes and will be non-weight-bearing for prolonged periods, visiting nurses, home health aides, and physical therapists have become vital members of the multidisciplinary team. When less than adequate support for these services exists at home, admission to a rehabilitative center or transitional care unit should be considered. These factors should be identified early in the course of the patient's hospitalization so discharge planning can proceed in a timely and stress-free manner.

ANESTHESIA TECHNIQUES

The presence of profound peripheral sensory neuropathy and the localized nature of many of these procedures make local anesthesia with monitored intravenous sedation ideal. Epidural or general anesthesia should only be contemplated when more extensive surgery is being considered. This includes most major rearfoot procedures. It should be remembered, however, that either of these techniques increases the perioperative morbidity and mortality *(20)*. The final choice of anesthesia should be made following discussion with the anesthesiologist and the patient's primary medical doctor and with a clear understanding of the procedure being performed.

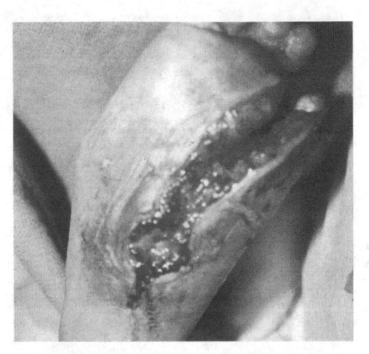

Fig. 1. An appropriate incision and drainage of infection should allow dependant drainage as the patient lies recumbent in bed.

SURGICAL APPROACH

Prior to definitive surgery or correction of an underlying deformity, the foot must be free of any acute infection. This implies that any areas of undrained sepsis be adequately drained and all necrotic tissue debrided to healthy granular tissue. The proper technique for draining wounds is to incise the wound in such a fashion to promote dependent drainage. Because the patient lies recumbent in bed with the extremity elevated, this implies the wound will presumably drain from distal to proximal *(10)* (Fig. 1). Multiple stab incisions with the use of Penrose drains should be avoided as they do not promote dependant drainage. Any tissue that appears to be infected or necrotic should be sharply excised at this time, including any exposed or infected bone. The wound is then packed widely open and inspected daily for the resolution of sepsis, cellulitis, and the development of healthy granulation tissue. The goal of this initial surgical debridement is to convert an acute infection into a chronic wound. Although negative cultures following initial debridement are preferred, they are not a prerequisite for definitive surgery and wound closure, as additional surgical debridement is performed at the time of wound closure.

Forefoot Procedures

First Ray

Although there are no studies showing the incidence of ulcers and their locations, ulcerations of the first ray (hallux and first metatarsal) are clearly among the most common ulcers treated. Common sites of ulcerations include (1) plantarmedial aspect of the hallux; (2) distal tip of the hallux; (3) directly plantar to the interphalangeal joint of

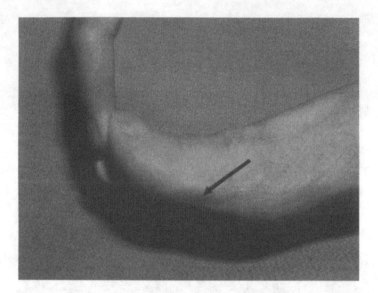

Fig. 2. A common location for ulcerations of the great toe is on the plantarmedial aspect of the interphalangeal joint of the hallux. The most common reason for these ulcerations is a hallux limitus.

the hallux; (4) directly plantar to the metatarsophalangeal joint; (5) directly plantar to the first metatarsal head; and (6) medial aspect of the first metatarsal head. The primary reason probably relates to the combination of increased weight-bearing forces across this joint and faulty biomechanics, leading to excessive pronation *(11–13)*. Additionally, any structural deformities such as osteoarthritis, hallux limitus/rigidus, or severe plantarflexion will increase the susceptibility of this joint to ulceration. Assessing the underlying structural or mechanical cause of the ulceration is vital to selecting the most appropriate procedure.

Ulcerations of the hallux, either plantarmedial or directly plantar to the interphalangeal joint, are most commonly related to abnormal biomechanics of the first ray. This can include excessive pronation with the development of callus on the medial aspect of the hallux ("medial pinch" callus) or limitation of motion at the first metatarsophalangeal joint (i.e., hallux limitus) (Fig. 2). This will result in hyperextension of the interphalangeal joint to compensate for this lack of motion *(14,15)*. Other less common causes of ulceration are an enlarged medial condyle on the distal phalanx or the presence of an interphalangeal sesamoid bone, in which case the ulceration is typically directly plantar to the interphalangeal joint.

The surgical treatment of this entity clearly depends on the underlying cause. When the cause of the ulceration is related lack of adequate motion, it can be addressed by either an arthroplasty of the hallux interphalangeal joint or of the first metatarsophalangeal joint (MTPJ). By resecting the head of the proximal phalanx, further motion is available to the first ray, and the ulceration should resolve *(16)*. This procedure can also be employed when osteomyelitis of the proximal phalanx is suspected. Occasionally, resection of an enlarged medial condyle can be effective in eliminating the callus. This, however, can result in instability of the joint and development of Charcot joint disease.

When there are significant degenerative changes at the level of the first MTPJ or complete lack of dorsiflexion, it is best to resect the base of the proximal phalanx and increase motion at this joint.

Surgical treatment of ulcerations directly plantar to the first metatarsal head can be addressed with excision of one or both sesamoid bones. During the propulsive phase of gait, the sesamoids will migrate distally and more plantarly, thus becoming more prominent. In the intrinsic minus foot this could serve as a potential pressure point and site of ulceration.

The basic indication for sesamoidectomy is the presence of a chronically recurrent ulceration directly plantar to the first metatarsal head without clinical or radiographic evidence of osteomyelitis of the first metatarsal head *(17,18)*. Contraindications for the procedure are significant degenerative changes of the first MTPJ or osteomyelitis of the first MTPJ. These are best treated with a Keller or first MTPJ arthroplasty. Additionally, the presence of a rigid plantarflexed first ray may be a relative contraindication to sesamoidectomy.

When the ulceration is found to extend to the level of the joint, osteomyelitis should be clinically suspected. Treatment must involve complete resection of the infected bone and joint. The procedure of choice is resection of the first MTPJ with excision of the ulceration. Although there may be alternate methods for addressing this problem surgically, there are clear advantages to utilizing this approach rather than allowing the ulcer to heal by secondary intention. By excising the ulceration, all infected, nonviable tissue is removed. It also allows for excellent exposure of all potentially infected tissues, such as the flexor hallucis longus tendon and the sesamoids, which are commonly involved. Wounds that are closed primarily heal more predictably. As a rule, these wounds will heal in 3–4 weeks. The healing rates of wounds that are allowed to heal by secondary intention depend on size and depth. The longer these wounds remain open, the greater the risk of secondary infection, as patient compliance often becomes an issue. Although disadvantages exist to closing these wounds primarily, it is our philosophy that the benefits of primary closure outweigh the risks.

The indication for first MTPJ resection with ulcer excision is the presence of an ulcer directly plantar to the first MTPJ with direct extension into the joint. This is best determined by the ability to pass a blunt sterile probe through the ulceration and palpate bone. Additionally, the presence of clear, viscous drainage is indicative of synovial fluid. This is an ominous sign, as it can only be coming from the joint itself (suggesting a tear in the joint capsule) or from the sheath of the flexor hallucis longus tendon (Fig. 3; *see* Color Plate 5, following p. 178). Even in the presence of negative x-rays, this is sufficient to make the diagnosis of clinical osteomyelitis *(19)*.

An elliptical incision is made that completely excises the ulceration. It is recommended that the ratio of incision length to incision width be at least 3:1 so that wound closure can be achieved with as little tension as possible. This incision is full-thickness and is carried down to the first metatarsal joint (Fig. 4; *see* Color Plate 6, following p. 178). This should excise all necrotic, infected tissue. At this point the flexor hallucis longus tendon will be visible. Typically, focal necrosis immediately plantar to the first MTPJ will be present, indicating infectious involvement. It is therefore best to sacrifice the tendon to prevent recurrence of the infection.

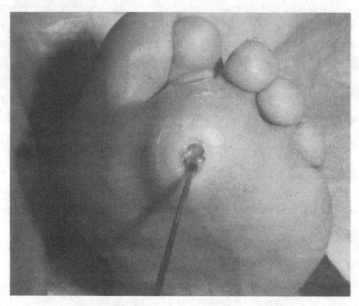

Fig. 3. The presence of synovial drainage from an ulceration is indicative of joint involvement and requires resection of that joint.

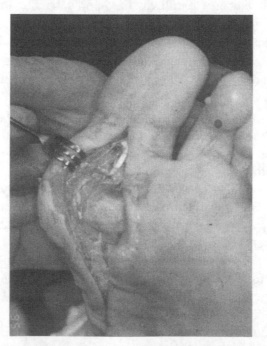

Fig. 4. Osteomyelitis of the first metatarsophalangeal joint is best addressed by elliptical excision of the ulcer with resection of the joint. Adequate resection of the first metatarsal should be performed to ensure complete eradication of infected bone.

Once the tendon is removed, the sesamoids will be visualized. These should also be sacrificed, as they are considered intraarticular structures and are in direct communication with the first MTPJ. The base of the proximal phalanx and the cartilage of the first metatarsal head are now resected. Although it is preferred to leave as much of the

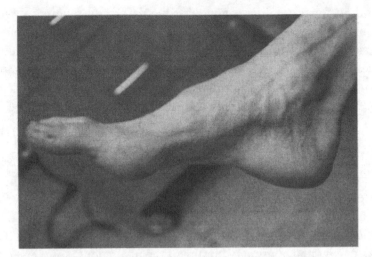

Fig. 5. Motor neuropathy is characterized by wasting of the instrinsic musculature in the arch of the foot. This typically results in deformities such as hammertoes, clawtoes, or plantarflexed metatarsals.

first metatarsal behind as possible to maintain function, enough metatarsal head should be resected so as to remove all focus of osteomyelitis.

The wound is closed by using full-thickness nonabsorbable sutures. Prolene is generally a good choice as it is nonabsorbable and monofilament. Sutures should be placed evenly and used to coapt skin edges with as little tension as possible. It is best to avoid using any deep sutures since these can serve as a potential focus of infection and may be difficult to retrieve at a later date if necessary. It is advisable to pack the proximal 1 cm of the wound with a 2 × 2 gauze sponge to promote drainage and avoid the development of a hematoma. This is usually removed after 24–48 hours, and the wound should heal uneventfully. The postoperative care mandates a period of total non-weight-bearing of at least 4 weeks. Early ambulation will result in wound dehiscence, persistent drainage, postoperative infection, and possible hypertrophic scar. The sutures are left in place this entire time.

Lesser Digits

Wasting of the intrinsic muscles of the foot commonly occurs with the development of motor neuropathy. This can result in forefoot deformities such as hammertoes and clawtoes *(20,21)* (Fig. 5). When sensory neuropathy is also present, ulcerations develop over the proximal interphalangeal joint, at the distal tip of a toe, or on adjacent sides of toes. Amputation of a lesser toe rarely results in long-term complications, with the exception of loss of the second toe. This can precipitate a hallux valgus deformity. When an ulceration is discovered early enough and treated aggressively, amputation of a toe can be avoided, thus maintaining appearance as well as function.

Hammertoes can be classified as either reducible or nonreducible. A reducible hammertoe implies that the deformity is being held by contractures of the soft tissues; a nonreducible deformity suggests there has been joint adaption and extensive soft tissue contractures. A reducible deformity is often amenable to correction by a tenotomy of the corresponding flexor tendon; a nonreducible deformity requires resection of the phalangeal head as well as release of the soft tissue *(21)*. A proximal interphalangeal joint arthroplasty can be combined with excision of the ulcer. In long-standing hammer-toe deformities, there may be a concomitant contracture at the level of the metatarso-phalangeal joint, often indicative of a subluxation or even a dislocation. When dislocated, an area of high focal pressure can develop on the ball of the foot under the corresponding metatarsal head. This is often manifested as callus or even ulceration. Failure to recognize this fact can lead to incomplete correction of the deformity and failure to resolve the ulceration. The contracture at the MTPJ often requires a tenotomy and capsulotomy of the joint. If the joint cannot be relocated following release of the soft tissue alone, a shortening osteotomy of the metatarsal may be necessary to relocate the joint and relieve the plantar pressure.

Osteomyelitis of the tip of the distal phalanx can often be treated by local excision of the distal phalangeal tuft and primary closure of the ulceration. If, however, there is any concern of residual infection, the wound may be left open and closed at a later date.

Lesser Metatarsal Procedures

The area under the metatarsal heads represents the next most common location of diabetic foot ulcerations. Common causes of high foot pressures include abnormal foot mechanics, plantarflexed metatarsals, limited joint mobility, and prior surgical intervention *(21–23)*. There are no definite studies on ulcer incidence and location. Empirically, however, it appears that the second metatarsal is more susceptible to ulceration, probably because of the second metatarsal's dependence on the mechanics of the first ray. When excessive pronation of the medial column occurs, there is increased weight transfer and pressure to the lateral metatarsals *(24,25)*. This is most often manifested by the development of callus under the second metatarsal head. After the second metatarsal, the typical order of ulcer development is the third metatarsal and then the fifth and fourth.

Selection of surgical procedures for ulcerations under the metatarsal heads requires careful evaluation of the ulcer. A critical determinant in the surgical management of these ulcerations is whether osteomyelitis is present.

Lesser Metatarsal Osteotomy

The primary goal of surgical procedures for metatarsal head ulcerations is to alleviate areas of high focal pressure. A metatarsal osteotomy can serve as a valuable adjunct in the management and resolution of these ulcerations *(26)*. The primary indication is the presence of a chronically recurrent ulceration under a metatarsal head without direct extension into bone. An incision is made dorsally over the involved metatarsal. Once the surgical neck is identified, a through and through osteotomy is made. Although varying techniques have been described, the preferred technique is a V-type osteotomy with the apex directed toward the joint (Fig. 6). This provides a stable bone cut resistant to medial or lateral dislocation. The metatarsal head is then elevated to the same level of the adjacent metatarsals. Fixation of the osteotomy with a 0.045 Kirschner wire is preferred. However, in the presence of an open ulceration, this is contraindicated. Fixation and stability are achieved by impacting the head onto the shaft. The patient is then maintained non-weight-bearing for 4–6 weeks to allow for early bone healing.

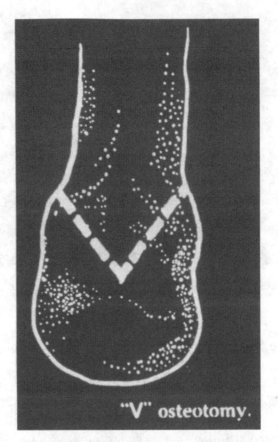

"V" osteotomy.

Fig. 6. A dorsal to plantar V-osteotomy through the surgical neck of the lesser metatarsal allows for adequate relief of plantar pressure overlying an ulceration. The medial and lateral wings of the V decrease the risk of medial or lateral dislocation of the metatarsal head.

Complications following this procedure may include transfer calluses or ulcerations and stress fractures of adjacent metatarsals. These most commonly result when the metatarsal head is elevated above the plane of the adjacent metatarsals. The risk of transfer problems can be reduced if the patient is fitted with an accommodative custom orthosis postoperatively. This will allow for more even distribution of weight-bearing forces across all metatarsal heads. Shoegear modification may also assist in this role.

LESSER METATARSAL HEAD RESECTION WITH ULCER EXCISION

An alternative approach for relieving plantar pressure is to resect the offending metatarsal head entirely. Although this will result in resolution of the ulceration, it carries a high incidence of transfer lesion or ulceration. For this reason, it is preferred to perform this procedure when osteomyelitis of the metatarsal head is suspected and there is no alternative but to resect the offending metatarsal head.

Resection of the metatarsal head can be approached through a dorsal linear incision centered directly over the metatarsal head. It should be remembered that the base of the corresponding proximal phalanx should also be resected, as this structure is also involved. The ulcer is then allowed to heal by secondary intention.

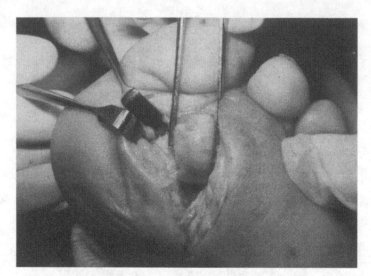

Fig. 7. An osteomyelitic lesser metatarsal head can be resected through a plantar elliptical incision, excising the ulceration in toto.

An alternate approach is to resect the metatarsal head through a plantar approach while excising the ulceration. The advantage of this approach is that all necrotic and infected tissue can be excised and all tissue be directly inspected (Fig. 7). Following resection of the metatarsal head, the wound can be closed primarily as described for first MTPJ resection.

Postoperative care requires that sutures be left in place for a minimum of 3 weeks and the patient kept totally non-weight-bearing for 3–4 weeks. The patient is maintained on oral antibiotics until the sutures are removed. Long-term complications include possible transfer lesions or ulcerations and stress fractures due to the altered weight-bearing surface. It is therefore recommended that patients be fitted with an appropriate orthotic device to distribute pressures evenly.

PANMETATARSAL HEAD RESECTION

Weight-bearing forces are designed to be evenly dispersed across all metatarsal heads. This weight-bearing interdependence between the metatarsal heads has been previously described, first by Morton *(11)* and later by Cavanagh et al *(12)*. Disruption of this relationship will alter normal weight distribution. This can occur from trauma to the metatarsals (resulting in dorsiflexed or shortened metatarsals, as seen in stress fractures), the atrophic form of Charcot joint (resulting in dissolution of metatarsal heads), or prior surgical resection of metatarsal heads for osteomyelitis.

The recidivistic nature of diabetic foot disease makes multiple metatarsal procedures common in this patient population. Osteomyelitis of multiple metatarsal heads was previously treated by transmetatarsal amputation. This procedure was popularized by Dr. Leland McKittrick of the New England Deaconess Hospital and was responsible for saving thousands of limbs *(27)*. It is not without complications. Ulcerations at the distal stump and equinovarus contractures are common long-term complications (Fig. 8). Patients have difficulty psychologically accepting this procedure because it will often require special shoegear, drawing attention to the fact they have had an amputation.

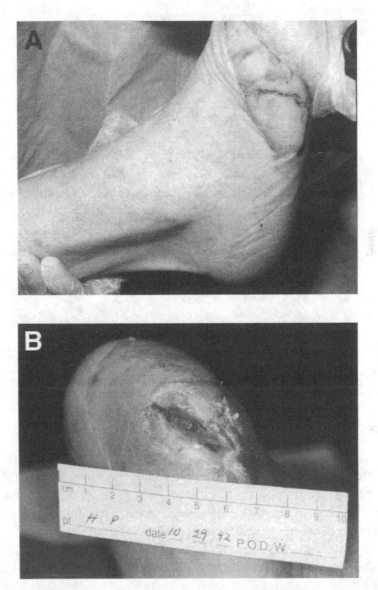

Fig. 8. **(A)** A common complication following transmetatarsal amputation is contracture of the Achilles tendon and subsequent equinus deformity. This can lead to characteristic lesions at the distal end of the transmetatarsal. **(B)** A distal lateral ulceration of a transmetatarsal with an underlying equinovarus deformity.

The panmetatarsal head resection and its variations were originally described for the treatment of painful lesions in patients with rheumatoid arthritis *(28–31)*. Jacobs *(32)* first described the use of the panmetatarsal head resection for the successful treatment of chronic neuropathic ulcerations. Subsequently Giurini et al. *(33)* studied a larger series of patients and described an alternate technique. Similar success rates were cited. Over the years, the panmetatarsal head resection has replaced transmetatarsal resection as the procedure of choice in patients with recurrent ulcerations following prior surgical resection of metatarsal heads *(34)*.

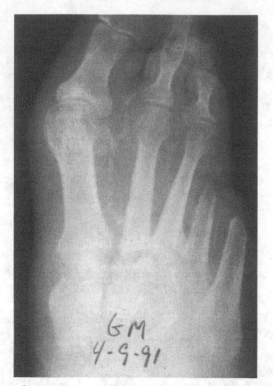

Fig. 9. Prior resection of two metatarsal heads and the presence of osteomyelitis of a remaining metatarsal head are indications for panmetatarsal head resection.

The primary indication for panmetatarsal head resection is the presence of chronically recurrent neuropathic ulcerations on the plantar aspect of the foot following prior metatarsal head resections or ray amputations. It is our belief that if two or more metatarsals have already been resected or need to be resected to eliminate osteomyelitis, the patient would then be best served by a panmetatarsal head resection (Fig. 9). At first this may appear to be a drastic recommendation. However, experience has shown that this approach may actually spare patients additional trips to the operating room for transfer ulcerations.

Various surgical approaches have been described for panmetatarsal head resection. Dorsal approaches, plantar approaches, or a combination of the two have been performed with equal success (35). When possible, the preferred approach is the four-incision dorsal approach: one incision directly over the first metatarsal, one between the second and third metatarsals, one directly over the fourth metatarsal, and one directly over the fifth metatarsal. This approach has the advantages of allowing adequate exposure of all metatarsal heads, decreasing the potential for retraction injury on the skin edges, and maintaining adequate skin islands so as not to affect vascular supply. Because the primary indication for this procedure is the presence of an open ulceration with osteomyelitis, the most common approach is to combine a dorsal incision with a plantar incision that excises the ulceration. The plantar wound and all necrotic tissue can then be excised, the involved metatarsal head(s) can be resected, and the wound can be closed primarily as previously described.

The surgical technique for resection of the metatarsal heads has already been described. The most important technical point to remember in performing this procedure is to maintain the metatarsal parabola. This typically means that the first and second metatarsals are approximately the same length, whereas the third, fourth, and fifth metatarsals are each sequentially shorter. Failure to maintain this relationship can lead to recurrent ulceration and additional surgery. If a prior metatarsal head resection or ray amputation has already been performed, then a perfect parabola may not be achievable. In that case the metatarsal parabola should be recreated with the remaining metatarsals. Additionally, the extensor tendons are identified and retracted. This will maintain the function of these tendons during the gait cycle affording this procedure a prime advantage over transmetatarsal resection.

Midfoot Procedures

Surgery in this region of the foot is usually necessary following foot deformities resulting from neuroarthropathic (Charcot) joint disease. The most common location of Charcot joint involves the tarsometatarsal (Lisfranc's) joints, but other joints in the midfoot may also be affected *(36,37)*. Instability of Lisfranc's joint often results in a rocker bottom deformity of the midfoot and plantarmedial ulceration, primarily because of subluxation of the first metatarsal and medial cuneiform, creating a plantar prominence. Ulcerations on the plantar and lateral aspect of the foot are not uncommon. These result from plantar extrusion of the cuboid from a Charcot process at the calcaneocuboid joint *(36)*. They pose a significant management problem as they are typically recalcitrant to conservative measures. No one surgical procedure can be applied to all ulcers in this location. Therefore, a flexible approach to these lesions is required. Surgical approaches may involve simple ostectomy with or without fasciocutaneous flap or primary arthrodesis of unstable joints.

Ostectomy

This is the simplest approach to chronic ulcerations of the midfoot. It is reserved for those deformities that have their apex directly plantar to the first metatarsal-medial cuneiform joint and where the midfoot is not hypermobile.

The depth of the ulceration will dictate the best surgical approach. A direct medial incision centered over the joint is preferred when the ulceration is superficial and not involving bone. This will allow for excellent visualization of the joint and the prominent bone. The prominence can then be resected from medial to lateral, either with an osteotome or with a saw. The goal should be to remove an adequate amount of bone to alleviate the plantar pressure and not create a new bony prominence, which could create a new source of irritation and ulceration, thus negating the benefits of the procedure.

Ulcerations that communicate with bone and show signs of osteomyelitis clinically are best managed by excision of the ulceration with bone resection and primary closure of the ulceration. This is performed as previously described. In addition to removing the infected bone, the ability to close the ulceration without tension is an additional goal. The use of closed suction irrigation is also recommended to prevent hematoma formation, which can lead to wound dehiscence or infection.

This approach can be used when the ulcer is located either plantar central or plantar lateral in the midfoot. The most likely etiology for these ulcerations is plantar displacement

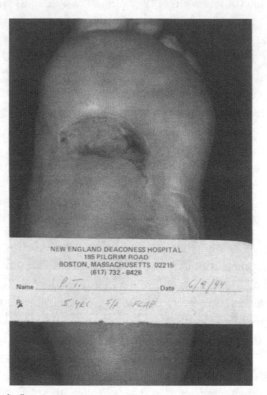

Fig. 10. Patient who is 5 years status post cuboid exostectomy with an interpositional muscle flap and a rotational fasciocutaneous flap.

of the cuboid. When the ulceration measures less than 2.5 cm, this surgical approach can be used. For ulcerations greater than 2.5 cm in diameter, an alternate approach should be employed. This will often require some form of rotational or fasciocutaneous flap. The flexor digitorum brevis muscle is well suited for this purpose because of its anatomic location and ease of dissection. The muscle is rotated laterally to cover the cuboid. A full-thickness fasciocutaneous flap based on the medial plantar artery is then rotated from medial to lateral to cover the actual ulcer site. A split-thickness skin graft is then used to cover the donor site in the medial arch (Fig. 10).

Six weeks of total non-weight-bearing is required for adequate healing and incorporation of the flap. This is followed by an additional 2–4 weeks of protected weight bearing in a healing sandal. Long-term care will require the use of Plastizote orthoses and modified shoegear.

Medial Column Fusion

When resolution of the Charcot joint process has resulted in significant bone loss such that there is significant instability at the first metatarsal-medial cuneiform joint, primary fusion of this joint should be considered. Simple exostectomy in the presence of instability will often fail owing to continued collapse of this segment, resulting in a new bony prominence. Stabilization of this joint therefore is the better alternative.

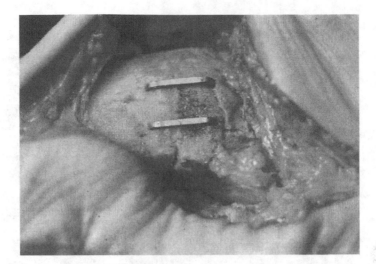

Fig. 11. Fusion of the first metatarsal-medial cuneiform joint for an unstable Charcot joint complicated by recurrent ulceration can be achieved by use of staples.

The joint can be approached surgically through a direct medial incision. This will afford adequate exposure of the dorsum of the joint as well as the plantar surface. The articular cartilage on both sides of the joint can be resected with a sagittal saw. It is recommended that the bone cut on the first metatarsal side be slightly angulated from dorsal-proximal to plantar-distal. This will plantarflex the first metatarsal slightly, restoring the weight-bearing function of the first ray. In addition, it is recommended that any plantar bony prominence also be resected from medial to lateral.

Fixation of the joint can be achieved in a variety of ways. Although crossed 0.062 Kirschner wires and staples are acceptable means of fixation, the authors prefer the use of a medial plate with an interfragmentary screw to provide rigid internal fixation and compression (Figs. 11 and 12). It is advisable to insert a Jackson-Pratt drain to prevent the accumulation of an hematoma.

The postoperative course requires immobilization and non-weight-bearing. Although there are no standard periods of immobilization and non-weight-bearing, the patient can expect to be non-weight-bearing on average 3 months. Partial weight-bearing may begin when serial x-rays show early trabeculation across the first metatarsal-medial cuneiform joint. Continued resumption of weight-bearing is allowed as long as both clinical and radiographic evaluation suggest continued healing of the fusion site.

Exostectomy with Fasciocutanous Flap

Ulcers located centrally in the midfoot secondary to plantar subluxation of the cuboid bone are among the more difficult to manage. This is the type 5 in the Harris and Brand classification of Charcot joint disruption (pattern II in the Sanders classification) and has been described as being very resistant to conservative care *(36,37)*. Resolution of these ulcerations often requires surgical intervention of some type. As previously discussed, when ulcerations of this type exceed 2.5 cm in diameter, primary excision with closure is often not possible, and an alternate technique must be sought *(38)*.

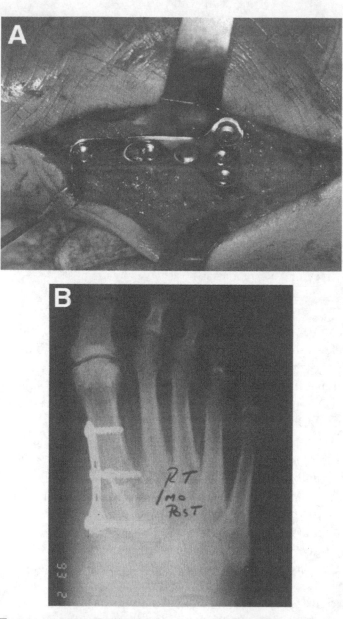

Fig. 12. (A) A T-plate with an interfragmentary screw is another acceptable form of fixation of the first metatarsal-medial cuneiform joint in the presence of unstable Charcot joint. **(B)** Radiograph of patient with T-plate and interfragmentary screw across the first metatarsal-medial cuneiform joint.

Ulcerations of this size are typically excised circumferentially to the level of the cuboid bone. This will allow removal of all necrotic, infected tissue as well as any hyperkeratotic margins bordering the ulcer. The joint capsule and periosteum of the cuboid are next encountered, which are reflected off the underlying cuboid. This will expose the peroneal groove of the cuboid bone. The peroneus longus will often be found running in the groove. When possible, this should be retracted so as to protect it from

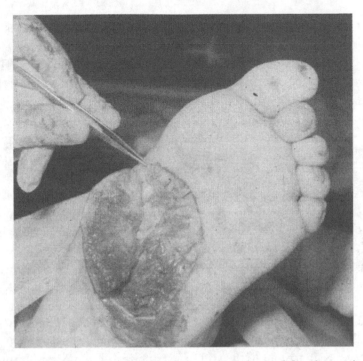

Fig. 13. The flexor digitorum brevis muscle is commonly used for closure in large plantar ulcerations following ulcer excision and exostectomy of the offending bone.

inadvertent injury. On rare occasions, however, it may be necessary to sacrifice the peroneus longus to gain adequate exposure of the bony prominence. The peroneal groove is next resected with the use of an osteotome and mallet. Once surgery is completed, the wound should be carefully inspected for any remaining bony prominence or spicules that can serve as a new point of pressure and possible ulceration.

This procedure will often leave a relatively large dead space, which can serve for the collection of a hematoma. It is best to fill this dead space with a muscle flap, which will serve two purposes: (1) it will decrease the dead space following the bony resection; and (2) it will provide a layer of soft tissue between the underlying bone and the overlying skin (Fig. 13).

Rearfoot Procedures

Surgical procedures of the rearfoot are most commonly performed for reconstruction of unstable Charcot joint disease and can be truly classified as limb salvage procedures. These include partial or subtotal calcanectomy, triple arthrodesis, and pantalar arthrodesis.

Indications for these reconstructive procedures include chronic, nonhealing ulcerations with underlying rearfoot deformity or instability, severe instability of the rearfoot making ambulation difficult at best, or chronic heel ulcerations with underlying osteomyelitis. Because of the high-risk nature of these procedures, all conservative measures should be attempted prior to intervening surgically or when the only alternative is a major limb amputation.

Calcanectomy

Heel ulcerations are not an uncommon event in patients with diabetes. Owing to the comorbid conditions most diabetic patients display, periods of prolonged bed rest are not unusual. Without proper protection, decubitus ulcerations can occur. However, other causes for heel ulcers include blisters from shoe or cast irritation and heel fissures resulting from dry skin or puncture wounds. Regardless of the precipitating cause, the end result is prolonged disability and morbidity. In cases of bone involvement (i.e., osteomyelitis), below-knee amputation can be the final outcome. Attempts to save this extremity to provide a limb capable of functional ambulation can involve excision of the ulceration and the calcaneus, either partial or subtotal.

The goals of the calcanectomy should include excision of all necrotic and infected soft tissue, resection of any and all infected bone, and primary closure of the wound whenever possible. Additional bone resection may be necessary to achieve primary closure. Hindrances to primary closure can include the lack of mobility of the surrounding soft tissue and severe tissue loss from infection. In these cases, a more creative approach may be necessary. This can include rotational skin flaps or free tissue transfers.

The second goal of this procedure is resection of the calcaneus. This procedure is usually performed for osteomyelitis. It is therefore critical that adequate bone be removed to eliminate the infection. It is also important that no plantar prominence be left behind that could serve as an irritant to the soft tissue and result in ulceration. In resecting the calcaneus, the Achilles tendon is often encountered. Depending on the extent of infection, it may need to be debrided or even released. Although one may be tempted to reattach the tendon, it is rarely advisable to do so. Advancement of the Achilles tendon would require the introduction of foreign materials such as screws or anchors, which could serve as a possible source of recurrent infection. When the Achilles tendon is detached, it will often fibrose to the surrounding tissues and provide some degree of plantarflexion (Fig. 14).

Triple Arthrodesis

The incidence of Charcot joint disease involving the tarsal joints—talonavicular, calcaneocuboid or subtalar—ranges from 1.8 to 37%, depending on the reports *(39–41)*. Clinically, these feet may appear with a rocker bottom deformity from plantar subluxation of the talonavicular joint or the calcaneocuboid joint that can lead to chronic ulceration. When faced with a significant degree of instability from this destructive process, the approach should include surgical stabilization of the involved joint or joints. This often requires fusion of the talonavicular joint, calcaneocuboid joint, and subtalar joint, i.e., triple arthrodesis.

The goal of a triple arthrodesis is to stabilize the foot and reduce the deformity, thereby reducing the risk of recurrent ulceration. The surgery should be delayed until the acute phase has resolved and the Charcot joint has entered the coalescent phase. If an open ulceration is present, surgery should be delayed until all acute signs of infection are resolved.

The triple arthrodesis is performed in the standard manner *(42)*. The calcaneocuboid joint is approached through a lateral incision just inferior to the lateral malleolus and extending distally to the base of the fourth and fifth metatarsals. Although it is possible

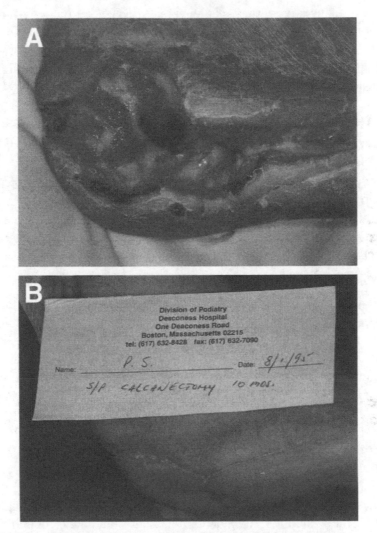

Fig. 14. (A) Osteomyelitis of the calcaneus with resultant soft tissue loss is a common cause of lower limb amputation. **(B)** Patient in following partial calcanectomy with excision and debridement of infected, necrotic tissue and primary closure. Succesful eradication of infected bone resulted in limb salvage.

to obtain adequate exposure of the talonavicular joint through this incision, one should not hesitate to make a separate incision medially if this affords better exposure.

The cartilage is resected off all joint surfaces until bleeding bone is exposed. The joints are then reapproximated. If significant deformity exists, wedge resections through the joints may be required to reduce the deformity adequately. Additionally, significant bone resorption may have occurred as a result of the destructive process. In these cases bone graft may be necessary to fill the gaps between joint surfaces. This can be obtained from the iliac crest or from the bone bank.

The method of fixation is the surgeon's choice. Typically, the posterior subtalar joint is fixated with a 6.5-mm cancellous screw through the talar neck. Although screws are preferred for the talonavicular and calcaneocuboid joints, staples can also be used.

Adequate apposition of joints and accurate placement of fixation devices is achieved by the use of intraoperative x-rays. The goal of surgery is correction of the deformity with good apposition of all joint surfaces. Minimal to no gapping should be present. This should always be confirmed with a final intraoperative x-ray to assess the final position of all fixation devices, adequate joint apposition, and appropriate foot position. The position of the calcaneus should be neutral to slight valgus.

Postoperatively, the patient is initially placed in a posterior splint to immobilize the fusion site. This is replaced with a below-the-knee fiberglass cast usually 4–5 days following surgery. Total non-weight-bearing is maintained for a minimum of 3–4 months. Serial x-rays are obtained to evaluate bone healing and maintenance of postoperative correction and alignment. The patient is then advanced to gradual protected weight-bearing when x-rays show signs of bony union. Anecdotal reports suggest that the likelihood and rate of fusion may be improved with the use of electrical bone stimulation, although prospective, randomized, double-blind trials are needed to determine overall efficacy *(43)*.

Pantalar Arthrodesis

The ankle joint that has undergone severe destruction from Charcot joint disease is particularly problematic. This typically will result in an ankle joint so flail that ambulation is extremely difficult if not impossible. This deformity may result from total collapse of the talar body or fractures through the medial malleolus, lateral malleolus, or both. Patients with these type of fractures will often be found ambulating directly on either the medial or lateral malleolus. This inherent instability will result in the development of chronic ulcerations that are extremely difficult to control with conservative care alone. The prognosis for these deformities is poor. In order for limb salvage to be achieved, primary fusion of the ankle and subtalar joints is necessary.

The surgical approach depends on the level and degree of destruction. If the primary level of instability and destruction involves the tibiotalar joint, isolated fusion of this joint may be sufficient. However, if destruction of the other rearfoot joints is present, then fusion of the ankle and talonavicular, subtalar, and calcaneocuboid joints (i.e., pantalar fusion) should be performed. All surgical intervention should be delayed until all signs of acute Charcot joint disease have resolved. Attempted fusion during the active, hyperemic phase of this disorder will not only make fusion technically difficult but may also result in failure to fuse.

A lateral incision that begins approximately at the midfibula and extends to the tip of the lateral malleolus offers adequate exposure of the ankle joint. If a pantalar fusion is to be performed, this incison can be extended distally to the calcaneocuboid joint. The fibula is typically osteotomized just proximal to the ankle joint line. The anterior aspect of the fibula is dissected free and reflected posteriorly. This preserves the vascular supply to the fibula and will allow the fibula to be used as a vascularized strut graft on the lateral side of the ankle joint. The ankle joint is now well visualized.

The articular cartilage is resected down to bleeding cancellous bone from the distal tibial articular surface and the talar dome. The ankle joint is repeatedly reapproximated so as to realign the foot. The joint surfaces are continually remodeled until optimal bone apposition and foot alignment is achieved. If a pantalar fusion is being performed, the remaining rearfoot joints can be addressed at this time in the same manner as in a triple arthrodesis.

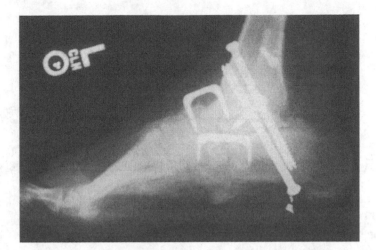

Fig. 15. Severe instability of the rearfoot due to Charcot joint often requires major reconstructive surgery of the hindfoot and ankle. A pantalar fusion was performed in this patient for severe cavoadductovarus deformity and chronic ulceration resulting from Charcot joint. Two 7.0-mm cannulated screws were used to fuse the subtalar and ankle joints.

After all articular surfaces have been resected, the foot should be positioned so that all bone surfaces are in good apposition with minimal to no gapping. Care should also be taken to avoid any interposition of soft tissue. If the foot cannot be aligned properly or bone surfaces do not appose adequately, further remodeling of the bone should be performed. Once optimal alignment has been achieved, the ankle joint is ready for fixation. This is typically performed with the introduction of two 7.0-mm cannulated screws. These are typically inserted from a plantar to dorsal direction through the body of the calcaneus and across the resected ankle joint. This will also fixate the posterior subtalar joint (Fig. 15). Ideally, the tips of the screw should purchase the cortex of the tibia. When bone quality precludes the use of internal fixation, external devices for fixation are appropriate alternatives. The use of intraoperative imaging is critical in the placement of temporary fixation. This can be achieved with fluoroscopy or intraoperative radiographs. It is critical that the calcaneus be positioned either in neutral or in slight valgus position. Any degree of varus should be avoided. After fixation of the ankle joint, the remaining rearfoot joints can be fixated as previously described.

As with triple arthrodesis, postoperative care is critical to successful limb salvage. Wound infection, dehiscence, and nonunion are the major complications seen with this procedure. Immobilization of the extremity immediately postoperatively can decrease the risks of these complications. Total non-weight-bearing in a fiberglass below the knee cast is required for a minimum of 4–6 months. The fusion site must be protected with cast immobilization, and casts must be changed frequently to prevent abrasions or cast irritations. Once it is felt fusion is sufficient to support weight bearing, this should be instituted in a gradual protected manner. A return to protected weight bearing will be dictated by serial x-rays. The use of adjunctive modalities to promote fusion, such as electrical bone stimulation, should be considered in this patient population as these patients and procedures are considered at high risk for nonunion.

REFERENCES

1. Reiber GE, Boyko EJ, Smith DG. Lower extremity foot ulcers and amputations in diabetes, in *Diabetes in America*, 2nd ed. NIH Publication no. 95–1468. National Institutes of Health, Bethesda, MD, 1995, pp. 409–428.
2. Centers for Disease Control and Prevention. *Diabetes Surveillance, 1993*. US Department of Health and Human Services, Atlanta, GA, 1993, pp. 87–93.
3. Jiwa F. Diabetes in the 1990s—an overview. *Stat Bull Metropolitan Life Insurance Co* 1997;78:2–8.
4. DHHS. *Diabetes and Chronic Disabling Conditions*, in *Healthy People 2000*. DHHS Publication no. PHS 91–50212. US Department of Health and Human Services, Public Health Service, Washington, DC, 1991, p. 442.
5. Edmonds ME, Blundell MP, Morris HE, et al. Improved survival of the diabetic foot: the role of the specialist foot clinic. *Q J Med* 1986;232:763–771.
6. Thomson FJ, Veves A, Ashe H, et al. A team approach to diabetic foot care—the Manchester experience. *Foot* 1991;1:75–82.
7. Frykberg RG. Diabetic foot ulcerations, in *The High Risk Foot in Diabetes Mellitus* (Frykberg RG, ed.), Churchill Livingstone, New York, 1991, p. 151.
8. Caputo GM, Cavanagh PR, Ulbrecht JS, Gibbons GW, Karchmer AW. Assessment and management of foot disease in patients with diabetes. *N Engl J Med* 1994;331:854–860.
9. Gibbons GW. Vascular evaluation and long-term results of distal bypass surgery in patients with diabetes. *Clin Podiatr Med Surg* 1995;12:129–140.
10. Gibbons GW. The diabetic foot: amputations and drainage of infection. *J Vasc Surg* 1987; 5:791–793.
11. Morton DJ. *The Human Foot*. Columbia University Press, New York, 1935.
12. Cavanagh PR, Rodgers MM, Iiboshi, A. Pressure distribution under symptom-free feet during barefoot standing. *Foot Ankle* 1987;7:262–276.
13. Ctercteko GC, Chanendran M, Hutton WC, Lequesne LP. Vertical forces acting on the feet of diabetic patients with neuropathic ulceration. *Br J Surg* 1981;68:608–614.
14. Dannels E. Neuropathic foot ulcer prevention in diabetic American Indians with hallux limitus. *J Am Podiatr Med Assoc* 1989;76:33–37.
15. Downs DM, Jacobs RL. Treatment of resistant ulcers on the plantar surface of the great toe in diabetics. *J Bone Joint Surg [Am]* 1982;64:930–933.
16. Rosenblum BI, Giurini JM, Chrzan JS, Habershaw GM. Preventing loss of the great toe with the hallux interphalangeal joint arthroplasty. *J Foot Ankle Surg* 1994;33:557–560.
17. Giurini JM, Chrzan JS, Gibbons GW, Habershaw GM. Sesamoidectomy for the treatment of chronic neuropathic ulcerations. *J Am Podiatr Med Assoc* 1991;81:167–173.
18. Frykberg RF, Giurini JM, Habershaw GM, Rosenblum BI, Chrzan JS. Prophylactic surgery in the diabetic foot, in *Medical and Surgical Management of the Diabetic Foot* (Kominsky, SJ, ed.), Mosby-Year Book, St. Louis, MO, 1994, pp. 399–439.
19. Grayson ML, Gibbons GW, Balogh K, Levin E, Karchmer AW. Probing to bone in infected pedal ulcers: a clinical sign of underlying osteomyelitis in diabetic patients. *JAMA* 1995; 273:721–723.
20. Young MJ, Coffey J, Taylor PM, Boulton AJM. Weight bearing ultrasound in diabetic and rheumatoid arthritis patients. *Foot* 1995;5:76–79.
21. Masson EA, Hay EM, Stockley I, et al. Abnormal foot pressures alone may not cause ulceration. *Diabet Med* 1989;6:426–428.
22. Giurini JM, Rosenblum BI. The role of foot surgery in patients with diabetes. *Clin Podiatr Med Surg* 1995;12:119–127.
23. Fernando DJ, Masson EA, Veves A, Boulton AJM. Relationship of limited joint mobility to abnormal foot pressures and diabetic foot ulceration. *Diabetes Care* 1991;14:8–11.

24. Root M, Weed J, Orien W. *Normal and Abnormal Function of the Foot*. Clinical Biomechanics, Los Angeles, 1977, p. 211.
25. Veves A, Sarnow MR, Giurini JM, et al. Differences in joint mobility and foot pressures between black and white diabetic patients. *Diabet Med* 1995;12:585–589.
26. Tillo TH, Giurini JM, Habershaw GM, Chrzan JS, Rowbotham JL. Review of metatarsal osteotomies for the treatment of neuropathic ulcerations. *J Am Podiatr Med Assoc* 1990; 80:211–217.
27. McKittrick LS, McKittrick JB, Risley T. Transmetatarsal amputation for infection or gangrene in patients with diabetes mellitus. *Ann Surg* 1949;130:826.
28. Kates A, Kessel L, Kay A. Arthroplasty of the forefoot. *J Bone Joint Surg [Br]* 1967;49B: 552.
29. Hoffman P. Operation for severe grades of contracted or clawed toes. *Am J Orthop Surg* 1912;9:441–449.
30. Marmor L. Resection of the forefoot in rheumatoid arthritis. *Clin Orthop* 1975;108:223.
31. Clayton, ML. Surgery of the forefoot in rheumatiod arthritis. *Clin Orthop* 1960;16:136–140.
32. Jacobs RL. Hoffman procedure in the ulcerated diabetic neuropathic foot. *Foot Ankle* 1982; 3:142–149.
33. Giurini JM, Habershaw GM, Chrzan JS. Panmetatarsal head resection in chronic neuropathic ulcerations. *J Foot Surg* 1987;26:249–252.
34. Giurini JM, Basile P, Chrzan JS, Habershaw GM, Rosenblum BI. Panmetatarsal head resection: a viable alternative to the transmetatarsal amputation. *J Am Podiatr Med Assoc* 1993; 83:101–107.
35. Hodor L, Dobbs BM. Pan metatarsal head resection: a review and new approach. *J Am Podiatr Assoc* 1983;73:287–92.
36. Harris JR, Brand PW. Patterns of disintegration of the tarsus in the anesthetic foot. *J Bone J Surg [Br]* 1966;48B:4–16.
37. Sanders LJ, Frykberg RG. Diabetic neuropathic osteoarthropathhy: the Charcot foot, in *The High Risk Foot in Diabetes Mellitus* (Frykberg RG, ed.), Churchill Livingstone, New York, NY, 1990, pp. 297–338.
38. Rosenblum BI, Giurini JM, Miller LB, Chrzan JS, Habershaw GM. Neuropathic ulcerations plantar to the lateral column in patients with Charcot foot deformity: a flexible approach to limb salvage. *J Foot Ankle Surg* 1997;36:360–363.
39. Miller DS, Lichtman WF. Diabetic neuropathic arthropathy of feet. *Arch Surg* 1955;70:513.
40. Sinha S, Munichoodappa C, Kozak GP. Neuroarthropathy (Charcot joints) in diabetes mellitus. Clinical study of 101 cases. *Medicine* 1972;52:191.
41. Cofield RH, Morison MJ, Beabout JW. Diabetic neuroarthropathy in the foot: patient characteristic and patterns of radiographic change. *Foot Ankle* 1983;4:15.
42. Banks AS, McGlamry ED. Charcot foot. *J Am Podiatr Med Assoc* 1989;79:213–235.
43. Bier RR, Estersohn HS. A new treatment for Charcot joint in the diabetic foot. *JAMA* 1987; 77:63–69.

16
Amputations and Rehabilitation

Ronald A. Sage, DPM, Michael Pinzur, MD,
Rodney Stuck, DPM, and Coleen Napolitano, DPM

INTRODUCTION

Amputation of the foot may be indicated when neuropathy, vascular disease, and ulcerative deformity have led to soft tissue necrosis, osteomyelitis, uncontrollable infection, or intractable pain.

Amputations of the lower extremity are often considered either a failure of conservative management or an unpreventable outcome of diabetes. The patient sees amputation as the end of productivity and the start of significant disability. Amputation should be viewed as a procedure leading to rehabilitation and return to productivity for the patient disabled by an ulcerated, infected, or intractably painful extremity. The patient needs assurance, and efforts should be made to follow up the procedure with efforts to return him or her to productive community activity. This may involve consultation among the specialties of medicine, podiatry, orthopedics, vascular surgery, physiatry, and prosthetics. As the patient is rehabilitated and returns to the activities of daily living, the residual limb and the contralateral limb must be protected. Revision amputation and amputation of the contralateral limb remain a significant problem, occurring in as many as 20% of amputee cases (1).

The goal of any limb salvage effort is to convert all patients' diabetic feet, from Wagner grades 1 to 4, back to grade 0 extremities. Those patients with grade 5 feet will require an appropriately higher level of amputation. If salvage is not feasible, then all efforts are made to return the patient to some functional level of activity after amputation. The more proximal the amputation, the higher the energy cost of walking. This problem is most significant in our patients who have multisystem disease and limited cardiopulmonary function. These factors may negatively impact the patient's postoperative independence.

Patients may require several surgical treatments prior to definitive amputation. Incision and drainage or open amputation is frequently required to stabilize acute infection. The parameters of healing, to be mentioned later, may not apply at that time. The goal of the first stage of a multistaged procedure is simply to eradicate infection and stabilize the patient. If medical review of the patient suggests an inability to tolerate multiple operations, a higher initial level of amputation may be indicated, foregoing attempts at distal salvage. However, if salvage is possible, and the patient is medically stable, then a systematic approach to limb salvage should be pursued.

From: *The Diabetic Foot: Medical and Surgical Management*
Edited by: A. Veves, J. M. Giurini, and F. W. LoGerfo © Humana Press Inc., Totowa, NJ

LIMB SALVAGE VERSUS LIMB AMPUTATION

The enlightened orthopedic care of the new millennium has changed the focus from results to outcomes. Burgess taught us that amputation surgery is the first step in the rehabilitation of a patient with a nonfunctionally reconstructable limb *(2)*. He taught us to focus on the reentry of the amputee into normal activities, setting achievable functional goals.

Lower extremity amputation is performed for gangrene, infection, trauma, neoplastic disease, or congenital deformity. Irrespective of the diagnosis, the following questions should be addressed before undertaking either an attempt at limb salvage or performing an amputation:

1. Will limb salvage outperform amputation and prosthetic limb fitting? If all transpires as one could reasonably predict, will the functional independence of the patient following limb salvage/reconstruction be greater, or less than, amputation and prosthetic limb fitting? This will vary greatly with age, vocational ability, medical health, lifestyle, education, and social status.
2. What is a realistic expectation of functional capacities at the completion of treatment? A realistic appreciation of functional end results should be made with respect to both limb salvage and amputation. Consultation with Physical Medicine and Rehabilitation, Social Work, and Physical Therapy can assist in determining reasonable outcome expectations.
3. What is the time and effort commitment required for both the treatment team and the patient? Both the physician and patient must have a reasonable understanding of the duration of the rehabilitation process, the inherent risks involved with revascularization, and the effort required for both.
4. What is the expected financial cost to the patient and resource consumption of the health care system? In the current medical-economic climate, one must realistically address these issues from both the patient and health care system perspective *(3,4)*.

Physical and Metabolic Considerations

Metabolic Cost of Amputation

The metabolic cost of walking is increased with proximal level amputations, being inversely proportional to the length of the residual limb and the number of joints preserved. With more proximal amputation, patients have a decreased self-selected, and maximum, walking speed. Oxygen consumption is increased. From an outcomes perspective, functional independence (functional independence measure [FIM score]) is directly correlated with amputation levels. Distal level amputees achieve proportionally higher FIM scores (Fig. 1) *(5–7)*.

Cognitive Considerations

It is suggested that many individuals with long-standing diabetes have cognitive and perceptual deficits *(8–12)*. Certain specific cognitive capacities are necessary for individuals to become successful prosthetic users: (1) memory, (2) attention, (3) concentration, and (4) organization. For patients with these deficiencies to become successful prosthetic users, they require either specific, successful education and training, or the physical presence of a caregiver who can provide substitute provision of these skills.

Load Transfer and Weight Bearing

Our feet act as uniquely adapted end organs of weight bearing. Following amputation, the residual limb must assume the tasks of load transfer, adapting to uneven terrain,

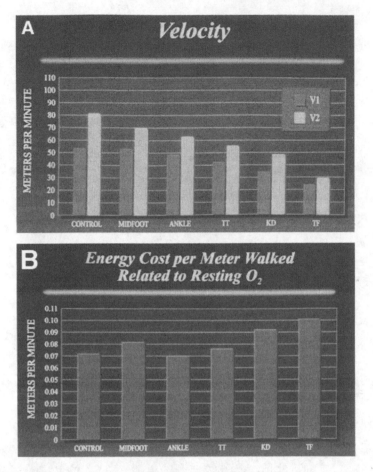

Fig. 1. (**A**) Walking velocity compared with surgical amputation level. V1 is self-selected walking speed. V2 is maximum walking speed. (**B**) Oxygen consumption per meter walked compared with surgical amputation level. Note that the metabolic cost of walking is increased with a more proximal level amputation.

and propulsion, utilizing tissues that are not biologically engineered for that purpose. The weight-bearing surfaces of the long bones are wider than the corresponding diaphysis. This increased surface area dissipates the force applied during weight bearing over a larger surface area, and the more accommodative articular cartilage and metaphyseal bone allow cushioning and shock absorption during weight bearing.

Direct load transfer, i.e., end bearing, which is achieved in disarticulation amputations at the knee and ankle joint levels, takes advantage of the normal weight bearing characteristics of the terminal bone of the residual limb. The overlying soft tissue envelope acts to cushion the bone, much as the heel pad and plantar tissues function in the foot.

Indirect load transfer, or total contact weight bearing, is necessary in diaphyseal transtibial and transfemoral amputation levels, in which the surface area and stiffness of the terminal residual limb require unloading. The weight-bearing load must be applied to the entire surface area, with the soft tissue envelope acting as a cushion *(5)* (Fig. 2).

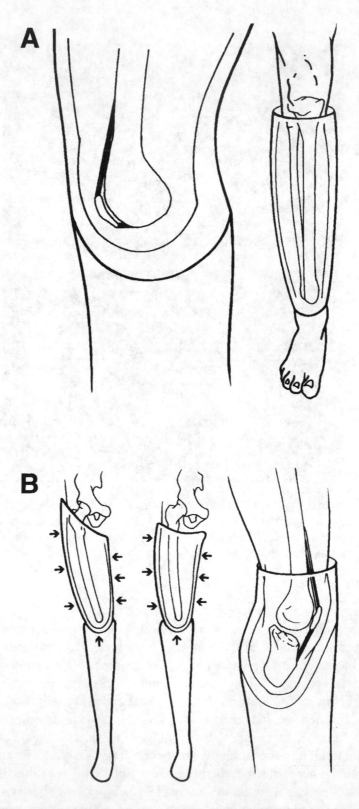

Fig. 2. (A) Direct load transfer (end-bearing) is accomplished in knee disarticulation and Syme's ankle disarticulation amputation levels. **(B)** Indirect load transfer (total contact) is accomplished in transtibial and transfemoral amputation levels.

Soft Tissue Envelope

The soft tissue envelope acts as the interface between the bone of the residual limb and the prosthetic socket. It functions both to cushion the underlying bone and to dissipate the pressures and forces applied during weight bearing. Ideally, it should be composed of a mobile, nonadherent muscle mass and full-thickness skin. If the soft tissue envelope is adherent to bone, the shear forces will produce skin blistering, ulceration, and tissue breakdown. It should be durable enough to tolerate the direct pressures and pistoning within the prosthetic socket.

Healing Parameters

Vascular Perfusion

Amputation wounds generally heal by collateral flow, so arteriography is rarely a useful diagnostic tool to predict wound healing. Doppler ultrasound has been utilized to assess blood flow in the extremity prior to amputation. An ankle-brachial index of 0.45 in the diabetic has been considered adequate for healing as long as the systolic pressure at the ankle was 70 mmHg or higher. These values are falsely elevated (and nonpredictive) in at least 15% of patients with peripheral vascular disease, owing to the noncompressibility and noncompliance of calcified peripheral arteries (13). The transcutaneous partial pressure of oxygen ($TcPO^2$) is the present gold standard measure of vascular inflow. It actually records the oxygen-delivering capacity of the vascular system to the skin at the proposed level of surgery (14,15). Values of 30 mmHg or higher have a 90% healing rate. Values between 20 and 29 mmHg have a 70% healing rate, and values less than 20 mmHg are associated with failure rates greater than 50%. Edema and cellulitis may falsely lower the oxygen values and make this exam invalid (16). Peripheral vascular consultation should be obtained for patients who do not have adequate inflow on these exams.

Nutrition and Immunocompetence

Preoperative review of nutritional status is obtained by measuring the serum albumin and the total lymphocyte count (TLC). The serum albumin should be at least 3.0 g/dL, and the TLC should be greater than 1500. The TLC is calculated by multiplying the white blood cell count by the percent of lymphocytes in the differential. When these values are suboptimal, nutritional consultation is helpful prior to definitive amputation. If possible, surgery in patients with malnutrition or immunodeficiency should be delayed until these issues can be adequately addressed. When infection or gangrene dictate urgent surgery, then surgical debridement of infection (or open amputation at the most distal viable level) followed by open wound care can be accomplished until wound healing potential can be optimized (17–19). At times, such as with severe renal disease, the nutritional values will remain suboptimal, and distal salvage attempts may still be pursued, but at known higher risk for failure.

Glucose control is also important, as high glucose levels will deactivate macrophages and lymphocytes and may impair wound healing. High glucose levels have also been associated with other postoperative infections including those of the urinary tract and respiratory system. Ideal management involves maintenance of glucose levels below 200 mg/dL (20). However, caution must be exercised in managing the perioperative patient's glucose with calorie reduction, as this process may lead to significant protein depletion and subsequent wound failure. A minimum of 1800 calories daily should be provided to avoid the negative nitrogen balance that could accompany depletion of protein stores.

It has been shown that when the combined wound healing parameters of vascular inflow and nutritional status are satisfactory, markedly improved healing rates are seen for pedal amputations. Attempting to normalize these parameter values preoperatively, when medically possible, will limit the risk of wound complications and failure.

Perioperative Considerations

Pedal amputations may be performed under local or regional anesthesia. The effectiveness of local anesthetics may be impaired by the presence of infection and may need to be administered proximal to any cellulitis. When amputating above the ankle, spinal or general anesthesia will be necessary. Spinal anesthesia is contraindicated in the patient with sepsis, demonstrated by fever over 100°F.

Culture-specific antibiotic therapy should be continued perioperatively. If the focus of infection is completely removed with amputation, then the antibiotics may be discontinued 24 hours after surgery. If, however, infection remains a concern, then antibiotics are continued for a soft tissue course of 10–14 days, or 6–8 weeks for bone infection.

Tourniquets may be needed to control bleeding at surgery. The surgeon must ensure that the tourniquet is not placed over a vascular anastomosis site or distal to an area of infection. The patient with severe vascular compromise will not require a tourniquet.

Preoperative Summary

Preoperative planning including vascular and nutritional review is necessary for final amputation level selection. Measurements of serum albumin, TLC, and tissue perfusion are helpful in assessing the healing potential for procedures distal to the malleoli. With satisfactory values in all three categories, healing rates of 90% may be attainable. This suggests that 10% of even ideal cases may require revision surgery. The patient needs to understand this risk, and efforts should be made to use this information to plan procedures that will limit exposure to yet another surgical intervention.

RAY AMPUTATIONS

Indications

Single toe amputation or ray resection may be performed for irreversible necrosis of a toe without medial or lateral extension. Deep infection of the phalanx to bone is also an appropriate indication for toe amputation. If uncontrollable infection extends to the metatarsal phalangeal joint or metatarsal head, then ray resection is appropriate. This procedure is also useful for infection or necrosis of the toe, requiring more proximal resection to obtain viable wound margins.

Ray resection is an excellent method of decompressing deep fascial infection limited to one compartment of the plantar structures of the foot, be that medial, lateral, or central. In such cases the wound is always left open to allow continued drainage, and a more proximal, definitive procedure may follow when the acute infection is stable, if healing parameters are acceptable for a distal limb salvage procedure *(21)*.

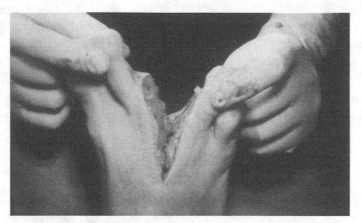

Fig. 3. Patient after third ray amputation for a diabetic ulcer and osteomyelitis. Note that the plantar ulcer was also excised.

Procedure

Ray resections are performed at our institution as a wedge excision of the involved toe and metatarsal. Longitudinal incisions are made parallel to the involved ray, converging on the dorsal and plantar surfaces of the foot. If ulceration is present, as frequently occurs plantar to the metatarsal head, the ulcer is resected along with the wedge of soft tissue that includes the affected toe. The initial incisions are carried to bone, and the toe is disarticulated at the metatarsophalangeal joint. The periosteum of the metatarsal is reflected as far proximally as necessary down the shaft of the bone to ensure that the resection is performed at a level of viable, noninfected bone. The bone is usually cut at the proximal diaphysis, or the diaphyseal metaphyseal junction. It is rarely necessary to do the extensive dissection required to disarticulate the metatarsal cuneiform joint.

Once the bone is removed from the wound, the foot is compressed from proximal to distal to ensure that there is no remaining ascending purulent drainage. If the flexor or extensor compartments reveal pus on compression, then they are opened and irrigated to clean out any remaining apparent infection. If the ray resection was performed for metatarsal or plantar space infection, it is usually left open to facilitate drainage and allow for healing by second intention. This usually occurs in 6 weeks with patients who exhibit acceptable healing parameters, and avoid full weight bearing on the operated foot (Fig. 3).

Postoperative Care

The only ray resection that should be closed primarily is that performed for infection localized to the toe, with clearly viable wound edges, and no suggestion of proximal infection. In this case a gauze dressing is applied and the patient is maintained in a postoperative shoe until healed. A cane or walker is utilized for protected weight bearing.

When the wound is left open, culture-directed antibiotics should be administered for soft tissue or bone infection depending on the extent of the infection. Infectious Disease Service consultation is advisable. The wound itself should be treated according to the surgeon's preferred protocol. If a significant space is present, this should be packed with saline-soaked gauze or alginate dressings. Packing should be sufficient to absorb excess drainage but not aggressive enough to interfere with wound contraction. The amount of packing should decrease each week as the wound contracts and granulates. The foot should be protected from full weight bearing during this time with crutches, a walker, or wheelchair with a leg lift as necessary.

Once healing has been achieved, the patient should have a prescription for protective foot gear. If there is evidence of pressure keratosis developing adjacent to the ray resection site, the patient should be seen in clinic as necessary to pare the callus, in order to prevent transfer ulceration. Such visits may be necessary every 1, 2, or 3 months.

Complications

Persisting infection is rare if the wound was adequately debrided at the time of the ray resection. However, if residual infection is suspected, follow-up surgical debridement should be done. Wound failure may be caused by inadequate healing parameters, such as impaired blood flow or abnormal serum albumin. Such metabolic wound failures may require more proximal amputation to obtain healing.

The most common late complication of ray resection is transfer lesion and reulceration. If pressure keratosis cannot be managed with debridement and prescription shoes, then resection of the remaining metatarsal heads or more proximal amputation may become necessary *(22)*.

TRANSMETATARSAL AND LISFRANC AMPUTATION

Indications

The indications for amputation in a diabetic foot include irreversible necrosis of a significant portion of bone or tendon, uncontrollable infection, or intractable pain. If ulceration is present for a prolonged period, is not responsive to nonsurgical treatment, and is causing significant disability, then amputation of the ulcerated part may be a necessary step to rehabilitation. If the amputation is to be at the level of the toes, foot, or ankle, attention should be directed at well-established vascular and metabolic parameters to ensure a reasonable chance for healing success.

In 1949, McKittrick et al. *(23)* advocated transmetatarsal amputation for infection or gangrene of the toes in diabetic patients. In 1977, Wagner *(24)* subsequently recommended its use in patients with diabetic foot complications, advocating preoperative vascular review. He advised that Doppler studies demonstrating an ankle brachial artery index greater than 0.45 could predict healing of the procedure with 90% accuracy. The present authors' group reviewed 64 transmetatarsal and Lisfranc amputations in 1986 *(25)*. These amputations were performed for gangrene of the forefoot or for forefoot ulcers resistant to nonsurgical attempts at healing. Their results indicated that patients with Doppler ankle-brachial artery index above 0.5, combined with serum albumin levels greater the 3.0 g/dL and TLC greater than 1500/cm^3, healed at a rate of 92%. Those patients lacking one or more of these three indicators healed at a rate of 38%.

Amputation of a single toe or metatarsal may be successfully performed for patients with a localized ulceration if preoperative healing indices are satisfactory. However, there can be significant transfer ulceration following such procedures, leading to later complications, even if early healing is achieved *(21)*.

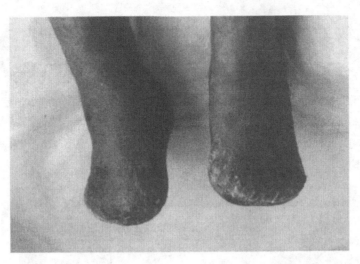

Fig. 4. Bilateral transmetatarsal amputation. The wounds are well healed at 6 weeks.

This experience suggests that transmetatarsal amputation may be a more definitive procedure for the management of forefoot ulceration. Transmetatarsal amputation may be considered for patients with more than one ulceration or site of necrosis of the forefoot. Likewise, this procedure may be considered in cases with a significant nonhealing ulceration and other foot deformity that is likely to lead to subsequent ulcer. However, transmetatarsal amputation, in itself, does not ensure that no further ulceration of the foot is likely.

In our long-term review of midfoot amputations, including transmetatarsal and Lisfranc procedures, 9 of 64 feet sustained new ulcerations within the first year after healing the primary procedure *(26)*. The source of these ulcerations included hypertrophic new bone formation and subsequent varus or equinus deformity. These dynamic deformities were more likely in Lisfranc amputations, in which muscle imbalance was likely to occur because of loss of the attachments of the peroneals and extensors (Figs. 4 and 5).

Plantar ulceration under the metatarsals may deter the surgeon from a transmetatarsal amputation, favoring a more proximal, yet more poorly functional, procedure because of the inability to preserve a long plantar flap for closure of the procedure. However, Sanders *(27)* has demonstrated that a V-shaped excision of the ulceration, with the apex proximal and the base at the junction of the dorsal and plantar flaps, allows conversion of the wound from a simple transverse incision to a T-shaped closure. This produces a longer, ulcer-free flap that can be closed over a transmetatarsal procedure, rather than requiring a more proximal Lisfranc operation to eliminate the plantar ulcer.

The specific indications for transmetatarsal amputation remain similar to those indicated by McKittrick, ulcer or gangrene of the toes. Thanks to Sanders' plantar flap modification (Fig. 6), metatarsal head ulceration is also an appropriate indication for this procedure when the ulceration is not responding to nonsurgical treatment. Ulceration or infection of a single toe may be treated by an isolated ray resection, with the understanding that a risk of transfer ulceration exists. If that risk is increased by obvious

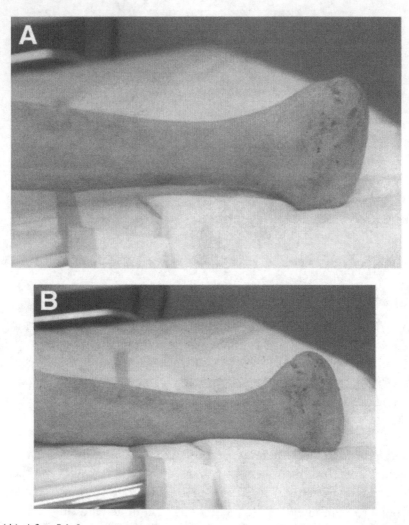

Fig. 5. (**A**) After Lisfranc amputation, equinus may develop and lead to reulceration at the distal stump. (**B**) Percutaneous tendo-Achilles lengthening was performed on this patient to improve ankle dorsiflexion and reduce the risk of ulcer.

ulcerative deformity in other parts of the foot, then transmetatarsal or the slightly more proximal Lisfranc amputation becomes more appropriate. All these procedures are most likely to heal when albumin, lymphocyte count, and arterial inflow meet the recognized minimal standards described above. Prior to definitive midfoot amputation, acute infection should be stabilized by incision, drainage, debridement, or ray resection. Residual infected tissue present at the time of the definitive procedure can be expected to compromise success and should be eliminated in a staged procedure, if necessary. If these criteria cannot be met, then higher amputation may be more appropriate.

Technique

This procedure can be performed with monitored anesthesia care and spinal or ankle block. General anesthesia is rarely necessary. Appropriate medical clearance should be obtained regarding glycemic management and cardiovascular risks.

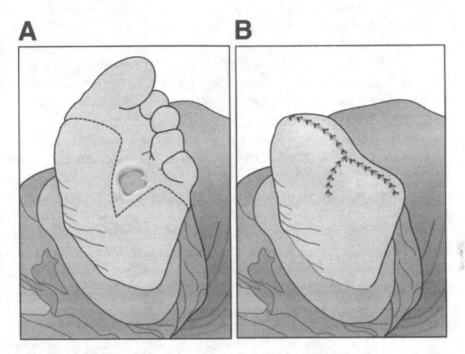

Fig. 6. (**A**) The Sanders technique for plantar flap revision with transmetatarsal amputation in the presence of a distal plantar ulcer. (**B**) The margins of the ulcer site are then approximated with closure as shown.

The transmetatarsal and Lisfranc amputations differ in technique mainly at the point of detachment of the forefoot from the hindfoot. The transmetatarsal procedure is osteotomized through the metatarsal bases, leaving the insertion of the tibialis anterior, peroneus longus, and peroneus brevis intact. The metatarsal osteotomy should be performed through the proximal metaphysis, to avoid long plantar metatarsal shafts and irregular parabola that might later result in plantar stump ulceration. The Lisfranc amputation requires disarticulation at the metatarsal cuneiform and cuboid joints, resulting in loss of the tendon insertions mentioned before. The authors have made occasional attempts to preserve the base of the fifth metatarsal and peroneus brevis insertion, but this is not always practical.

The procedure begins with a dorsal incision across the metatarsal bases, from the medial to the lateral side of the foot, deferring the plantar incision for the time being. If no tourniquet is used, staging the incision like this avoids dealing with bleeding from both the top and bottom of the foot at the same time. The incision is carried to bone through the dorsal tendons and neurovascular structures. Significant vessels, such as the dorsalis pedis, are identified and ligated. The periosteum of the metatarsal bases is incised and reflected using an elevator to expose either the site of the intended osteotomy or the metatarsal tarsal articulation.

If a transmetatarsal amputation is to be performed, the osteotomies are now initiated. The first metatarsal is cut with a power saw, directing the plane slightly medially and plantarly. The second, third, and fourth metatarsals are cut, taking care to produce a smooth parabola, leaving no stump particularly longer than the adjacent bone. The fifth metatarsal is cut last, directing the plane slightly lateral and plantar. At this point the plantar incision is made, initiated at an angle of 90° to the dorsal incision, carried distally to the sulcus, around the metatarsal heads, and then posteriorly along the lateral side of the foot to the fifth metatarsal base. The incision should be carried to bone as much as possible. If a plantar metatarsal head ulceration is present, it should be excised using a V-shaped wedge, directing the apex distally and the base proximally at the level of the distal transverse incision. When this is closed, a T-shaped flap results (Fig. 3).

The metatarsals may now be lifted from the plantar flap from proximal to distal, dissecting along the metatarsal shafts to preserve as much of the soft tissue structures in the plantar flap as possible. The remaining distal attachments of the metatarsal heads are cut, and the forefoot is removed. Significant vascular structures should be ligated. The entire wound should be thoroughly irrigated. Remaining fibrous, ligamentous, and exposed tendinous structures should be cleanly cut from the flap. Minimal debulking of remaining intrinsic muscle structures may be performed if necessary to obtain approximation. However, as much of the viable tissue of the plantar flap as possible should be preserved.

The technique is similar for a Lisfranc amputation, except that the metatarsal cuneiform and cuboid articulations are detached instead of the metatarsal osteotomy. The first cuneiform is invariably long and needs to be ronguered or cut proximally to a smooth parabola with the remaining metatarsals. This cut should be directed slightly medially and plantarly. Articular cartilage from the remaining tarsals is ronguered to bleeding cancellous bone. Since adapting the Sanders plantar flap technique, the present author perform very few Lisfranc procedures because of the obvious functional disadvantage of varus and equinus associated with this procedure. If a Lisfranc is the only option, the tibialis anterior is released from the medial side of the first cuneiform, and a percutaneous tendo-Achilles lengthening is performed.

Prior to closure, the wound should be thoroughly irrigated. If a tourniquet was used, it should be released and significant hemorrhaging vessels ligated. Since the procedure leaves relatively little dead space, drains are rarely necessary. The wound is closed in two to three layers, starting with sutures placed in the middle of the planar flap musculature and approximated to the intermetatarsal or intertarsal ligamentous structures. Then subcutaneous sutures are passed from the distal deeper layers of the flap to the dorsal retinaculum. Finally, the skin is closed with mattress or simple interrupted sutures of 3-0 nylon as needed to obtain a satisfactory incision line.

Postoperative Care

Mild compression and protection of the flap from tension are the authors' objectives in immediate postoperative wound care. Thus a soft gauze roll dressing is applied from the foot to the ankle. Moderated compression is applied, with minimal force directed from plantar to dorsal to protect the plantar flap from undue stress on the incision line. Then two to three layers of cast padding are applied from the foot to the tibial tuberosity, maintaining the foot and ankle in neutral position, neither dorsiflexed or plantarflexed. Finally, several layers of 5 × 30-inch plaster of Paris splints are applied posteriorly from the tip of the stump to the calf, proximal to the knee. The splints are wrapped with another two layers of cast padding, and then an Ace wrap secures the entire dressing.

This resembles a Jones dressing, protecting the wound from any contusions and from any dorsal or plantar tension.

This dressing is left in place for approximately 48 hours before the wound is inspected. A similar dressing is maintained for 2–4 weeks until the incision line is clearly stable. During this time the patient is instructed in the use of crutches, a walker, or wheel chair with leg elevation. Little or no weight bearing on the operated foot is allowed until the wound is clearly stable and free of risk of major dehiscence. Occasional superficial dehiscence may occur, especially in high-risk patients. This is treated like any other grade I ulcer with cleansing, debridement, and topical wound care measures until it is healed. Major postoperative dehiscence, infection, or necrosis of the plantar flap will probably require revision surgery.

Complications

Wagner *(24)* has stated that distal amputations can be expected to heal up to 90% of the time in diabetics who exhibit adequate circulation as determined by Doppler examination demonstrating ankle-brachial artery index of 0.45 or better. The present authors' group confirmed that healing can be achieved in over 90% of diabetics undergoing midfoot amputation if the ankle-brachial artery index is over 0.5, serum albumin is greater than 3.0 g/dL, and TLC is over 1500/cm3 *(25)*. However, we have also noted that up to 42% of midfoot amputations may suffer some form of complication, even though in most their surgical wounds may ultimately heal *(26)*. Complications include early wound dehiscence and late reulceration, which can be treated successfully with resulting limb salvage in most cases. Patients most likely to suffer wound dehiscence include those with marginal vascular indices and low serum albumin. This is especially true in renal failure patients. These prognostic indicators should be taken into consideration in preoperative planning and discussed with the patient. Those at high risk for failure may be better served by a higher amputation that is more likely to heal with one operation.

Biomechanical abnormality resulting from muscle imbalance can result in dynamic varus, producing lateral foot ulceration. This is particularly true in Lisfranc amputations because of the varus pull of an unopposed tibialis anterior. Tibialis anterior tendon transfer can successfully treat problem in some cases. Armstrong and associates *(28)* noted that bone regrowth after partial metatarsal amputation resulted in a significantly increased risk of reulceration. This regrowth was likely to occur in metaphyseal procedures, in males, when manual bone cutting equipment was utilized. In our experience, these reulcerations can be treated with aggressive exostectomy of the underlying bone and standard subsequent wound care.

Long-Term Follow-up Needs

Patients with a history of ulceration remain at high risk for reulceration, even after the foot has been returned to grade 0 by a surgical procedure. The patient who has undergone any form of partial foot amputation should be placed in a high-risk foot clinic for regular follow-up visits. Both short- and long-term complications have been recognized. Even though the benefits of distal limb salvage are well accepted, biomechanical review and management visits must be included in after care for the amputation to be successful

(29). Early on, the wound should be protected with a posterior splint or cast and limited weight bearing. Rehabilitation should include crutch or walker training, if feasible. If the patient cannot use gait-assistive devices, a wheel chair with leg lift and instruction in wheel chair mobility and transfer techniques should be provided. These protective measures should be continued until the wound is clearly healed.

Later, protective foot care, or even a Plastizote-lined ankle foot orthosis may need to be prescribed for adequate protection. Although many patients may function well with an oxford shoe and anterior filler, others may need more elaborate orthotic management. Custom-made short shoes, rocker bottom shoes with a steel shank and anterior filler, or conventional shoes with an ankle-foot orthosis have all been advocated. Each patient should be observed carefully during the return to full ambulation to determine the need for orthotic management. Computer-assisted pressure mapping may be helpful in determining the success of any device in off-loading residual pressure points. If keratotic lesions should develop, these should be considered preulcerative and debrided regularly before ulceration can occur *(30,31)*.

Transmetatarsal and Lisfranc amputation have the benefit of improved function and patient acceptance over higher amputation for individuals suffering from serious forefoot infection, ulceration, or gangrene. However, these operations must be recognized as high-risk procedures. Nevertheless, with appropriate preoperative planning, meticulous surgical technique, protective postoperative care, and long-term follow up, midfoot amputations can be successful limb salvage techniques for most patients undergoing these procedures.

CHOPART AMPUTATION

Indications

François Chopart described disarticulation through the midtarsal joint while working at the Charité Hospital in Paris in the 1800s *(32)*. The operation has been thought to have limited applications because the residual partial foot is susceptible to progressive equinovarus deformity. The Chopart amputation is gaining new favor because the length of the limb is retained and the potential complications of the procedure are frequently successfully addressed *(33–36)*.

Amputation levels are usually chosen on the basis of tissue viability and residual limb function. A Chopart level amputation may be considered when the longer transmetatarsal or Lisfranc amputation level is not an option because of the extent of forefoot tissue destruction. Half of all patients undergoing an initial nontraumatic amputation will probably require an amputation of the contralateral limb *(37)*. There is a higher metabolic requirement for ambulation in those patients who undergo more proximal amputations. Therefore the decision on amputation level should attempt to maximize the patient's mobility and independence by preserving length whenever possible, thus making the Chopart amputation useful when more distal foot procedures are not feasible.

An open Chopart amputation is useful to provide resection of grossly infected forefoot structures, as a stage I procedure, anticipating a higher definitive procedure such as a Boyd or Syme's amputation. The open Chopart amputation procedure disarticulates the foot at the level of the calcaneocuboid and talonavicular joints, leaving the articular surfaces intact. The proximal spread of infection may be less likely with the cancellous spaces unopened *(38)*. During the open Chopart procedure, care must be taken to visualize and resect all necrotic and/or nonviable tissue. Compression of the limb proximal to the open amputation site is done manually to identify purulent drainage from the compartments of the leg. If purulence is expressed with compression, then the affected compartment must be incised and irrigated to provide adequate drainage. Once the acute infection is resolved and the healing parameter indices are reviewed, the open Chopart may be revised to a definitive level. If the surgeon anticipates that the acute infection may be stabilized and that healing at the Chopart level is likely to occur, then care must be taken during the open Chopart procedure to retain sufficient skin and subcutaneous tissue to account for shrinkage and provide coverage of the stump.

The prerequisite for a definitive Chopart amputation is that the plantar heel pad and ankle/subtalar joint articulations not be compromised *(39)*. A closed or definitive Chopart amputation is considered if the forefoot infection extends proximal to the metatarsal bases and neither a transmetatarsal nor Lisfranc amputation can be salvaged. Reyzelman et al. *(40)* suggest that a Chopart amputation is more advantageous then a short transmetatarsal or a Lisfranc amputation because it does not disrupt the transverse arch of the foot. The disruption of the transverse arch creates an overpowering of the tibialis anterior, tibialis posterior, and gastrocnemius muscles to the peroneus brevis muscle. The muscle imbalance created in the short transmetatarsal or Lisfranc amputation may lead to a varus rotation of the residual foot. A frontal plane rotation of the weight-bearing surface of a Chopart amputation is less likely to occur, unless the calcaneus or ankle is structurally in varus *(40)*. The Chopart amputation does, however, lead to an equinus deformity because of the unopposed pull of the Achilles tendon. An Achilles lengthening and/or a tibialis anterior transfer at the time of the definitive closure may address this.

Technique

The dorsal incision begins from the tuberosity of the navicular extending dorsolateral to the midcuboid level. The medial and lateral incisions are carried distally to the midshaft level of the first and fifth metatarsal and continued transversely at this level along the plantar aspect of the foot. These incisions form a fishmouth, with dorsal and plantar flaps. The incisions are deepened to expose the talonavicular and calcaneocuboid joints. The tibialis anterior should be identified and preserved for later transfer to the talar neck. The remaining soft tissue structures are incised to complete the disarticulation of the forefoot from the rearfoot. The articular cartilage of the talus and calcaneus should be resected, creating a flush surface when the definitive procedure is being performed. The tibialis anterior tendon may be attached to the talar neck at this time with either a drill hole or suture. If a tourniquet has been utilized, it is deflated and hemostasis is achieved. The skin edges are then reapproximated and secured with the suture or staples. A drain is necessary only if significant loose soft tissue is present or if excessive bleeding is anticipated, to prevent hematoma formation. The Achilles tendon is lengthened by either double or triple hemisection technique or by tenotomy after the wound is closed, to limit later equinus deformity (Fig. 7). A sterile compressive dressing and a posterior splint are applied to the lower extremity.

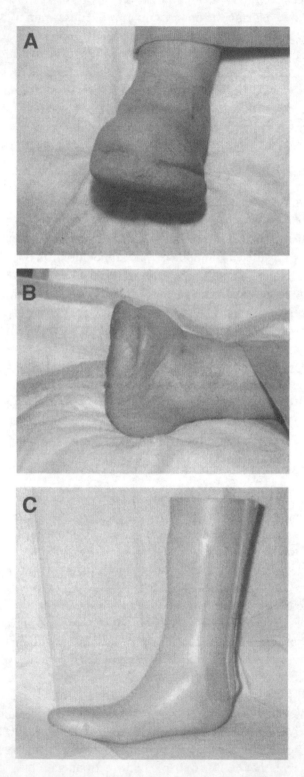

Fig. 7. (A, B) A Chopart level amputation that was primarily closed. A percutaneous Achilles tenotomy was also performed to reduce the high risk of equinus deformity. **(C)** A variety of Chopart prostheses have been advocated. This prosthesis has a posterior closure.

Postoperative Care

The patient is maintained non-weight-bearing in a posterior splint or below-knee cast until the wound is healed, for up to 6 weeks if necessary. The Chopart amputee without equinus is capable of ambulating in an extra inlay depth shoe with a forefoot filler but functions best with a polypropylene solid ankle foot orthosis (AFO) prosthesis with a foam filler *(41)*. The prosthesis helps to eliminate or minimize the pistoning motion of the distal amputation in a normal shoe. If the Chopart amputee has an equines, then he or she should be fitted for a clamshell prosthesis *(42)* (Fig. 5C).

Complications

The usual potential complications of infection or wound failure may occur with this procedure, as with any distal amputation. These are more likely if the procedure is preformed on patients who do not meet the generally accepted vascular and nutritional parameters described earlier. Care must be taken to fashion the flaps to provide adequate coverage for the residual stump without closing under excessive tension, as this may lead to wound dehiscence. Equinus deformity can still occur over time even if Achilles lengthening is performed. The development of a plantar ulceration in an equinus positioned stump is a common occurrence and may lead to revision surgery. As always, close postoperative follow-up and early intervention may minimize these problems.

In spite of these shortcomings, the Chopart amputation remains useful as an early incision and drainage procedure to stabilize acute infection. It is also useful as a definitive procedure in select cases because of its advantage of limb length and tissue preservation.

TRANSMALLEOLAR AMPUTATION: THE SYME PROCEDURE

Indications

Hindfoot amputation, to be successful, must produce a reliable result with a long-lasting and functional residual limb. A Chopart amputation at the talonavicular and calcaneal-cuboid joints creates significant muscle imbalance, frequently resulting in ankle equinus and ulceration. The Boyd amputation has also been advocated *(43)*. This procedure involves fusion of a portion of the calcaneus to the distal tibia. The advantage is that the heel pad remains well anchored to the calcaneus. An additional problem becomes evident in attaining union of the tibia to calcaneus. There may also be difficulty in prosthetic fitting. The residual limb remains long, and there is inadequate space to place a dynamic response prosthetic foot without raising the height of the contralateral limb to compensate for this addition. It is unknown whether this height difference results in gait problems for the diabetic patient.

The Syme amputation is performed through the malleoli and results in physiologic weight bearing throughout the residual limb. The fat pad takes the load directly and transfers it directly to the distal tibia *(44)*. With the use of dynamic response feet, this amputation level results in decreased energy expenditure with ambulation, compared with higher procedures or midfoot amputation *(45–48)*. Contraindications include local infection or gangrene at the level of the amputation, as well as inadequate nutritional and vascular parameters to sustain distal healing. Heel ulceration has been considered a contraindication to a Syme procedure in the past. However, a recent report suggested that an anterior flap may be useful in patients with a nonviable heel pad *(47)*. A long-term review of this procedure modification in a significant series of patients has not yet been performed.

Procedure

The incision is placed anteriorly across the ankle mortise and then in a stirrup fashion across the anterior heel at the level of the malleoli. The incision is deepened at the anterior ankle, and the ankle capsule is incised transversely. The ankle ligaments are released sharply, and the talus is displaced anteriorly in the mortise. A bone hook is placed into the talus and used to distract the talus anteriorly so that soft tissues may be freed from the talus and the calcaneus. Care is exercised at the posterior calcaneus to prevent buttonholing of the skin while releasing the soft tissues. Once free, the residual foot is removed from the wound, which is thoroughly irrigated. The residual tendons are gently distracted 0.5–1.0 cm and sectioned. If needed, the anterior ankle vessels may be ligated with appropriate suture. Anterior and posterior margins of the distal tibia may require debridement to diminish excessive spurring. Two drill holes may be placed in the posterior and/or anterior tibia. A heavy absorbable suture (0) may be utilized through the drill holes to anchor the plantar fascia to the distal tibia. The anterior aspect of the residual plantar fascia is sewn into the anterior ankle capsule, and the subcutaneous tissues and skin are closed in layers. A medium Hemovac drain is placed prior to closure. A posterior splint or a short leg cast is placed. The drain is removed 24–48 hours after surgery.

Postoperative Care

The patient may begin assisted/partial weight bearing at 3–5 days and is maintained in a short leg cast for 3–6 weeks. The patient is then advanced to a fiberglass cast temporary prosthesis with a rubber bumper distally. Once the limb has matured and there is minimal residual edema, the patient is fitted for a Canadian Syme prosthesis with a dynamic response foot (Figs. 8 and 9). Full activity is resumed. The need for physical therapy gait training is unusual.

Complications

Healing rates for this level vary from 70 to 80%. Early complications with the wound may occur in up to 50% of the patients. Most of these problems may be treated with local wound care, total contact casting, and culture-specific antibiotic therapy. Other problems include heel pad migration and new bone formation. Heel pad migration has become less frequent with anchoring of the fascia. Should new bone formation become significant or cause ulceration, exostectomy may become necessary *(44)*.

TRANSTIBIAL OR BELOW-KNEE AMPUTATION

Indications

Individuals with transtibial amputation provide the largest population of patients that are capable of achieving meaningful rehabilitation and functional independence following lower extremity amputation. The most predictable method of obtaining a durable residual limb is with a posterior myofasciocutaneous flap *(3)*. This level takes advantage of the plastic surgical tissue transfer technique of a composite tissue flap without dissection between layers, thus minimizing the risk for devascularization of the overlying skin.

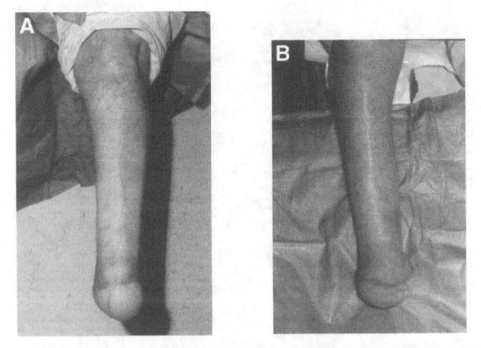

Fig. 8. (A) A well-performed Syme's amputation with tapered stump and heel pad. **(B)** A more bulbous residual limb with medial and lateral flairs is a typical appearance. If these lateral prominences become problematic, wedge excision of these tissues may become necessary.

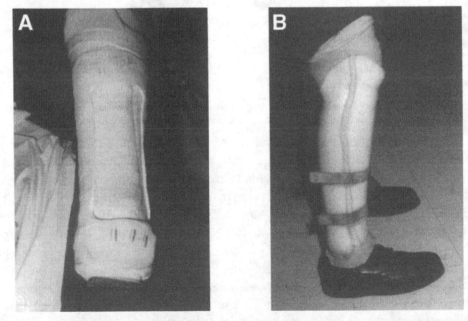

Fig. 9. (A) A fiberglass cast with a distal rubber bumper and a medial window is used as a temporary prosthesis to allow early ambulation for the Syme's amputation patients. **(B)** A thermoplastic variation of a temporary prosthesis with a prosthetic foot attached. In a patient with very limited ambulation, this may also serve as a permanent prosthesis.

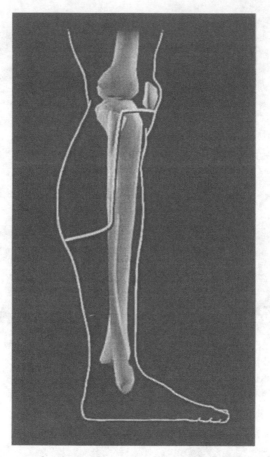

Fig. 10. Posterior myofasciocutaneous flap used in transtibial amputation level.

Procedure

The optimal length of the tibial bone cut is the junction between the proximal and middle quarters of the tibia. A simple rule of thumb is 5 inches (12–15 cm) distal to the knee joint. The length of the posterior flap should be the length of the diameter of the limb at the level of the amputation, plus 1 cm. The longitudinal component of the flap should be between one-third and one-half of the width of the limb, depending on the size of the patient. Thinner patients require more bulk to create a functional residual limb (Fig. 10).

The muscle of the flap should be beveled to obtain good soft tissue padding without being too bulky. The tibia is transected with a power saw, taking careful attention to beveling the anterior surface. The fibula is cut just proximal to the tibia, to provide an optimal bony surface for load transfer. The posterior gastrocnemius muscle fascia should be sutured to the anterior-distal residual tibia via drill holes or to the enveloping periosteum of the tibia. The lateral aspect of the flap is secured to the transected anterior compartment fascia. Securing the gastrocnemius muscle flap to the tibia serves two purposes: (1) it creates a cushioned soft tissue interface to alleviate the shear forces of weight bearing in a prosthesis; and (2) control of the residual tibia positions the tibia in optimal alignment for effective load transfer to the prosthesis *(49)*. A suction drain is generally used under the flap, and the skin is reapproximated without tension.

Postoperative Care

Postoperatively, a rigid plaster dressing is applied *(50)*. Weight bearing with a prosthesis is initiated at 5–21 days, based on the experience and resources of the rehabilitation team (Fig. 11).

KNEE DISARTICULATION

Indications

Knee disarticulation is generally performed in patients with the biologic capacity to heal a surgical wound at the transtibial level but who are not considered able to walk with a prosthesis *(51,52)*. In selected patients, it provides an excellent direct load transfer residual limb for weight bearing in a prosthesis. In limited household walkers, or in feeble amputees with limited ambulatory capacity, this level takes advantage of the intrinsically stable polycentric four-bar linkage prosthetic knee joint. The enhanced inherent stability of this prosthetic system decreases the risk for falls in this limited ambulatory population.

Procedure

The currently recommended technique takes advantage of the accepted transtibial posterior myofasciocutaneous flap *(53)*. The skin incision is made transversely midway between the level of the inferior pole of the patella and the tibial tubercle, at the approximate level of the knee joint. The length of the posterior flap is equal to the diameter plus 1 cm (as with transtibial). The width of the flap again varies with the size of the patient, ranging between the posterior and middle thirds of the circumference of the leg (Fig. 12). The patellar ligament is detached from the tibia, and the capsule of the knee joint is incised circumferentially. The cruciate ligaments are detached from the tibia. A full-thickness posterior myofasciocutaneous flap is created along the posterior surface of the tibia. The soleus muscle is generally removed, unless it is needed to provide bulk. The gastrocnemius muscle is transected at the level of the posterior skin incision, with no creation of a tissue plane between the muscle and skin layers. The patellar ligament is then sutured to the distal stumps of the cruciate ligaments with nonabsorbable suture. The posterior gastrocnemius fascia is then sutured to the patellar ligament and retained knee joint retinaculum. The skin is reapproximated, and a rigid postoperative plaster rigid dressing is applied.

Postoperative Care

Early weight bearing with a preparatory prosthesis or pylon can be initiated when the tissues of the residual limb appear secure. A locked knee or polycentric four-bar linkage prosthetic knee joint can be used, depending on the walking stability of the patient.

TRANSFEMORAL, OR ABOVE-KNEE AMPUTATION

Indications

Gottschalk has clearly shown that the method of surgical construction of the transfemoral residual limb is the determining factor in positioning the femur for optimal load transfer *(54)*. Standard transfemoral amputation with a fishmouth incision disengages

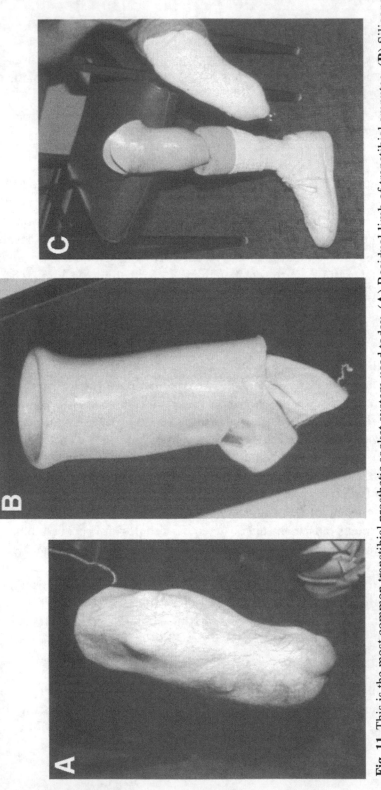

Fig. 11. This is the most common transtibial prosthetic socket system used today. (**A**) Residual limb of transtibial amputee. (**B**) Silicone suspension sleeve. The silicone sleeve fits the residual limb snugly, much like a condom. The bolt at the bottom locks into the (**C**) prosthesis.

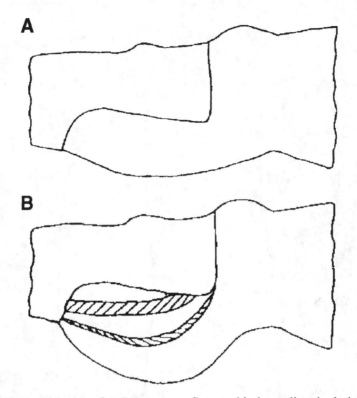

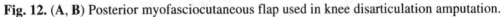

Fig. 12. (A, B) Posterior myofasciocutaneous flap used in knee disarticulation amputation.

the action of the adductor musculature. By disengaging the adductor muscles, the femur assumes an abducted, nonfunctional position. This relative functional shortening of the abductors produces an apparently weak abductor gait pattern. By using an adductor-based myocutaneous flap, the adductor muscles can be secured to the residual femur, allowing the femur to be appropriately prepositioned within the prosthetic socket *(55)*.

Procedure

Using the rule of thumb, the bone cut is 5 inches above the knee joint. The soft tissue envelope is composed of a medial-based myofasciocutaneous flap (Fig. 13). The flap, including adductor magnus insertion, is dissected off the femur. After securing hemostasis and cutting the bone, the adductor muscles are secured to the lateral cortex of the femur via drill holes, under normal resting muscle tension. The anterior and posterior muscle flaps are also secured to the residual femur via drill holes. Careful attention is paid to secure the muscles to the residual femur with the hip positioned at neutral flexion-extension, so as to avoid an iatrogenic hip flexion contracture, which is often produced by repairing the soft tissues with the residual limb propped on bolsters during wound closure.

Postoperative Care

An elastic compression dressing is applied, and weight bearing with a preparatory prosthesis is initiated when the wound appears secure.

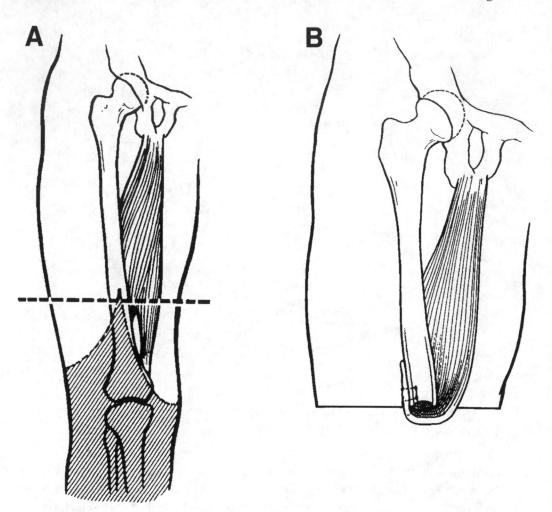

Fig. 13. (A) Skin incision for adductor myofasciocutaneous transfemoral amputation technique. **(B)** Schematic of muscle attachment.

HIP DISARTICULATION

Few hip disarticulation amputees become functional prosthetic users. Whether sitting in a chair or sitting in a prosthetic socket, the weight-bearing platform can be enhanced by retaining the femoral head within the socket.

REHABILITATION

Amputation surgery should be considered as reconstructive surgery following removal of a nonfunctional organ of locomotion. Thus the concept of rehabilitation should begin prior to surgery. It cannot be sufficiently stressed that optimal functional outcomes can generally be achieved when the treatment team establishes reasonable goals. If functional walking is not reasonable, possibly independent wheelchair transfer for ambulation is most appropriate. The treatment team should have a reasonable expectation of goal outcomes at the end of treatment, before initiating treatment. When one measures results from an ambulatory perspective or from a measure of achieving activities of daily living, amputees with more proximal level amputations are less functional or independent. Unilateral ankle disarticulation amputees walk and functional at a level very comparable to their age- and disease-matched counterparts. Although 87% of transtibial amputees will be functional walkers at 2 years, 36% will have died *(56)*. Ambulatory knee disarticulation amputees fare somewhat less well from both ambulatory and independence perspectives. Very few diabetic, dysvascular transfemoral amputees or bilateral amputees will become functional walkers.

Residual limb care in the early postoperative period can enhance or detract from good surgical technique. Specific wound care is related to the circumstances of the surgery. The use of rigid postoperative plaster dressings in transtibial or knee disarticulation amputations controls swelling, decreases postoperative pain, and protects the limb from trauma. The rigid plaster dressing is changed at 5–7-day intervals, with early postoperative prosthetic limb fitting and weight bearing being initiated between 5 and 21 days following surgery. Immediate postoperative prosthetic fitting should be reserved for patients with very stable, secure residual limbs. Generally, the residual limb of the transfemoral amputee is managed with a suspended compression dressing. Weight bearing with a prefabricated or custom prosthetic socket and training pylon can be initiated when the wound appears secure. Patients who have multiple organ disease and more proximal level amputations, are more likely to require walking aids, with almost all dysvascular diabetic amputees requiring the use of a walker or crutches for their limited range of walking.

When the treatment team develops reasonable, realistic goals, patients are capable of achieving the highest level of functional walking compatible with their multiple organ system disease.

CONCLUSIONS

Partial foot amputations are frequently used to accomplish limb salvage successfully. If below-knee or higher amputation is required to achieve healing, many patients return to community ambulation, still utilizing and stressing the remaining limb. Once any form of amputation has occurred, the patient must be considered at high risk for further amputation *(30)*. The principles of managing any high-risk foot must be applied, and regular review and management services are essential for preserving the salvaged and contralateral limb.

Patient education, shoe review with appropriate prescription or recommendation, and regular professional foot exams are the mainstay of any preventive program *(30)*. Regular follow-up must be initiated after healing has been accomplished. The patient should be instructed in regular self-exams of the foot, as well as the effects of sensory neuropathy. Potentially ulcerative pressure points should be identified and accommodated with orthotics and/or shoes as needed. Recurring pressure keratosis should be acknowledged as a potential ulceration and debrided as necessary to prevent the callus from becoming hemorrhagic or ulcerative. This may require intervals as little as every 4 weeks *(31)*.

It has been the authors' experience that no surgical procedure is effective in itself for preventing subsequent foot ulcers. The patient with any form of lower extremity amputation must be considered at high risk for further ulceration. Careful clinical follow-up, orthotic care, and debridement of chronic focal pressure keratosis are far more effective in preventing ulceration or further amputation than any operation.

REFERENCES

1. Adler AI, Boyko EJ, Ahroni JH, Smith DG. Lower extremity amputation in diabetes. The independent effects of peripheral vascular disease, sensory neuropathy and foot ulcers. *Diabetes Care* 1999;22:1029–1035.
2. Burgess EM, Romano RL, Zettl JH. *The Management of Lower Extremity Amputations.* US Government Printing Office, Washington, DC, 1969.
3. Pinzur MS, Bowker JH, Smith DG, Gottschalk FA. Amputation surgery in peripheral vascular disease. *Instructional Course Lectures, The American Academy of Orthopaedic Surgeons* 1999;48:687–692.
4. Pinzur MS, Sage R, Stuck R, Ketner L, Osterman H. Transcutaneous oxygen as a predictor of wound healing in amputations of the foot and ankle. *Foot Ankle* 1992;13:271–272.
5. Waters RL. The energy expenditure of amputee gait, in *Atlas of Limb Prosthetics* (Bowker J, Michael J, eds.), Mosby Year Book, St. Louis, MO, 1992, pp. 381–387.
6. Pinzur MS, Gold J, Schwartz D, Gross N. Energy Demands for walking in dysvascular amputees as related to the level of amputation. *Orthopaedics* 1992;15:1033–1037.
7. Waters RL, Perry J, Antonelli D, et al. Energy cost of walking of amputees: the influence of level of amputation. *J Bone Joint Surg [Am]* 1976;58A:42–46.
8. Worral G, Moulton N, Briffett E. Effect of type II diabetes mellitus on cognitive function. *J Fam Pract* 1993;36:639–643.
9. Kruger S, Guthrie D. Foot care knowledge retention and self-care practices. *Diabetes Educ* 1992;18:487–490.
10. Thompson FJ, Masson EA. Can elderly diabetic patients cooperate with routine foot care? *Age Aging* 1992;21:333–337.
11. Pinzur MS, Graham G, Osterman H. Psychological testing in amputation rehabilitation. *Clin Orthop* 1988;229:236–240.
12. Pinzur MS. New concepts in lower-limb amputation and prosthetic management. *Instructional Course Lectures The American Academy of Orthopaedic Surgeons* 1990;39:361–366.
13. Emanuele MA, Buchanan BJ, Abraira C. Elevated leg systolic pressures and arterial calcification in diabetic occlusive vascular disease. *Diabetes Care* 1981;4:289–292.
14. Misuri A, Lucertini G, Nanni A, et al. Predictive value of trancutaneous oximetry for selection of the amputation level. *J Cardiovasc Surg* 2000;41:83–87.
15. Wyss CR, Harrington R, Burgess EM, et al. Transcutaneous oxygen tension as a predictor of wound healing in amputations of the foot and ankle. *J Bone Joint Surg [Am]* 1988;70:203.
16. Pinzur M, Stuck R, Sage R, et al. Transcutaneous oxygen tension in the dysvascular foot with infection. *Foot Ankle* 1993;14:254–256.
17. Dickhaut SC, Delee JC, Page CP. Nutrition status: importance in predicting wound healing after amputation. *J Bone Joint Surg [Am]* 1984;64:71–75.
18. Haydock DA, Hill GL. Improved wound healing response in surgical patients receiving intravenous nutrition. *Br J Surg* 1987;74:320–323.
19. Jensen JE, Jensen TG, Smith TK, et al. Nutrition in orthopaedic surgery. *J Bone Joint Surg [Am]* 1982;64:1263–1272.
20. Mowat AG, Baum J. Chemotaxis of polymorphonuclear leukocytes from patients with diabetes mellitus. *N Engl J Med* 1971;248:621–627.
21. Gianfortune P, Pulla RJ, Sage R. Ray resection in the insensitive or dysvascular foot: a critical review. *J Foot Surg* 1985;24:103–107.
22. Pinzur MS, Sage R, Schwaegler P. Ray resection in the dysvascular foot. *Clin Orthop* 1984;191:232–234.
23. McKittrick LS, McKittrick JB, Risley TS. Transmetatarsal amputation for infection or gangrene in patients with diabetes mellitus. *Ann Surg* 1949;130:826–831.
24. Wagner FW. Amputations of the foot and ankle. *Clin Orthop* 1977;122:62–69.

25. Pinzur M, Kaminsky M, Sage R, Cronin R, Osterman H. Amputations at the middle level of the foot. *J Bone Joint Surg [Am]* 1986;68–A:1061.

26. Sage R, Pinzur MS, Cronin R, Preuss HF, Osterman H. Complications following midfoot amputation in neuropathic and dysvascular feet. *J Am Podiatr Med Assoc* 1989;79:277.

27. Sanders LJ. Transmetatarsal and midfoot amputations. *Clin Podiatr Med Surg* 1997;14:741–762.

28. Armstrong DG, Hadi S, Nguyen HC, Harkless LB. Factors associated with bone regrowth following diabetes-related partial amputation of the foot. *J Bone Joint Surg* 1999;81:1561–1565.

29. Mueller MJ, Sinacore DR. Rehabilitation factors following transmetatarsal amputation. *Phys Ther* 1994;74:1027–1033.

30. Mayfield JA, Reiber GE, Sanders LJ, Janisse D, Pogach L. Preventive foot care in people with diabetes. *Diabetes Care* 1998;21:2161–2177.

31. Sage RA, Webster JK, Fisher SG. Out patient care and morbidity reduction in diabetic foot ulcers associated with chronic pressure ulcers, presented at *2000 CDC Diabetes Translation Conference: Reducing the Burden of Diabetes*, April 17–20, New Orleans, LA, 2000.

32. Christie J, Clowes CB, Lamb DW. Amputation through the middle part of the foot. *J Bone Joint Surg [Br]* 1980;24:473–474.

33. McDonald A. Choparts amputation. *J Bone Joint Surg [Br]* 1955;37:468–470.

34. Lieberman JR, Jacobs RL, Goldstock L, et al. Chopart amputation with percutaneous heel cord lengthening. *Clin Orthop* 1993;296:86–91.

35. Chang BB, Bock DE, Jacob RL, et al. Increased limb salvage by the use of unconventional foot amputations. *J Vasc Surg* 1994;19:341–349.

36. Bingham J. The surgery of partial foot amputation, in *Prosthetics and Orthotic Practice* (Murdoch, ed.), Edward Arnold, London, 1970, p. 141.

37. Roach JJ, Deutscsh A, McFarlane DS. Resurrection of the amputations of Lisfranc and Chopart for diabetic gangrene. *Arch Surg* 1987;122:931–934.

38. Wagner FW. The dysvascular foot: a system for diagnosis and treatment. *Foot Ankle* 1981; 2:64–122.

39. Early JS. Transmetatarsal and midfoot amputations. *Clin Orthop* 1999;361:85–90.

40. Reyzelman AM, Suhad H, Armstrong DG. Limb salvage with Chopart's amputation and tendon balancing. *JAPMA* 1999;89:100–103.

41. Cohen-Sobel E. Advances in foot prosthetics, in *Advances in Podiatric Medicine and Surgery* (Kominsky SJ, ed.), Mosby, St. Louis, MO, 1995, pp. 261–273.

42. Cohen-Sobel E, Cuselli M, Rizzuto J. Prosthetic management of a Chopart amputation variant. *JAPMA* 1994;84:505–510.

43. Grady JF, Winters CL. The Boyd amputation as a treatment for osteomyelitis of the foot. *JAPMA* 2000;90:234–239.

44. Stuck RM. Syme's ankle disarticulation: the transmalleolar amputation. *Clin Podiatr Med Surg* 1997;14:763–774.

45. Pinzur M, Morrison C, Sage R, et al. Syme's two-stage amputation in insulin requiring diabetics with gangrene of the forefoot. *Foot Ankle* 1991;11:394–396.

46. Pinzur M. Restoration of walking ability with Syme's ankle disarticulation. *Clin Orthop Related Research* 1999;361:71–75.

47. Robinson KP. Disarticulation at the ankle using an anterior flap: a preliminary report. *J Bone Joint Surg [Br]* 1999;81:617–620.

48. Waters RL, Perry J, Antonelli D, et al. Energy cost of walking of amputees: the influence of level of amputation. *J Bone Joint Surg [Am]* 1976;58:42.

49. Pinzur MS, Reddy N, Charuk G, Osterman H, Vrbos L. Control of the residual tibia in transtibial amputation. *Foot Ankle Int* 1996;17:538–540.

50. Pinzur MS. Current concepts: amputation surgery in peripheral vascular disease. *Instructional Course Lectures, The American Academy of Orthopaedic Surgeons* 1997;46:501–509.

51. Pinzur MS, Smith DG, Daluga DG, Osterman H. Selection of patients for through-the-knee amputation. *J Bone Joint Surg [Am]* 1988;70A:746–750.
52. Pinzur MS. Knee disarticulation: surgical procedures, in *Atlas of Limb Prosthetics* (Bowker JH, Michael JW, eds.), Mosby Year Book, St. Louis, MO, 1992, pp. 479–486.
53. Bowker JH, San Giovanni TP, Pinzur MS. North American experience with knee disarticulation with use of a posterior myofasciocutaneous flap. Healing rate and functional results in seventy-seven patients. *J Bone Joint Surg [Am]* 2000;82A:1571–1574.
54. Gottschalk F, Kourosh S, Stills M. Does socket configuration influence the position of the femur in above-knee amputation? *J Prosthet Orthot* 1989;2:94–102.
55. Gottschalk F. Transfemoral amputation, in *Atlas of Limb Prosthetics* (Bowker JH, Michael JW, eds.), Mosby Year Book, St. Louis, MO, 1992, pp. 501–507.
56. Pinzur MS, Gottschalk F, Smith D, et al. Functional outcome of below-knee amputation in peripheral vascular insufficiency. *Clin Orthop* 1993;286:247–249.

17

Reconstruction of Soft Tissue Defects of the Foot

Nancy Falco Chedid, MD

INTRODUCTION

Management of soft tissue defects of the foot demands attention to specific features of regional anatomy and function as well as general principles of wound repair. In diabetes mellitus, devotion to these basic principles is crucial: the effects of neuropathy, peripheral vascular disease, and susceptibility to infection manifest as increased risk of skin ulceration and decreased capacity for wound healing. The complex wounds encountered in patients with diabetes may contain exposed bone or tendon, or they may lie in weight-bearing areas of the foot.

Certain factors in wound healing can be altered through surgical intervention. In principle, the primary benefit of reconstructive surgery for nonhealing wounds is the introduction of tissue with good vascular supply, to deliver oxygen, nutrients, and growth factors. The placement of a flap or graft also can reduce wound tension and provide mechanical and thermal protection, as well as hydration. In theory, recurrent ulceration may be forestalled by placement of a sensory-innervated flap. A goal of reconstructive surgery is to replace lost tissue with "like" tissue, or with tissue that can fulfill the functional requirements of the original.

The surgeon approaching a wound with the goal of repair must weigh several issues, especially the location and dimensions of the wound and the availability of local tissues. The complexity of a planned procedure, the likelihood of initial success and long-term stability, and the risks to the patient must also be considered. Options for reconstruction are limited in the lower extremity, which has the conformation of a peninsula with the foot at its far end and no tissue available for transfer from a distal direction.

It is helpful to imagine the surgical options in a hierarchical arrangement, from local to distant and from simple to complex: linear repair/skin graft/local flap/regional flap/distant flap/free tissue transfer. Sometimes it is appropriate to bypass consideration of simple techniques outright in favor of complex ones, as in the setting of a foot wound that cannot be repaired except by using a free flap with a remote arterial source.

The distant flap—specifically the cross-leg flap—will be mentioned only briefly, as it has largely been displaced by free tissue transfer. The cross-leg flap is awkward and distressing to the patient since it requires immobilization of the two lower limbs together for at least several days, prior to flap division. However, some authors have argued that an updated version of the cross-leg flap, designed as a fasciocutaneous flap, is relatively

From: *The Diabetic Foot: Medical and Surgical Management*
Edited by: A. Veves, J. M. Giurini, and F. W. LoGerfo © Humana Press Inc., Totowa, NJ

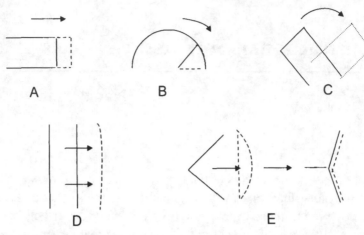

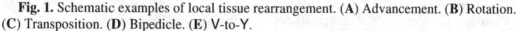

Fig. 1. Schematic examples of local tissue rearrangement. (**A**) Advancement. (**B**) Rotation. (**C**) Transposition. (**D**) Bipedicle. (**E**) V-to-Y.

less morbid and more reliable than its predecessor *(1)*. Certainly this option should be considered for soft tissue repair of the foot, if a shortage of equipment or technical expertise precludes the use of a free flap.

The above-named procedures all are examples of primary repair. Secondary repair, namely, delayed closure or healing by secondary intention, also has a place in the surgical repertoire. Furthermore, although advances in surgical techniques have improved prospects for limb salvage generally, not every wound should be subjected to repair. If reconstruction entails a heroic treatment course with a small likelihood of success, and particularly if a patient is unable to maintain postoperative restrictions, then amputation may be the better alternative.

Definitions: Grafts and Flaps

A graft is a piece of tissue that has been detached from its native blood supply and that depends on nourishment from a recipient site to survive. A flap, on the other hand, is transferred along with its vasculature. In an island flap, the tissues to be moved are incised circumferentially, leaving the flap attached only by its blood supply; a peninsular pedicled flap retains skin and/or deeper soft tissue at the base of the flap. In the case of a free flap, the arteriovenous pedicle accompanies the transferred tissue but is severed at its origin and anastomosed to recipient blood vessels.

Skin grafts retain an important role in reconstructive surgery, either as a primary means of repair or to mend the donor site of a flap. Tendon and bare cortical bone will not support a skin graft, but healthy paratenon, periosteum, and even cancellous bone will do so. Most skin grafts are harvested with split (or partial) thickness, leaving residual dermis at the donor site that will epithelialize spontaneously.

Skin flaps have traditionally been categorized as either axial pattern or random. Axial pattern flaps have in their longitudinal axis an identifiable arteriovenous system arising from a vascular pedicle. Random flaps do not have such a recognizable arrangement of pedicle and tributaries. The familiar advancement, rotation, and transposition flaps are examples of random skin flaps (Fig. 1). According to conventional wisdom, a random flap should not exceed 3:1 in its length-to-width ratio. However, current opinion holds that the pattern of viability in a flap depends on the specific vasculature incorporated within its bounds *(1,2)*.

Territorial Blood Supply: Implications for Flap Design

Vascular anatomy is the foundation for flap design. Segmental anastomotic vessels run deep to skeletal muscles. Perforator vessels travel within a connective tissue framework, supplying overlying cutaneous vessels either directly or by nourishing the intervening muscle tissue. Perforator branches form a plexus just deep to the fascia and also give off radiating arteries superficial to the fascia, but the pattern is variable from one region to another. Blood is sent to the dermis through a dermal and subdermal plexus. These patterns of distribution are the basis for the various common types of flaps: muscle, musculocutaneous, and fasciocutaneous.

Through a series of elaborate injection studies, Taylor and Palmer *(3)* have delineated the blood supply to the skin and adjoining tissues throughout the body. They introduced the term *angiosome*, to denote the three-dimensional territory (including the skin surface) supplied by any named source artery. These and subsequent studies have inspired the creation of numerous perforator-based skin flaps.

Muscle flaps, which are widely used in reconstructive surgery, bring increased blood flow and improved resistance to bacterial infection to the wound site. These hardy flaps can be grafted with skin, if necessary. An alternative is the musculocutaneous flap, which is a composite of skin, muscle, and subcutaneous tissue. Precise knowledge of the flap's vascular anatomy is essential for proper planning and preservation of the overlying skin.

Where only skin is needed to cover a wound, fasciocutaneous flaps are less bulky and easier to transfer than musculocutaneous flaps. The advantages of applying a thin, conforming flap to restore the contours of the foot are considerable. However, this type of flap shows relatively less collagen deposition and relatively less resistance to bacterial inoculation. The donor site usually requires repair with a skin graft and may have a residual contour defect; the rate of complications at both the recipient site and the donor site is higher than that with musculocutaneous flaps.

Free Tissue Transfer: General Considerations

The free flap, on the top rung of the reconstructive ladder, is often considered after other options have been exhausted. However, free tissue transfer should sometimes be the primary choice, particularly in attempts at limb salvage when there is insufficient local tissue for coverage of exposed vital structures, bone, or tendon (Fig. 2). For large wounds that would otherwise require prolonged conservative treatment, alone or in preparation for a skin graft, use of a free flap may allow for primary healing and a reduced period of disability for the patient. Moreover, a free flap may be the best choice when specialized tissue, such as a sensate flap, is desired.

There are many, if not limitless, options in selecting a free-flap donor site. As a general rule, donor tissue from above the waist is preferred, as atherosclerotic changes usually are less prominent there. The "workhorse" muscle flaps, rectus abdominis and latissimus dorsi, are easily harvested and are useful for filling large defects, especially those with exposed bone. They may also be transferred as composite, musculocutaneous flaps, but in this guise they tend to be too thick. In the foot, smaller muscle flaps such as the gracilis or serratus anterior may be more appropriate.

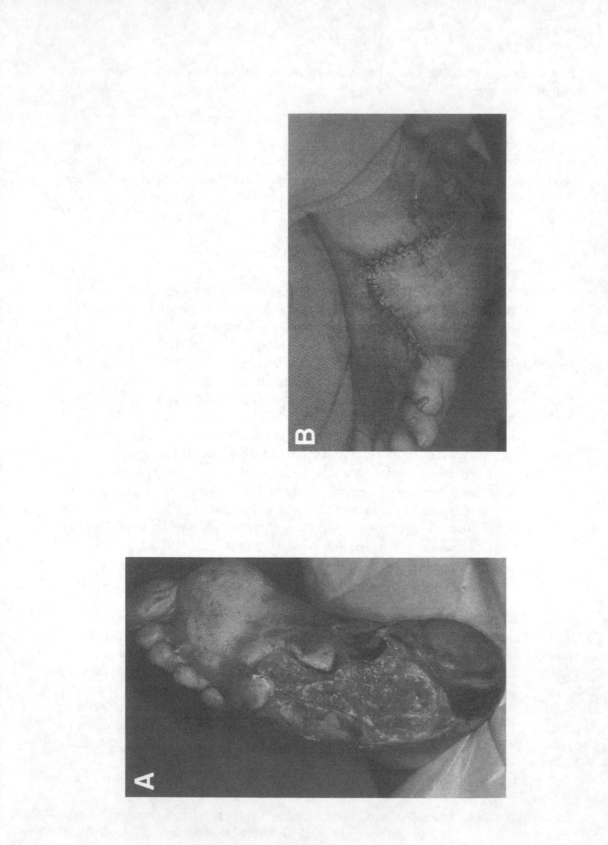

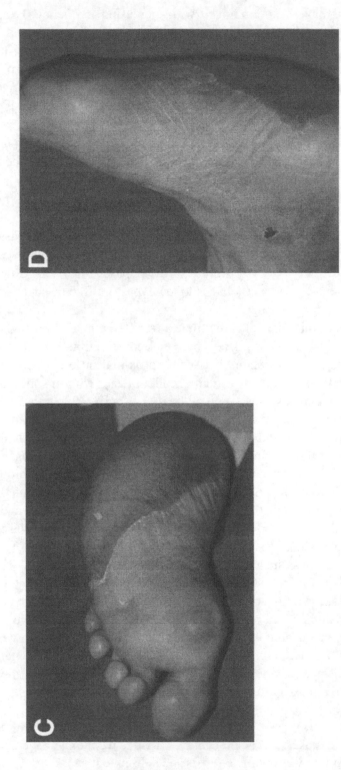

Fig. 2. Free-tissue transfer for resurfacing of plantar surface of left foot. (**A**) Preoperative view: massive infection resulted in necrosis of majority of plantar skin and subcutaneous tissue. (**B**) Dorsal/lateral view after transfer of latissimus dorsi musculocutaneous flap. (**C, D**) Plantar and medial view 5 months after surgery. Later revisions were required for flap debulking and for debridement of residual osteomyelitis of posterior calcaneus, but the weight-bearing surface has remained intact over a 4-year follow-up period.

349

Fasciocutaneous flaps have been employed with increasing frequency. Examples are the scapular and parascapular flaps, which tend to be rather bulky, and the dorsalis pedis artery flap, which is relatively contraindicated in patients with diabetes frequently accompanied by vascular disease. The lateral arm, deltoid, and radial forearm areas have the potential to be harvested as sensate flaps. The radial forearm flap may provide excellent tissue for foot reconstruction, but the donor site can be unsightly and is prone to complications, especially with regard to healing of skin graft over exposed flexor tendons. This flap should be used only if the surgeon has confirmed good flow through the ulnar artery and an intact palmar arch; Allen testing must be negative. Sacrifice of the radial artery should not be undertaken lightly in a patient with diabetes.

The use of distal bypass grafts in combination with free-tissue transfer has greatly expanded opportunities for limb salvage. In this way well-vascularized tissue may be introduced to a relatively ischemic area of the foot that may contain no "bypassable" arteries. The flap (donor) artery should be anastomosed to the best available vessel—either the native artery distal to the bypass graft, or the bypass graft itself. Colen and Mathes (3a) have found end-to-side anastomosis to the bypass graft to be superior from a technical standpoint.

The logical extension of this concept is to utilize a free flap for salvage of an ischemic limb whose arterial system is considered to be unreconstructible. This procedure involves the use of a long venous conduit between a proximal inflow vessel and the flap donor artery. Shestak and others (4) had an excellent result with this method and reported evidence of indirect revascularization of the foot after free-flap transfer. However, this experience has not been universal. Others have observed poor healing at the interface of flap and native tissue and/or eventual need for amputation (5,6). Although further documentation is still forthcoming, the severity of the ischemia at presentation may be a significant factor in determining the success or failure of this technique.

The question often arises of whether free-tissue transfer for limb salvage can be performed safely in this group of diabetic patients, many of whom are elderly and have intercurrent disease. The important study by Chick and others (7) of free flaps in the elderly showed that advanced age alone was not a risk factor for complications of surgery. However, comorbid disease was such a risk factor.

A series of 21 free flaps for limb salvage diabetic patients was reported by Karp et al. (8). Hospitalization was lengthy and costly, the rate of minor recipient-site complications was high (33%), and 26% of patients required proximal amputation during the 5-year study period. In general, amputation was required for progression of underlying vascular disease and not for flap failure per se. Since patients in the study began with nonhealing wounds and since all whose flaps survived went on to ambulate, the combined technique of distal bypass graft and microvascular free flap transfer was highly recommended, in spite of any associated morbidity.

In Colen and Musson's (9) series of 10 patients with severe peripheral vascular disease who had free-tissue transfer as a salvage procedure, only one went on to have a below-knee amputation. This failure was owing to sepsis and subsequent cardiovascular compromise. The author followed a routine of wound debridement at the time of the vascular bypass procedure, with flap repair of the wound performed 5–7 days later. In this way both cleanliness of the wound and anastomotic patency of the graft could be ensured.

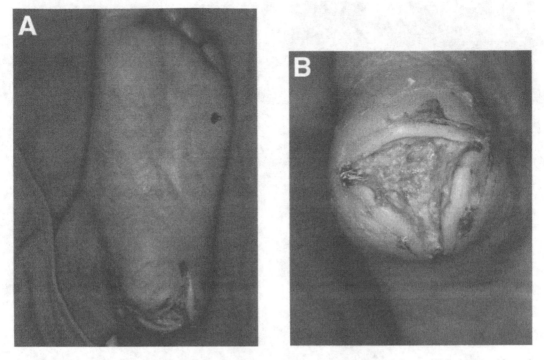

Fig. 3. Neglected infection of non-weight-bearing heel required incision and drainage. (**A** and **B**) Tripartite, stellate design of incisions resulted in retraction of skin edges, precluding repair using local tissue. Patient also had occlusion of the posterior tibial artery.

GENERAL GUIDELINES FOR WOUND CARE

Preoperative Management

Preparation of a wound for surgical repair requires attention to the several factors that may be contributing to impaired healing. These include infection, vascular insufficiency, neuropathy, and edema. Systemic factors such as inadequate control of blood glucose or nutritional deficits should also be addressed. Ideally a multidisciplinary team will manage the patient in concert.

As with any wound, a foot wound in a patient with diabetes should be debrided of infected and necrotic tissue. This is usually accomplished most efficiently by sharp excision. Occasionally an enzymatic debridement agent may be useful if the interface between viable and nonviable tissue is not well defined, or if a patient has an intercurrent problem that delays surgery.

Whether the initial debridement is performed by the reconstructive surgeon or by another team member, the prospective wound repair should be kept in mind. For example, in obtaining access for drainage of an abscess or for ostectomy of an ulcer, incisional orientation can be modified to facilitate skin closure at a later date. As long as exposure is not compromised, "stellate" incisions should be avoided. This traditional design was intended to keep a wound open and draining, as it produces multiple small skin flaps that contract out and away from the wound's center (Fig. 3). Alternatively, if

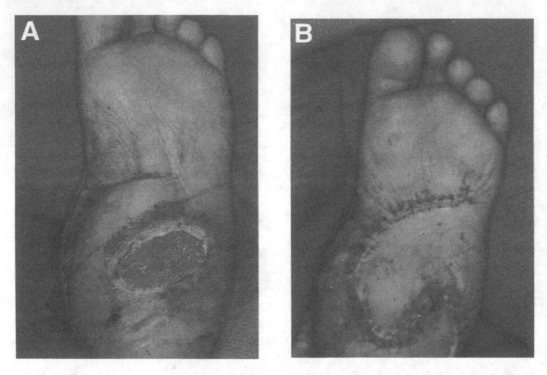

Fig. 4. (A) Midfoot ulcer of 13 months' duration. Following ostectomy through a remote incision, ulcer size decreased and pliability of surrounding tissue increased. **(B)** Following debridement and repair of ulcer with intrinsic muscle flap, skin was closed with minimal tension using two opposing suprafascial skin rotation flaps, one large and one small.

a pair of curvilinear incisions (both clockwise, or both counterclockwise) are made from opposite sides of the wound, then repair can then be accomplished by rotation of the two opposing skin flaps (Fig. 4).

If a wound is unsuitable for immediate repair after debridement, generally because of infection, swelling, or incomplete demarcation, then initial debridement and closure are performed as staged procedures. The wound is further prepared during this interval with dressing changes, the standard of care being a medium with a hydrated interface. A hydrated environment provides a favorable milieu for healing in general, but when tissues are prone to dessication, it is critical. Specifically if debridement results in exposure of tendon, bone, or a large area of subcutaneous fat, then the appropriate dressing must be placed immediately, that is, on the operating table. This is conveniently accomplished by application of a wound gel followed by a saline-moistened dressing. If adequate debridement has been performed but the wound has not responded to optimization of contributing factors (vascular insufficiency, infection, and so on), then topical application of a growth factor preparation may be appropriate. As of this writing, becaplermin (Regranex, Ortho-McNeil Pharmaceuticals) is the only type that is commercially available, and indications for usage are still being defined.

Another device that deserves mention is the Vacuum-Assisted Closure (VAC) apparatus (Kinetic Concepts). This has been particularly helpful in the management of large or deep, draining wounds, or in wounds with exposed tissue such as fascia that tend to dry out with conventional dressing techniques. The device produces a local area of negative atmospheric pressure, which promotes growth of small blood vessels; the occlusive nature of the dressing and the suction mechanism that controls secretions are additional features that enhance the wound healing environment.

The peripheral vascular evaluation is paramount in the diabetic patient with a non-healing foot wound. As a general rule, a palpable pedal pulse indicates pulsatile flow that is adequate to support healing. However, this rule may not apply when there is regional vascular insufficiency. The frequently encountered posterior heel ulcer, which may result from a variable combination of pressure, ischemia, and infection, is typically attended by disease in the posterior tibial artery. A bypass graft to the dorsalis pedis artery—which, not surprisingly, may be the patient's only reconstructible vessel in the foot—may still not produce adequate local perfusion of the heel.

Besides palpation and bedside Doppler evaluation of pulses, the clinical examination should include a standard assessment of skin color, turgor, and temperature. Edema may be present, which thwarts a thorough physical examination of pulses. A "Dopplered" pedal pulse should be at least biphasic, to support healing. If there is any doubt about the adequacy of perfusion, then noninvasive studies should be obtained. The ankle-brachial index (ABI) may be unreliable in patients with noncompressible lower-leg vessels. In general, however, an ABI of less than 0.5 in the setting of a nonhealing wound indicates a need for vascular reconstruction. According to Colen and Musson (9), an ABI of 0.7 or greater is appropriate if a free flap with a distal arterial anastomosis is planned.

The same author has utilized a combination of noninvasive techniques (directional Doppler and duplex ultrasonography) in the preoperative assessment of patients who will receive free-tissue transfers. Although dependent on the technical skill and experience of the operator, this method can provide detailed information about local arterial flow and may even permit selection of the best site for anastomosis to the recipient artery. Miller and others (10) also documented the utility of duplex scanning in the planning of perforator-based skin flaps.

Traditional or magnetic resonance arteriography remains the gold standard for preoperative vascular evaluation. Unless there is a strong contraindication, it is reasonable to obtain an angiogram in any diabetic patient being prepared for free-tissue transfer. This study effectively provides a map for the surgeon who must plan an anastomosis to a vessel that is likely to be diseased. Unsuspected anatomic variations or areas of stenosis may become apparent. In patients with diabetes and evidence of advanced peripheral vascular disease, angiography may be appropriate even if a local or regional flap is planned.

Preoperative assessment should include a peripheral neurologic examination. An incision on the foot may damage cutaneous sensory nerves. Ironically, in a patient with dense neuropathy, the design of incisions may be less critical in this regard. Also there is no point in considering transfer of a sensate free flap if the patient's neuropathy extends proximal to the level of the planned anastomosis. Moreover, the presence of tarsal tunnel syndrome should be considered, as this may be amenable to surgical decompresssion.

Determining when a wound is ready for closure in reality is usually an exercise in clinical judgment, although bacterial cultures showing sterility or sparse growth may be reassuring. The wound base should be pink, may bleed readily when manipulated, and should be well hydrated but free of excessive drainage or odor. The presence of granulation tissue is often taken as a sign of a wound's ability to heal.

Intraoperative Management

Great care must be taken in the operating room, even before an incision is made. The patient should be positioned and draped so as to avoid pressure points, neurapraxias, and heat loss. The anesthesiologist has an important role in helping to maintain an adequate arterial pressure head, not only for the patient's general well-being, but for the sake of local tissue perfusion.

The choice of anesthetic technique must be individualized to each patient and each wound. This decision is made in consultation with the anesthesiologist and logically is influenced by the patient's medical condition. In patients with dense neuropathy, procedures that are confined to the foot may be performed with local anesthesia—or in some instances without anesthesia. If a skin graft is planned, a thigh donor site, for example, may be effectively anesthetized by local infiltration, but in this case monitored sedation adds greatly to the patient's comfort. For most local and regional flaps, and for nearly all free flaps, a general or spinal anesthetic is preferred. Procedures of longer duration, disparate location of donor and recipient sites, and the need for a tourniquet are all factors that may favor the use of general anesthesia. Furthermore, neuropathic patients, while having no awareness of incisional pain, in the awake state may exhibit involuntary movements of the lower extremity that significantly hamper procedures requiring a delicate technique. These sometimes dramatic tremors may be exaggerated in the twilight condition of intravenous sedation.

Utilization of a tourniquet, whether a prudently applied Esmarch bandage on the lower leg or a pneumatic tourniquet on the thigh, should be considered carefully. Certainly peripheral vascular disease is a relative contraindication to tourniquet use, and a recent bypass graft in the field is a strong contraindication. However, the risks of a finite period of ischemia should be weighed against the advantages of decreased blood loss, enhanced visualization of small vital structures, and (often) reduced operating time.

General principles of surgical technique should be applied with particular diligence in diabetic patients, who demonstrate impaired healing and increased risk of infection. Hemostasis should be obtained with care. Closed suction drains may be used to control and monitor postoperative drainage from a wound and to apply a vacuum to wounds with a substantial dead space. Any residual nonviable areas should be debrided. Pulsatile irrigation may help to dislodge loose, necrotic tissue and reduce the surface bacterial load, following sharp debridement (Fig. 5).

The importance of careful tissue handling cannot be overemphasized. In diabetes, the tissues are especially intolerant of the ischemia produced by tension on a wound. If, despite thoughtful planning and selection of the optimal surgical method, there is a small gap between opposing skin edges at the end of the procedure, then the skin should not be hauled together. It is better to apply a small skin graft or allow the wound to close secondarily than to create stresses that result in necrosis of the skin.

Eversion of skin edges and approximation of the dermis are accepted principles of plastic surgical technique for wound closure. These goals are surprisingly elusive when inflammation of a chronic ulcer has produced fibrosis and immobility of the soft tissues, especially on the plantar surface of the foot, where the skin may be grossly hyperkeratotic.

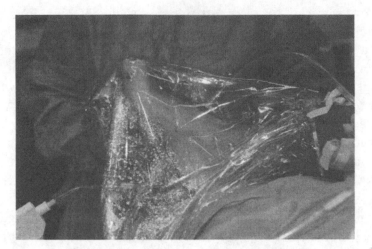

Fig. 5. Example of use of pulsatile irrigation system for infected foot wound, following thorough mechanical debridement. To control spray and drainage, a transparent isolation bag is placed over the foot, and irrigation and suction catheters are introduced through separate openings.

Where possible, scarred tissue should be excised. In extreme cases the skin may be conditioned preoperatively through a period of non-weight-bearing with local care, such as shaving of callus and application of moisturizers; antibiotic ointment may be used as the moisturizer if there is a concern about introduction of bacteria. At operation, secure closure of the dermis with imperfect epidermal approximation is preferable to the converse situation.

Effective dressing and immobilization of the foot and ankle should be considered a basic component of the operation. Most suture lines are covered with dry dressings only, to reduce the risk of maceration. Skin grafts are usually secured with bolsters. A bolster made from adhesive-backed foam rubber may cause less trauma to the surrounding skin than the traditional tie-over design. Nearly every type of wound repair to the foot should be protected with a padded, posteriorly based, lower-leg splint. For some wounds about the mobile ankle, casting may be the only method capable of reducing shear forces to a graft or a flap. The cast must be applied carefully to avoid constriction or focal pressure, and it may be windowed to allow subsequent inspection and local care of the operative site.

Postoperative Management

In the early postoperative period, the repaired site should be elevated and kept immobilized to reduce edema, drainage, and excessive motion. The duration of splinting varies, but commonly the repair is not secure until 2 or 3 weeks postoperatively. Likewise, in the case of most plantar wounds, all weight bearing is prohibited for a minimum of 6 weeks. It is eminently difficult for many patients to adhere to these guidelines.

Skin grafts are usually inspected at postoperative day 5—earlier if there are signs of infection. Flaps should be evaluated by physical examination for venous congestion and for arterial insuffiency, which may be exacerbated by excess tension on the suture line. Particularly in the case of a free flap, a monitoring device may track temperature, blood flow, pO_2, or pH.

The index of suspicion for secondary infection should be high. Intraoperative and postoperative wound cultures should guide specific antibiotic therapy. Infection with opportunistic organisms such as *Pseudomonas* is a particular risk in wounds with macerated, necrotic tissue and in patients who have been treated with systemic antibiotics for a prolonged period (Fig. 6). Multiple-antiobiotic resistance is seen with increasing frequency in bacteria such as *Staphylococcus aureus*, *Enterococcus*, and *Xanthomonas*.

In individuals with neuropathy, pressure ulcers and injuries caused by unrecognized trauma are genuine dangers even in the postoperative period. Moreover, many patients who initially achieve a healed wound eventually develop new or recurrent ulceration. This tendency should be regarded as a chronic disease, and prevention of skin breakdown is of paramount importance. Assuming that an appropriate method of soft tissue reconstruction was employed, the fate of the repaired wound depends largely on patient education and follow-up. The podiatrist has a particularly important role in recommending footwear and providing preventive maintenance care.

OPTIONS FOR SOFT TISSUE REPAIR

It is convenient and practical to consider the various methods of reconstruction separately, as applied to different regions of the foot. These areas are distinguished by both anatomic location and functional requirements. The dorsum, the distal plantar area, the midfoot, the proximal plantar area, and lastly the Achilles region and non-weight-bearing heel along with the medial and lateral malleoli, will be discussed in turn.

Dorsum of the Foot

In repairing defects of the dorsal aspect of the foot, skin grafting is the technique that should always be considered first. Skin grafts to this area do not have the same requirements of resistance to pressure and shearing forces as those to the weight-bearing surfaces of the foot. Grafts are usually split thickness and most conveniently harvested from a broad, flat area such as the thigh.

Skin grafts are appropriate for partial-thickness wounds or for deeper wounds that are well perfused (Fig. 7). Since a graft, in contrast to a flap, does not derive its blood supply from the donor site, it must depend on the vascularity of the recipient site. As noted, even tendon with intact paratenon and bone with intact periosteum will "take" a skin graft, but in reality, once these structures have been exposed, it is difficult to prevent dessication and loss of viability.

Standard methods of local tissue rearrangement, such as bipedicle and rotation flaps, are applicable in repair of smaller defects (Fig. 8). The greater laxity and mobility of the dorsal skin, compared with that of the plantar surface, facilitates transfer of these skin flaps. The intrinsic abductor hallucis and abductor digiti minimi muscles are useful for repair only of small, distal defects. A reverse dorsal metatarsal artery flap has been described for reconstruction of the distal foot *(11)*, but again, it offers a limited amount of coverage and its viability depends on adequate flow from the plantar system through the distal communicating artery. The extensor digitorum brevis muscle flap may be appropriate for repair of deeper dorsal wounds, especially those containing exposed bone (Fig. 9). Following wound repair with either a graft or a flap, it is particularly important in this area to reduce motion of the underlying tendons by immobilization of the ankle.

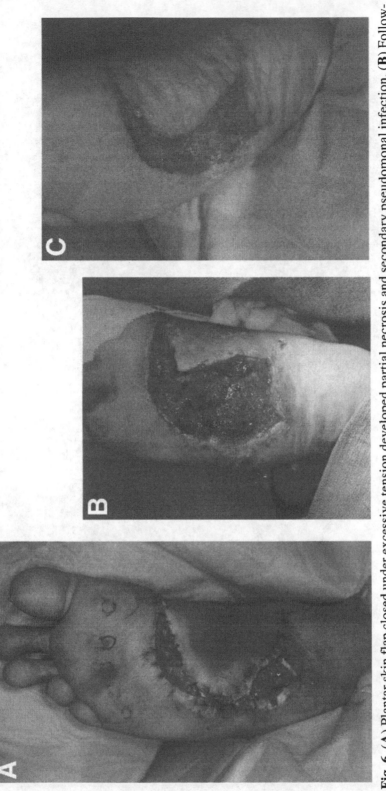

Fig. 6. (A) Plantar skin flap closed under excessive tension developed partial necrosis and secondary pseudomonal infection. (B) Following debridement, local care, and appropriate antibiotic therapy. Underlying muscle flap remained viable. (C) Despite delayed healing of the lateral border, the entire wound eventually closed after secondary repair with a skin graft.

357

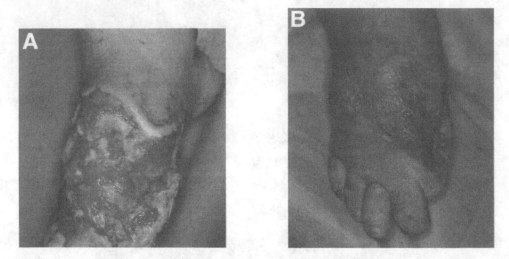

Fig. 7. (A) Large, full-thickness dorsal foot wound. The surface developed a generous amount of granulation tissue following revascularization of the limb. **(B)** Wound covered with split-thickness skin graft. Repair remained intact when patient was admitted 1 year later with an ulcer of the opposite foot.

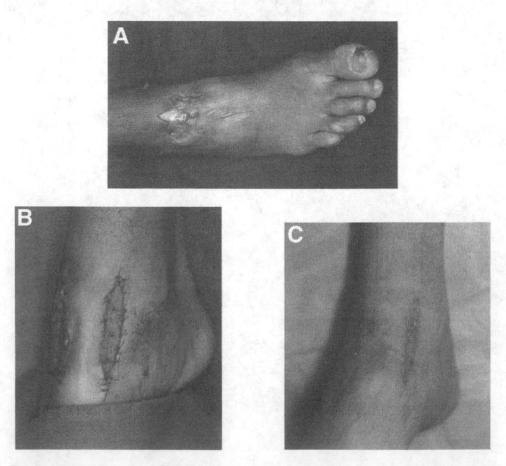

Fig. 8. (A) Chronic nonhealing area of dorsal foot and ankle with exposed extensor tendon. **(B)** Immediately after repair with bipedicle flap and skin graft. **(C)** Three months postoperatively.

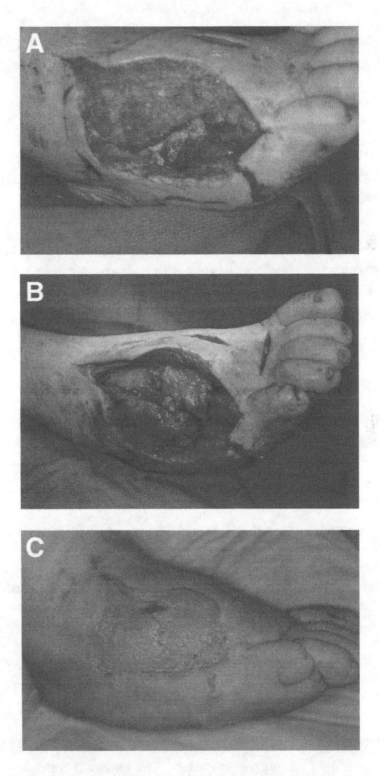

Fig. 9. (**A**) Unusual deep dorsal wound after debridement of infected tissue, including portions of fourth and fifth metatarsals. (**B**) Bone was covered with a distally based flap of extensor digitorum brevis muscle, and the wound was skin-grafted. (**C**) One month postoperatively. The skin went on to complete healing and has remained intact for 7 months.

A special feature of this dorsal region is that tendons with long excursion lie close to the surface and are easily exposed. For wounds with a large surface area where preservation of mobile tendons is to be attempted, free-tissue transfer is indicated. In general, only fasciocutaneous flaps or skin-grafted fascial flaps are sufficiently thin to be used in this area. Donor sites for fascial free flaps include the temporoparietal fascia and the dorsal thoracic fascia *(11a)*. A free dorsalis pedis artery flap from the contralateral foot, of course, would provide perfectly suited tissue, but this is rarely a good choice in patients with diabetes, who are prone to vascular disease.

There are several series of distally based fasciocutaneous flaps from the leg for use in dorsal foot defects, the superficial sural flap, the lateral supramalleolar artery flap, and the medial or posterior tibial flap among them *(12–14)*. This type of flap may be rotated or used in "turnover" fashion and deepithelialized with the exposed surface covered by a skin graft. As noted, a fasciocutaneous flap may also be donated from the opposite limb as a cross-leg flap. Reported complication rates with skin/fascia flaps have been high among patients with diabetes. Perforator-based flaps must be used with caution as their viability rests with the integrity of the respective underlying tibial or peroneal vessel.

Distal Plantar Area

Among the lesions that occur in this region, the most frequently encountered in diabetic patients is the submetatarsal ulcer. Neuropathy with consequent intrinsic paralysis focuses pressure on the metatarsal heads. Decreased sensibility also increases the risk of injury from external causes, such as a hot surface or foreign body.

The functional demands of replacement tissue are high in this weight-bearing area, yet local options for repair are few. Proximally based flaps generally will not reach anterior defects, and those based distally may be tenuously perfused. Free-tissue transfer is usually necessary for repair of wounds that are more than a few centimeters in diameter.

Common methods of local tissue rearrangement such as rotation of a random skin flap are occasionally useful for coverage of modest peripheral defects, but in a sensate foot, incisions may interrupt important cutaneous innervation (Fig. 10). For small wounds, the V-to-Y advancement technique is effective. Careful dissection with preservation of perforating vessels can enhance the viability of this flap *(15,16)*.

A reverse-flow flap based on the first dorsal metatarsal artery, and island flaps based on digital vessels in the plantar webspace, have also been described *(17,18)*. These may be used if preoperative and intraoperative evaluation indicates adequate perfusion to the flap axial vessels. Amarante and others *(19)* designed a distally based median plantar flap to overcome the limited arc of rotation of the proximally based flap; sensibility was achieved by anastomosing the nerve branch of the flap to a proximal dorsal cutaneous nerve.

Finally, the toe flap should not be overlooked as a reconstructive option. Although most surgeons and patients are hesitant to sacrifice a toe that is not already destined for amputation, a filleted toe can provide a moderate quantity of tissue and a favorable match to the forefoot skin. The morbidity of loss of the first toe can be substantial, but this toe may donate a flap from its lateral aspect and still maintain functional integrity.

The Plantar Midfoot:
Special Considerations in the Treatment of Charcot Ulcers

Defects of the non-weight-bearing arch can be closed with skin grafts. As a general rule, flaps for repair of this area should not be taken away from adjacent weight-bearing tissue as long as the instep has a normal contour. In fact, however, most diabetic midfoot ulcers appear in the setting of neuropathy, arthropathy, and loss of the arch. Therefore areas that normally are non-weight-bearing can become weight bearing. The best effort should be made to offload an ulcer through surgical techniques and/or using orthotics, and methods for soft tissue repair must emulate those used in regions that normally bear weight—flaps containing skin, or muscle flaps covered with skin graft (Fig. 11; *see* Color Plate 7, following p. 178).

The central plantar skin ulcer that follows collapse of the bony midfoot is emblematic of Charcot arthropathy. Edema and fibrosis typically accompany the ulceration, and the surrounding tissues are grossly stiff and thickened. Initial care includes standard methods of debridement and appropriate antibiotic therapy. Although vascular status should be assessed, it is unusual to find arterial insufficiency as a significant contributing factor in nonhealing of Charcot ulcers. Special attention should be given to treatment of edema, primarily through conservative methods of leg elevation and distal-to-proximal wrapping with Ace bandages. It is paradoxical that swelling may impair wound healing, but the inflammatory process contributing to the swelling will not resolve completely until after the wound has been closed.

Preliminary treatment of bony deformity by the podiatrist and/or orthopedist is a prerequisite for soft tissue repair. Although weight-bearing distribution has been irrevocably altered in Charcot arthropathy, an attempt should be made to restore bony architecture and relieve pressure from the ulcer. Techniques range from simple planing of the cuboid to complex fusions. Bony restoration may produce dramatic alterations in the overlying soft tissue, with reduction of local edema and even changes in the size and orientation of an ulcer. The resulting increase in soft tissue redundancy and malleability facilitates the wound closure and increases the likelihood of successful repair.

Operative repair begins with complete tangential excision of the ulcer, to remove contaminated and fibrotic tissue. A muscle flap is best suited to fill the resulting defect and introduce well-vascularized tissue. In the central plantar area, the flexor digitorum brevis muscle is often the most convenient and efficacious for this purpose. The plantar aponeurosis is opened for exposure of the muscle, which is detached distally and transposed into the wound. Access is usually obtained through gentle sigmoid extensions of the skin opening, in both anterior and posterior directions; this also permits subsequent closure over the muscle flap by rotation of the two resulting skin flaps toward the center of the defect. If the skin cannot be closed without tension, then a second choice is to skin-graft the exposed portion of the muscle flap. Although native plantar skin is the preferred surface for ambulation, a skin graft over muscle may provide durable coverage and will contract substantially during healing.

When choosing a method for soft tissue reconstruction, the surgeon may be concerned that the flexor brevis muscle or other intrinsic muscle of the foot lies within the zone of disease of the Charcot ulcer. However, in this practice it has been consistently observed that the defect, no matter how deep, does not involve these muscles (Fig. 12).

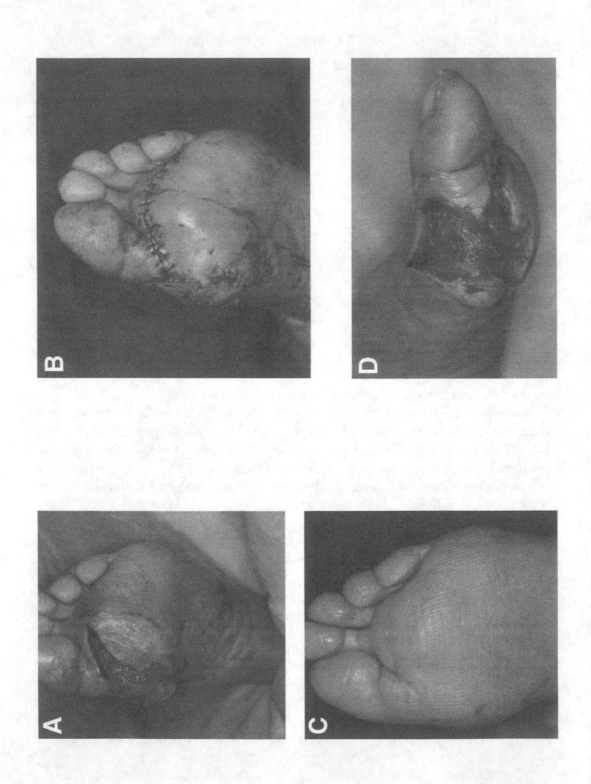

362

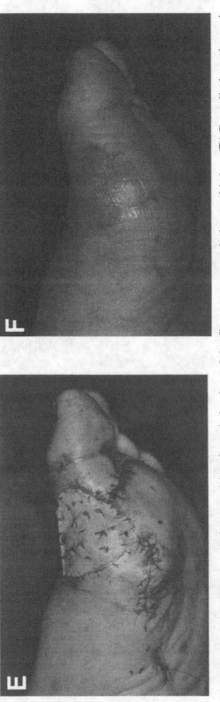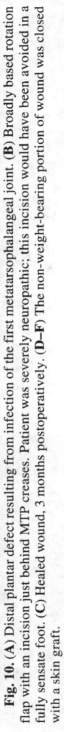

Fig. 10. (A) Distal plantar defect resulting from infection of the first metatarsophalangeal joint. **(B)** Broadly based rotation flap with an incision just behind MTP creases; this incision would have been avoided in a fully sensate foot. **(C)** Healed wound, 3 months postoperatively. **(D–F)** The non-weight-bearing portion of wound was closed with a skin graft.

363

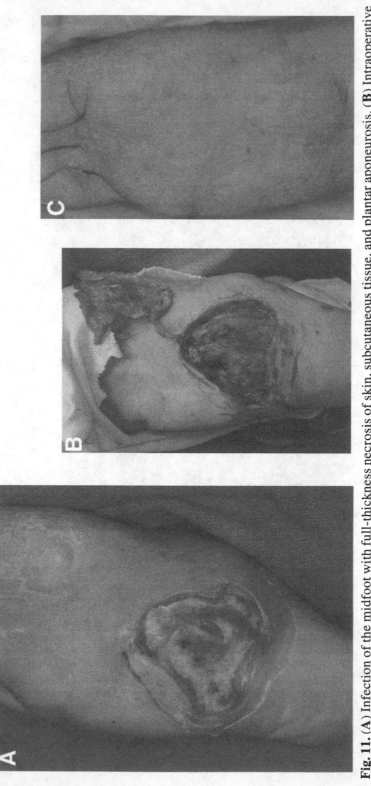

Fig. 11. (A) Infection of the midfoot with full-thickness necrosis of skin, subcutaneous tissue, and plantar aponeurosis. (B) Intraoperative view showing excised plantar fascia and intact flexor digitorum brevis muscle. (C) Skin grafted directly to muscle provided stable coverage.

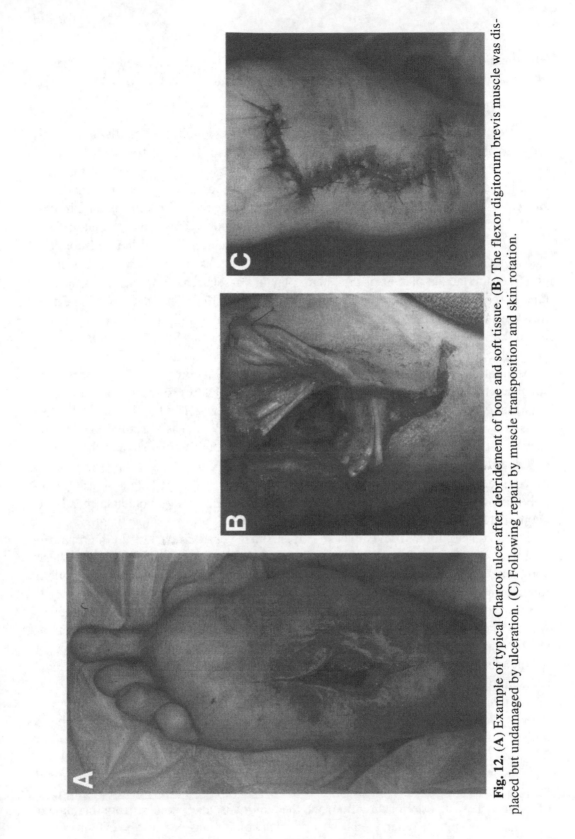

Fig. 12. (**A**) Example of typical Charcot ulcer after debridement of bone and soft tissue. (**B**) The flexor digitorum brevis muscle was displaced but undamaged by ulceration. (**C**) Following repair by muscle transposition and skin rotation.

365

The flexor digitorum brevis is often grossly displaced by the adjacent ulcer and has an oblique rather than a vertical orientation, but its appearance is otherwise normal

Proximal Plantar Area/Weight-Bearing Heel

In reconstruction of the foot, the proximal plantar region is arguably the most challenging and important anatomic area. Although defects here occur frequently and can be quite extensive, options for local tissue transfer are limited. Free flaps to this area must be selected carefully and tailored with precision, to have a reasonable chance of success. Any repair must be designed for durability in the face of weight-bearing forces.

The instep island flap may used either for local or for free transfer (the latter from the opposite foot). The donor site is the non-weight-bearing arch of the midfoot. The flap is harvested full thickness to include fascia or both fascia and muscle and is based on either the medial plantar or the lateral plantar vessels. This flap has the disadvantage of requiring a deep dissection and leaving a substantial donor defect and anesthetic areas in the foot. Necrosis of the perimeter of the skin island can be seen, especially in smokers with vascular disease; a corollary observation is that no substantial arterial perforators traverse the fascia into the overlying skin of the midfoot (Fig. 13).

An alternate choice is the suprafascial plantar skin rotation flap *(20)*. Dissection is superficial, at the level of the plantar aponeurosis, and allows for preservation of sensory innervation from the medial and lateral plantar nerves. The flap is quite robust as long as it is broadly based and transferred without tension. The vascular basis of the flap is a subcutaneous plexus with contributions from both the dorsal and the plantar circulation (Fig. 14), as well described by Hidalgo and Shaw *(21,22)*. This flap can be based either laterally or medially, but the latter is preferred if the heel is sensate. Distally, the skin incision should lie at least 3 cm posterior to the metatarsal heads, to avoid disturbing cutaneous nerves as they become progressively superficial.

The flexor digitorum brevis muscle (Fig. 15) has been quite useful in the repair of heel wounds. The excursion of this muscle flap includes the entire weight-bearing heel, and sometimes beyond. The straightforward dissection of the flap may begin with a longitudinal incision approximately in the center of the plantar axis of the foot, extending from the heel defect anteriorly to a point behind the metatarsal heads. However, when there is a need to rotate a skin flap at the same setting (or when the potential exists for such a need in the future), the skin can be incised in a broad arc and dissected off the plantar aponeurosis (Fig. 16; *see* Color Plate 8, following p. 178). The fascia is divided longitudinally and peeled back to reveal the underlying flexor brevis muscle; alternatively, a segment of fascia may be left attached to the muscle and transferred with it. Care should be taken to dissect all four muscle slips, as the slip to the fifth toe may be found deep as well as lateral to that of the fourth toe. The flexor digitorum longus is tendinous in this region but immediately underlies the flexor brevis and can be confused with the brevis in the distal part of the dissection. The flexor brevis muscle is retracted, and its tendons are divided. Blunt dissection (primarily) facilitates transfer of the muscle in a posterior direction, and the major vascular pedicles from the plantar vessels are left intact. When the posterior "reach" of the muscle must be extended, the dissection is carried to the level of the posterior tibial artery. If skin closure with a local rotation flap over the muscle is not feasible, a split-thickness skin graft can be applied to the muscle surface.

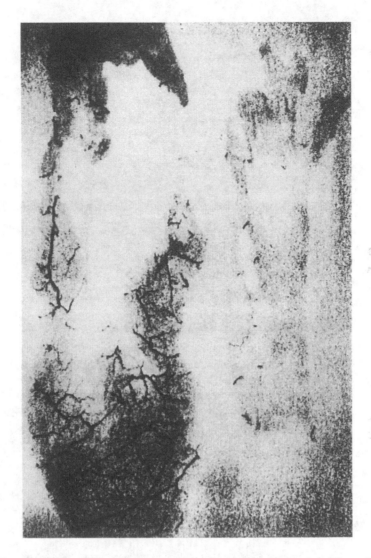

Fig. 13. Blood vessels of plantar aspect of foot, visualized after injection of radioopaque material via the tibial arteries. Vessels are numerous in the subcutaneous tissue (left), but are strikingly absent at the level of the plantar fascia (right). (Reproduced with permission from Colen LB, Replogle MD, Mathes SJ. The V-Y plantar flap for reconstruction of the forefoot. *Plast Reconstr Surg* 1988;81: 221.)

The abductor hallucis and abductor digiti minimi muscles are also available but have sufficient tissue to fill only small defects (Fig. 17). These muscles may be approached directly through plantar incisions and are raised from distal to proximal, leaving intact the medial plantar and lateral plantar vascular pedicles, respectively. The abductor digiti minimi has a greater posterior and lateral excursion if accessed through a lateral incision.

Free tissue transfer is generally required for repair of heel defects with a large surface area (Fig. 18). Moreover, local flaps are dependent on the posterior tibial artery and should not be undertaken unless the surgeon is confident of adequate antegrade flow through this vessel. Several authors have addressed the question of which type of

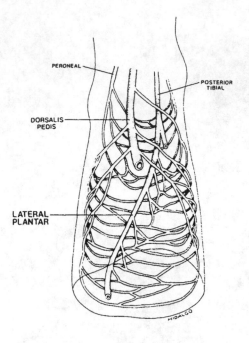

Fig. 14. Schematic representation of the proximal plantar subcutaneous plexus, as viewed through the dorsum of the foot. This depicts a substantial contribution from the dorsal circulation as well as the lateral plantar artery. (Reproduced with permission from Hidalgo DA, Shaw WW. Anatomic basis of plantar flap design. *Plast Reconstr Surg* 1986;78:633.)

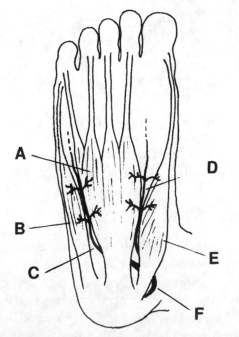

Fig. 15. Schematic drawing of plantar intrinsic muscles, deep to plantar fascia. A, Flexor digitorum brevis. B, Abductor digiti minimi. C, D, Lateral and medial plantar arteries, respectively, course between the flexor and abductor muscles and provide their blood supply. E, Abductor hallucis. F, Posterior tibial artery.

free flap is best suited and most durable for resurfacing of the sole—musculocutaneous, fasciocutaneous, or muscle with a skin graft *(23–25).*

Among these investigators a consensus has emerged that composite, musculocutaneous flaps are relatively contraindicated. These flaps have too much bulk and permit excessive lateral shear; therefore they are prone to breakdown. Similar complications were reported with fasciocutaneous flaps until thin flaps, such as the radial forearm, became commonplace. Fasciocutaneous flaps can be very successful and the need for revision minimized, if inset at the time of initial repair is close to ideal. Excellent contour restoration and lack of skin redundancy are goals of the reconstruction.

Muscle flaps surfaced with a skin graft are generally favored for repair of the weight-bearing heel. Muscle tissue conforms well to irregular defects and can be tailored to the dimensions of a wound. May and others *(26)*, in a clinical and gait analysis study of free muscle flaps, described shear planes that formed between skin graft and muscle and between muscle and bone. During ambulation these planes may allow for limited soft tissue motion, which is believed to protect against the abrasive forces that cause breakdown of skin grafted directly to bone. Analysis of ambulation showed reduction in vertical forces after free-flap repair; it was concluded that deep sensibility through the flap was sufficient for patients to make unconscious alterations in their gait and that cutaneous sensation perhaps was not necessary. Based on available data, it seems that the sensibility of a flap is not as important as the degree to which it conforms to the normal contour of the foot. Well-crafted but insensate flaps on the weight-bearing surface of the foot have proved to be durable, with a low incidence of ulceration.

Non-Weight-Bearing Heel, Achilles Region, and Malleoli

Soft tissue defects about the ankle and posterior heel are challenging to repair even though these areas are non-weight-bearing. Often bone or mobile tendon is exposed, local perfusion is poor, and few regional flaps are available. Frequently there is no satisfactory alternative to free-tissue transfer.

The most common lesion of the non-weight-bearing heel occurring in diabetic patients is the posterior decubitus ulcer (Fig. 19). Although pressure is usually the immediate cause, sensory impairment is a risk factor, and infection may complicate the ulcer. Typically the posterior tibial artery is diseased; often it is not reconstructible. Unfortunately, the posterior heel ulcer often arises secondary to bed rest in a hospital or nursing facility and is highly preventable by frequent inspection and use of protective devices such as the Multipodus splint (Restorative Care of America).

If the ulcer consists of a dry eschar and is not obviously infected, then there is no urgent need to debride it. The surgeon should not embark on unroofing the ulcer without being prepared to repair the wound imminently. Debridement usually exposes poorly perfused, subcutaneous fat that dessicates readily, thus expanding the zone of nonviable tissue. The calcaneus, even if not initially involved in the ulcer, can rapidly become exposed. Only occasionally will the aggressive use of a hydrating dressing, instituted immediately after debridement, be effective in counteracting this process.

Nonhealing wounds and ulcers in the Achilles region often present as full-thickness defects with dried, exposed tendon. If the tendon is clearly necrotic or nonviable, there should be no hesitation in debriding the involved tissue. Partial loss of the Achilles tendon, particularly if it involves less than the full width of the tendon, rarely results in

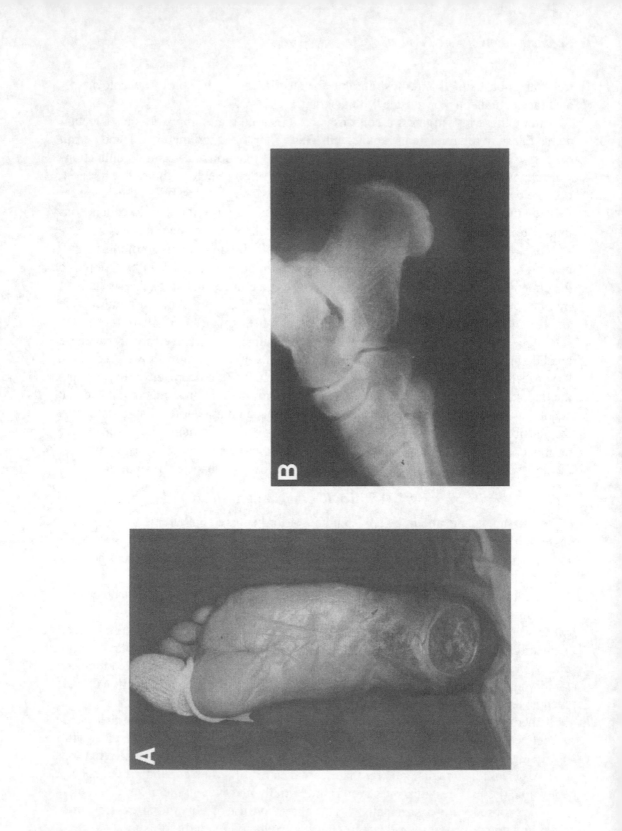

370

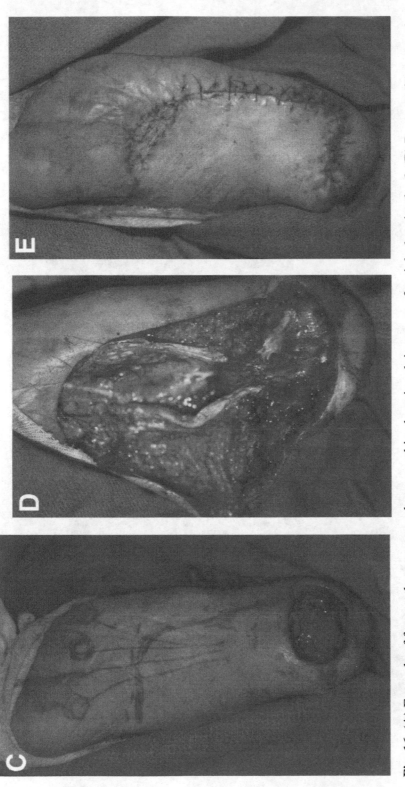

Fig. 16. (**A**) Example of frequently encountered neuropathic ulcer, involving most of weight-bearing heel. (**B**) Preoperative x-ray shows prominence of plantar surface of calcaneus. (**C**) After debridement of bone and soft tissue, a thin skin flap was designed for rotation; the distal incision is at least 3 cm posterior to the metatarsal heads. (**D**) Skin flap elevated, and flexor brevis muscle transposed into ulcer. (**E**) Closed wound, with skin graft applied to flap donor site.

371

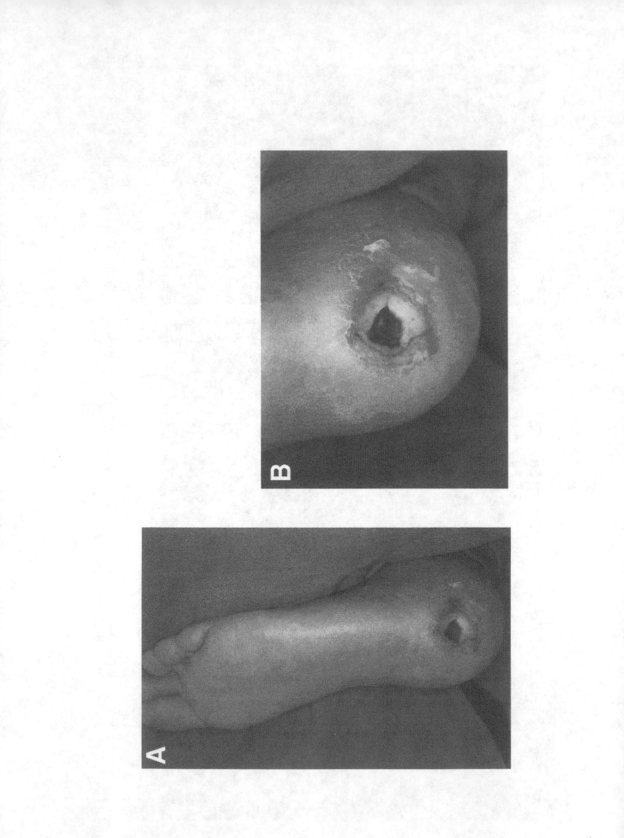

372

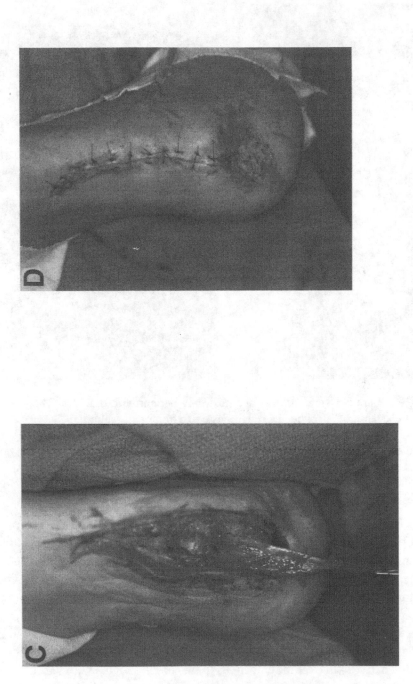

Fig. 17. (**A, B**) Lateral, plantar heel ulcer in patient with neuropathy. Abductor digit minimi muscle (**C**) transposed and (**D**) covered with skin graft.

373

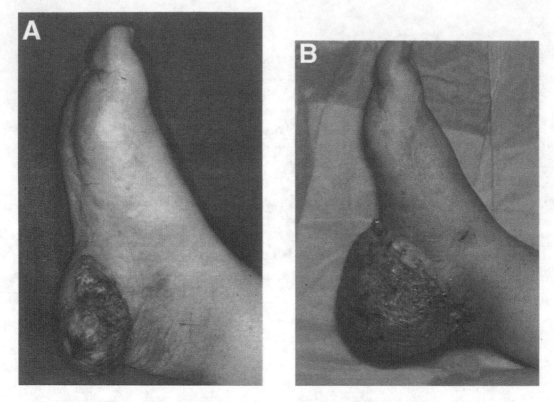

Fig. 18. (**A**) Preoperative view of large heel lesion in patient with diabetes. The mass was radically excised because of suspicion of squamous cell carcinoma; pathology showed verruca (wart). (**B**) Three months after excision and repair: heel has been resurfaced with latissimus dorsi muscle flap and skin graft. The course was complicated by early postoperative infection requiring debridement and repeat skin grafting, but the muscle flap was unaffected. Despite (expected) atrophy of flap, debulking was required at a later date.

perceptible difficulty with ambulation that would require use of a brace postoperatively. The scarring and fibrosis that occur with the inflammatory response to the wound and with wound healing usually prevent instability at the ankle. If preservation of exposed but viable tendon is desired, then coverage with a flap is mandatory.

Upton and colleagues *(27)* reported on a series of patients with defects of the Achilles tendon that were treated with free fascial flaps. The surgical procedures were technically demanding, but complications were few; these included separation between the flap skin graft and the native skin over the calcaneus in two older patients with vascular insufficiency. The authors suggest that this technique should be used with caution in patients with diabetes and/or peripheral vascular disease.

The lateral calcaneal artery flap (Figs. 20 and 21) is used for repair of lateral ankle, posterior heel, or Achilles defects *(28)*. This axial pattern skin flap is based on a branch or terminal portion of the peroneal artery. Sensibility may be maintained in the flap if the sural nerve is included. The base of the flap is approximately 4.5 cm wide, beginning just posterior to the lateral malleolus and just anterior to the border of the Achilles tendon. The shorter, more consistent version of the flap is dissected in a plantar direction along

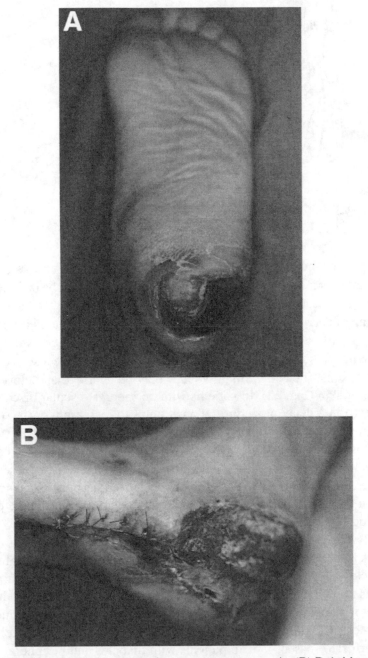

Fig. 19. (A) Posterior heel ulcer secondary to pressure necrosis. **(B)** Debridement and rotation flap were undertaken, but posterior tibial circulation was severely compromised and was insufficient for any type of repair using local tissue. Moreover, the zone of ischemic injury extended well into calcaneal bone. After failure of the ill-advised repair, below-knee amputation was performed.

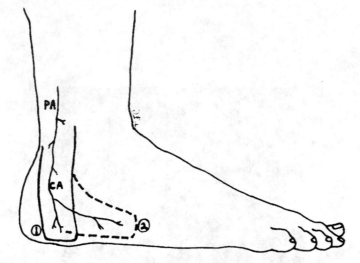

Fig. 20. Axial pattern skin flap based on lateral calcaneal artery, (1) shorter and (2) longer version (see text). PA, peroneal artery; CA, lateral calcaneal artery.

the lateral aspect of the foot and is about 8 cm long. In the longer version, the flap is extended toward the base of the fifth metatarsal; this portion should be included only if the Doppler signal of the lateral calcaneal artery can be found through the length of the flap.

In the setting of neuropathy, ulcers of the medial and lateral malleoli often appear with minor trauma—particularly with pressure from rigid devices such as the AFO brace, prescribed for patients with foot drop. Defects about the ankle are also seen in association with venous insufficiency. Small wounds may be debrided and closed with local rotation flaps of skin (Fig. 22). In patients with peripheral vascular disease, it may be prudent to perform a delay procedure in an attempt to increase the survival length of the flap: At the time of ulcer debridement the flap is incised but left *in situ*, and then several days (usually 2 weeks) later it is transferred. Use of this technique has had unexpected results in a few patients at this institution. Following excision of a small lateral malleolar ulcer, a skin graft was applied directly to cancellous bone as a "biologic dressing." The skin graft healed and in fact provided stable coverage, and the delayed flap was not needed (Fig. 23).

The distally based soleus muscle may reach defects of the lower leg or about the ankle, but this flap is often not reliable, even in adult patients with normal vasculature. Reverse-flow lower-leg skin flaps based on the septocutaneous perforating vessels may also reach this area. Examples are the sural flap, the saphenous flap, and the posterior-tibial perforator flap. Preoperative assessment at a minimum should include noninvasive vascular testing, with mapping of perforators using a Doppler device. Experience with these perforator-based flaps in patients with diabetes and peripheral arterial disease is still limited.

Based on the lateral tarsal and its parent the dorsalis pedis artery, the extensor digitorum brevis muscle (Figs. 24 and 25) can provide a moderate amount of tissue for repair of wounds about the ankle measuring up to 5–7 cm *(29)*. If used as an island flap with dissection carried to the anterior tibial artery, it may reach the posterior heel, lower Achilles region, and even the distal one-third of the leg. Unfortunately, this flap, as well

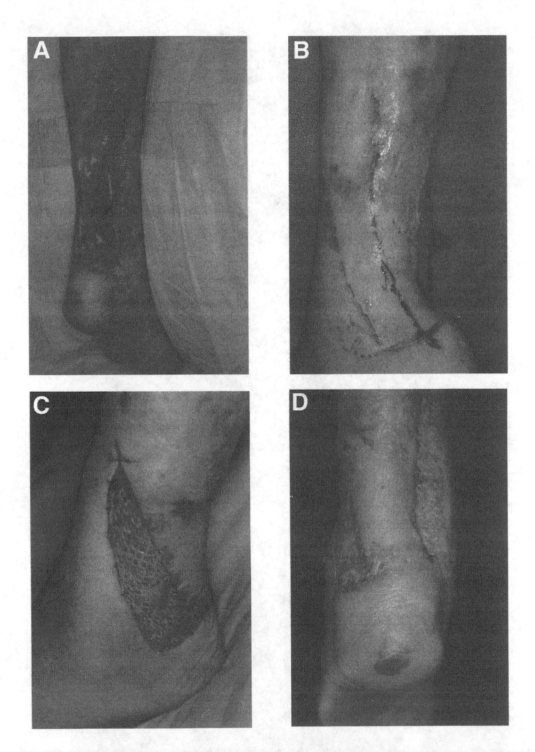

Fig. 21. (A) A revascularized extremity had an extensive posterior and medial defect resulting from preoperative ischemia; the wound was complicated by exposed superior edge of calcaneus and partial loss of Achilles tendon. **(B)** Design of rotation flap with distribution of lateral calcaneal artery in its distal portion. **(C)** After transfer of skin flap, skin grafts were applied to flap donor site and medial aspect of wound. **(D)** Healed wound 1 month postoperatively. Shortly afterward, the bypass graft thrombosed and below-knee amputation was required.

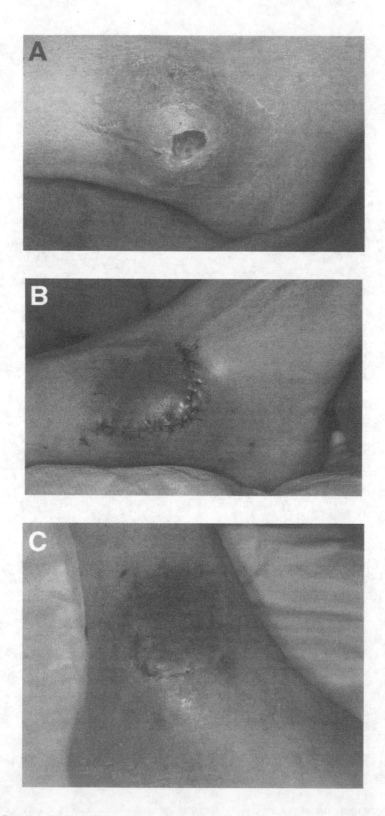

Fig. 22. Small lateral malleolar ulcer secondary to pressure from a rigid brace (**A**). Ulcer was closed with simple rotation flap, shown (**B**) at operation and (**C**) 2 months postoperatively.

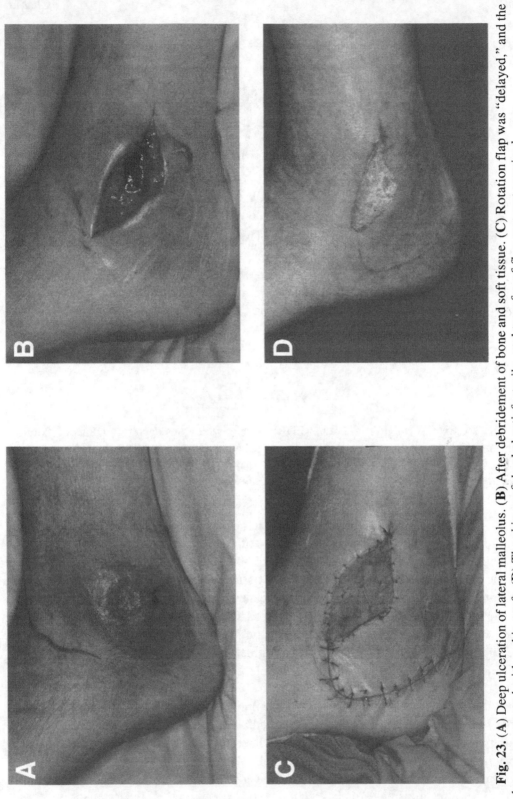

Fig. 23. (**A**) Deep ulceration of lateral malleolus. (**B**) After debridement of bone and soft tissue. (**C**) Rotation flap was "delayed," and the ulcer was protected with a skin graft. (**D**) The skin graft healed satisfactorily, and transfer of flap was not required.

379

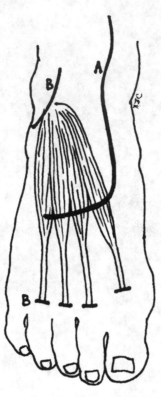

Fig. 24. Extensor digitorum brevis (EDB) muscle, which lies deep to tendons of extensor digitorum longus. A, Recommended, medial dorsal incision, shown with optional lateral extension over the muscle bellies of the EDB. B, Alternate or supplemental incisions, often used in free-tissue transfer, near origin and insertion of muscle.

as the dorsalis pedis fasciocutaneous flap, can be used only very selectively in the population of patients with diabetes, as division of the dorsalis pedis artery is required.

The extensor digitorum brevis muscle originates from the lateral and superior aspect of the calcaneus and adjacent ligamentous tissue. The lateral three slips insert on the tendons of the extensor digitorum longus; the medial slip inserts on the proximal phalanx of the first toe and is sometimes considered as a separate muscle, the extensor hallucis brevis. Dissection of the flap requires retraction of the extensor longus tendons, which lie superficial to the extensor brevis, and great care should be taken to preserve the vascular pedicle as it enters deep to the muscle. The usual pattern of arterial supply consists of the lateral tarsal artery—which by itself may be sufficient to support the flap— entering 1 cm distal to the extensor retinaculum, and the lateral metatarsal or arcuate artery entering 1–2 cm further distal. A medially based dorsal incision may preserve skin perfusion better than an incision that is laterally based *(30)*. However, small accessory incisions just anterior to the lateral malleolus and proximal to the toes (i.e., at the origin and insertion) may facilitate dissection and reduce trauma to the skin from retraction. The latter incisions are also recommended for harvest of the extensor digitorum brevis as a free muscle flap *(31)*.

Partial calcanectomy should be remembered as a simple technique that may permit linear closure of small defects of the non-weight-bearing heel. For completeness, the flexor digitorum brevis and the abductor muscles should be included in a discussion of

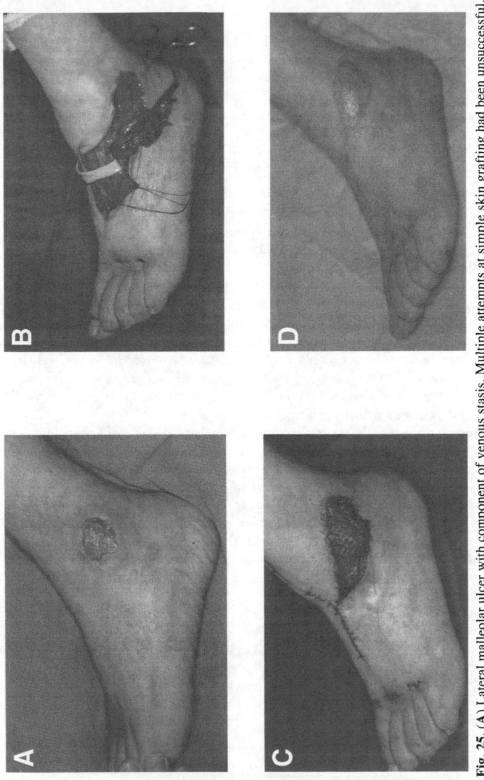

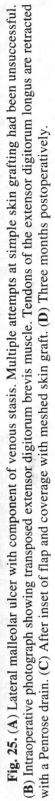

Fig. 25. (**A**) Lateral malleolar ulcer with component of venous stasis. Multiple attempts at simple skin grafting had been unsuccessful. (**B**) Intraoperative photograph showing transposed extensor digitorum brevis muscle. Tendons of the extensor digitorum longus are retracted with a Penrose drain. (**C**) After inset of flap and coverage with meshed skin graft. (**D**) Three months postoperatively.

malleolar and non-weight-bearing heel defects. The abductor hallucis and abductor digiti minimi muscles may sometimes reach medial and lateral heel defects, respectively, but these muscles provide only small amounts of tissue. Similarly, the flexor digitorum brevis muscle cannot always be relied on to reach wounds of the posterior heel except those that are located toward the plantar aspect.

CONCLUSIONS:
CURRENT LIMITATIONS AND FUTURE POSSIBILITIES

The modern reconstructive surgeon must be a student of vascular anatomy. Skin grafts must be applied to recipient beds with adequate circulation, and free flaps require satisfactory recipient vessels to survive. The design of a local, regional, or distant flap calls for general knowledge of the blood supply to the skin and specific knowledge of the flap's arterial and venous anatomy.

Advances in wound care, control of infection, general physiologic management, and peripheral vascular surgery have created new scenarios for the plastic and reconstructive surgeon. In particular, the success of distal bypass grafts has expanded applications for limb-preserving soft tissue reconstruction and at the same time has defined its limits. Many microvascular surgeons with increasing skill have performed free-tissue transfers but are still limited by the quality and availability of both arterial and venous recipient conduits. Furthermore, as some have observed, a well-executed flap may still not be sufficient to salvage a globally ischemic foot.

Progress in the care of the diabetic foot wound may be made in an incremental fashion, by physicians in practice: Ideally, patients will be managed by a team that includes endocrinologists, vascular and plastic surgeons, podiatrists, and orthotic technicians. The challenging and mundane aspects of patient education and compliance with non-weight-bearing status, weight reduction, and smoking cessation, must be confronted.

Those conducting clinical research have numerous avenues to pursue. More experience is needed with perforator-based flaps and sensate flaps in the patient with diabetes. The pathophysiology and treatment of the soft tissue changes accompanying Charcot arthropathy deserve further scrutiny, and the indications for use of topical growth factors need to be refined.

Innovations with broader application are expected in the foreseeable future from basic research in wound healing, angiogenesis, and tissue engineering. Improved treatments for peripheral neuropathy and methods of bolstering the intrinsic immune system to battle infection will be welcome. Finally, advances in the prevention and treatment of diabetes mellitus may succeed in making all the aforementioned obsolete.

REFERENCES

1. Batchelor JS, McGuiness A. A reappraisal of axial and nonaxial lower leg fascial flaps: an anatomic study in human cadavers. *Plast Reconstr Surg* 1996;97:993–1000.
2. Milton SH. Pedicled skin flaps: the fallacy of the length: width ratio. *Br J Surg* 1970;57: 502–508.
3. Taylor GI, Palmer JH. The vascular territories (angiosomes) of the body—experimental study and clinical applications. *Br J Plast Surg* 1987;40:113–141.
3a. Colen LB, Mathes SJ. Foot, in *Plastic Surgery: Principles and Practice*, vol 2 (Jurkiewicz MJ, Krizek TJ, Mathes SJ, Ariyan SA, eds.), Mosby, St. Louis, 1990, pp. 1003–1050.

4. Shestak KC, Hendricks DL, Webster MW. Indirect revascularization of the lower extremity by means of microvascular free-muscle flap—a preliminary report. *J Vasc Surg* 1990; 12:581–585.
5. McDaniel MD, Zwalak RM, Schneider JR, et al. Indirect revascularization of the lower extremity by means of microvascular free-muscle flap—a preliminary report [Letter]. *J Vasc Surg* 1991;14:829–830.
6. Serletti JM, Deuber MA, Guidera PM, et al. Atherosclerosis of the lower extremity and free-tissue reconstruction for limb salvage. *Plast Reconstr Surg* 1995;96:1136–1144.
7. Chick LR, Walton RL, Reus W, Colen L, Sasmor M. Free flaps in the elderly. *Plast Reconstr Surg* 1992;90:87–94.
8. Karp NS, Kasabian AK, Siebert JW, Eidelman Y, Colen S. Microvascular free-flap salvage of the diabetic foot: a five-year experience. *Plast Reconstr Surg* 1994;94:834–840.
9. Colen L, Musson A. Preoperative assessment of the peripheral vascular disease patient for free tissue transfers. *J Reconstr Microsurg* 1987;4:1–14.
10. Miller JR, Potparic Z, Colen LB, Sorrell K, Carraway JH. The accuracy of duplex ultrasonography in the planning of skin flaps of the lower extremity. *Plast Reconstr Surg* 1995; 95:1221–1227.
11. Hayashi A, Maruyama Y. Reverse first dorsal metatarsal artery flap for reconstruction of the distal foot. *Ann Plast Surg* 1993;31:117–122.
11a. Colen LB, Pessa JE, Potparic Z, Reus WF. Reconstruction of the extremity with the dorsal thoracic fascia free flap. *Plast Reconstr Surg* 1998;101:738–744.
12. Rajacic N, Darweesh M, Jayakrishnan K, Gang K, Kojic S. The distally based superficial sural flap for reconstruction of the leg and foot. *Br J Plast Surg* 1996;49:383–389.
13. Masquelet AC, Beveridge J, Romana C, Gerber C. The lateral supramalleolar flap. *Plast Reconstr Surg* 1988;81:74–81.
14. Jones EB, Cronwright I, Lalbahadur A. Anatomical studies and five years clinical experience with the distally based medial fasciocutaneous flap of the lower leg. *Br J Plast Surg* 1993;46:639–643.
15. Colen LB, Replogle MD, Mathes SJ. The V-Y plantar flap for reconstruction of the forefoot. *Plast Reconstr Surg* 1988;81:220–227.
16. Sakai S, Terayama I. Modification of the island subcutaneous pedicle flap for reconstruction of defects of the sole of the foot. *Br J Plast Surg* 1991;44:179–182.
17. Sakai S. A distally based island first dorsal metatarsal artery flap for coverage of a distal plantar defect. *Br J Plast Surg* 1993;46:480–482.
18. Granick MS, Newton ED, Futrell JW, Hurwitz D. The plantar digital webspace island flap for reconstruction of the distal sole. *Ann Plast Surg* 1987;19:68–74.
19. Amarante J, Martins A, Reis J. A distally based median plantar flap. *Ann Plast Surg* 1988; 20:468–470.
20. Shaw WW, Hidalgo DA. Anatomic basis of plantar flap design: clinical applications. *Plast Reconstr Surg* 1986;78:637–649.
21. Hidalgo DA, Shaw WW. Anatomic basis of plantar flap design. *Plast Reconstr Surg* 1986; 78:627–636.
22. Hidalgo DA, Shaw WW. Reconstruction of foot injuries. *Clin Plast Surg* 1986;13:663–680.
23. Sommerlad BC, McGrouther DA. Resurfacing the sole: long-term follow-up and comparison of techniques. *Br J Plast Surg* 1978;31:107–116.
24. Noever G, Bruser P, Kohler L. Reconstruction of heel and sole defects by free flaps. *Plast Reconstr Surg* 1986;78:345–352.
25. Meland NB. Microsurgical reconstruction of the weightbearing surface of the foot. *Microsurgery* 1990;11:54–58.
26. May JW Jr, Halls MJ, Simon SR. Free microvascular muscle flaps with skin graft reconstruction of extensive defects of the foot: a clinical and gait analysis study. *Plast Reconstr Surg* 1985;75:627–641.

27. Upton J, Baker TM, Shoen SL, Wolfort F. Fascial flap coverage of Achilles tendon defects. *Plast Reconstr Surg* 1995;95:1056–1059.
28. Grabb WC, Argenta LC. The lateral calcaneal artery skin flap (the lateral calcaneal artery, lesser saphenous vein, and sural nerve flap). *Plast Reconstr Surg* 1981;68:723–730.
29. Landi A, Soragni O, Monteleone M. The extensor digitorum brevis muscle island flap for soft-tissue loss around the ankle. *Plast Reconstr Surg* 1985;75:892–897.
30. Giordano PA, Argenson C, Pequignot J-P. Extensor digitorum brevis as an island flap in the reconstruction of soft-tissue defects in the lower limb. *Plast Reconstr Surg* 1989;83: 100–109.
31. Strauch B, Yu H-L. *Atlas of Microvascular Surgery*. Thieme, New York, 1993, pp. 314–385.

ADDITIONAL READING

Atiyeh BS, Sfeir RE, Hussein MM, Husami T. Preliminary arteriovenous fistula for free-flap reconstruction in the diabetic foot. *Plast Reconstr Surg* 1995;95:1062–1069.

Barclay TL, Sharpe DT, Chisholm EM. Cross-leg fasciocutaneous flaps. *Plast Reconstr Surg* 1983;72:843–847.

Buncke HJ Jr, Colen LB. An island flap from the first web space of the foot to cover plantar ulcers. *Br J Plast Surg* 1980;33:242–244.

Carriquiry C, Aparecida Costa M, Vasconez LO. An anatomic study of the septocutaneous vessels of the leg. *Plast Reconstr Surg* 1985;76:354–361.

Clark N, Sherman R. Soft tissue reconstruction of the foot and ankle. *Orthop Clin N Am* 1993; 24:489–503.

Colen LB. Limb salvage in the patient with severe peripheral vascular disease: the role of microsurgical free tissue transfer. *Plast Reconstr Surg* 1987;79:389–395.

Colen LB, Buncke HJ. Neurovascular island flaps from the plantar vessels and nerves for foot reconstruction. *Ann Plast Surg* 1984;12:327–332.

Colen LB, Reus WF III, Kalus R. Posterior hindfoot reconstruction. *J Reconstr Microsurg* 1990;6:143–149.

Cormack GC, Lamberty BGH. *The Arterial Anatomy of Skin Flaps*, 2nd ed. Churchill Livingstone, Edinburgh, 1994, pp. 258–267.

Leitner DW, Gordon L, Buncke HJ. The extensor digitorum brevis as a muscle island flap. *Plast Reconstr Surg* 1985;76:777–780.

Masquelet AC, Romana MC, Wolf G. Skin island flaps supplied by the vascular axis of the sensitive nerves: anatomic study and clinical experience in the leg. *Plast Reconstr Surg* 1992; 89:1115–1121.

McCraw JB. Selection of alternative local flaps in the leg and foot. *Clin Plast Surg* 1979;6:227–246.

Miyamoto Y, Ikuta Y, Shigeki S, Yamura M. Current concepts of instep island flap. *Ann Plast Surg* 1987;19:97–102.

Morain WD, Colen LB. Wound healing in diabetes mellitus. *Clin Plast Surg* 1990;17:493–501.

Rautio J. Resurfacing and sensory recovery of the sole. *Clin Plast Surg* 1991;18:615–626.

Saltz R, Hochberg J, Given KS. Muscle and musculocutaneous flaps of the foot. *Clin Plast Surg* 1991;18:627–638.

Searles JM Jr, Colen LB. Foot reconstruction in diabetes mellitus and peripheral vascular insufficiency. *Clin Plast Surg* 1991;18:467–483.

Thorne CHM, Siebert JW, Grotting JC, et al. Reconstructive surgery of the lower extremity, in *Plastic Surgery*, vol 6 (McCarthy JG, ed.), WB Saunders, Philadelphia, 1990, pp. 4081–4088.

Vasconez HC, Vasconez LO. Fasciocutaneous flaps of the leg and foot, in *Fasciocutaneous Flaps* (Hallock GG, ed.), Blackwell Scientific, Boston, 1992, pp. 119–130.

18

Role of Growth Factors in the Treatment of Diabetic Foot Ulceration

David L. Steed, MD

PRINCIPLES OF WOUND HEALING AND GROWTH FACTOR THERAPY

Wound healing is the process of tissue repair and the tissue response to injury. It is a complex biologic process involving chemotaxis, cellular reproduction, matrix protein, neovascularization, and scar remodeling *(1)*. Much progress has been made in our understanding of the cellular and molecular biology of wound repair and remodeling in recent years, yet many aspects about wound healing remain unclear. Growth factors are polypeptides that control the growth, differentiation, and metabolism of cells and regulate the process of tissue repair *(2,3)*. The role of growth factors in wound healing and specifically in diabetic ulcer healing is the subject of this chapter.

The three phases of wound healing (inflammation, fibroplasia, and maturation) are all controlled by growth factors, which, though present in only small amounts, exert a powerful in their influence on wound repair. There is great interest in manipulating the cellular environment of the wound with proteins, growth factors, and gene therapy.

The first phase of wound healing is the inflammatory response, initiated immediately after the injury *(4)*. Vasoconstriction limits hemorrhage to the site of wounding. As blood vessels are damaged and blood leaks from within the lumen, platelets come into contact with collagen in the wall of the vessel beneath the endothelium. Platelets are activated by the collagen and initiate coagulation. Serotonin and thromboxane are released and enhance vasoconstriction locally, keeping the healing factors within the wound. Simultaneously, vasodilation occurs, allowing new factors to be brought into the wound. Vasodilation is mediated by histamine, released by the platelets, mast cells, and basophils. There is also an increase in vascular permeability, allowing blood-borne factors to enter this area. Arachidonic acid is produced and serves as an intermediate for production of prostglandins and leukotrienes. These proteins are intense vasodilators that increase vascular permeability, along with histamine, bradykinin, and complement. Thromboxane also increases platelet aggregation and local vasoconstriction.

Platelets control hemorrhage by initiating clotting through the coagulation system. The intrinsic system is activated by Hageman factor (factor XII) as it comes into contact with collagen. In the presence of kininogen, a precursor of bradykinin and prekallikrein, factor XII activates factor XI, then factor IX, and then factor VIII. Thromboplastin

From: *The Diabetic Foot: Medical and Surgical Management*
Edited by: A. Veves, J. M. Giurini, and F. W. LoGerfo © Humana Press Inc., Totowa, NJ

triggers a response in the extrinsic system. Thromboplastin is formed as phospholipids and glycoproteins are released by blood coming into contact with the injured tissues. Factor VII is activated in the presence of calcium. Both the intrinsic and extrinsic systems activate the final common pathway, producing fibrin and leading to fibrin polymerization. To balance the coagulation cascade, the fibrinolytic system is activated. This system monitors clotting to prevent coagulation from extending beyond the wound. It is activated by the same factors that initiate coagulation and thus regulates the process.

The complement cascade is activated by platelets and neutral proteases. This system produces potent proteins known as anaphylotoxins, which cause mast cells to degranulate and release histamine. Substances released by the inflammatory process are chemoattractants for neutrophils. This causes margination of white blood cells and then migration of these white blood cells into the wound. The neutrophils are phagocytes for bacteria. Wounds can heal without white blood cells, but the risk of infection is increased. Neutrophils produce free oxygen radicals and lysosomal enzymes for host defense. The neutrophils are later removed from the wound by tissue macrophages.

Monocytes enter the wound space and become tissue macrophages. They take over control of the wound environment by the third day. Wounds cannot heal without the macrophage. These cells regulate the production of growth factors including platelet-derived growth factor (PDGF), tumor necrosis factor (TNF), and transforming growth factor-β (TGF-β); thus they control protein production, matrix formation, and remodeling. Extracellular matrix is a group of proteins in a polysaccharide gel made up of glycosaminoglycans and proteoglycans produced by the fibroblast. These proteins are structural, such as collagen and elastin, or are involved in controlling cell adhesion, such as fibronectin and laminin (5). Thrombospondin and von Willebrand factor are other adhesion molecules. Fibronectin is also a chemoattractant for circulating monocytes and stimulates their differentiation into tissue macrophages.

The second phase of wound healing is fibroplasia; it begins with macrophages and fibroblasts increasing in number in the wound, while the number of white blood cells decrease as fewer enter the wound. The inflammatory response ends as the mediators of inflammation are no longer produced and those already present are inactivated or removed by diffusion or by macrophages. Fibroplasia begins around the fifth day following injury and may continue for 2 weeks. This begins the process of matrix formation, especially collagen synthesis.

Angiogenesis is the process of rebuilding the blood supply to the wound (6). Fibroblasts are attracted to the wound and replicate in response to fibronectin, PDGF, fibroblast growth factor (FGF), TGF-β and C5a, a product of the complement system. Fibroblasts produce proteoglycans and structural proteins. The cellular matrix is composed of hyaluronate and fibronectin, which allow for cellular migration through chemotactic factors formed in the wound. Fibronectin binds proteins and fibroblasts in the matrix and provides a pathway along which fibroblasts can move. Fibronectin also plays a role in epithelialization and angiogenesis.

Collagen is the most common protein in the mammalian world and is produced by the fibroblast. It is a family of at least 12 proteins, rich in glycine and proline and bound in a tight triple helix. Crosslinking between the three strands of collagen provides for a highly stable molecule, resistant to breakdown. Macrophages control the release of collagen from fibroblasts through growth factors such as PDGF, epidermal growth factor (EGF), FGF, and TGF-β. Collagen is remodeled for several years in a healing wound. Elastin is the other major structural protein and contains proline and lysine. It is present as random coils, allowing both stretch and recoil, in much smaller amounts than collagen.

Angiogenesis occurs by the budding of existing capillaries after stimulation by FGF. Endothelial cells proliferate and migrate through the healing wound, allowing connections between the capillaries to form a vascular network in the wound space. This capillary network provides an avenue of access for new healing factors into the wound and ends when the wound has an adequate blood supply. Hypoxia triggers angiogenesis; thus it appears as if this process is controlled by oxygen tension *(7,8)*.

Epithelialization occurs as cells migrate from the edge of the wound over a collagen-fibronectin surface. This process results in mature skin covering the wound. Scar contracture then occurs as the wound matures.

The final phase of wound repair is maturation or scar remodeling. Wound remodeling involves a number of proteins including hyaluronidase, collagenase, and elastase. Hyaluronate in the matrix is replaced by dermatan sulfate and chondroitin sulfate. These proteins reduce cell migration and allow cell differentiation. Plasmin, which is formed from plasminogen, degrades fibrin. Urokinase, produced by leukocytes, fibroblasts, endothelial cells, and keratinocytes, activates collagenase and elastase. Collagenase, which allows collagen remodeling, is secreted by macrophages, fibroblasts, epithelial cells, and white blood cells. It is able to break the collagen triple helix to allow remodeling. The scar becomes less hyperemic and less red in appearance as blood supply is reduced. The scar remodels and wound strength increases for up to 2 years following injury, yet the total collagen content of the wound does not change.

GROWTH FACTORS

Growth factors are polypeptides that initiate the growth and proliferation of cells and stimulate protein production *(2,3)*. They are named for their tissue of origin, their biologic action, or the cell on which they exert their influence. Growth factors may have paracrine or autocrine function whereby they affect not only adjacent cells but also have a self-regulating effect. Some are transported (plasma bound) to large carrier proteins and thus serve an endocrine function. They are produced by a variety of cells including platelets, macrophages, epithelial cells, fibroblasts, and endothelial cells. Growth factors are chemoattractants for neutrophils, macrophages, fibroblasts, and endothelial cells. Growth factors bind to specific receptors on the cell surface to stimulate cell growth. Although they are present in only minute amounts, they exert a powerful influence on wound repair.

The growth factors involved in wound healing include PDGF, TGF-β, EGF, FGF, and insulin-like growth factor (IGF). The platelet, which is critical to the initiation of the wound healing process, is rich in growth factors. Growth factors initially released in the wound space by platelets are subsequently degraded by proteases. Other cells that have been drawn into the wound space such as inflammatory cells, fibroblasts, and epithelial cells are also involved in growth factor production. Macrophages also release factors such as TNF. Keratinocytes are stimulated by EGF, IGF-1, TGF-α, and interleukin-1 (IL-1). Wound remodeling occurs under the control of collagenase, produced in response to EGF, TNF, IL-1, and PDGF. Thus all wound healing is under the direct or indirect control of growth factors. It is reasonable then to speculate that exogenous growth factors applied to the wound may influence healing.

Platelet-Derived Growth Factor

PDGF has been studied more widely than any other growth factor and is approved for clinical use. PDGF has a molecular weight of 24,000. It is a potent chemoattractant and mitogen for fibroblasts, smooth muscle cells, and inflamatory cells. PDGF is produce by platelets, macrophages, vascular endothelium, and fibroblasts (9). It is composed of two chains, an A and a B chain, held together by disulfide bonds in three dimeric forms, AA, AB, and BB. There is a 60% amino acid homology between the two chains. Human platelets contain all three forms of PDGF in a ratio of about 12% AA, 65% AB, and 23% BB. The B chain is quite similar to the transforming gene of the simian sarcoma virus, an acute transforming retrovirus. The human protooncogene C-*cis* is similar to the viral oncogene V-*cis* and encodes for the B chain of PDGF.

There are two PDGF receptors, an α and a β receptor. The α receptor recognizes both the A and B chains of PDGF and thus can bind to the AA, AB, and BB forms. The β receptor recognizes only the B chain and thus binds to the BB form and weakly to the AB form. Most cells have many times more β receptors than α receptors. Cells with PDGF receptors include fibroblasts, vascular smooth muscle cells, and some microvascular endothelial cells. PDGF acts with TGF-β and EGF to stimulate mesenchymal cells. Although PDGF is produced by endothelial cells of the vascular system, the endothelial cells do not respond to PDGF, rather, they work in a paracrine manner to stimulate adjacent smooth muscle cells. Smooth muscle cells also act in an autocrine fashion and produce PDGF.

PDGF is stable to extremes of heat, a wide range of pH, and degradation by proteases. The principle cells involved in the early stages of wound healing all synthesize and secrete PDGF. Platelets, among the first cells to enter the wound, are the largest source of PDGF in the human body. Circulating monocytes are attracted to the wound and become tissue macrophages. These cells also produce PDGF. PDGF stimulates the production of fibronectin and hyaluronic acid, proteins that are important components of provisional matrix. Collagenase, a protein important in wound remodeling, is also produced in response to PDGF. There are no reported cases of a human deficient in PDGF, suggesting that PDGF is critical to the survival of the individual.

PDGF, has been manufactured by recombinant DNA technology. In animal models, it has been shown to improve the breaking strength of incisional wounds when applied topically as a single dose. It also accelerated acute wound healing. By 3 months, however, there was no difference in wound healing compared with untreated wounds, suggesting that although PDGF accelerated wound healing, the wound healing was quite similar to normal healing. Wounds treated with PDGF had a marked increase in inflammatory cells entering the wound, including neutrophils, monocytes, and fibroblasts. As a result of this cellular response, granulation tissue production was also increased. Even though PDGF does not directly affect keratinocytes, wounds in animals were shown to have an increased rate of epithelialization. This is probably owing to the influence from macrophages and fibroblasts attracted into the wound space by PDGF. Wounds

Table 1
Results of Trials of Platelet-Derived Growth Factor
in the Treatment of Diabetic Foot Ulcers

Author	Treatment	Patients Healed No./total	%
Steed *(12)*	Placebo gel	14/57	25
	Becaplermin gel 30 µg/g	29/61	48
Wieman et al. *(12a)*	Placebo gel	44/127	35
	Becaplermin gel 30 µg/g	48/132	36
	Becaplermin gel 100 µg/g	62/123	50
Wieman et al. *(12b)*	Good wound care	15/68	22
	Placebo gel	25/70	36
	Becaplermin gel 100 µg/g	15/34	44
Total	Good wound care	15/68	22
	Placebo gel	83/254	33
	Becaplermin gel 30 µg/g	29/61	48
	Becaplermin gel 100 µg/g	77/157	49
	Becaplermin (total)	106/218	49

treated topically with PDGF have an increase in neovascularization, although PDGF does not directly stimulate endothelial cells. Thus it appears as if PDGF accelerates wound healing by accelerating the normal sequences of healing. The healed wounds appear to be normal in all aspects.

PDGF has been studied extensively in clinical trials (Table 1). The effectiveness of recombinant human PDGF-BB in healing was first studied in decubitus ulcers *(10,11)*. Patients were treated with PDGF topically and followed for 28 days. There was a greater amount of wound closure in patients treated with the highest dose of PDGF. The lower doses had little effect. In another trial, patients with decubitus ulcers were treated with 100 or 300 µg/mL or placebo, again for 1 month. The ulcer volume was significantly reduced in the PDGF-treated patients. No significant toxicity related to PDGF was noted. Complete wound closure was not an end point in either study, and thus the question as to whether PDGF could accomplish complete wound healing in humans was not answered.

A randomized prospective double-blind trial of recombinant PDGF-BB was performed in patients with diabetic neurotrophic foot ulcers *(12)*. Patients were treated with PDGF at a dose of 2.2 µg/cm^2 of wound in vehicle, carboxymethylcellulose, or vehicle alone for 20 weeks or until complete wound closure occurred. Patients had wounds of at least 8 weeks' duration, were considered to be free of infection, and had an adequate blood supply as demonstrated by a transcutaneous oxygen tension (TcPO$_2$) of at least 30 mmHg. All wounds were debrided by completely excising the wound prior to entry into the study and as needed during the trial. In these patients with chronic nonhealing wounds, 48% healed following treatment with PDGF, whereas only 25% healed with vehicle alone ($p < 0.01$). The median reduction in wound area was 98.8% for PDGF-treated patients but only 82.1% for those treated with vehicle. There were no significant differences in the incidence or severity of adverse events in either group. This was the first clinical trial to suggest that a growth factor, PDGF, could be applied topically and be effective and safe in accelerating the healing of chronic wounds in humans.

In another trial using recombinant human PDGF in the treatment of similar patients with diabetic foot ulcers, those patients treated with PDGF-BB had an increase in the incidence of complete wound closure of 43% compared with placebo ($p = 0.007$). PDGF also decreased the time to achieve complete wound closure by 32% ($p = 0.013$) compared with placebo.

In reviewing patients treated with PDGF or vehicle alone, it was noted that those patients receiving the best wound care healed better whether PDGF or vehicle was applied. Debridement proved to be critically important. The benefits from PDGF will be minimized if the wounds are not treated properly. The vehicle, carboxymethylcellulose, was tested to determine whether it was inert in wound healing. It did provide a moist environment for wound healing but did not improve healing significantly. PDGF was recently approved for use in the United States and is sold as Regranex.

Transforming Growth Factor

The growth factor studied most extensively after PDGF is TGF-β. TGFs are composed of two polypeptide chains, α and β. TGF-α has a 30% amino acid homology with EGF. It is named because of its ability to stimulate the growth of cells reversibly. Cancer cells do this also. TGF-α is produced by many different cells including macrophages, keratinocytes, hepatocytes, and eosinophiles *(13)*. TGF-α and EGF are mitogens for keratinocytes and fibroblasts, but TGF-α is a more potent angiogenesis factor. Both TGF-α and EGF bind to the EGF receptor, but their specific actions may be different, partly owing to differences in their binding. As yet there have been no clinical trials of wound healing with TGF-α.

TGF-β has no amino acid homology with TGF-α or any other group of growth factors. TGF-β is a group of proteins that can reversibly inhibit growth of cells, especially those of ectodermal origin. TGF-β is produced by a variety of cells including platelets, macrophages, fibroblasts, keratinocytes, and lymphocytes. Nearly all cells have receptors for TGF-β and have the potential to respond to it. TGF-β can stimulate or inhibit the growth or differentiation of many different cells. It appears as if TGF-β is the most widely acting group of growth factors.

Three forms of TGF-β have been isolated, TGF-β1, TGF-β2, and TGF-β3. The actions of the three different forms of TGF-β are very similar. TGF-βs have a molecular weight of about 25,000. They reversibly stimulate growth of fibroblasts and thus received their name. TGF-βs are potent stimulators of chemotaxis in inflammatory cells and trigger cells to produce extracellular matrix and therefore are important in wound healing. TGF-β was tested in three different doses in a collagen sponge, with a standard care arm in the trial *(14)*. There was a significant improvement in the healing of diabetic ulcers treated with each of the three doses of TGF-β compared with collagen sponge. In this study, the patients treated with standard care healed better than those patients treated with TGF-β. The role of TGF-β in treating patients with chronic wounds remains undetermined.

Vascular Endothelial Growth Factor

Vascular endothelial growth factor (VEGF) is quite similar to PDGF. It has a molecular weight of 45,000. It has a 24% amino acid homology to the B chain of PDGF. VEGF, however, binds different receptors than PDGF and has different actions. Although it is a potent mitogen for endothelial cells, it is not a mitogen for fibroblasts or vascular smooth muscle cells, as is PDGF. VEGF is angiogenic and may play a role in wound healing by way of this property. There has been interest in using VEGF to stimulate the development of collateral arteries in patients with vascular disease, but as yet there are no clinical trials to suggest whether it will be of benefit clinically in wound healing.

Epidermal Growth Factor

EGF is a small molecule similar to TGF-α. EGF is produced by the platelet and is found in high quantities in the early phase of wound healing. The active form has a molecular weight of 6,200. EGF is produced by the kidney, salivary glands, and lacrimal glands and thus is found in high concentrations in urine, saliva, and tears. EGF promotes epidermal regeneration in pigs and corneal epithelialization in rabbits. It also increases the tensile strength of wounds in animals. EGF increases wound healing by stimulating the production of proteins such as fibronectin. Although EGF does not stimulate collagen production, it increases the number of fibroblasts in the wound. These cells produce collagen and improve the wound strength. EGF shares a receptor with TGF-α.

EGF has been studied in a randomized trial of healing of skin graft donor sites *(15)*. Donor sites treated with silver sulfadiazine containing EGF had an accelerated rate of epidermal regeneration compared with patients treated with silver sulfadiazine alone. EGF reduced the healing time by 1.5 days. These results did not have clinical significance; however, this was the first trial to demonstrate a benefit from treatment with a single growth factor in human wounds. In another trial, EGF was used in an open-label study with a crossover design in patients with chronic wounds *(16)*. Patients with chronic wounds were treated with silver sulfadiazine. In those who did not heal, silver sulfadiazine containing EGF was then used. Improvement was noted in many of these patients. The results of these studies suggest that EGF may be of benefit in wound healing, although as yet there are not enough data to confirm this.

Fibroblast Growth Factor

FGFs form a group of heparin-bound growth factors. There are two forms: acidic FGF (aFGF) and basic FGF (bFGF). Both molecules have molecular weights of 15,000. There is a 50% amino acid homology between the two molecules. They are commonly bound to heparin or to heparan sulfate, which protects them from enzymatic degradation. FGF can be produced by fibroblasts, endothelial cells, smooth muscle cells, and chondrocytes. In addition to endothelial cells, FGFs can stimulate fibroblasts, keratinocytes, chondrocytes, and myoblasts. At least four different FGF receptors have been identified thus far. They appear to have a similar function. Both aFGF and bFGF are found in the extracellular matrix in the bound form. Matrix degradation proteins then acts to release aFGF or bFGF. Acidic FGF is similar to endothelial cell growth factor, whereas bFGF is similar to endothelial cell growth factor II. Both aFGF and bFGF are similar to keratinocyte growth factor. These proteins are mitogens for cells of meso-dermal and neuroectodermal origin. FGFs are potent mitogens for endothelial cells and function as angiogenesis factors by stimulating growth of new blood vessels through proliferation of capillary endothelial cells. To date, no clinical trials have proved FGF to be of benefit in clinical wound healing.

Keratinocyte Growth Factor

Keratinocyte growth factor (KGF) is closely related to the FGFs. It is a protein with a molecular weight of 28,00 and a significant amino acid homology with the FGFs. Although KGF is found only in fibroblasts, it stimulates keratinocytes, not fibroblasts. It may share a receptor with FGF. KGF-2 was used in a randomized prospective blinded trial of patients with venous stasis ulcers *(17)*. There appeared to be a benefit from treatment with KGF-2. The role of KGF-2 in wound healing is still, however, unclear.

Insulin-Like Growth Factor

IGFs, or somatomedins, are proteins that have a 50% amino acid homology with proinsulin and have insulin-like activity *(18)*. There are two forms of this growth factor, IGF-1 and IGF-2. IGF-1 and IGF-2 are anabolic hormones that can stimulate the synthesis of glycogen and glycosaminoglycans. They can also increase the transport of glucose and amino acids across cell membranes. They increase collagen synthesis by fibroblasts. At this time, no clinical trials have been reported using IGFs. Both are secreted as large precursor molecules that are then cleaved to an active form. IGF-1 is identical to somatomedin-C, and IGF-2 is similar to somatomedin. These growth factors are found in the liver, heart, lung, pancreas, brain, and muscle. IGF-2 is also synthesized by many different tissues but is particularly prominent during fetal development and plays a significant role in fetal growth. IGF-1 and IGF-2 have separate receptors. The actions of pituitary growth hormone may be mediated through IGF-1. IGF-1 then causes cell division. IGF-1 is produced predominantly in the liver. It is found in high concentrations in platelets and is released into the wound when clotting occurs. Levels of IGF-1 and IGF-2 depend on many different factors, such as age, gender, nutritional status, and hormone level. Growth hormone is a regulator of IGF-1 and IGF-2, as are prolactin, thyroid hormone, and sex hormones. Elevated levels of somatomedins are found in patients with acromegaly.

Platelet Releasates

In the first 2 days following injury, growth factors are produced and released by platelets. Thereafter, growth factor production is taken over by macrophages. Within the α granules of the human platelet are multiple growth factors that are released when platelets are activated and degranulate. These include PDGF, TGF-β, FGF, EGF, platelet factor four, platelet-derived angiogenesis factor, and β-thromboglobulin. A purified platelet releasate can be prepared by stimulating platelets to release the contents of their α granules by using thrombin. Use of a platelet releasate in wound healing has theoretical advantages. The growth factors that are released are identical to and in the same proportion as those factors normally brought into the wound by the platelet. Preparation of a platelet releasate is simple and inexpensive since the platelets can be harvested from peripheral blood. Platelets readily release the contents of their α granules when stimulated with thrombin. Growth factors are preserved in banked blood. Thus, large quantities of growth factors can be retrieved from the platelets of pooled human blood. There may, however, be disadvantages to using a platelet releasate. Not all growth factors promote wound healing. There is a signal for wound healing to stop. A platelet releasate might concentrate factors that heal the wound as well as those that signal the wound healing process to end. There is also the possibility of transmission of an infectious agent if the platelet releasate applied to the wound is from another individual. This risk could be reduced if the releasate were harvested from a single donor or from the patient.

There has been considerable experience with the use of platelet releasates in wound healing. A preliminary report described the use of an autologous platelet releasate in six patients with chronic lower extremity ulcers from connective tissue diseases. A homologous platelet releasate was used to treat 11 patients with leg ulcers from diabetes and 8 patients with leg ulcers secondary to chronic venous insufficiency *(19)*. No benefit was observed from using the platelet releasate; however, this study pointed out the importance of topical growth factor application only in the context of good wound care and in a narrowly defined group of patients. Growth factors cannot be expected to have a positive influence on wound healing unless they are applied in a comprehensive wound care program. The underlying etiology of these wounds, such as venous hypertension, diabetic neuropathy, or ischemia, must be addressed. In another trial, 49 patients with chronic wounds were treated with an autologous platelet releasate *(20)*. There appeared to be a correlation with complete wound healing and initial wound size. This was the first clinical trial to suggest a benefit from a platelet releasate applied topically.

A randomized trial of platelet releasate versus a platelet buffer was conducted in patients with ulcers secondary to diabetes, peripheral vascular disease, venous insufficiency, or vasculitis *(21)*. This study suggested a benefit from the treatment of leg ulcers in these 32 patients from a topically applied growth factor preparation. The growth factor preparation was added to microcrystalline collagen, a potent stimulator of platelets. The exact contribution from the collagen to the healing of these wounds was not defined.

Two other trials suggested a benefit from a platelet releasate. In one trial, patients were treated for 3 months with silver sulfadiazine *(22)*. Only 3 of the 23 lower extremity wounds healed; however, when the platelet releasate was then applied, the remaining ulcers healed. Another study of 70 patients suggested a similar benefit from a platelet releasate *(23)*. Despite evidence that platelet releasates are of benefit, another trial observed a very different result. In a randomized prospective double-blind, placebo-controlled trial, topical platelet releasate was applied to the leg ulcers of 26 patients. The ulcers were secondary to diabetes, peripheral vascular disease, or chronic venous insufficiency *(24)*. Wounds treated with the platelet releasate increased in size (that is, worsened), whereas wounds in the control group improved. This study suggested that a platelet releasate might be detrimental to wound healing.

Thirteen patients with diabetic neurotrophic ulcers were enrolled in a randomized trial of a platelet releasate versus saline placebo *(25)*. A benefit was seen in those treated with the platelet releasate. By 20 weeks of therapy, five of seven patients healed using the platelet releasate, whereas while only two of six patients healed using the saline placebo. By 24 weeks of treatment, three additional patients in the control group healed, suggesting that the platelet releasate stimulated more rapid healing but did not result in a greater proportion of healed wounds.

Although there is some evidence to suggest that a platelet releasate may be of benefit when applied topically to lower extremity wounds, the inconsistency of the results as well as the concern about transmission of infectious agents in using a homologous preparation leaves their role in human wound healing undefined.

In summary, growth factors exert a powerful influence over wound healing, controlling the growth, differentiation, and metabolism of cells. Only a few studies have reported that growth factors applied topically can exert a positive influence on wound repair; however, there is no doubt that they control wound healing. It is likely that their actions will be defined in the future, and we will thus be able to control the wound environment to achieve complete and durable wound healing.

REFERENCES

1. Edington HE. Wound healing, in *Basic Science Review for Surgeons* (Simmons RL, Steed DL, eds.), WB Saunders, Philadelphia, 1992, pp. 41–55.
2. McGrath MH. Peptide growth factors and wound healing. *Clin Plast Surg* 1990;17:421–432.
3. Rothe MJ, Falanga V. Growth factors and wound healing. *Clin Dermatol* 1992;9:553–559.
4. Steed DL. Mediators of inflammation, in *Basic Science Review for Surgeons* (Simmons RL, Steed DL, eds.), WB Saunders, Philadelphia, 1992, pp. 12–29.
5. Grinnel F. Fibronectin and wound healing. *Am J Dermatopathol* 1982;4:185–192.
6. Folkman T, Lansburn M. Angiogenic factors. *Science* 1987;235:442–447.
7. Knighton DR, Hunt TK, Schewenstuhl A. Oxygen tension regulates the expression of angiogenesis factor by macrophages. *Science* 1983;221:1283–1290.
8. Knighton DR, Silver IA, Hunt TK. Regulation of wound healing angiogenesis: effect of oxygen gradients and inspired oxygen concentration. *Surgery* 1981;90:262–269.
9. Lynch SE, Nixon JC. Role of platelet-derived growth factor in wound healing: synergistic effects with growth factors. *Proc Natl Acad Sci USA* 1987;84:7696–7697.
10. Robson M, Phillips L. Platelet-derived growth factor BB for the treatment of chronic pressure ulcers. *Lancet* 1992;339:23–25.
11. Mustoe T, Cutler N. A phase II study to evaluate recombinant platelet-derived growth factor- BB in the treatment of stage 3 and 4 pressure ulcers. *Arch Surg* 1994;129:212–219.
12. Steed DL. Diabetic Ulcer Study Group: clinical evaluation of recombinant human platelet-derived growth factor for the treatment of lower extremity diabetic ulcers. *J Vasc Surg* 1995;21:71–81.
12a. Wieman TJ, Smiell JM, Su, Y. Efficacy and safety of a topical gel formulation of recombinant human platelet-derived growth factor-BB (becaplermin) in patients with chronic neuropathic diabetic ulcers. A phase III randomized placebo-controlled double-blind study. *Diabetes Care* 1998;21:822–827.
12b. Wieman TJ. Clinical efficacy of becaplermin (rhPDGF-BB) gel. Becaplermin Gel Studies Group. *Am J Surg* 1998;176(Suppl 2A):74S–79S.
13. Sporn MB, Robert AB. Transforming growth factor. *JAMA* 1989;262:938–941.
14. McPherson J, Pratt B, Steed D, Robson M. Healing of diabetic foot ulcers using transforming growth factor-beta in collagen sponge, in *Abstracts of the Meeting of the European Tissue Repair Society*, August, 1999.
15. Brown GL, Curtsinger L, Nanney LB. Enhancement of wound healing by topical treatment with epidermal growth factor. *N Engl J Med* 1989;321:76–80.
16. Brown GL, Curtsinger L. Stimulation of healing of chronic wounds by epidermal growth factor. *Plast Reconstr Surg* 1991;88:189–194.

17. Robson M, Steed D, Jensen J. Keratinocyte growth factor 2 in the treatment of venous leg ulcers, in *Abstracts of the World Congress of Wound Healing*, September, 2000.

18. Spencer EM, Skover G, Hunt TK. Somatomedins: do they play a pivotal role in wound healing?, in *Growth Factors and Other Aspects of Wound Healing: Biological and Clinical Implications* (Barbul A, Pines E, Caldwell M, eds.), Alan R Liss, New York, 1988, pp. 103–106.

19. Steed DL, Goslen B, Hambley R, et al. Clinical trials with purified platelet releasate, in *Clinical and Experimental Approaches to Dermal and Epidermal Repair: Normal and Chronic Wounds* (Barbul A, ed.), Alan R Liss, New York, 1990, pp. 103–113.

20. Knighton DR, Ciresi KF. Classifications and treatment of chronic nonhealing wounds. *Ann Surg* 1986;104:322–330.

21. Knighton DR, Ciresi K. Stimulation of repair in chronic, nonhealing, cutaneous ulcers using platelet-derived wound healing formula. *Surg Gynecol Obstet* 1990;170:56–60.

22. Atri SC, Misra J. Use of homologous platelet factors in achieving total healing of recalcitrant skin ulcers. *Surgery* 1990;108:508–512.

23. Holloway GA, Steed DL, DeMarco MJ, et al. A randomized controlled dose response trial of activated platelet supernatant topical CT-102 (APST) in chronic nonhealing wounds in patients with diabete melitus. *Wounds* 1993;5:198–206.

24. Krupski WC, Reilly LM. A prospective randomized trial of autologous platelet-derived wound healing factors for treatment of chronic nonhealing wounds: a preliminary report. *J Vasc Surg* 1991;14:526–532.

25. Steed DL, Goslen JB, Holloway GA. CT-102 activated platelet supernatant, topical versus placebo: a randomized prospective double blind trial in healing of chronic diabetic foot ulcers. *Diabetes Care* 1992;15:1598–1604.

19

Living Skin Equivalents for Diabetic Foot Ulcers

Hau T. Pham, DPM, Thanh L. Dinh, DPM, and Aristidis Veves, MD

INTRODUCTION

Basic Principles of Wound Healing

Wound healing has posed a concern to the medical community since the early Stone Age and has since evolved through many ideologies. The ancient healers were cognizant of the importance of basic wound healing principles, such as eradicating necrotic tissue to promote healing, maintaining a moist wound environment, and preserving adequate wound coverage to prevent infection (1). The process of excising dead tissue evolved from the crude method of pouring hot oil into the wound to the more refined use of sharp debridement in vogue today. Preservation of a moist wound bed is a universally accepted standard that can be accomplished through a variety of means (2). The most commonly employed method involves the use of saline-moistened gauze. Although this technique is simple and economical, a number of technologically advanced dressings and modalities are available today that offer additional advantages to improve wound healing. Maintaining coverage of a wound has been more difficult to achieve, but with recent technologic advances, that problem may have a variety of solutions.

Wound Healing in Diabetes

The wounds of patients with diabetes are particularly difficult to manage, and they fail to heal for several reasons discussed elsewhere in this book. The cost of treating diabetic foot ulcers (DFUs) carries a high economic and social burden for many health care systems (3–5). In the United States, the direct cost of diabetic foot ulcers alone has been estimated at 150 million dollars in 1986 (ICD-9 CM 704). Each year, diabetic foot pathology affects approximately 7% of individuals with diabetes and is the leading complication resulting in hospitalization (6,7).

Owing to the staggering costs associated with DFU, adherence to a comprehensive wound care regimen has been instituted in an attempt to enhance healing time. A recent metaanalysis demonstrated that with good wound care, 24% of DFUs healed after 12 weeks, and 31% healed after 20 weeks (8). Although proper wound care has been shown to aid healing in DFU, efforts to develop better methods continue, largely because, disturbingly, failure to heal a DFU can lead to lower extremity amputation (9). DFUs are

From: *The Diabetic Foot: Medical and Surgical Management*
Edited by: A. Veves, J. M. Giurini, and F. W. LoGerfo © Humana Press Inc., Totowa, NJ

the single major risk factor for lower extremity amputation, with approximately 84% of the annual 500,000 amputations performed annually preceded by an ulcer. A multidisciplinary team approach to treating DFU has been found to be the most cost effective and successful in preventing the potentially devastating complication of amputation *(10)*. Unfortunately, the battle with DFU continues to be a losing one, despite many new treatment modalities, as evidenced by the continuing rise in diabetic lower extremity amputation rates over the last decade.

DFUs and Skin Grafting

The skin is an important organ of the body, providing the first line of defense against a number of potential pathogens. Human skin is composed of two layers: the outermost epidermis that is contiguous with the environment and the more inner dermis. The epidermis is structured by an ordered arrangement of keratinocytes cells responsible for the production of keratin, a complex filamentous protein that forms the surface coat of the skin. The principal component of the dermis is collagen, a fibrous protein synthesized by the fibroblast cell. Both keratinocytes and fibroblasts are essential to skin integrity and also play an important role in wound healing. Minor loss of skin integrity in the form of a cut or scrape may lead to cellulitis, abscess, or other skin infection. More major loss of skin can lead to a deeper and more severe infection, with major disability or even death resulting.

Poor wound healing in diabetic patients has been blamed on comorbidities such as peripheral neuropathy and macrovascular diseases. Neuropathy has been well documented as a major risk factor in the development of DFU. Vascular disease in the diabetic patient has been demonstrated to be at the posttibial vessels rather than at the microvasculatures *(11)*. There are functional defects at the small vessels that affect the blood flow to the area of injury *(12,13)*. Defects at the cellular level have also been implicated in delayed wound healing. For example, fibroblasts from chronic diabetic foot wounds have been shown to proliferate more slowly than in normal controls and also to express a different morphology *(14)*. Response to wound healing in diabetic patients had also been shown to be arrested at the inflammation phase.

Skin grafting affords one method of providing coverage to a chronic wound. Sir Astley Cooper is credited with performing the first successful skin graft *(15)* in 1817. Skin grafting has undergone considerable modification and improvement since its inception and has found use in challenging DFUs. Although skin grafting offers immediate availability, harvesting of the donor site may create a secondary wound with problematic healing. Furthermore, as discussed previously, the donor skin from a diabetic patient demonstrates defective cellular activity and may additionally lack the necessary growth factors essential for adequate wound healing. Because skin grafting provides the benefits of a biologic wound coverage and stimulation of wound healing, efforts have been made to find a suitable substitute for the epidermis, the dermis, or both layers.

For many decades, medical researchers sought methods to grow sheets of natural or synthetic human skin to treat many skin injuries. Research was mainly focused on the cellular components of the skin. Starting from small skin biopsies, researchers were able to grow sheets of keratinocytes in vitro. This was first reported in 1975 *(16)*, and scientists have since refined the process of growing skin cells. The technology of living skin equivalents (LSEs), the first product to emerge after years of research in tissue engineering, was born. Soon after, scientists were able to culture fibroblasts in vitro, and then the combination of natural, animal, and synthetic products, imparting stability to these in vitro skin cells. In many clinical studies, LSEs have demonstrated promise as adjunctive therapy for the treatment of burns and acute and chronic wounds. This chapter focuses on LSEs and their applications in DFU.

LIVING SKIN EQUIVALENTS

Cadaveric Allograft

Cadaveric allograft skin has been used successfully in providing temporary coverage of full-thickness burn wounds (17). The cadaver skin functions by closing and protecting the wound, thereby preventing life-threatening infections in already compromised burn patients. The cadaver skin is often removed at a later date, leaving behind a well-vascularized wound base that makes autografting more likely to take. Although this technique has proved life saving in many cases, the demand for cadaver skin is high and therefore it is not often available. Other serious drawbacks include the possibility of graft rejection and transmission of disease (18,19). Transmission of disease can occur owing to the lack of effectiveness in screening capabilities. Furthermore, at the time of graft harvesting, some transmittable diseases may not be fully expressed, causing further difficulty in screening procedures. The cadaveric allograft can be treated chemically to eradicate the possibility of infectious agents; however, the process itself results in an inert acellular dermal matrix with limited viability. The process of cryopreservation presents a second alternative to rid cadaver allograft of transmittable pathogens (20). Cryopreservation affords the allograft a longer storage life and availability but also makes the allograft more susceptible to sloughing off the wound bed.

Epidermal Replacements

Cultured epidermal grafts have been used successfully in the treatment of burn and chronic wounds (21–23). A cultured epithelial autograft technique is available for use in the United States (Epicel, Genzyme Tissue Repair, Cambridge, MA). The disadvantages with this technique include its high cost, a mandatory biopsy prior to application, and a 2–3-week delay in grafting to allow for sufficient epithelium to be cultured.

In contrast to the cultured epithelial autograft, cultured keratinocyte allografts were developed to be readily available with no inherent time delay prior to grafting. Keratinocyte allografts can be cryopreserved, allowing for a longer shelf life and increased availability (24,25). Cultured from neonatal foreskin cells, they can be placed in both acute and chronic wounds. Keratinocyte allografts have been used successfully to provide temporary wound coverage and stimulate wound healing (26–28). In some chronic wounds, it was found that the cultured cells stimulated the wound to heal from the edge, a normal healing process known as wound contraction. The disadvantages to these allografts include their expense and the additional risk of disease transmission owing to their allograft nature. Another major disadvantage with keratinocyte sheets is that they are fragile and very difficult to handle. They may fall apart if not held onto backing material. For this reason epidermal replacements are not suitable for use in full-thickness wounds. A dermal bed to support the epidermal component may add to the stability and durability of the cultured skin.

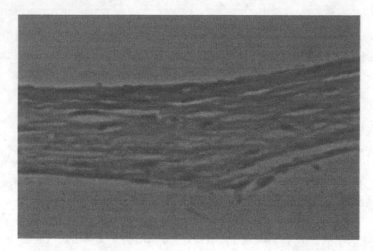

Fig. 1. Cross-section of Dermagraft showing collagen fibers in parallel bundles.

Dermal Replacements

As evidenced by the epidermal replacements, the epidermis is fragile when not supported by a dermal layer. Therefore, the cultivation of an adequate dermal substitute was initiated. The dermal element plays an important role in wound healing. It can have positive effects on epithelial migration, differentiation, attachment, and growth *(29)*. The first dermal graft utilized a collagen-based dermal analog of bovine collagen and chondroitin 6-sulfate with an outer Silastic cover (Integra, Integra Life Sciences, Plainsboro, NJ) This composite graft was used primarily in burn patients *(30)*.

Dermagraft

A variation in the preliminary composite graft gave rise to Dermagraft. In place of the bovine collagen, fibroblasts from neonatal foreskin were grown on a nylon mesh and covered with an outer silicone layer (Dermagraft-Transitional Covering, Advanced Tissue Sciences, La Jolla, CA). Dermagraft was designed to replace the dermal layer of the skin and to provide stimulus to improve wound healing. Histologic cross-sections of Dermagraft show collagen fibers arranged in parallel bundles, in a similar configuration to human skin (Fig. 1).

Dermagraft contains dermal fibroblasts cultured in vitro situated on a three-dimensional bioabsorbable mesh. The human fibroblasts are procured from newborn foreskin that is typically discarded following surgical circumcision. Supporting the fibroblasts is a mesh composed of polyglactin 910, a product commonly used in surgical suture and wound support. To ensure safety of the product, maternal blood samples are screened for exposure to infectious diseases. Maternal blood samples are tested for exposure to HIV, herpes simplex virus, hepatitis virus, and numerous other potential pathogens. The fibroblasts themselves are examined extensively for infectious agents prior to culturing and again at several stages during and after the manufacturing process. A closed bioreactor system used in the manufacturing process maintains sterility of the entire process. The Dermagraft is then cryopreserved for extended shelf life and availability. As a result of cryopreservation, the cells may lose some viability and therapeutic effect *(31)*.

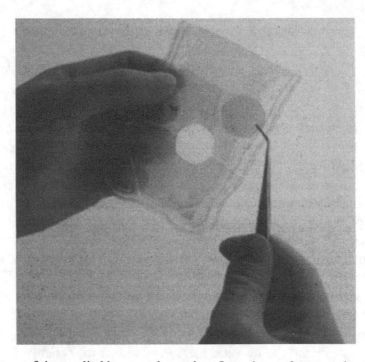

Fig. 2. Dermagraft is supplied in a translucent bag. It can be used to trace the ulcer and then the specimen can be cut to fit.

Dermagraft acts on a wound through cell colonization and provision of growth factors and cytokines. Following placement of Dermagraft into a wound, the fibroblasts proliferate across the mesh, secreting human dermal collagen, fibronectin, glycosaminoglycans (GAGs), growth factors, and other proteins in a self-produced dermal matrix. The final structure is comparable to the metabolically active papillary dermis of neonatal skin. Dermagraft boasts platelet-derived growth factor A, insulin-like growth factor (IGF), mitogen for keratinocytes, heparin-binding epidermal growth factor, transforming growth factors, vascular endothelial growth factor, and secreted protein acidic rich in cysteine. The matrix proteins and growth factors remain active after implantation onto the wound bed *(32,33)*. No exogenous human or animal collagen, GAG, or growth factors are added. The presence of the numerous growth factors appears to stimulate angiogenesis by upregulating cellular adhesion molecules *(34)*. Preclinical studies in animals indicated that Dermagraft incorporates quickly into the wound bed and vascularizes considerably during this process. Preclinical data also suggested that Dermagraft may present the additional benefit of limiting wound contraction and scarring.

Dermagraft is supplied as a 2 × 3-inch graft in a sealed plastic bag (Fig. 2) on dry ice. Storage at −70°C is necessary to preserve the integrity of the product, and this also affords the longer shelf life. Prior to application, Dermagraft must be rapidly thawed, warmed, and rinsed with sterile saline. The wound can be traced through the translucent packaging, with the Dermagraft cut to the exact wound dimensions and size. Following application to the wound, secondary dressings are used to keep the Dermagraft in place and maintain a moist wound environment.

402 Pham, Dinh, and Veves

CLINICAL APPLICATION

Dermagraft was initially proved useful in excised burn wounds (35). The prevalence of diabetic wounds prompted a study to investigate its therapeutic efficacy for DFUs. A small pilot study was performed on diabetic foot ulcers over a 12-week period (36). Fifty patients were enrolled and divided into four different treatment groups. Three of the four treatment groups received Dermagraft in a variety of applications in addition to conventional wound care over a 12-week period, whereas the control group received only conventional wound care. Patients in all groups were matched for similar demographic characteristics. After 12 weeks, the group treated with Dermagraft in eight separate applications achieved considerably more wound healing than the other three groups. The percentage of wound closures in this group was also significantly better than the control group. The Dermagraft-treated patients had no ulcer recurrence over a 14-month follow-up period.

After this promising pilot study, a large, multicenter, prospective study was conducted to investigate the effectiveness of Dermagraft for DFUs (37,38). A total of 281 patients were enrolled at 20 centers. Patients were randomized to receive either Dermagraft weekly for a total of eight applications or conventional dressing therapy alone. The control group, consisting of 126 patients, was treated with standard care and exhibited a 32% healing rate by the end of week 12. One-hundred nine patients received Dermagraft treatment, achieving a 39% healing rate by the end of week 12, a statistically nonsignificant result. Additionally, there was no significant difference with regard to adverse events, infection, or surgical intervention during the study.

After the completion of the above study, it was realized that a considerable number of patients had received application of Dermagraft with cells that were not in the indicated metabolic range. A retrospective analysis revealed that healing was most associated with a specific range of metabolic activity inherent in the graft itself. Thus, in the 76 patients who received metabolically active products for at least at the first application, 49% of the wounds healed by week 12. The 61 patients who received metabolically active products at the first two applications and with many subsequent applications had a 51% complete wound closure, whereas the highest healing rate of 54% was achieved in the 37 patients who received the correct metabolically active products at all applications (Fig. 3).

As a result of the above observations, a follow-up study was conducted to examine whether these results could be duplicated in a prospective (39). Thirty-nine patients at 12 centers completed the 12-week evaluation in this nonrandomized clinical study, and they all received Dermagraft with the appropriate metabolic range that ensured fibroblast recovery and new protein synthesis after implantation. The results showed that these patients had a 51% complete wound healing, very similar to the group that received metabolically active product in the previous study. Smaller, noncontrolled studies have also shown similar success for Dermagraft (40).

The producing company has also recently conducted a large, multicenter, randomized, placebo-controlled clinical trial. An initial data analysis has shown a 30% complete healing rate in the Dermagraft-treated patients compared with 18% in the control group. Dermagraft is under consideration for application in DFU.

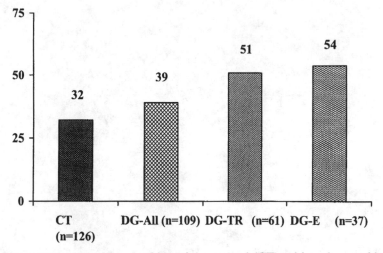

Fig. 3. Results of Dermagraft study. 32% of the control (CT) achieved wound healing compared with 39% of patients who received Dermagraft (DG-All) treatment ($p = 0.14$). Patients who received metabolically active products at the first two applications and most of the following application (DG-TR) achieved a 51% healing rate by week 12 ($p = 0.006$). Patients who received metabolically active products at all times (DG-E) achieved a 54% healing rate ($p = 0.007$).

Composite Replacements

Composite replacements incorporate both epidermal and dermal components. They are allogeneic, bilayered skin equivalents consisting of a well-differentiated human epidermis and a dermal layer of bovine collagen containing human fibroblasts. The first composite replacement (developed, cultured skin; CSS, Ortec International, New York, NY), integrated neonatal keratinocytes and fibroblasts cultured in a distinct bovine type I collagen layer *(41)*. This skin replacement was found to have limited use, was confined primarily to burns, and showed some efficacy for epidermolysis bullosa.

Graftskin (Apligraf)

Owing to the limitations of the initial composite replacement, a composite graft with multiple applications was developed for the coverage of full-thickness wounds. Apligraf is a bioengineered, allogeneic composite graft consisting of human epidermal cells, human fibroblasts, and type I bovine collagen (Graftskin, Organogenesis, Canton, MA). Simulating both epidermis and dermis, Apligraf features four components: epidermal keratinocytes, well-differentiated stratum corneum, extracellular matrix, and viable allogenic dermal fibroblasts.

Forming the epidermis, the keratinocytes also generate growth factors to encourage wound healing and achieve biologic wound closure. The keratinocytes initially multiply and then differentiate to replicate the architecture of the human epidermis. The stratum corneum imparts a natural barrier to mechanical damage, infection, and wound desiccation. The extracellular matrix incorporates type I bovine collagen organized into fibrils and fibroblast-produced proteins. This matrix promotes the ingrowth of cells, supports the scaffold for the three-dimensional structure of Apligraf, and grants

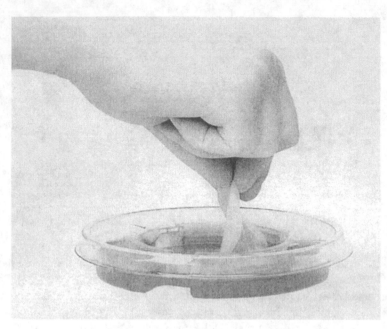

Fig. 4. Apligraf is manufactured in a culture medium disk approximately 3 inches in diameter. It looks and feels like human skin. It can be lifted off the disc and transferred to the wound.

mechanical stability and flexibility to the finished product. The dermal fibroblasts produce growth factors to stimulate wound healing, contribute to the formation of new dermal tissue, and provide factors that help to maintain the overlying epidermis.

Apligraf is manufactured under aseptic conditions. The manufacturing cycle is approximately 20 days. Both the dermal fibroblasts and keratinocytes are derived from discarded infant human foreskin. To ensure safety, blood samples of the maternal parent of the foreskin donor are screened and compared with normal ranges. Tests for a large number of infectious agents are performed, including anti-HIV virus antibody, HIV antigen, hepatitis, rapid plasma reagin, glutamic pyruvic transaminase, Epstein-Barr virus, and herpes simplex virus. Similarly, the donor cells are also scrutinized for any possible infectious pathogens and also for tumorigenic potential. Type I bovine collagen is extracted from the digital extensor tendon. The tendon is frozen, washed, ground, acid-extracted, salt-precipitated, and acid-treated again. The final product is a sterile, purified collagen. Each batch of collagen is tested rigorously by both in-house and outside certified testing facilities. All bovine material is obtained from countries free from bovine spongiform encephalopathy.

Apligraf is supplied as a circular sheet approximately 3 inches in diameter (44 cm^2) in a plastic container with gel-cultured medium. It looks and feels like human skin (Fig. 4). It contains all the matrix proteins and cytokines present in human skin (Table 1), but it does not contain Langerhans cells, melanocytes, lymphocytes, macrophages, blood vessels, sweat glands, and hair follicles (Fig. 5). The final product is delivered in a ready-to-use form on nutrient agarose in a sealed plastic bag that can be kept at room temperature for up to 5 days. Once the bag is opened, the product must be applied within 30 min-

Table 1
Cytokine Expression in Apligraf and Human Skin[1]

	Human keratinocytes	Human dermal fibroblasts	Apligraf	Human skin
FGF-1	+	+	+	+
FGF-2	–	+	+	+
FGF-7	–	+	+	+
ECGF	–	+	+	+
IGF-1	–	–	+	+
IGF-2	–	+	+	+
PDGF-AB	+	+	+	+
TGF-α	+	–	+	+
IL-1α	+	–	+	+
IL-6	–	+	+	+
IL-8	–	-	+	+
IL-11	–	+	+	+
TGF-β1	–	+	+	+
TGF-β3	–	+	+	+
VEGF	+	–	+	+

[1]Apligraf contains all the cytokines present in human skin. FGF, fibroblast growth factor; ECGF, endothelial cell growth factor; IGF, insulin-like growth factor; PDGF, platelet-derived growth factor, TGF, transforming growth factor; IL, interleukin; VEGF, vascular endothelial growth factor.

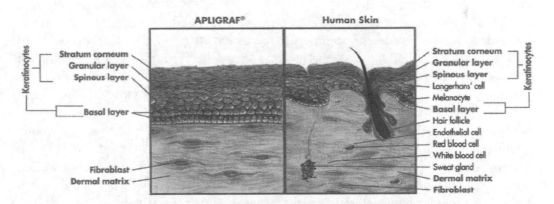

Fig. 5. Histology comparison between Apligraf and human skin showing that they are very similar. Apligraf lacks Langerhans cells and melanocytes at the epidermis level. At the dermis level, Apligraf contains no hair follicle, sweat glands, endothelial cells, or blood cells.

utes. The color of the agarose medium will change to indicate when the product is no longer usable. Located closest to the lid of the plastic container, the epidermal layer has a matt or dull finish. The dermal layer rests on the gel medium and demonstrates a glossy appearance. Application of Apligraf is both simple and quick. Prior to application, the wound bed should be debrided extensively of all necrotic tissue. The graft is then removed from its container and positioned with the dermal layer in direct contact with the wound bed. Apligraf can be trimmed to size, but overlap of the graft over the wound edge onto healthy surrounding tissues will not cause any harm. "Meshing" of the graft material allows for coverage of larger wounds and has the additional benefit of permitting drainage during the incorporation process. This can be done with a tissue expander or simply a scalpel. Although not necessary, suturing of Apligraf in place may be performed to ensure that the implant does not shift from the target wound. Secondary nonadhesive dressings are used to maintain the position of the implant and to sustain a moist wound environment.

CLINICAL APPLICATION

Apligraf first gained approval from the Food and Drug Administration for the treatment of venous leg ulcers *(42–44)*. Following its success in venous stasis ulcers, a prospective, multicenter, randomized, controlled clinical trial study was conducted to evaluate the efficacy of Apligraf in the treatment of chronic diabetic foot ulcers *(45)*. A total of 208 patients were enrolled in 24 centers across the country. Enrollment criteria included full-thickness diabetic neuropathic ulcers of greater than 2 weeks' duration with adequate circulation as evidenced by Doppler audible posterior tibial and dorsalis pedis pulses. Patients were excluded from the study if there was any evidence of clinical infection at the ulcer site, significant lower extremity ischemia, active Charcot disease, or an ulcer of nondiabetic pathophysiology. The patients were followed for 12 weeks, with an additional 3-month follow-up period to assess for any potential adverse side effects.

Of the 208 patients, 96 were randomized to the control group, receiving currently available state-of-the-art treatment. This treatment consisted of saline-moistened gauze changed twice daily. Additionally, all patients were instructed to avoid bearing weight on the affected foot and to use crutches or a wheelchair. The remaining 112 patients were randomized to the treatment group. In the treatment group, the ulcer was debrided and Apligraf applied in the customary aseptic technique. Apligraf treatment continued on a weekly basis until wound coverage occurred or the maximum of five applications was reached. After the fourth week, both treatment and control groups received identical state-of-the-art wound care regimens.

Apligraf-treated patients demonstrated significantly higher rates of complete wound healing compared with patients treated with the standard state-of-the-art care (Fig. 6). Improved wound healing in the Apligraf group was demonstrated as early as 4 weeks, with 20% of patients reaching complete wound healing compared with 3% in the control group. This trend continued throughout the 12-week study period, with 56% of Apligraf-treated patients attaining complete wound closure compared with 39% of the controls by the end of week 12. Complete wound closure in the Apligraf treatment group required an average of 3.9 applications per patient. The median time to 100% wound closure was also reduced to 65 days in the Apligraf group compared with 90 days for the control group.

In addition to enhanced wound closure, the wounds treated with Apligraf showed improvement in wound characteristics such as diminished undermining, maceration, exudate, eschar, and fibrin slough. Furthermore, the rates of osteomyelitis and lower limb amputations were significantly lower in the Apligraf group. This encouraging ancillary discovery may indicate that Apligraf, through augmented wound coverage, can prevent the deep tissue infection that leads to amputation. Ulcer recurrence rate

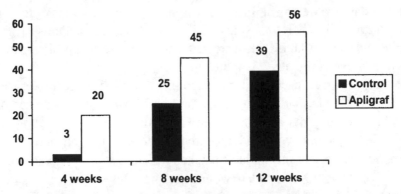

Fig. 6. Results of Multicenter Apligraf study. The difference between the control and Apligraf treatment is apparent early in the study. At week 4, 3% of patients who received control treatment had wound healing compared with 20% of patients who received Apligraf once a week for the first 4 weeks. At week 8, 25% of control patients achieved wound healing compared with 45% of the Apligraf-treated patients. By week 12, 39% of the control patients achieved complete wound healing compared with 56% of the patients who received Apligraf treatment ($p = 0.0026$).

was observed to be slightly less in the Apligraf treatment group but not significantly different. This finding suggests that wound healing with Apligraf results in a closure with comparable viscoelastic properties to healing via secondary intention.

Adverse events such as wound infection and cellulitis were also not significantly different in either the treatment or control groups. Previous studies have demonstrated that Apligraf does not elicit an immunologic response from the host, and therefore rejection of Apligraf is not a concern. This study also confirmed that finding, as there was no observable antibody or T-cell-specific responses against bovine type I collagen, human fibroblasts, or human keratinocytes. It is postulated that an immunologic response does not occur because the neonatal fibroblasts lack the HLA-DR surface antigens, the antigens responsible for generating allograft rejection *(43)*.

The healing rate in Apligraf-treated patients was highest in the center with the best recruitment *(46)*, indicating the existence of a learning curve in the clinical use of Apligraf. In addition, the healing rate in the control group in the whole study was higher in a metaanalysis of 10 other control groups. This reflects the benefits derived from centers with a multidisciplinary approach to DFU using standard state-of-the-art care. When the standard wound care regimen was supplemented with Apligraf, healing rates were enhanced.

In an effort to identify the patients who proceed to heal their ulcers, the healing rates for both control and treatment groups were calculated using weekly wound tracings. The first four weekly measurements were used. In the patients who did not heal their ulcer, the healing rate was 0.05 cm/week for the control-treated and 0.06 cm/week for the Apligraf-treated patients. In contrast, in the healed patients, the closure rate was 0.11 cm/week for the control and 0.14 cm/week for the Apligraf-treated patients. These results indicate that Apligraf should not be expected to increase the healing rate to levels considerably higher than those observed in patients who are going to heal their ulcers while on standard treatment. Instead, it should be expected that Apligraf increases the healing rate from the levels that were observed in nonhealing patients to the levels of the healing wounds and sustained this increased healing rate for the prolonged period that is required to achieve complete wound healing.

Apligraf has also been used with considerable success for the treatment of burn wounds, epidermolysis bullosa in newborns, acute surgical wounds, and as a donor site for split-thickness skin graft *(47–50)*. Apligraf may also aid wound healing in difficult wounds in diabetic patients with end-stage renal disease. Unpublished data from the authors' experience suggests that diabetic patients with end-stage renal disease on hemodialysis were able to achieve complete wound healing of chronic ulcers using Apligraf in addition to normal good wound care and off-loading technique.

LSE IN CLINICAL PRACTICE

The exact mechanism of action of living skin equivalents is still being considerably discussed and researched. The specific mechanism of action is unclear, but it is believed that cultured epidermal cells provide a temporary coverage for the wound until the host cells can play an active role in wound healing. It is hypothesized that stimulation of host cells to proliferate occurs owing to the release of growth factors and cytokines by the neonatal epidermal cells. Additionally, the wound is filled with an extracellular matrix that has been described as a smart matrix, recruiting cells necessary for healing to the wound site.

Although LSEs have demonstrated improved wound healing rates, improved wound closure, and reduced median time to closure, their use carries a considerable cost and should therefore be reserved for chronic foot ulcers that have failed to respond with standard care. However, the exorbitant cost of foot ulceration suggests that even expensive new modalities may be cost-effective when evaluated over the long term *(51,52)*. Until cost analysis studies are performed, LSEs remain a useful adjunct for the management of DFUs resistant to the currently available standard of care. Our healing rate analysis demonstrates that if a wound does not show significant progress (closing at less than 0.1 cm/week after 4 weeks of good standard wound care), then the use of proven adjunctive therapy such as LSEs can enhance the healing potential.

REFERENCES

1. Peacock JL, Lawrence WT, Peacock EE, Jr. Wound healing, in *The Physiologic Basis of Surgery* (O'Leary JP, Capote LR, eds.), Williams & Wilkins, Baltimore, 1993.
2. Field FK, Kerstein MD. Overview of wound healing in a moist environment. *Am J Surg* 1994;167:2S–6S.
3. Ramsey SD, Newton K, Blough D, et al. Incidence, outcomes and cost of foot ulcers in patients with diabetes. *Diabetes Care* 1999;22:382–387.
4. Apelqvist J. Wound healing in diabetes. Outcomes and costs. *Clin Podiatr Med Surg* 1998; 15:21–39.
5. Reiber GE, Lipsky BA, Gibbons GW. The burden of diabetic foot ulcers. *Am J Surg* 1998; 176(2A Suppl):5S–10S.
6. Harrington C, Zagari MJ, Corea J, Klitenic J. A cost analysis of diabetic lower-extremity ulcers. *Diabetes Care* 2000;23:1333–1338.
7. Reiber GE. Diabetic foot care: financial implications and guidelines. *Diabetes Care* 1992; 15(Suppl 1):29–31.

8. Margolis DJ, Kantor J, Berlin JA. Healing of diabetic neuropathic foot ulcers receiving standard treatment: a meta-analysis. *Diabetes Care* 1999;22:692–695.

9. Reiber GE, Boyko EJ, Smith DG. Lower extremity foot ulcers and amputations in diabetes, in *Diabetes in America*, 2nd ed (National Diabetes Data Group, ed.), National Institutes of Health, Washington 1995, pp. 409–428.

10. Apelqvist J, Larson J. What is the most effective way to reduce the incidence of amputation in the diabetic foot? *Diabetes Metab Res Rev* 2000;16(Suppl 1):S75–S83.

11. LoGerfo FW, Coffman JD. Vascular and microvascular disease of the foot in diabetes: implications for foot care. *N Engl J Med* 1984;311:1615–1618.

12. Veves A, Akbari CM, Primavera J, et al. Endothelial dysfunction and the expression of endothelial nitric oxide synthetase in diabetic neuropathy, vascular disease, and foot ulceration. *Diabetes* 1998;47:457–463.

13. Pham HT, Economides PA, Veves A. The role of endothelial function on the foot. Microcirculation and wound healing in patients with diabetes. *Clin Podiatr Med Surg* 1998;15:85–93.

14. Loots MAM, Lamme JR, Mekkes JR, Bos JD, Middlekoop E. Cultured fibroblasts from chronic diabetic wounds on the lower extremity (non-insulin-dependent diabetes mellitus) show disturbed proliferation. *Arch Dermatol Res* 1999;291:93–99.

15. McCarthy JG (ed.). *Introduction to Plastic Surgery*. WB Saunders, Philadelphia, 1990, pp. 1–68.

16. Rheinwald JG, Green H. Serial cultivation of strains of human epidermal keratinocytes: the formation of keratinizing colonies from single cells. *Cell* 1975;6:331–344.

17. Greenleaf G, Hansbrough JF. Current trends in the use of allograft skin for burn patients and reflections on the future of skin banking in the United States. *J Burn Care Rehabil* 1995;15:428.

18. Greenleaf G, Cooper ML, Hansbrough JF. Microbial contamination in allografted wound beds in patients with burns. *J Burn Care Rehabil* 1991;12:442.

19. Kealey GP. Disease transmission by means of allografts. *J Burn Care Rehabil* 1997;18:10–11.

20. Kolenik SA III, Lefell DJ. The use of cryopreserved human skin allografts in wound healing following Mohs surgery. *Dermatol Surg* 1995;21:615–620.

21. Phillips TJ, Gilchrest BA. Clinical applications of cultured epithelium. *Epithelial Cell Biol* 1992;1:39–46.

22. Odyssey R. Multicenter experience with cultured epidermal autografts for treatment of burns. *J Burn Care Rehabil* 1992;13:174–180.

23. Limova M, Mauro T. Treatment of leg ulcers with cultured epithelial autografts: treatment protocol and five year experience. *Wounds* 1995;7:170–180.

24. Teepe RGC, Koebrugge EJ, Ponec M, Vermeer BJ. Fresh versus cryopreserved allografts for the treatment of chronic skin ulcers. *Br J Dermatol* 1990;122:81–89.

25. Teepe RGC, Roseeuw DI, Hermans D, et al. Randomized trial comparing cryopreserved cultured epidermal allografts with hydrocolloid dressings in healing chronic venous ulcers. *J Am Acad Dermatol* 1993;29:982–988.

26. Phillips T. Cultured epidermal allografts: a temporary or permanent solution? *Transplantation* 1991;51:937–941.

27. Phillips T, Ghawan J, Leigh IM, et al. Cultured epidermal allografts: a study of differentiation and allograft survival. *J Am Acad Dermatol* 1990;23:189–198.

28. Phillips TJ, Kehinde O, Green H, Gilchrest BA. Treatment of skin ulcers with cultured epidermal allografts. *J Am Acad Dermatol* 1989;21:191–199.

29. Clark RAF. Basics of cutaneous wound repair. *J Dermatol Surg Oncol* 1993;19:693–706.

30. Burke JF, Yannas IV, Quinby WC, et al. Successful use of physiologically acceptable artificial skin in the treatment of extensive burn injury. *Ann Surg* 1981;194:413–428.

31. Mansbridge J, Liu K, Patch R, Symons K, Pinney E. Three-dimensional fibroblast culture implant for the treatment of diabetic foot ulcers: metabolic activity and therapeutic range. *Tissue Eng* 1998;4:403–411.

32. McColgan M, Foster A, Edmonds M. Dermagraft in the treatment of diabetic foot ulcers. *Diabet Foot* 1998;1:75–78.
33. Landeen LK, Zeigler FC, Halberstadt C, et al. Characterisation of a human dermal replacement. *Wounds* 1992;5:167–175.
34. Jiang WG, Harding KG. Enhancement of wound tissue expansion and angiogenesis by matrix-embedded fibroblasts (Dermagraft), a role of hepatocyte growth factor. *Int J Mol Med* 1998; 2:203–210.
35. Perdue GF. Dermagraft-TC pivotal safety and efficacy study. *J Burn Care Rehabil* 1996; 18:S13–S14.
36. Gentzkow GD, Iwasaki SD, Hershon KS, et al. Use of Dermagraft, a cultured human dermis, to treat diabetic foot ulcers. *Diabetes Care* 1996;19:350–354.
37. Pollak RA, Edington H, Jensen JL, Kroeker RO, Gentzkow GD, and the Dermagraft Diabetic Ulcer Study Group. A human dermal replacement for the treatment of diabetic foot ulcers. *Wounds* 1997;9:175–178.
38. Naughton G, Mansbridge J, Gentzkow G. A metabolically active human dermal replacement for the treatment of diabetic foot ulcers. *Artificial Organs* 1997;21:1203–1210.
39. Gentzkow GD, Pollak RA, Kroeker RO, et al. Implantation of a living human dermal replacement to heal diabetic foot ulcers. Presented at the 58th American Diabetes Association Scientific Sessions in Chicago, June 13–16, 1998.
40. Bowering CK. The use of Dermagraft in the treatment of diabetic foot ulcers. *J Cutan Med Surg* 1998;3(Suppl 1):S1–S29–S32.
41. Schwartz S. A new composite cultured skin product for treatment of burns and other deep dermal injury. Presented at the Bioengineering of Skin Substitute Conference, September 19, 1997, Boston, MA.
42. Sabolinski ML, Alvarez O, Auletta M, et al. Cultured skin as a "smart material" for healing wounds: experience in venous ulcers. *Biomaterials* 1996;17:311–320.
43. Falanga V, Margolis D, Alverez O, et al. Healing of venous ulcer and lack of clinical rejection with an allogenic cultured human skin equivalent. *Arch Dermatol* 1998;134:293–300.
44. Falanga V, Sabolinski M. A bilayered living skin construct (Apligraf) accelerates complete closure of hard-to-heal venous ulcers. *Wound Repair Regen* 1999;7:201–207.
45. Veves A, Falanga V, Armstrong DG, Sabolinski ML, for the Apligraf Diabetic Foot Ulcer Study Group. Graftskin, a human skin equivalent, is effective in the management of the non-infected neuropathic diabetic foot ulcers: a prospective, randomized, multicenter clinical trial. *Diabetes Care* 2001;24:290–295.
46. Pham HT, Rosenblum BI, Lyons TE, et al. Evaluation of Graftskin (Apligraf®), a human skin equivalent, for the treatment of diabetic foot ulcers in a prospective, randomized, clinical trial. *Wounds* 1999;11:79–86.
47. Falabella AF, Schachner LA, Valencia IC, Eaglstein WH. The use of tissue-engineering skin (Apligraf) to treat a newborn with epidermolysis bullosa. *Arch Dermatol* 1999;135: 1219–1222.
48. Eaglstein WH, Iriondo M, Laszlo K. A composite skin substitute (Graftskin) for surgical wounds. A clinical experience. *Dermatol Surg* 1995;21:839–843.
49. Eaglstein WH, Alverez OM, Auletta M, et al. Acute excisional wounds treated with a tissue-engineering skin (Apligraf). *Dermatol Surg* 1999;25:195–201.
50. Kirsner RS. The use of Apligraf in acute wounds. *J Dermatol* 1998;25:805–811.
51. Schonfeld WH, Villa KF, Fastenau JM, Mazonson PD, Falanga V. An economic assessment of Apligraf (Graftskin) for the treatment of hard-to-heal venous leg ulcers. *Wound Repair Regen* 2000;8:251–257.
52. Allenet B, Paree F, Lebrun T, et al. Cost-effectiveness modeling of Dermagraft for the treatment of diabetic foot ulcers in the French context. *Diabetes Metab* 2000;26:125–132.

20

Vascular Surgery for the Diabetic Foot

Frank B. Pomposelli, Jr., MD and David R. Campbell, MD

INTRODUCTION

Foot problems remain the most common reason for hospitalization of patients with diabetes mellitus (1,2). Approximately 20% of the 12–15 million diabetics in the United States can expect to be hospitalized for a foot problem at least once during their lifetime, and they account for an annual health care cost for this problem alone in excess of 1 billion dollars (3). The primary pathologic mechanisms of neuropathy and ischemia set the stage for pressure necrosis, ulceration, and multimicrobial infection, which, if improperly treated ultimately leads to gangrene and amputation (4). Understanding how the factors of neuropathy, ischemia, and infection are impacting on an individual patient with a foot complication and simultaneously effecting proper treatment for all factors present is essential to foot salvage. Although this chapter focuses on the treatment of ischemia caused by arterial insufficiency, it is important to remember that ischemia is accompanied by infection in approximately 50% of patients in our experience (5) and that most (if not all) patients will have peripheral neuropathy present as well. While focusing on correction of ischemia, often by arterial reconstruction, the vascular surgeon cannot ignore these other factors if foot salvage is ultimately to be successful.

Vascular Disease in Diabetics

A detailed discussion of vascular disease in diabetics can be found elsewhere in this book. The most important principle in treating foot ischemia in patients with diabetes is recognizing that the cause of their presenting symptoms is macrovascular occlusion of the leg arteries owing to atherosclerosis. In the past, many clinicians incorrectly assumed that gangrene, nonhealing ulcers, and poor healing of minor amputations or other foot procedures were caused by microvascular occlusion of the arterioles—so-called small vessel disease (6). This concept, although erroneous and subsequently refuted in several studies (7–11), persists to this day. In the minds of many clinicians and their patients, this concept has resulted in a pessimistic attitude toward treatment of ischemia that all too often leads to an unnecessary limb amputation without an attempt at arterial reconstruction. This attitude and approach is antiquated and inappropriate and must be discouraged in the strongest of terms. In the author's opinion, rejection of the small vessel theory alone could probably decrease the 40-fold increased risk of major limb amputation that those with diabetes face during their lifetime compared with nondiabetic counterparts.

From: *The Diabetic Foot: Medical and Surgical Management*
Edited by: A. Veves, J. M. Giurini, and F. W. LoGerfo © Humana Press Inc., Totowa, NJ

Atherosclerosis in Diabetes

Although histologically similar to disease in nondiabetics, atherosclerosis in the patient with diabetes has certain clinically relevant differences. Previous studies have confirmed that diabetes mellitus is a strong independent risk factor for atherosclerotic coronary *(12,13)*, cerebrovascular *(14)*, and peripheral vascular disease *(14)*. Patients with diabetes face a higher likelihood of cardiovascular mortality. In addition, generalized atherosclerosis is more prevalent and progresses more rapidly in diabetic patients. In those patients presenting with ischemic symptoms of the lower extremity, gangrene and tissue loss are more likely to be present compared with nondiabetics. Diabetic patients with coronary atherosclerosis are more likely to have so-called silent ischemia—absence of typical anginal symptoms or pain with myocardial infarction, particularly in those patients with significant polyneuropathy *(15)*.

These findings suggest that arterial reconstruction in these patients carries a higher risk of adverse outcome, particularly myocardial infarction and/or death. In fact, both Lee et al. *(16)* and Eagle et al. *(17)* have listed diabetes mellitus as an independent risk factor for adverse cardiac outcomes in patients undergoing major surgery. Our personal experience, however, in well over 3000 patients undergoing lower extremity arterial reconstruction in the last decade, refutes this position. In a recent study of nearly 800 lower extremity bypass procedures performed in patients with diabetes followed for a minimum of 5 years after surgery, the in-hospital mortality rate was 1% and the long-term graft patency, limb salvage, and patient survival rates were comparable or better than those of nondiabetic patients treated in the same time period *(18)* (Fig. 1). In our opinion, careful perioperative management, including an aggressive approach invasive cardiac monitoring in the early postoperative period, has been responsible for the low cardiac morbidity and mortality rate in these high-risk patients.

From the vascular surgeon's perspective, the most important difference in lower extremity atherosclerosis in diabetics is the location of atherosclerotic occlusive lesions in the artery supplying the leg and the foot *(8,10)*. In patients without diabetes, atherosclerosis most commonly involves the infrarenal aorta, iliac arteries, and superficial femoral artery with relative sparing of the more distal arteries. In patients with diabetes, however, the most significant occlusive lesion occurs in the crural arteries distal to the knee, the anterior tibial artery, peroneal artery, or posterior tibial artery, but with sparing of the arteries of the foot (Fig. 2). This pattern of occlusive disease, known as *tibial artery disease*, requires a different approach to vascular reconstruction and presents special challenges for the surgeon (see below). Moreover, diabetic patient who smoke may have a combination of both patterns of disease, making successful revascularization more complex.

PATIENT SELECTION

Many patients with diabetes will have evidence of peripheral vascular disease manifested by absence of palpable leg or foot pulses with either minimal or no symptoms. In these patients, disease is well compensated and no treatment is necessary other than education about vascular disease including signs and symptoms and reduction of associated risk factors, particularly cessation of smoking. Regular follow-up exams, usually at a 6–12-month interval, are reasonable. Many clinicians will obtain baseline noninva-

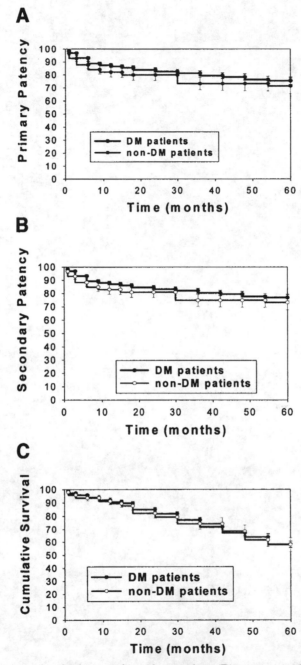

Fig. 1. Life table analysis of primary (**A**) and secondary (**B**) patency and survival (**C**) in 800 diabetic and nondiabetic patients undergoing lower extremity bypass at the Beth Israel Deaconess Medical Center since 1990, with a minimal follow-up of at least 5 years. No significant differences were noted.

sive arterial testing at this point, although this is not mandatory. Many such patients have associated coronary and carotid atherosclerosis, which may also be asymptomatic. Routine screening for disease in these territories in the absence of symptoms, purely based on evidence of lower extremity atherosclerosis, may be appropriate in individual patients but probably not cost-effective as a routine in all such patients.

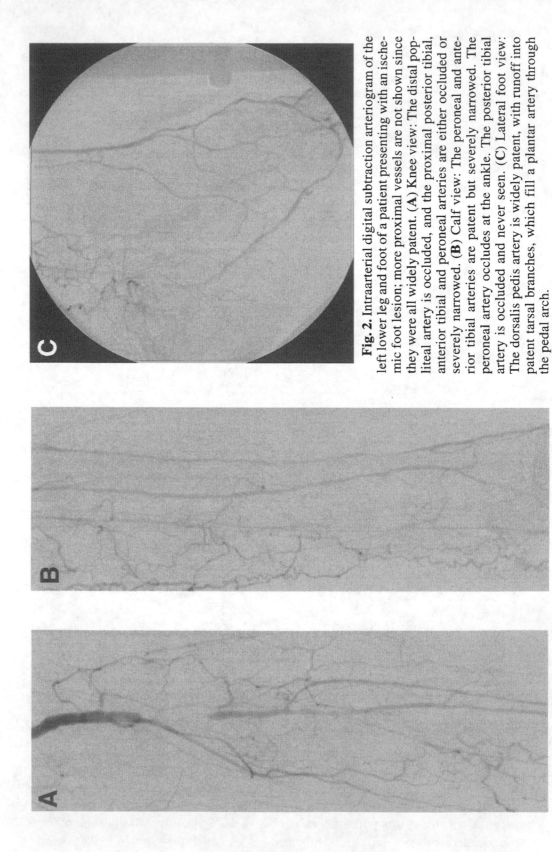

Fig. 2. Intraarterial digital subtraction arteriogram of the left lower leg and foot of a patient presenting with an ischemic foot lesion; more proximal vessels are not shown since they were all widely patent. (**A**) Knee view: The distal popliteal artery is occluded, and the proximal posterior tibial, anterior tibial and peroneal arteries are either occluded or severely narrowed. (**B**) Calf view: The peroneal and anterior tibial arteries are patent but severely narrowed. The peroneal artery occludes at the ankle. The posterior tibial artery is occluded and never seen. (**C**) Lateral foot view: The dorsalis pedis artery is widely patent, with runoff into patent tarsal branches, which fill a plantar artery through the pedal arch.

414

In patients presenting with typical symptoms mandating treatment, several factors must be taken into consideration. Certain patients may not be appropriate for arterial reconstruction, such as those with dementia and/or other organic brain syndromes who are nonambulatory or bedridden and have no likelihood of successful rehabilitation. Similarly, patients with severe flexion contractures of the knee or hip are poor candidates. Patients with terminal cancer with very short life expectancy or similar lethal comorbidities do poorly with vascular reconstruction and are also probably better served by primary amputations. Patients with an unsalvageable foot owing to extensive necrotizing infection, even when ischemic, likewise require primary amputation. However, in other patients presenting with infection complicating ischemia, proper control of spreading infection must be accomplished prior to arterial reconstruction. Broad-spectrum intravenous antibiotics to cover Gram-positive, Gram-negative, and anaerobic organisms should be started immediately after cultures are taken, since most infections in diabetics are multimicrobial *(1,19)*. Once culture data are available, antibiotics can then be appropriately adjusted. In addition, those patients with abscess formation, septic arthritis, necrotizing fasciitis, and so on should undergo prompt incision, drainage, and debridement including partial open toe, ray, or forefoot amputation *(20)* as indicated (Fig. 3).

In our series of pedal bypasses, secondary infection was present at the time of presentation in over 50% of patients *(21)*. Infection places an increased metabolic demand on already ischemic tissues and may accelerate and exacerbate tissue necrosis. Since many diabetic patients have a blunted neurogenic inflammatory response, typical inflammatory signs of infection may be absent or diminished. It is therefore imperative that all ulcers be carefully probed and inspected and superficial eschar unroofed to look for potential deep space abscesses, which are not readily apparent from visual inspection of the foot. The need to control spreading infection may delay vascular surgery for several days, but waiting longer than necessary to sterilize wounds is inappropriate and may result in further necrosis and tissue loss. Signs of resolving spreading infection include reduction of fever, resolution of cellulitis and lymphangitis, particularly in areas of potential surgical incisions, and return of glycemic control, which is probably the most sensitive indicator of improvement. During this period, which rarely extends beyond 4 or 5 days, contrast arteriography and other presurgical evaluations such as testing for coronary disease when necessary can be performed so that vascular surgery may be undertaken without subsequent delay.

In occasional patients infection cannot be totally eradicated prior to bypass. Patients with severe ischemia may have inadequate blood flow to distal sites to deliver adequate tissue penetration of antibiotics until arterial blood flow has been adequately restored. It is important in these patients to continue antibiotic coverage for several days following arterial reconstructive surgery. Occasionally, patients will seem to have worsening of their infection after revascularization owing to the enhanced inflammatory response that is possible once arterial blood flow has been restored.

It is important to realize that age alone is not a contraindication to arterial reconstruction. We have successfully performed these procedures in selected patients over the age of 90. When selecting patients for arterial reconstruction, the functional and physiologic status of the patient is far more important than chronologic age. In fact, a limb-salvaging arterial reconstruction may mean the difference for an elderly patient

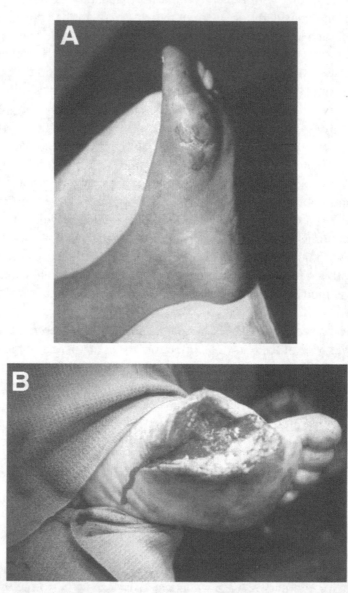

Fig. 3. Photographs of the right foot of a patient with diabetes who presented with a rapidly spreading infection as a result of a plantar ulcer over the first metatarsal. (**A**) Marked swelling and erythema of the medial forefoot is evident. There was palpable crepitus and malodorous drainage due to involvement of the bone, joint, and flexor tendon with gas-forming bacteria. (**B**) Control of this infection required an emergent open first ray amputation. Cultures grew multiple organisms including *Staph aureus*, *proteus*, and anaerobes.

between continued independent living and the need for permanent custodial nursing home care. We recently evaluated our results with arterial reconstruction in a cohort of patients who were 80 years of age or older at the time of arterial reconstruction, evaluating both the rate of success of the initial procedure and two important quality of life outcomes—the ability to ambulate and whether or not the patient returned to his or her own residence following surgery. At 1 year following surgery, the vast majority (>80%) was still ambulatory and residing in their homes either alone or with relatives *(22)*.

Patients with limb ischemia who present with signs and symptoms of coronary disease such as worsening angina, recent congestive heart failure, or recent myocardial infarction need to have stabilization of their cardiac disease prior to arterial reconstruction. Occasionally angioplasty or even coronary artery bypass grafting may be required prior to lower extremity surgery, although in our experience this has been unusual. Moreover, routine noninvasive cardiac evaluation in all patients has proved both costly and unnecessary. Virtually all diabetic patients with lower extremity ischemia have occult coronary disease *(23)*. Consequently, screening tests such as dipyridmole-thallium imaging are almost always abnormal to some degree. Attempting to quantify the degree of abnormality with such testing has occasionally proved useful in stratifying those patients at excessive risk for perioperative cardiac morbidity or mortality; however, most such patients with severely abnormal scans usually have obvious clinical signs or symptoms as well *(24)*. As a result, we rely mostly on the patient's clinical presentation and electrocardiogram in determining when further evaluation is needed, and we use imaging studies selectively in those patients with unclear or atypical symptoms. In asymptomatic patients who are reasonably active with no acute changes on an electrocardiogram, no further studies are generally undertaken. We have found that frequent use of invasive perioperative cardiac monitoring (including pulmonary arterial catheters along with anesthesia management by personnel accustomed to treating patients with ischemic heart disease and managing patients in a specialized, subacute, monitored unit with cardiac monitoring capabilities) in the early postoperative period has significantly reduced perioperative cardiac morbidity and mortality in our patients. Moreover, in a recent prospective randomized trial the type of anesthesia given (i.e., spinal, epidural, or general endotracheal) did not affect the incidence of perioperative cardiac complications *(25)* or graft thrombosis *(26)*.

Patients with renal failure present special challenges. When acute renal insufficiency occurs, most commonly following contrast arteriography, surgery is delayed until renal function stabilizes or returns to normal. Most such patients will demonstrate a transient rise in serum creatinine without other symptoms. It is rare that such patients will become anuric or require hemodialysis. Withholding contrast arteriography in patients with diabetes and compromised renal function is therefore generally inappropriate and unnecessary. If there are severe concerns about renal function, magnetic resonance angiography (see below) can usually provide adequate images to plan arterial reconstruction *(27)*.

Patients with chronic, dialysis-dependent renal function can safely undergo arterial recon-struction. Many such patients have severe, advanced atherosclerosis with target arteries that are often heavily calcified. Gangrene and tissue loss are frequently present, and the healing response in such patients is poor, even with restoration of arterial blood flow. Studies have demonstrated that graft patency and limb salvage (although reasonable) in these patients are less often successful than in patients without chronic renal failure *(28–31)*. Some such patients will require amputation even with patent arterial bypass grafts. Careful patient selection is therefore extremely important. Further study is clearly needed in this patient population to determine which patients with chronic renal failure are most likely to have a favorable outcome from arterial reconstructive surgery and which patients might be better treated with primary amputation.

EVALUATION AND DIAGNOSTIC STUDIES

Patients requiring surgical intervention for lower extremity arterial insufficiency usually present with severely disabling intermittent claudication or signs and symptoms of limb-threatening ischemia. Intermittent claudication is pain, cramping, or a sensation of severe fatigue in the muscles of the leg, which occurs with walking and is promptly relieved by rest. Many patients adjust their lifestyle to minimize or eliminate any significant walking. The location of discomfort can give hints to the location of the disease. Patients with aortoiliac atherosclerosis will often complain of buttock and thigh pain, whereas patients with femoral disease will typically have calf discomfort, although patients with aortoiliac occlusive disease can have calf claudication as their only presenting symptom. Patients with tibial arterial occlusive disease will also have calf claudication and may also complain of foot discomfort or numbness with walking. Nocturnal muscle cramping, which is a common complaint among patients with diabetes, is not a typical symptom of vascular disease, even though it may involve the calf muscles, and should not be mistaken for intermittent claudication.

Most patients with intermittent claudication do not require surgical intervention. Studies on the natural history of claudication have demonstrated that progression to limb-threatening ischemia is uncommon *(32,33)*. Many patients respond to conservative treatment measures such as cessation of tobacco use, correction of risk factors for atherosclerosis, weight reduction when necessary, and an exercise program involving walking *(34)*. Additionally, two medications are available; pentoxifilline, 400 mg orally three times daily, or cilostazol, 100 mg orally twice daily, which have been demonstrated to improve walking distance in patients with claudication caused by atherosclerosis *(35–37)*. Both drugs are generally well tolerated but need to be taken for several weeks before improvement in walking distance can be appreciated. In the authors' experience, pentoxifilline has been disappointing in relieving claudication symptoms. The more recently released cilostazol has been more effective, but it has more side effects and is contraindicated in patients with a history of congestive heart failure. In most cases, we start with exercise and risk factor reduction alone as a first step and add a medication later if necessary. Surgical intervention for claudication is reserved for those patients who are severely disabled, with a very limited functional capacity, unable to work owing to their symptoms, or who have not responded to more conservative treatment. In the authors' experience, patient noncompliance is the most common reason for failure of conservative treatment measures.

Most diabetic patients referred for vascular intervention have limb-threatening ischemic problems, which if not promptly treated are likely to result ultimately in amputation. The most common presenting problem is a nonhealing ulcer with or without associated gangrene and infection. Many patients will initially develop an ulcer as a result of neuropathy, which will then not heal in spite of proper treatment, owing to associated arterial insufficiency—the so-called neuropathic ischemic ulcer. Some patients are referred after a minor surgical procedure in the foot fails to heal due to ischemia. Patients with limb-threatening ischemia can also present with ischemic rest pain with or without associated tissue loss. Ischemic rest pain typically occurs in the distal foot, particularly the toes. It is exacerbated by recumbency and relieved by dependency. Patients often give a history of noticing pain, numbness, or paresthesias when retiring

Table 1
Distinguishing Features of Ischemic Rest Pain and Painful Neuropathy

Rest pain	Neuropathy
Usually unilateral	Often bilateral
Consistently present	Waxes and wanes
Relieved by dependency of foot	Not relieved by dependecy
Always associated with absent pulses	Pulses may be present and normal

for bed, which is then relieved by placing the foot in a dependent position. Patients often do not recognize that placing the foot in a dependent position is the cause of relief and may associate relief with other maneuvers such as walking and stamping the involved foot on the floor or getting up and taking an oral analgesic. It is important but occasionally difficult to differentiate rest pain from painful diabetic neuropathy, which may also be subjectively worse at night (Table 1). Neuropathic patients may also present with no rest pain in spite of overt severe foot ischemia owing to the complete loss of sensation. Nocturnal muscle cramps are a common complaint, but these are not caused by arterial insufficiency.

The noninvasive vascular laboratory *(38,39)* is particularly useful in those diabetic patients presenting with pain in the foot and absent pulses in whom the etiology is unclear and may be owing to either ischemia or painful diabetic neuropathy. Patients with severe ischemia will usually have ankle-brachial indices of <0.4. In patients with diabetes, however, care must be taken in interpreting ankle pressures since many patients will have unexpectedly elevated ankle pressures owing to calcification of the arterial wall, making vessels difficult to compress with a blood pressure cuff *(40)*. In fact, approximately 10% of patients will have incompressible vessels, making ankle pressures incalculable. Pulse volume recordings are useful in these patients since they are unaffected by calcification of vessels. Severely abnormal waveforms at the ankle or forefoot suggest severe ischemia (Fig. 4). Some centers have found toe pressures *(40)* and transcutaneous oxygen measurements *(41,42)* to be useful also in these patients, although we do not routinely use these two modalities in our practice.

Noninvasive arterial testing with exercise *(38,40)* is also useful in patients with claudication presenting with palpable distal pulses. Baseline studies are taken and then repeated with exercise, usually walking on a treadmill at a slight elevation until symptoms are reproduced. A subsequent reduction in arterial pressures or worsening of pulse volume waveforms suggests proximal stenotic lesions. In patients with development of claudication who do not have an associated change in their noninvasive testing, another cause for claudication such as spinal stenosis (so-called pseudoclaudication) may be present.

Following surgery, noninvasive testing can be used to quantify the degree of improvement in distal circulation. Arterial reconstructions with vein grafts are susceptible to the development of neointimal hyperplasia, which can lead to stricture and stenosis in vein grafts and ultimately graft thrombosis. Ultrasound evaluation of vein grafts with color flow duplex scanning is useful in detecting vein graft stenoses caused by intimal

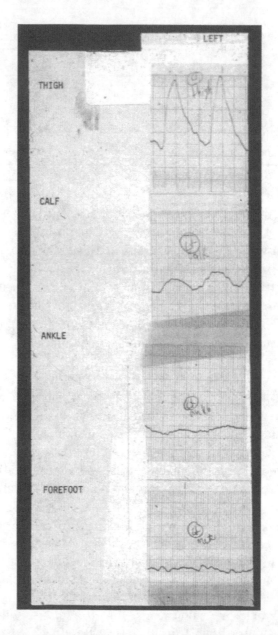

Fig. 4. A pulse volume recording (PVR) of the leg and foot obtained from a diabetic patient with a nonhealing foot ulcer and absent pulses. The ankle brachial index (ABI) was 0.7, usually indicative of mild ischemia (see text). Measurements were taken at the thigh, calf, ankle, and forefoot. The first waveform depicted is the thigh measurement and is normal. The more distal tracings are all abnormal. The lowest tracing is from the forefoot and is completely flat, indicating severe ischemia. The patient subsequently had an arteriogram and an arterial reconstruction.

hyperplasia *(43)*. When detected, significant stenoses can often be repaired by vein patch angioplasty or interposition grafts, prior to graft thrombosis *(44)*.

However, noninvasive testing adds little to the evaluation of patients presenting with obvious signs of foot ischemia and absent foot pulses. For most patients a careful history and physical examination will detect significant arterial insufficiency. The most important feature of the physical examination is the status of the foot pulses. If the posterior tibial and dorsalis pedis artery pulses are nonpalpable in patients presenting with typical signs and symptoms of ischemia, no further noninvasive testing is necessary, and contrast arteriography should be performed straight away.

The ultimate goal of lower extremity reconstruction is to restore perfusion pressure in the distal circulation by bypassing all major occlusions and (if possible) reestablish a palpable foot pulse. The outflow target artery (the point of the distal anastomosis) should be relatively free of occlusive disease and demonstrate unimpeded arterial flow into the arteries of the foot. In general, the most proximal artery distal to the occlusion meeting these two criteria is chosen. To make these determinations, the vascular surgeon needs a high-quality, comprehensive, contrast arteriogram of the entire lower extremity circulation extending from the infrarenal aorta to the base of the toes. It is crucial to visualize the entire tibial and foot circulation since the former is the most common location of the most significant occlusive lesions and the latter is an important potential site for placement of the distal anastomosis of the bypass graft. Iliac artery atherosclerosis accompanies lower extremity atherosclerosis in approximately 10–20% of patients with diabetes. When encountered and significant, balloon angioplasty of iliac lesions, with or without placement of a stent, is almost always possible and will improve arterial inflow for bypass. Moreover, this can be performed at the same time as the diagnostic arteriogram. For many years, our preference has been to use intraarterial digital subtraction arteriography *(45)* exclusively to evaluate the lower extremity arterial circulation. With currently available equipment, it is possible to obtain a complete survey from the infrarenal aorta to the base of the toes with approximately 100 mL of contrast or one-half of the amount required for conventional arteriography. Although conventional arteriography can provide excellent views of the lower extremity arterial anatomy, we have found cases in which it failed to demonstrate a suitable outflow vessel that was subsequently seen by the digital subtraction method.

Arteriography should never be withheld because of fear of exacerbating renal insufficiency. For patients with mild to moderate renal insufficiency (creatinine <2.5 mg/dL), hydration prior to angiography with normal saline will usually prevent significant deterioration of renal function. When renal function does worsen, it is usually asymptomatic and transient, with creatinine levels usually returning to normal within a few days. For patients with more marginal renal function, magnetic resonance arteriography (MRA) can provide adequate images of the distal circulation to plan the arterial reconstruction. Although some centers feel that this technique is superior to contrast arteriography *(27)*, we have found that intraarterial digital subtraction arteriography continues to provide the best quality images, and we reserve MRA for those patients in whom the administration of contrast is potentially harmful or contraindicated (Fig. 5).

VASCULAR RECONSTRUCTION

One of the most important developments in vascular surgery has been the demonstration that autogenous saphenous vein as opposed to prosthetic graft material gives the best short- and long-term results for distal bypass. In a large multicenter prospective randomized clinical trial, the 6-year patency rate of saphenous vein grafts was more than four times that of prosthetic grafts *(46)*.

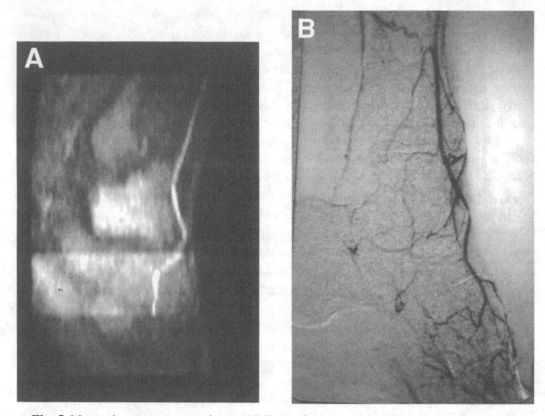

Fig. 5. Magnetic resonance arteriogram (MRA) of the lateral foot in a patient with diabetes mellitus being evaluated for arterial reconstruction. (**A**) The dorsalis pedis artery is patent, with a suggestion of a stenosis in its midportion. (**B**) The identical view as seen on an intraarterial digital subtraction arteriogram. The resolution and image quality is superior to the MRA study.

For more than 50 years, the standard procedure performed for lower extremity arterial revascularization has been the reversed saphenous vein bypass *(47)*. An inherent problem with reversing the vein, which is necessary to overcome the impediment of flow from valves, is a size discrepancy that results between the arteries and veins when they are connected. Vein grafts that are <4 mm in diameter at the distal end can thrombose when connected directly to the much larger common femoral artery at the groin, because of the size discrepancy. For many years, some vascular surgeons would routinely discard saphenous veins that were smaller than 4 mm at the distal end in order to prevent this cause of early graft thrombosis when performing an arterial bypass with a reversed saphenous vein. Methods were developed to render the valves incompetent in order to allow the vein to be used nonreversed or "in situ." However, no procedure was widely accepted until the late 1970s when Leather and associates *(48)* described a new technique using a modified Mills valvulotome that cut the valves atraumatically and quickly. Vascular surgeons enthusiastically embraced the Leather technique and began reporting improved results with the in situ bypass *(49–51)*. This led some to conclude that the in situ bypass possesses some inherent biologic superiority to the reversed saphenous vain graft *(52)*. However, evidence to support this concept is lacking *(53)*. Moreover, when in situ bypasses are compared with more contemporary series of reversed saphenous vein bypasses, no apparent superiority is evident *(54)*. In our own experience, we have frequently used both procedures and have observed essentially identical results with both vein configurations *(55)*. Nevertheless, the in situ technique is an important advance in lower extremity reconstructive surgery and continues to be widely used by most vascular surgeons.

In the 1980s Ascer and associates *(56)* reported the first series of bypass grafts with inflow (proximal anastomosis) taken from the popliteal artery. They showed equivalent results with the traditional approach of taking inflow from the common femoral artery. These results have been confirmed by other groups *(57)* including our own *(58)*, and the technique has proved to be another important advance in arterial reconstruction in patients with diabetes. Because atherosclerotic occlusive disease often spares the superficial femoral artery in diabetics, the popliteal artery can be readily used as a source of inflow for the distal vein graft. Doing so shortens the operative procedure and avoids potentially troublesome groin wound complications, which often accompany thigh and groin dissections. Short vein grafts are also advantageous in patients who have a limited quantity of adequate saphenous vein. Theoretically, shorter vein grafts should also have higher flow rates and possibly better long-term patency. Our recent experience with extreme distal arterial reconstructions has shown that popliteal artery inflow is possible in about 60% of diabetic patients undergoing vascular reconstruction in the lower extremity *(55)*.

When the saphenous vein is unavailable owing to previous harvesting or vein stripping, alternative sources of conduit must be used. Although some surgeons will use a prosthetic graft in these circumstances, alternative vein grafts including the contralateral saphenous vein, arm vein, or lesser saphenous vein can be used. We have generally not harvested the contralateral saphenous vein in diabetic patients without absent distal pulses in the opposite extremity. Our experience has demonstrated that in patients with a missing ipsilateral saphenous vein, the likelihood of requiring another arterial reconstruction in the opposite extremity approaches 40% at 3 years following the first operation *(59)*. Moreover, in our tertiary care practice, many such patients do not have an adequate available contralateral saphenous vein owing to its use for other vascular procedures or venous disease.

When the saphenous vein is unavailable, our conduit of choice has been the arm vein. Our recent results with arm vein grafts have been improved by examining the vein with the angioscope *(60)* to exclude segments with strictures or recanalization from trauma induced by previous venapuncture and thrombosis. Using the angioscope in this way to upgrade the quality of arm vein grafts has significantly improved our results with these grafts and further reduces the number of patients requiring a prosthetic conduit *(61)*. One potential disadvantage of arm vein grafts is their limited length, although the use of popliteal artery inflow makes shorter arm vein graft conduits possible in many patients. Moreover, the use of composite grafts made of various segments of the arm vein including the cephalic-basilic vein loop graft *(62)* can provide enough conduit length to reach from the groin to the distal tibial and even foot vessels in many patients. Our results with arm vein grafts in over 500 procedures have recently been reported *(63)*.

Patency and limb salvage rates were 57.5 and 71.5%, respectively, at 5 years. These results were inferior to those with de novo reconstructions done with saphenous vein; however, they were significantly better than those reported with prosthetic conduits.

A review at our institution of arteriograms imaging the entire lower extremity circulation in patients evaluated for vascular surgery has demonstrated that in 10% of cases a foot artery, usually the dorsalis pedis artery, is the only suitable outflow vessel. In another 15% of patients the dorsalis pedis artery will appear to be a better quality outflow target vessel than other patent but diseased tibial vessels. As a result, we began per-forming bypasses to the dorsalis pedis artery approximately 13 years ago when no other bypass option existed and we felt the patient was definitely facing amputation as the only alternative. Early results proved gratifying enough that we standardized our technique and indications to encompass all patients in whom we thought the dorsalis pedis artery was the best bypass option even if more proximal outflow target arteries were present (64). Our results with bypass to the dorsalis pedis artery have previously been reported (21); we demonstrated graft patency of 80% and limb salvage approaching 90% at 5 years. Moreover, we have demonstrated that even in the presence of foot infection, pedal bypass can be safely performed as long as spreading sepsis is controlled prior to surgery (5). These results have compared favorably with other reports of pedal level arterial reconstruction (65–69) and are comparable to or better than results now routinely reported for popliteal and tibial artery reconstructions. Although pedal arterial bypass represents the most "extreme" type of distal arterial reconstruction, it is almost always possible, particularly when the vascular surgeon is flexible in terms of how the vein graft is prepared and where the proximal anastomosis is placed.

Distal arterial reconstructions present special technical challenges for the vascular surgeon and require meticulous attention to detail. The target arteries are usually small (1.0–2.0 mm in diameter) and often calcified owing to medial calcinosis. Since long-term success requires the use of a venous conduit, harvesting an adequate venous conduit is essential and can often present problems, particularly when the ipsilateral saphenous vein is not available. In the early days of distal bypass surgery, many procedures were unsuccessful, resulting in amputation. Technical improvements in arteriography, surgical instruments and sutures, and techniques like the in situ bypass have significantly improved the outcome of distal arterial bypass, and outstanding results are often reported in more contemporary series. The improvements have proved to be especially beneficial to patients with diabetes mellitus, since their occlusive disease almost always requires a bypass to this level. In particular, the development and application of bypasses to the dorsalis pedis artery has had a direct effect in our own experience on the likelihood of amputation in patients with diabetes presenting with limb-threatening ischemia. Since its inception, pedal bypass has resulted in a significant decline in all amputations performed for ischemia (70). Currently bypasses to the dorsalis pedis artery constitute approximately 25% of all lower extremity arterial reconstructions in our patients with diabetes.

It is important to remember, however, that foot artery bypass is not the only procedure applicable to patients with diabetes. In general, the goal of treatment is to restore maximal arterial flow to the foot since this provides the best chance for healing. The diagnostic preoperative arteriogram is the key piece of information necessary in planning an appropriate surgical procedure. If a bypass to the popliteal or tibial artery will restore maximal arterial flow and restoration of palpable foot pulses, then bypasses need not extend to the level of the foot. Since the quality of the venous conduit is the most important determinant in long-term success, using the shortest length of high-quality venous conduit necessary to achieve this goal is the basic rule. Each operation must be individualized based on the patient's available venous conduit and arterial anatomy as demonstrated on the preoperative arteriogram.

Successful arterial reconstruction with restoration of maximal arterial flow does not end a vascular surgeon's responsibility to the patient. Often, significant wounds and/or ulcerations may still be present on the foot. Devising an appropriate treatment plan to close the wounds and heal the foot is the ultimate treatment goal. Until the skin envelope is intact, the patient is still susceptible to infection even with excellent arterial circulation. The methods involved in healing open wounds and ulcerations in the diabetic foot after restoration of arterial flow is complex and extends beyond the scope of this chapter. A variety of treatment methods are used and are individualized according to the patient's clinical circumstances. Although many small ulcers can be left to heal by secondary intention, some may require toe or partial forefoot amputations, especially when associated with gangrene and chronic osteomyelitis. For larger wounds, split-thickness skin grafts are used when the area involved is not a weight-bearing surface. For patients with complex wounds of weight-bearing surfaces, particularly the heel, or when bone or tendons need to be covered, more sophisticated plastic surgical reconstructions involving local rotational flaps and even free tissue transfers have been occasionally employed in our practice. Success in these procedures requires the expertise of plastic surgeons in conjunction with foot and ankle or podiatric surgeons.

CONCLUSIONS

This chapter has reviewed the principles of evaluation, diagnosis, and treatment of arterial disease in patients with lower extremity ischemia in diabetes. Rejection of the small vessel hypothesis and understanding the location of atherosclerotic occlusive disease in the lower extremity of patients with diabetes is key to effecting proper treatment. Understanding the interplay of neuropathy and infection with ischemia and providing proper treatment for this problem as well as for arterial insufficiency is essential to ultimate success. A thorough understanding of the pathophysiology of ischemia and a carefully planned approach, including the prompt control of infection when present, a high-quality digital subtraction arteriogram, and an extreme distal arterial reconstruction to maximize foot perfusion should lead to rates of limb salvage in patients with diabetes that equal or exceed those achieved in nondiabetic patients with lower extremity ischemia.

REFERENCES

1. Gibbons GW, Eliopoulos GM. Infection of the diabetic foot, in *Management of Diabetic Foot Problems* (Kozak G, ed.), WB Saunders, Philadelphia, 1984, pp. 1–18.
2. Edmonds ME. The diabetic foot: pathophysiology and treatment. *Clin Endocrinol Metab* 1986;15:889–916.
3. Grunfeld C. Diabetic foot ulcers: etiology, treatment, and prevention. *Adv Intern Med* 1992; 37:103–132.

4. Levin M. The diabetic foot: pathophysiology, evaluation and treatment, in *The Diabetic Foot* (Levin M, ed.), Mosby-Year Book, St. Louis, 1987, pp. 1–50.

5. Tannenbaum GA, Pomposelli FB Jr, Marcaccio EJ, et al. Safety of vein bypass grafting to the dorsal pedal artery in diabetic patients with foot infections. *J Vasc Surg* 1992;15:982–988.

6. Goldenberg SG AM, Joshi RA. Nonatheromatous peripheral vascular disease of the lower extremity in diabetes mellitus. *Diabetes* 1959;8:261–273.

7. Barner HB, Kaiser GC, Willman VL. Blood flow in the diabetic leg. *Circulation* 1971;43: 391–394.

8. Conrad MC. Large and small artery occlusion in diabetics and nondiabetics with severe vascular disease. *Circulation* 1967;36:83–91.

9. Irwin ST, Gilmore J, McGrann S, Hood J, Allen JA. Blood flow in diabetics with foot lesions due to 'small vessel disease.' *Br J Surg* 1988;75:1201–1206.

10. LoGerfo FW, Coffman JD. Current concepts. Vascular and microvascular disease of the foot in diabetes. Implications for foot care. *N Engl J Med* 1984;311:1615–1619.

11. Strandness DE PR, Gibbons GE. Combined clinical and pathological study of diabetic and nondiabetic peripheral arterial disease. *Diabetes* 1964;13:366–372.

12. Kannel WB, McGee DL. Diabetes and cardiovascular disease. The Framingham study. *JAMA* 1979;241:2035–2038.

13. Smith JW, Marcus FI, Serokman R. Prognosis of patients with diabetes mellitus after acute myocardial infarction. *Am J Cardiol* 1984;54:718–721.

14. Petersen CM KJ, Jovanovic L. Influence of diabetes on vascular disease and its complications, in *Vascular Surgery: A Comprehensive Review*, 5th ed. (Moore WS, ed.), WB Saunders, Philadelphia, 1998, pp. 146–167.

15. Zarich S, Waxman S, Freeman RT, et al. Effect of autonomic nervous system dysfunction on the circadian pattern of myocardial ischemia in diabetes mellitus [see comments]. *J Am Coll Cardiol* 1994;24:956–9962.

16. Lee TH, Marcantonio ER, Mangione CM, et al. Derivation and prospective validation of a simple index for prediction of cardiac risk of major noncardiac surgery. *Circulation* 1999; 100:1043–1049.

17. Eagle KA, Coley CM, Newell JB, et al. Combining clinical and thallium data optimizes preoperative assessment of cardiac risk before major vascular surgery. *Ann Intern Med* 1989; 110:859–866.

18. Akbari CM, Pomposelli FB Jr, Gibbons GW, et al. Lower extremity revascularization in diabetes: late observations. *Arch Surg* 2000;135:452–456.

19. Grayson ML, Gibbons GW, Habershaw GM, et al. Use of ampicillin/sulbactam versus imipenem/cilastatin in the treatment of limb-threatening foot infections in diabetic patients. *Clin Infect Dis* 1994;18:683–693.

20. Gibbons GW. The diabetic foot: amputations and drainage of infection. *J Vasc Surg* 1987;5: 791–793.

21. Pomposelli FB Jr, Marcaccio EJ, Gibbons GW, et al. Dorsalis pedis arterial bypass: durable limb salvage for foot ischemia in patients with diabetes mellitus. *J Vasc Surg* 1995;21: 375–384.

22. Pomposelli FB Jr, Arora S, Gibbons GW, et al. Lower extremity arterial reconstruction in the very elderly: successful outcome preserves not only the limb but also residential status and ambulatory function. *J Vasc Surg* 1998;28:215–225.

23. Nesto RW. Screening for asymptomatic coronary artery disease in diabetes [editorial; comment]. *Diabetes Care* 1999;22:1393–395.

24. Zarich SW, Cohen MC, Lane SE, et al. Routine perioperative dipyridamole ^{201}Tl imaging in diabetic patients undergoing vascular surgery. *Diabetes Care* 1996;19:355–360.

25. Bode RH Jr, Lewis KP, Zarich SW, et al. Cardiac outcome after peripheral vascular surgery. Comparison of general and regional anesthesia [see comments]. *Anesthesiology* 1996;84: 3–13.

26. Pierce ET, Pomposelli FB Jr, Stanley GD, et al. Anesthesia type does not influence early graft patency or limb salvage rates of lower extremity arterial bypass. *J Vasc Surg* 1997;25: 226–232; discussion 232–233.

27. Carpenter JP, Baum RA, Holland GA, Barker CF. Peripheral vascular surgery with magnetic resonance angiography as the sole preoperative imaging modality. *J Vasc Surg* 1994;20: 861–869; discussion 869–871.

28. Lumsden AB, Besman A, Jaffe M, MacDonald MJ, Allen RC. Infrainguinal revascularization in end-stage renal disease. *Ann Vasc Surg* 1994;8:107–112.

29. Carsten CG III, Taylor SM, Langan EM III, Crane MM. Factors associated with limb loss despite a patent infrainguinal bypass graft. *Am Surg* 1998;64:33–37.

30. Johnson BL, Glickman MH, Bandyk DF, Esses GE. Failure of foot salvage in patients with end-stage renal disease after surgical revascularization. *J Vasc Surg* 1995;22:280–285.

31. Korn P, Hoenig SJ, Skillman JJ, Kent KC. Is lower extremity revascularization worthwhile in patients with end-stage renal disease? *Surgery* 2000;128:472–479.

32. Dormandy J, Heeck L, Vig S. The natural history of claudication: risk to life and limb. *Semin Vasc Surg* 1999;12:123–137.

33. McDermott MM, McCarthy W. Intermittent claudication. The natural history. *Surg Clin North Am* 1995;75:581–591.

34. Hertzer NR. The natural history of peripheral vascular disease. Implications for its management. *Circulation* 1991;83:I12–I19.

35. Dawson DL, Cutler BS, Hiatt WR, et al. A comparison of cilostazol and pentoxifylline for treating intermittent claudication. *Am J Med* 2000;109:523–530.

36. Dawson DL, Cutler BS, Meissner MH, Strandness DE Jr. Cilostazol has beneficial effects in treatment of intermittent claudication: results from a multicenter, randomized, prospective, double-blind trial. *Circulation* 1998;98:678–686.

37. Gillings DB. Pentoxifylline and intermittent claudication: review of clinical trials and cost-effectiveness analyses. *J Cardiovasc Pharmacol* 1995;25:S44–S50.

38. Gahtan V. The noninvasive vascular laboratory. *Surg Clin North Am* 1998;78:507–518.

39. Raines J, Traad E. Noninvasive evaluation of peripheral vascular disease. *Med Clin North Am* 1980;64:283–304.

40. Weitz JI, Byrne J, Clagett GP, et al. Diagnosis and treatment of chronic arterial insufficiency of the lower extremities: a critical review. *Circulation* 1996;94:3026–3049.

41. White RA, Nolan L, Harley D, et al. Noninvasive evaluation of peripheral vascular disease using transcutaneous oxygen tension. *Am J Surg* 1982;144:68–75.

42. Hauser CJ, Klein SR, Mehringer CM, Appel P, Shoemaker WC. Superiority of transcutaneous oximetry in noninvasive vascular diagnosis in patients with diabetes. *Arch Surg* 1984; 119:690–694.

43. Bandyk DF, Seabrook GR, Moldenhauer P, et al. Hemodynamics of vein graft stenosis. *J Vasc Surg* 1988;8:688–695.

44. Cohen JR, Mannick JA, Couch NP, Whittemore AD. Recognition and management of impending vein-graft failure. Importance for long-term patency. *Arch Surg* 1986;121:758–759.

45. Blakeman BM, Littooy FN, Baker WH. Intra-arterial digital subtraction angiography as a method to study peripheral vascular disease. *J Vasc Surg* 1986;4:168–173.

46. Veith FJ, Gupta SK, Ascer E, et al. Six-year prospective multicenter randomized comparison of autologous saphenous vein and expanded polytetrafluoroethylene grafts in infrainguinal arterial reconstructions. *J Vasc Surg* 1986;3:104–114.

47. Kunlin J. Le traitment de l'arterité obliterante par la greffe veinuse. *Arch Mal Coeur Vaiss* 1949;42:371.

48. Leather RP, Powers SR, Karmody AM. A reappraisal of the in situ saphenous vein arterial bypass: its use in limb salvage. *Surgery* 1979;86:453–461.

49. Buchbinder D, Rolins DL, Verta MJ, et al. Early experience with in situ saphenous vein bypass for distal arterial reconstruction. *Surgery* 1986;99:350–357.

50. Hurley JJ, Auer AI, Binnington HB, et al. Comparison of initial limb salvage in 98 consecutive patients with either reversed autogenous or in situ vein bypass graft procedures. *Am J Surg* 1985;150:777–781.
51. Strayhorn EC, Wohlgemuth S, Deuel M, Glickman MH, Hurwitz RL. Early experience utilizing the in situ saphenous vein technique in 54 patients. *J Cardiovasc Surg (Torino)* 1988; 29:161–165.
52. Bush HL Jr, Corey CA, Nabseth DC. Distal in situ saphenous vein grafts for limb salvage. Increased operative blood flow and postoperative patency. *Am J Surg* 1983;145:542–548.
53. Cambria RP, Megerman J, Brewster DC, et al. The evolution of morphologic and biomechanical changes in reversed and in-situ vein grafts. *Ann Surg* 1987;205:167–174.
54. Taylor LM Jr, Edwards JM, Porter JM. Present status of reversed vein bypass grafting: five-year results of a modern series. *J Vasc Surg* 1990;11:193–205.
55. Pomposelli FB Jr, Jepsen SJ, Gibbons GW, et al. A flexible approach to infrapopliteal vein grafts in patients with diabetes mellitus. *Arch Surg* 1991;126:724–727.
56. Ascer E, Veith FJ, Gupta SK, et al. Short vein grafts: a superior option for arterial reconstructions to poor or compromised outflow tracts? *J Vasc Surg* 1988;7:370–378.
57. Cantelmo NL, Snow JR, Menzoian JO, LoGerfo FW. Successful vein bypass in patients with an ischemic limb and a palpable popliteal pulse. *Arch Surg* 1986;121:217–220.
58. Stonebridge PA, Tsoukas AI, Pomposelli FB Jr, et al. Popliteal-to-distal bypass grafts for limb salvage in diabetics. *Eur J Vasc Surg* 1991;5:265–269.
59. Holzenbein TJ, Pomposelli FB Jr, Miller A, et al. Results of a policy with arm veins used as the first alternative to an unavailable ipsilateral greater saphenous vein for infrainguinal bypass. *J Vasc Surg* 1996;23:130–140.
60. Miller A, Campbell DR, Gibbons GW, et al. Routine intraoperative angioscopy in lower extremity revascularization. *Arch Surg* 1989;124:604–608.
61. Stonebridge PA, Miller A, Tsoukas A, et al. Angioscopy of arm vein infrainguinal bypass grafts. *Ann Vasc Surg* 1991;5:170–175.
62. Balshi JD, Cantelmo NL, Menzoian JO, LoGerfo FW. The use of arm veins for infrainguinal bypass in end-stage peripheral vascular disease. *Arch Surg* 1989;124:1078–1081.
63. Faries PL, Arora S, Pomposelli FB Jr, et al. The use of arm vein in lower-extremity revascularization: results of 520 procedures performed in eight years. *J Vasc Surg* 2000;31:50–59.
64. Pomposelli FB Jr, Jepsen SJ, Gibbons GW, et al. Efficacy of the dorsal pedal bypass for limb salvage in diabetic patients: short-term observations [see comments]. *J Vasc Surg* 1990; 11:745–751.
65. Andros G, Harris RW, Salles-Cunha SX, et al. Bypass grafts to the ankle and foot. *J Vasc Surg* 1988;7:785–794.
66. Darling RC III, Chang BB, Shah DM, Leather RP. Choice of peroneal or dorsalis pedis artery bypass for limb salvage. *Semin Vasc Surg* 1997;10:17–22.
67. Levine AW, Davis RC, Gingery RO, Anderegg DD. In situ bypass to the dorsalis pedis and tibial arteries at the ankle. *Ann Vasc Surg* 1989;3:205–209.
68. Shanik DG, Auer AI, Hershey FB. Vein bypass to the dorsalis pedis artery for limb ischaemia. *Ir Med J* 1982;75:54–56.
69. Shieber W, Parks C. Dorsalis pedis artery in bypass grafting. *Am J Surg* 1974;128:752–755.
70. LoGerfo FW, Gibbons GW, Pomposelli FB Jr, et al. Trends in the care of the diabetic foot. Expanded role of arterial reconstruction. *Arch Surg* 1992;127:617–620.

21

Angioplasty and Other Noninvasive Surgical Procedures

David P. Brophy, MD, FFRRCSI, FRCR, MSCVIR

INTRODUCTION

Diabetes accounts for half of lower extremity amputations in the United States. It has been estimated that the relative risk of amputation is 40 times greater in patients with diabetes *(1,2)*. The management of gangrene and ulcers in diabetics is more difficult than in the nondiabetic patients, and the need for amputation for predominant ischemic disease in diabetics is many times greater. Eighty-five percent of diabetes-related amputations are preceded by foot ulcer. The management of diabetics with critical ischemia presents many challenges compared with that of nondiabetic atherosclerotic patients, as disease is both more diffuse and more severe. Recent improvements in limb salvage rates in diabetics with critical foot ischemia can be attributed to a multidisciplinary approach, including prevention, patient education, and multifactorial treatment. Although diabetics with peripheral vascular disease may present with claudication, they usually present with limb-threatening ischemia, usually chronic, which indicates surgical or endovascular intervention. Advances in vascular bypass surgery techniques, together with ancillary procedures such as angioplasty, stent placement, thrombolysis, and atherectomy, have played a role in reducing amputation rates by 43–85% *(3)*.

PERCUTANEOUS TRANSLUMINAL ANGIOPLASTY AND STENTING

In diabetics, endovascular intervention is only indicated in selected patients with critical ischemia in whom rest pain is debilitating and/or ulceration fails to heal despite appropriate conservative measures. As with nondiabetics, persistent debilitating intermittent claudication despite exercise treatment may also indicate intervention.

Image-guided catheter intervention was first described in 1964 *(4)*. Since then, advances in technology, together with refinements in techniques and more ubiquitous expertise, allow more widespread application of percutaneous techniques such as percutaneous transluminal angioplasty (PTA) and now stenting. Complication rates with angioplasty and stenting are generally low and rarely severe.

From: *The Diabetic Foot: Medical and Surgical Management*
Edited by: A. Veves, J. M. Giurini, and F. W. LoGerfo © Humana Press Inc., Totowa, NJ

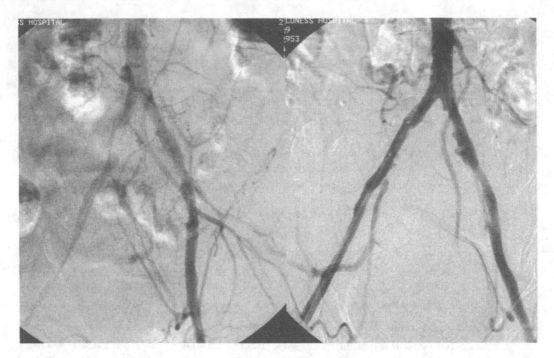

Fig. 1. A 46-year-old male smoker with insulin-dependent diabetes mellitus presents with a nonhealing right foot ulcer. Initial iliac digital subtraction arteriogram (DSA; left) shows a smooth though eccentric severe stenosis of the distal right common iliac artery, the eccentric nature of the lesion suggesting PTA failure and need for stent placement. However, after PTA with a 9-mm balloon, repeat arteriography (right) with a measuring catheter reveals a good-caliber vessel at the PTA site and no pressure gradient across the PTA site, arguing against the need for stent placement.

Aortoiliac PTA and Stenting

Indications

In contradistinction to nondiabetic patients, in whom claudication is invariably the presenting problem, foot ischemia is the most common indication for iliac PTA and stenting when diabetics present for intervention. Indeed, iliac percutaneous inflow procedure is not uncommonly performed in combination with a more distal vascular surgical graft placement (i.e., infrainguinal revascularization) to facilitate graft inflow and promote long-term patency rates. Aortoiliac revascularization by percutaneous intervention can improve lower extremity flow enough to allow ulcer/wound healing without the need for an ancillary infrainguinal procedure. PTA is the treatment of choice for a single smooth stenosis of <3 cm length involving either the common or external iliac artery (Fig. 1). For diffuse unilateral or bilateral iliac steno-occlusive disease, iliac stenosis with abdominal aortic aneurysm, or bilateral external iliac artery occlusions, surgical treatment is the option of choice and PTA should be avoided. For lesions between these extremes of disease, endovascular techniques are being increasingly utilized, but more evidence is required before endovascular techniques can be routinely recommended for such lesions. With the introduction of metal stents, the numbers of patients considered candidates for iliac PTA have now increased. Stenting is indicated after suboptimal

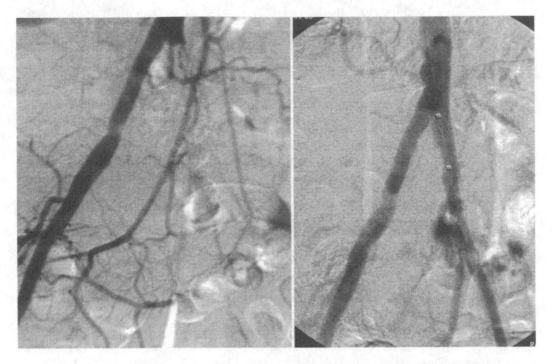

Fig. 2. A 59-year-old man with non-insulin-dependent diabetes mellitus presents with a nonhealing left foot ulcer and absent left femoral pulse on clinical exam. Total left common iliac artery occlusion is seen on DSA (left). Although the lesion was successfully transgressed with a wire and catheter system, PTA of the occlusive lesion failed, indicating placement of a stent to restore patency (right).

or complicated PTA. Primary stenting has been shown in a randomized study to have no benefit over PTA but rather to be less cost-effective than PTA *(5)*. However, in diabetics, iliac lesions are often eccentric and calcified, features that predict suboptimal PTA. With such lesions, primary stenting may prove to be justified. Iliac artery occlusions also require primary stenting, as PTA not only is likely to fail, but runs a significant risk of distal embolization *(6)* (Fig. 2).

Technique and Evaluation of Technical Outcome

The hemodynamic significance of a stenotic iliac lesion is determined by its angiographic appearance. For the iliac artery, at least an 80–85% area stenosis (i.e., approximately a 50–60% reduction in cross-sectional luminal diameter) is required for a significant pressure decrease to occur. The ability of angiographic appearance alone to provide information about functional significance of a stenotic lesion can be limited (e.g., inter- and intraobserver variation and inability to assess eccentric stenoses accurately) *(7)*. Therefore, pressure measurements with vasodilators or reactive hyperemia are required for determining the significance of borderline lesions and the success of percutaneous interventions. Although what constitutes a significant pressure gradient is the subject of some debate, a mean pressure gradient decrease of 5 mmHg across a lesion is considered significant; this usually corresponds to a systolic gradient in the region of 10–15 mmHg *(8)*. These angiographic and pressure parameters are also used to determine the technical success of PTA, need for stenting after PTA, and technical success of stenting. Agents that are commonly used for vasodilation include nitroglycerine (100–150 µg), tolazoline (25–40 mg), and papaverine (15–30 mg). Stenting is indicated following PTA if hemodynamic measurements indicate an unsatisfactory result, particularly if flow-limiting dissection is present either proximal or distal to the original lesion.

Ipsilateral common femoral artery access facilitates advantages in recanalizing an iliac artery, more accurate stent placement, less tortuosity, and less propensity for antegrade dissection. Some argue in favor of a contralateral approach for external iliac intervention because access in these cases is uncomplicated by proximity to the access site. Previous groin surgery, groin infection, or the presence of a femoral graft favor an opposite groin access.

Once access is achieved, a sheath is usually placed. Small and short (e.g., 5 French, 10-cm) sheaths are generally used for PTA, with larger and longer sheaths used for stent introduction. Stenotic and occlusive lesions are transgressed with a combination of a directing catheter and guidewire. Hydrophilic guidewires are particularly useful in this regard. The selection of appropriate balloon and stent dimensions can be facilitated by the use of a measuring catheter at the time of angiography.

Infrarenal aortic disease is amenable to PTA and stenting. An inferior mesenteric artery arising from the stenotic aortic segment is a relative contraindication to intervention, however.

Treatment of a common iliac origin lesion requires a kissing balloon technique to prevent plaques being displaced across the contralateral common iliac origin at the time of balloon inflation. Just as important, disease at the aortic bifurcation frequently involves the distal aorta. Similarly, bilateral common iliac origin stenoses require simultaneous balloon inflation from a right and left access. Kissing balloons treat the distal aorta as well as the common iliac lesions.

Although PTA and stenting of iliac bifurcation (i.e., distal common iliac and proximal external iliac artery) lesions run the risk of occlusion of the internal iliac artery, such lesions can be safely treated percutaneously, particularly if the contralateral internal iliac artery is patent.

Segmental iliac occlusion predicts the need for stent placement, as PTA of these lesions fails owing to stenosis recoil and can be associated with embolization of occluding material. The primary use of stents is preferred to reconstruct these occlusive lesions, particularly self-expanding stents. Predilation with a small balloon may be needed when using balloon-expandable stents. This predilation allows placement of the delivery system and protects the stent from being stripped off the balloon during passage through the stenotic segment.

Although heparin is routinely used for infrainguinal PTA, it is not required, as rapid flow through most iliac arteries is sufficient to maintain patency during and after iliac intervention. However, when the ipsilateral access system compromises flow, or with diffuse disease, heparin should be given at 50–100 U/kg, with additional doses hourly of 10–15 U/kg. It is not necessary to continue heparin after the procedure.

Platelet glycoprotein (GP) IIb/IIIa inhibitors such as abciximab (ReoPro, Centocor, Malpern, PA), tirofiban (Aggrastat, Merck, West Point, PA), or eptifibatide (Integrillin, Schering-Plough, Madison, NJ) are finding use after coronary stent placement. Given their cost, the potential for bleeding complications, and the low incidence of acute occlusion, the generalized use of these agents does not appear warranted after aortoiliac PTA and stenting at this time.

Patients should routinely take aspirin (81 mg daily) after arterial revascularization procedures. The antiplatelet effect of aspirin has the potential of preventing rethrombosis as well as myocardial infarction and stroke. More recent antiplatelet agents such as ticlopidine (Ticlid, Roche Laboratories, Nutley, NJ) and clopidogrel (Plavix, Sanofi Pharmaceuticals, New York, NY) may also find a similar role in the future.

Complications

Complication rates of aortoiliac percutaneous revascularization procedures are low, but complications can occur at the puncture site, the aortoiliac lesion site, or remotely distal to the site of intervention. Usually these complications can be recognized immediately or early post procedure. However, some occur late and make recognition more difficult. Many complications can be managed with endovascular techniques, but it must be realized that some complications can be devastating such as arterial rupture and stent infection.

Complication rates for aortoiliac percutaneous revascularization range between 6 and 19.4% (9–14). Determining the true rate of major complications is difficult owing to variations in definition, but 1.7% of patients have been reported to have complications requiring surgery (15). Systemic complications are far fewer than those associated with surgical revascularization (16). Complication rates are similar for stenting and PTA procedures, but stenting does allow higher technical success rates, and long-term patency rates may be improved with stenting (17).

The most common complications after iliac interventions are access site complications, which have an incidence between 0.2 and 15% of iliac interventions (9,13,15). Hemorrhage and hematoma are the most common access site complications and are readily recognized. Massive blood loss can occur, however, without obvious groin hematoma in cases of retroperitoneal extension of hemorrhage.

Pulsatile mass in the groin signifies a femoral pseudoaneurysm. Ultrasound-guided compression has been the preferred treatment, with 90% success rates possible. With antiplatelet and anticoagulation treatment, this success rate decreases to 62–73%. Ultrasound-guided thrombin injection appears to offer high treatment success rates even in these patients (18).

Arterial rupture at the site of intervention is a rare (0.1% [19]) but potentially serious complication. Although most ruptures described occur at the time of intervention, delayed rupture has been described as well as pseudoaneurysm formation at the site of intervention. Management requires acute recognition of the complications of the rupture, balloon tamponade, intravenous resuscitation, and operative repair. Successful treatment has been achieved with balloon tamponade alone. Endovascular grafts, which have already been used to treat ruptures in the setting of trauma, are likely to find a role in treating focal rupture (20).

Other complications can be related to devices used during the procedure and include balloon rupture, stent displacement or migration, stent collapse, or compression. On occasion snaring techniques are needed to retrieve some or all of such devices.

Acute occlusion is now rare with the advent of stents and was previously related to hemodynamically significant dissections after PTA. Risk factors for early stent thrombosis are increased when treating the following lesion types: an occlusive lesion, a lesion over 4 cm long, an external iliac lesion, and a lesion with poor runoff distally *(15)*.

Distal embolization can complicate PTA and stenting in as many as 3–7% of patients *(9,15)*. Emboli may consist of thrombus, plaque, or cholesterol. The success of thrombolysis is dependent on the embolus being thrombus rather than atheromatous plaque. Suction thrombectomy is an alternative technique that can treat plaque emboli *(20)*.

Infection at intervention sites appears to be an exceedingly rare although serious complication. Stent deployment appears more likely to be associated with the increasing incidence of infection than with PTA, possibly because the stent material acts as a nidus for bacteria (*Staphylococcus* invariably) to lodge. Given the large number of stents placed without sequelae, it is unclear whether antibiotics should be used routinely at the time of implantation *(20)*. The general susceptibility of diabetics to infection suggests a role for antibiotics at the time of stent deployment, particularly if stent grafts are being utilized. However, uncovered stents have been deployed with no antibiotic prophylaxis in many diabetics without complication.

Clinical Outcomes

Endovascular repair is generally performed on patients with less severe disease than those undergoing surgical repair, although percutaneous revascularization can have an important role in the management of high-risk surgical candidates. The risks of endovascular techniques are much lower than those of surgical treatment. However, PTA and stents offer less durability of the result compared with bifurcated graft surgery, with surgery consistently having a 5-year patency rate of over 85% *(21)*. The adjusted 4-year primary patency rate for endovascular treatment of chronic limb ischemia, with technical failures included, was 53% after PTA and 67% after stent placement *(17,22)*.

Outcomes (in terms of patency rates and limb salvage rates) for iliac intervention are comparable for diabetic and nondiabetic patients who undergo current methods of percutaneous iliac intervention and infrainguinal reconstruction *(23)*. Diabetic patients with critical ischemia are more likely to have poorer runoff, a documented poor prognostic indicator for response. Consequently, diabetics are more likely to undergo peripheral reconstruction than nondiabetics, and it is possible that the effects of the peripheral reconstruction, when performed around the time of the iliac intervention, contribute to these comparable patency rates. The critical nature of limb ischemia may be reversed by iliac percutaneous intervention alone. This is especially evident in patients with large pressure gradients across the iliac lesion before iliac intervention, and such patients may show sufficient improvement in distal flow to obviate the need for infrainguinal reconstruction. This has important implications for diabetic patients with high operative risks or in whom there is limited vein for grafts.

Femoropopliteal and Infrapopliteal PTA and Stenting

Indications

The purpose of PTA in patients with chronic limb ischemia is to allow ulcer healing and to salvage a functioning foot. Late restenosis or occlusion after PTA may result in recurrent ulceration but rarely precludes subsequent surgery or compromises additional vascular segments. Indeed, PTA can spare saphenous vein for subsequent use in the limb or coronary circulation.

Indications for infrainguinal PTA are severe claudication, rest pain, and tissue loss. For patients with rest pain and tissue loss, a combination common to diabetics, severe steno-occlusive disease invariably involves both femoropopliteal and infrapopliteal vessels. For this reason, PTA of femoropopliteal and infrapopliteal vessels can be considered together, as effective treatment of both segments may be required to alleviate symptoms and signs of ischemia *(24,25)*. Indeed, some consider that restoration of tibioperoneal flow improves the durability of femoropopliteal PTA *(26)*. However, few series have evaluated PTA of femoropopliteal and infrapopliteal vessels together *(27–29)*. Although with recent advances in technology, virtually all short lesions can be technically recanalized *(30–32)*, appropriate selection of anatomically suitable lesions remains the key to acceptable results in patients with infrainguinal steno-occlusive disease and chronic limb ischemia.

PTA is most effective for single, short stenotic lesions <3 cm in length involving the superficial femoral and above the knee popliteal artery, provided there is good runoff via tibioperoneal vessels. However, for patients with critical limb ischemia, this scenario is rarely evident. Indeed, lack of continuity is to be expected between the popliteal artery and the pedal arch, with either occlusion or severe stenotic disease involving all three runoff vessels. PTA can be effectively utilized to restore adequate flow in one or two of these tibioperoneal vessels if the stenoses are short (<1 cm long) and less than five in number *(32)*. This favorable distribution of disease for PTA appears in <20% of diabetics presenting with nonhealing foot ulceration or foot gangrene, however.

PTA can also be utilized to improve inflow to a more distal surgical graft, particularly when limited vein graft is available. The Transatlantic Inter-Society Consensus Committee recommends surgery for complete femoral or popliteal and trifurcation occlusions *(33)*. For the spectrum of disease in between these two extremes, more evidence is needed to make any firm recommendation for endovascular treatment. Future studies should determine whether endovascular repair of single lesions 3–10 cm long or multiple 3–5-cm steno-occlusive lesions can replace surgery as a first-line treatment.

Femoropopliteal stenting as a primary approach to interventional treatment of intermittent claudication or chronic limb ischemia is not indicated. However, stents have a limited role in salvage of acute PTA failures or complications *(33)*.

Technique and Evaluation

High-quality diagnostic arteriography, with biplane imaging of branching/vessel overlap sites, is required if PTA of infrainguinal arteries is to be effective. Ipsilateral antegrade puncture is the most favorable approach via the ipsilateral common femoral artery. Placement of a sheath (usually 5 or 6 French) is essential for balloon passage and facilitates injection of contrast while wire access across the PTA site is maintained. For tibioperoneal PTA, 0.014–0.018-inch guidewires are preferred and low-profile balloons.

Heparin is advised with infrainguinal PTA, as well as judicious use of vasodilators such as nitroglycerine, to lower peripheral resistance, improve flow, and overcome vasospasm. Pressure measurements are of no benefit in PTA of infrainguinal vessels as the catheters used to measure the pressures interfere with accurate pressure measurement by virtue of being partially occlusive. Technical success can be expected in >90% of appropriate selected patients *(25,26,32)*.

As with any lower extremity percutaneous intervention, distal pulses should be checked at the end of the procedure to ensure that distal embolization and catheter complications have not been overlooked. Monitoring post procedure includes bed rest, vital sign monitoring, and hydration. Patients should be closely monitored for occult retroperitoneal, groin, or thigh hemorrhage after antegrade puncture in particular. Such hemorrhage can have serious consequences for patients with limited cardiac reserve. Serial hematocrits and urine output measurement can help facilitate earlier diagnosis. If there is suspicion of occult bleeding, a computed tomography scan of the pelvis and thigh accurately diagnose and determine the severity of such hemorrhage.

Aspirin is recommended for reducing thrombotic events in all patients with peripheral vascular disease. Particularly after endovascular procedures, such antiplatelet therapy should be continued indefinitely *(34)*. More recently, a role has been suggested for antiplatelet agents such as ticlopidine and clopidogrel after surgical bypass *(35)*, but use of both these agents has been associated with the side effects of thrombocytopenia *(36,37)*.

Complications

The types of procedure-related complications are similar to those that can occur after aortoiliac endovascular interventions. Complications have been reported in 3–14% of femoropopliteal and tibioperoneal PTA cases *(30,38–43)*. Most commonly these are related to access site hematoma/hemorrhage, thrombosis, distal vessel embolization, pseudoaneurysm and arteriovenous fistula formation, and renal failure. Many of the reported cases of distal embolism were successfully treated by percutaneous catheter-directed thrombolysis.

Clinical Outcomes

As with other interventions in critical limb ischemia, the purpose of PTA is to salvage the foot. Late restenosis of occlusion can result in recurrent ulceration but rarely compromises additional vascular segments or future surgery. Effective restoration of continuity of flow in the tibioperoneal segment is believed to increase the durability of femoropopliteal PTA. Few studies, however, have analyzed PTA of the femoropopliteal and tibioperoneal segments together *(27–29)*.

Appropriate selection of anatomically suitable cases is the key to obtaining acceptable results.

Long lesion length is considered one of the factors detracting from both technical success and durability of femoropopliteal PTA *(39,40,42,44)*. PTA of lesions longer than 7–10 cm offers little benefit (23% patency of femoropopliteal PTA at 6 months *[39]*), whereas those <3 cm in length do well *(40,45)*. Although occlusive lesions limit technical success, these lesions can be expected to have the same patency as that of a stenosis of the equivalent length *(38,40,42)*. Concentric lesions appear to respond better than eccentric and/or calcified lesions *(40,42)*. This is an especially important consideration in diabetics with renal failure, a subgroup of patients who tend to have profound vascular calcification.

Probably the most important predictor of long-term success of PTA for patients with critical limb ischemia is the status of the runoff circulation. Two- or three-vessel runoff has at least a two times greater femoropopliteal patency rate than those with zero to one-vessel runoff at 3 and 5 years. Three and 5-year PTA patency rates for patients with good runoff have been reported up to 78 and 53%, respectively, compared with up 37 and 31%, respectively, for patients with poor runoff *(41,44,45)*.

Although diabetes and critical ischemia are believed to influence the outcome of PTA adversely, this association is probably related to poor runoff vessels, vessel calcification, and the presence of end-stage renal disease. Diabetics with good tibioperoneal runoff can benefit from iliac and femoropopliteal PTA *(46)* as well as diabetics with good inflow, in whom continuous flow to the pedal arch can be restored by tibioperoneal PTA *(47)*. Dilation of proximal lesions when a distal artery is severely diseased will not impart clinical benefit *(43,47,48)*. The importance of anatomic selection is highlighted by a 2-year 80% limb salvage rate in patients with "straight line flow" to the foot in at least one tibial vessel compared with 0% when distal flow was obstructed *(47)*.

It should be remembered that the 5-year survival for patients presenting with limb salvage indications for endovascular or surgical repair is only approximately 50%, with mortality usually attributed to coronary heart disease or stroke *(24)*. The low morbidity and mortality of PTA should be weighed against poor outcomes of PTA in anatomically unsuitable diffuse disease with poor runoff when deciding between endovascular repair and surgical approach.

OTHER ENDOVASCULAR TECHNIQUES FOR TREATMENT OF LOWER LIMB ISCHEMIA

Catheter-directed thrombolysis has the theoretical advantages over surgical thromboembolectomy of decreasing damage to the endothelium and also revealing the underlying lesions that caused the acute limb ischemia presentation. Other forms of percutaneous treatment for limb ischemia, such as percutaneous aspiration thrombectomy with large lumen catheters, and percutaneous mechanical thrombectomy, which utilizes non-recirculation devices that function by clot fragmentation, have limited clinical experience, and further study is needed to determine their therapeutic role.

The details of thrombolytic therapy and the limited role of percutaneous atherectomy are discussed here with reference to their roles in treating diabetics with limb ischemia.

Thrombolysis

Indications

Thrombolytic therapy has a role for patients with acute/subacute onset of worsening ischemic symptoms related to thrombosis (superimposed on atherosclerotic disease), embolism, or bypass graft occlusion. The potential benefits of intervention with thrombolysis as opposed to alternative treatment modalities must always be balanced against the potential risk of thrombolytic intervention.

With acute embolic or thrombotic occlusion in diabetics, this occlusion is invariably superimposed on chronic disease, indicated by the presence of numerous collateral vessels, and therefore tends to result in a relatively moderate deterioration in hemodynamics. This deterioration, however, may be enough to overwhelm compensatory flow and can result in limb-threatening ischemia nonetheless. This is in contradistinction to patients without underlying arterial steno-occlusive disease and therefore undeveloped collateral flow, who tend to present more rapidly with more profound ischemia and are more likely to have a nonviable limb at presentation.

The use of thrombolytic therapy for aortoiliac or infrainguinal disease should be based on the clinical history. An acute deterioration (<14 days) suggests a role for thrombolysis to unmask the causative lesion and prevent distal embolization with PTA (Fig. 3).

Similarly, with an occluded peripheral bypass graft of <14 days' duration associated with threatened limb loss, thrombolysis is the preferred option to restore patency *(49,50)*. Some patients with early graft occlusion may not be symptomatic at the time of occlusion but later develop new ischemic symptoms such as tissue loss. Potentially salvageable grafts may be lost if not treated promptly. This is particularly relevant in patients with limited vein for a new distal bypass or patients with previous episodes of graft loss and delayed onset of ischemic symptoms. An exception is early postoperative graft failure within 14 days of the primary operation: thrombolysis should not be used.

Before thrombolytic therapy can be undertaken, careful consideration should to be given to the severity of ischemia, allowing time for thrombolysis and indeed clinical findings that can contraindicate such treatment. Viable (no muscle or sensory loss) and marginally threatened limbs (no muscle weakness and minimal sensory loss) *(51)* are often chosen for thrombolytic therapy first. Absolute contraindications include an established intracranial event (trauma, surgery, stroke, transient ischemic attack), active bleeding diathesis, and recent gastrointestinal bleed (within 10 days). Relative contraindications include major surgery or cardiopulmonary resuscitation within the previous 10 days and uncontrolled hypertension. Relative minor contraindications include diabetic hemorrhagic retinopathy. Many diabetic patients presenting with critical limb ischemia will give a history of retinopathy, and this should be a contraindication to thrombolytic therapy if it has been associated with hemorrhage within the 3 months before proposed thrombolytic therapy *(52)*.

Technique and Evaluation

Once thrombolytic therapy has been decided on, success of such therapy depends on the ability to pass a wire and infusion catheter to a position that allows infusion of thrombolytic agent directly into the clot. If infusion catheter placement within the clot fails, regional infusion (dripping thrombolytic agent proximal to occlusion) can be performed with a view to passing the catheter distally within clot to achieve a more optimal position within 6 hours.

After successful thrombolysis in atherosclerotic disease or occluded grafts, the underlying lesion should be identified. This lesion (atherosclerotic steno-occlusive plaque, graft, or anastomotic stenosis/occlusion) should then be treated by the most appropriate percutaneous or surgical technique.

Patients undergoing thrombolytic therapy need expert clinical and nursing care in appropriate facilities with staff who are familiar with thrombolytic therapy and its inherent risks. It is not unusual for thrombolytic therapy to be associated with an initial clinical deterioration in terms of peripheral ischemia. This is related to thrombolysis producing peripheral embolization of fragmented clot, and clinical improvement can be expected with continued thrombolysis. Although measurement of fibrinogen levels is controversial, regular estimation of hemoglobin and hematocrit can help detect occult minor hemorrhage, and daily renal function and urinary output is considered prudent *(53)*.

Postprocedural anticoagulation should be continued until endovascular or surgical intervention corrects the underlying stenosis or occlusion. Long-term anticoagulation

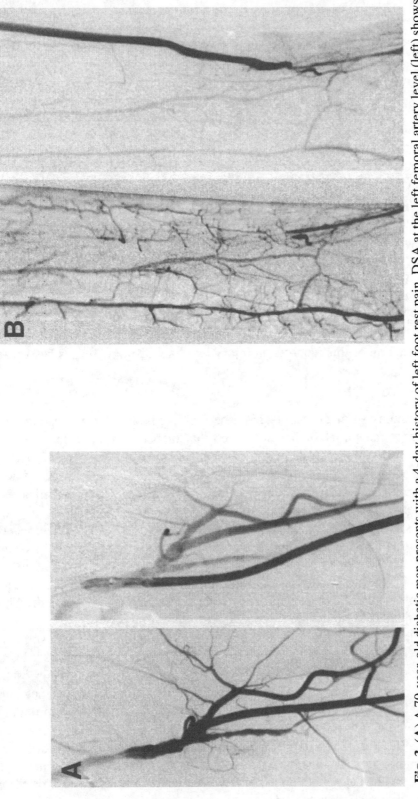

Fig. 3. (A) A 70-year-old diabetic man presents with a 4-day history of left foot rest pain. DSA at the left femoral artery level (left) shows total occlusion of the left femoral-distal anterior tibial vein graft, which had been placed 2 years previously, and occlusion of the left superficial femoral artery. The good-caliber left profunda femoris in part explains the subacute presentation. After 14 hours of thrombolysis (right), the graft appears widely patent. (B) At the calf level, of the same patient, initially a diseased posterior tibial artery (which occludes before the plantar origin), a peroneal artery, and a distally reconstituted anterior tibial artery are seen (left). After 14 hours of thrombolysis (right), the graft is patent and a stenosis at the distal anastomosis is revealed. Continuity to a good dorsalis pedis was demonstrated on examination of the foot. This anastomotic lesion was treated surgically, and patency of the graft is maintained at 9-month follow-up.

should be considered if no underlying steno-occlusive lesion has been determined or corrected.

Complications

Severe systemic or intracranial bleeding is the most significant clinical risk associated with thrombolytic therapy. The overall risk of stroke is reported to be between 1 and 2.3%, with major and minor bleeding reported in 5.1 and 14.8%, respectively *(50,54,55)*.

Most commonly, bleeding complications are at the puncture site, with occasional pseudoaneurysm formation. Retroperitoneal and intraabdominal bleeding can occur spontaneously and manifest as abdominal or back pain. Irrespective of the site of bleed, management follows a standard pattern: stop thrombolytic and anticoagulation treatment, consider replenishing coagulation factors, and perform surgery if bleeding continues or if hematoma pressure phenomenon produces significant clinical deterioration.

Thrombolytic therapy can cause a sudden return of oxygenated blood to acutely ischemic muscle, which can in turn cause the release of free radicals and subsequent cell damage. Failure to anticipate or recognize this reperfusion injury complication can lead to rapid development of compartment syndrome and myonecrosis, necessitating fasciotomy. Prevention of this reperfusion injury by pharmacologic means has yet to be determined.

Outcome

The most common use of thrombolysis in the diabetic population is treatment of occluded bypass grafts. Initial studies suggested that diabetics respond less well to graft and native vessel thrombolysis, with technical success of thrombolysis reported in 80% of nondiabetics and 52% of diabetics *(56,57)*. More recently, the presence of diabetes has been found not to affect technical success adversely (76% for diabetics and 67% for nondiabetics) or to significantly affect long-term outcome in terms of graft patency or limb salvage when compared with nondiabetics *(58)*. Technical success is more common in patients with acute ischemia, short duration of occlusion favoring clot lysis, and reestablishment of antegrade flow *(58,59)*. Furthermore, the STILE investigators *(54)* found that thrombolysis was more efficacious than surgery in patients with symptoms of <14 days' duration. These investigators also found that patients with chronic ischemia had better outcomes with surgery than thrombolysis.

Patients with underlying lesion, revealed by thrombolysis and treatable by surgery, have the most favorable prognosis. Thrombolysis of infrapopliteal bypass grafts is technically as successful as more proximal graft thrombolysis with an underlying lesion suitable for graft revision in more than 50% of patients. The cumulative patency and limb salvage results, however, are worse for distal graft thrombolysis than for proximal graft thrombolysis. Reported cumulative patency for proximal grafts (mainly femoropopliteal) are 56% at 1 year *(60)* and 46% at 18 months *(61)* compared with 36% at 1 year and 32% at 18 months for distal (infrapopliteal) grafts *(58)*. Limb salvage rates at 1 (51%) and 3 years (42%) appear to be lower for distal grafts *(58)* than those of more proximal grafts (84% at 30 months) *(61)*.

Atherectomy

The concept of debulking plaque was initially directed at the limitations of PTA for treating eccentric calcified lesions. These catheter devices are introduced through per-

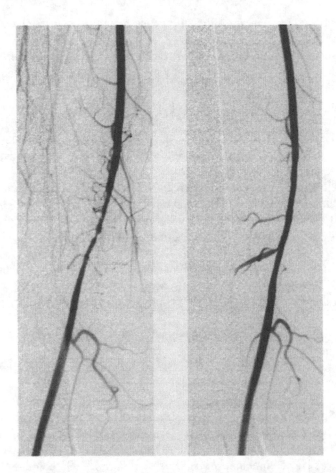

Fig. 4. A 32-year-old insulin-dependent diabetic man presents with intermittent claudication. At the level of previous surgical superficial femoral artery endarterectomy and vein patch angioplasty performed a year previously, DSA (left) now shows a recurrent severe stenosis. Because intimal hyperplasia is probably contributing to this stenotic lesion, atherectomy is performed with a 6 French atherectomy catheter (right), with restoration of patency and relief of symptoms reported at 6-month follow-up.

cutaneous sheaths and passed over a wire. Despite actual removal and debulking of plaque and/or intimal hyperplasia lesions, the invariable vessel wall trauma produced by the device still induces intimal hyperplasia, which subsequently results in recurrent stenosis. Although encouraging clinical results for treatment of infrainguinal disease were shown initially, the results after 6 months are similar to those reported with PTA *(62)*. Atherectomy devices have failed to reduce the incidence of restenosis that occurs with other endovascular procedures such as PTA. Until such time as intimal hyperplasia restenosis can be solved, atherectomy is limited to cases in which PTA is ineffective or contraindicated (Fig. 4). Such cases might include recurrent intimal hyperplastic stenotic lesions in failing lower extremity bypass grafts *(63,64)*.

REFERENCES

1. Nathan DM. Long-term complications in diabetes mellitus. *New Engl J Med* 1993;328: 1676–1685.

2. American Diabetes Association. Clinical practice recommendations, 1992–1993. *Diabetes Care* 1993;16:1–118.
3. Larsson J, Apequist J, Agardh CD, Stenstrom A. Decreasing incidence of major amputation in diabetic patients: a consequence of a multidisciplinary foot care management team approach? *Diabet Med* 1995;12:770–776.
4. Dotter CT, Judkins MP. Transluminal treatment of atherosclerotic obstructions: description of a new technique and preliminary report of its application. *Circulation* 1964;30:654–670.
5. Tetteroo E, Haaring C, Van der Graaf Y, et al. Randomised comparison of primary stent placement versus primary angioplasty followed by selective stent placement in patients with iliac-artery occlusive disease. *Lancet* 1998;341:1153–1159.
6. Ring EJ, Freiman DB, McLean GK. Percutaneous recanalization of common iliac artery occlusions: an unacceptable complication rate? *AJR* 1982;139:587–589.
7. Kinney TB, Rose SC. Intraarterial pressure measurements during angiographic evaluation of peripheral vascular disease: techniques, interpretation, applications and limitations. *AJR* 1996;166:277–284.
8. Bonn J. Percutaneous vascular intervention: value of hemodynamic measurements. *Radiology* 1996;201:18–20.
9. Palmaz JC, Laborde JC, Rivera FJ, et al. Stenting of the iliac arteries with the Palmaz stent: experience in a multicenter trial. *Cardiovasc Intervent Radiol* 1992;15:291–297.
10. Murphy TP, Khwaja AA, Webb MS. Aortoiliac stent placement in patients treated for intermittent claudication. *J Vasc Intervent Radiol* 1998;9:421–428.
11. Dyet JF, Gaines PA, Nicholson AA, et al. Treatment of chronic iliac artery occlusions by means of percutaneous endovascular stent placement. *J Vasc Intervent Radiol* 1997;8:349–353.
12. Ballard JL, Sparks SR, Taylor FC, et al. Complications of iliac artery stent deployment. *J Vasc Surg* 1996;24:545–555.
13. Martin EC, Katzen BT, Benenati JF, et al. Multicenter trial of the Wallstent in the iliac and femoral arteries [see comments]. *J Vasc Intervent Radiol* 1995;6:843–849.
14. Gardiner GA Jr, Meyerovitz MF, Stokes KR, et al. Complications of transluminal angioplasty. *Radiology* 1986;159:201–208.
15. Strecker EP, Boos IB, Hagen B, et al. Flexible tantalum stents for the treatment of iliac artery lesions; long-term patency, complications, and risk factors. *Radiology* 1996;199:641–647.
16. Ballard JL, Bergan JJ, Singh P, et al. Aortoiliac stent deployment versus surgical reconstruction: analysis of outcome and cost. *J Vasc Surg* 1998;28:94–103.
17. Bosch JL, Hunick MG. Meta-analysis of the results of percutaneous transluminal angioplasty and stent placement for aortoiliac occlusive disease. *Radiology* 1997;204:87–96.
18. Brophy DP, Sheiman RG, Amatulle P, Akbari C. Iatrogenic femoral pseudoaneurysms: thrombin injection after failed US-guided compression. *Radiology* 2000;214:278–282.
19. Belli AM, Cumberland DC, Knox AM, et al. The complication rate of percutaneous peripheral balloon angioplasty. *Clin Radiol* 1990;41:380–383.
20. Darcy M. Complications of iliac angioplasty and stenting. *Techn Vasc Intervent Radiol* 2000;3:226–239.
21. Group TW. Aortoiliac disease-surgical treatment. *J Vasc Surg* 2000;31:S205–S206.
22. de Vries SO, Hunick MG. Results of aortic bifurcation grafts for aortoiliac occlusive disease: a meta-analysis. *J Vasc Surg* 1997;26:558–569.
23. Spence LD, Hartnell GG, Reinking G, et al. Diabetic versus nondiabetic limb-threatening ischemia: outcome of percutaneous intervention. *AJR* 1999;172:1335–1341.
24. Veith FJ, Gupta SK, Wengerter KR, et al. Changing atherosclerotic disease patterns and management strategies in lower-limb-threatening ischemia. *Ann Surg* 1990;212:402–414.
25. Bakal CW, Cynamon J, Sprayregen S. Infrapopliteal percutaneous transluminal angioplasty: what we know. *Radiology* 1996;200:36–43.

26. Horvath W, Oertl M, Haidinger D. Percutaneous transluminal angioplasty of crural arteries. *Radiology* 1990;177:565–569.
27. Matsi PJ, Manninen HI, Suhonen MT, Pirenen AE, Soimakaillio S. Chronic critical limb ischemia: prospective trial of angioplasty with 1-36 month follow-up. *Radiology* 1993;188:381–387.
28. Sivanathan UM, Browne TF, Thorley PJ, Rees MR. Percutaneous transluminal angioplasty of the tibial arteries. *Br J Surg* 1994;81:1282–1285.
29. Wagner HJ, Starck EE, McDermott JC. Infrapopliteal percutaneous transluminal revascularization: results of a prospective study on 148 patients. *J Vasc Intervent Radiol* 1993;8:81–90.
30. Morgenstern BR, Getrajdman GI, Laffey KJ, Bixon R, Martin EC. Total occlusion of the femoropopliteal artery: high technical success rate of conventional balloon angioplasty. *Radiology* 1989;172:937–940.
31. Hartnell GG, Jones AM, Murphy P. Do hydrophilic guidewires affect the technical success rates of percutaneous angioplasty? *Angiology* 1995;46:229–234.
32. Schwarten DE, Cutcliff WB. Arterial occlusive disease below the knee: treatment with percutaneous transluminal angioplasty performed with low-profile catheters and steerable guide wires. *Radiology* 1988;169:71–74.
33. Group TW. Infrainguinal disease-endovascular treatment. *J Vasc Surg* 2000;31:S226–S233.
34. Collaboration AT. Collaborative overview of randomised trials of antiplatelet therapy. II: Maintenance of vascular grafts or arterial patency by antiplatelet therapy. *BMJ* 1994;308:159–168.
35. Becquemin JP. Effect of ticlopidine on the long term patency of saphenous vein bypass grafts in the legs. *N Engl J Med* 1997;337:1726–1731.
36. Bennett CL, Connors JM, Carwile JM, et al. Thrombotic thrombocytopenic purpura associated with clopidogrel. *N Engl J Med* 2000;342:1773–1777.
37. Steinhubl SR, Tan WA, Foody JM, Topol EJ. Incidence and clinical course of thrombotic thrombocytopenic purpura due to ticlopidine following coronary stenting. *JAMA* 1999;281:806–810.
38. Matsi PJ, Manninen HI, Vanninen RL, et al. Femoropopliteal angioplasty in patients with claudication: primary and secondary patency in 140 limbs with 1–3 year follow-up. *Radiology* 1994;191:727–733.
39. Murray RR, Hewes RC, White RI, et al. Long segment femoropopliteal stenoses: is angioplasty a boon or a bust? *Radiology* 1987;162:473–476.
40. Krepel VM, Van Andel GJ, Van Erp WF, Breslau PJ. Percutaneous transluminal angioplasty of the femoropopliteal artery: initial and long term results. *Radiology* 1985;156:25–28.
41. Johnson KW. Femoral and popliteal arteries: reanalysis of results of balloon angioplasty. *Radiology* 1992;183:767–771.
42. Capek P, McLean GK, Berkowitz HD. Femoropopliteal angioplasty: factors influencing long term success. *Circulation* 1991;83:I-70–I-80.
43. Brown KT, Moore ED, Getrajdman GI, Saddekni S. Infrapopliteal angioplasty: long-term follow up. *J Vasc Intervent Radiol* 1993;4:139–144.
44. Gallino A, Mahler F, Probst P, Nachbur B. Percutaneous transluminal angioplasty of the arteries of the lower limbs: a 5 year follow-up. *Circulation* 1984;70:619–623.
45. Jeans WD, Armstrong S, Cole SE, Horocks M, Baird RN. Fate of patients undergoing transluminal angioplasty for lower limb ischemia. *Radiology* 1990;177:559–564.
46. Stokes KR, Strunk HM, Campbell DR, et al. Five-year results of angioplasty of iliac and femoropopliteal angioplasty in diabetic patients. *Radiology* 1990;174:977–982.
47. Bakal CW, Sprayregen S, Scheinbaum K, Cynamon J, Veith FJ. Percutaneous transluminal angioplasty of the infrapopliteal arteries: results in 53 patients. *AJR* 1990;154:171–174.
48. Bull PG, Mendel H, Hold M, Schlegl A, Denck H. Distal popliteal and tibioperoneal transluminal angioplasty: long term follow-up. *J Vasc Intervent Radiol* 1992;3:45–53.

49. Camerota AJ, Weaver FA, Hosking JD, et al. Results of prospective, randomized trial of surgery versus thrombolysis for occluded lower extremity bypass grafts. *Am J Surg* 1996; 172:105–112.

50. Ouriel K, Veith FJ, Sasahara AA, et al. Thrombolysis or peripheral arterial surgery (TOPAS): phase 1 results. *J Vasc Surg* 1996;23:64–75.

51. Rutherford RB, Baker JD, Ernst C, et al. Recommended standards for reports dealing with lower limb ischemia: revised version. *J Vasc Surg* 1997;26:517–538.

52. NIH Consensus Development Conference. Thrombolytic therapy in thrombosis. *BMJ* 1980; 280:1585–1587.

53. Working Party on Thrombolysis in the Management of Limb Ischemia. Thrombolysis in the management of lower limb peripheral arterial occlusion—a consensus document. *Am J Cardiol* 1998;81:207–218.

54. The STILE Investigators. Results of a prospective randomised trial evaluating surgery versus thrombolysis for ischemia of the lower extremity. *Ann Surg* 1994;220:251–268.

55. Berridge DC, Niakin GS, Hopkinson BR. Local low-dose intra-arterial thrombolytic therapy, the risk of major stroke and haemorrhage. *Br J Surg* 1989;76:1230–1232.

56. Ouriel K, Shortell CK, Azodo MV, Guiterrez OH, Marder VJ. Acute peripheral arterial occlusion: predictors of success in catheter-directed thrombolytic therapy. *Radiology* 1994; 193:561–566.

57. Shortell C, Ouriel K. Thrombolysis in acute peripheral arterial occlusion: predictors of immediate success. *Ann Vasc Surg* 1994;8:59–65.

58. Spence LD, Hartnell GG, Reinking G, et al. Thrombolysis of infrapopliteal bypass grafts: efficacy and underlying angiographic pathology. *AJR* 1997;169:717–721.

59. Durham JD, Geller SC, Abbott WM, et al. Regional infusion of urokinase into occluded lower-extremity bypass grafts: long-term clinical results. *Radiology* 1989;172:83–87.

60. Sullivan KL, Gardiner GA, Kandarpa K, et al. Efficacy of thrombolysis in infrainguinal bypass grafts. *Circulation* 1991;83:99–105.

61. Hye RJ, Turner C, Valji K, et al. Is thrombolysis of occluded popliteal and tibial bypass grafts worthwhile? *J Vasc Surg* 1994;20:588–597.

62. Vroegindeweij D, Tielbeek AV, Buth J, et al. Directional atherectomy vs. balloon angioplasty in segmental femoropopliteal artery disease: 2-year follow-up with color flow duplex scanning. *J Vasc Surg* 1995;21:255–269.

63. Porter DH, Rosen MP, Skillman JJ, Kent KC, Kim D. Mid-term and long-term results with directional atherectomy of vein graft stenoses. *J Vasc Surg* 1995;23:554–567.

64. Dolmatch BL, Gray RJ, Horton KM, Rundback JH, Kline ME. Treatment of anastomotic bypass graft stenosis with directional atherectomy: short-term and intermediate results. *J Vasc Intervent Radiol* 1995;6:105–113.

22

Footwear in the Prevention of Diabetic Foot Problems

Luigi Uccioli, MD

INTRODUCTION

Diabetes represents the primary cause of non-traumatic amputation in the western world *(1)*. It is estimated that approximately 25% of subjects with diabetes will, over the course of their lives, experience problems with their feet and that one-third of these patients will undergo amputation *(2–4)*. Although these data highlight the extent of this problem in the diabetic population, they do not necessarily predicate inevitability: on the contrary, they serve to demonstrate that simple and relatively inexpensive measures may be able to reduce the number of amputations by up to 85% *(5–9)*. Some clinical conditions put the diabetic patient "at risk of ulceration." An awareness of these conditions and the identification of subjects at risk may permit the introduction of suitable preventive strategies *(10–13)*.

Although peripheral vascular disease is only rarely a precipitating factor in ulcer formation *(3)*, neuropathy has a central role in the mechanisms underlying the lesion, and represents a predisposing factor; other external factors may precipitate the situation and determine the appearance of ulcers *(14–16)*. Among the latter, a decisive role is played by footwear: indeed, unsuitable footwear may not sufficiently protect the foot and in some cases may even be dangerous. Given that the interaction between foot and footwear is crucial in the mechanism of ulceration, it is important that the health provider not only be aware of the importance of the selection of suitable footwear but that he or she be able to make a professional evaluation in this regard, as correct footwear may represent a valid means of prevention. Moreover, it is important to focus attention on the role of footwear and loading characteristics in repair mechanisms insofar as a neuropathic ulcer may heal spontaneously simply through an appropriate unloading at the site of the lesion.

Neuropathic complications may pose a risk of foot ulceration through two different mechanisms. The first is related to sensory neuropathy *(17)*. The insensitivity of the feet to painful stimuli makes them particularly vulnerable in terms of external forces such as very high temperatures (water, sand, heaters, and so on) or to foreign bodies in the shoe (pebbles, coins, and so on) or even to very worn shoes or to those containing

From: *The Diabetic Foot: Medical and Surgical Management*
Edited by: A. Veves, J. M. Giurini, and F. W. LoGerfo © Humana Press Inc., Totowa, NJ

contusive particles (e.g., tacks), or to unsuitable footwear in terms of size and/or shape. The footwear may be too tight or incorrectly sized, or unsuitable for deformed toes (with ensuing friction between the foot and shoe); in any case, painful symptoms are absent and are therefore unable to protect the foot from detrimental external factors *(18)*. Numerous prospective studies demonstrate the relationship between neuropathy and ulceration. The determination of the vibratory perception threshold using biotesiometry or tactile sensitivity with monofilaments allows an evaluation of the degree of risk encountered by patients owing to neuropathic complications *(14,19–23)*.

The other mechanism through which neuropathy is responsible for foot lesions is related to the presence both of sensory and motor neuropathies *(24)*. The latter, owing to the ensuing imbalance between the flexor and extensor muscles, cause deformities such as clawtoe, hammertoe, bunions, and arched feet *(25,26)*. Although not exclusive to diabetic neuropathy, clawtoe, hammertoe, and bunions, are all particularly dangerous conditions when associated with peripheral neuropathy. On the one hand, they generate friction with footwear (e.g., clawtoe not adequately accommodated in insufficient space in the frontal region and ensuing friction with the surface of the foot); on the other, they are associated with a lack of sense perception (and consequently of sensitivity) and a reduced defense capacity from the point of view of mechanical damage. Furthermore, these deformities result in areas of hyperpression, particularly at the level of the metatarsal heads, where reactive hyperkeratosis first appears, followed by ulceration *(20,27,28)*.

In the presence of neuropathy, foot deformities are responsible for the frontal shift of the submetatarsal adipose pads, following which the metatarsal heads come into direct contact with the ground *(29)*. It is in this situation that the development of hyperkeratosis, which is a response mechanism to the overload, is in itself responsible for further hyperpression. (Indeed, it has been ascertained that the removal of a hyperkeratosis is able to reduce hyperpression by up to 30% *[30]*). Some prospective studies have also demonstrated the relationship between areas of hyperpression and the subsequent development of ulceration *(31)*. It should also be borne in mind that an increase in pressure associated with insensitivity represents an increased risk; indeed, subjects who have rheumatoid arthritis with comparable hyperpression do not experience ulceration *(32)*. Therefore, it is fairly evident that a reduction in hyperpression represents a means of reducing the risk of ulceration.

Another important aspect to bear in mind is related to the role of footwear in the mechanisms associated with the pathogenesis and/or prevention of lesions; it is fairly obvious that, given their vulnerability, diabetic subjects must select footwear that does not pose a further threat of risk and that ideally serves as a form of protection. It is important that the physician, conscious of the importance of the role of footwear, be fully informed in order to make suitable recommendations. In turn, the patient must be made aware of the potential risk of lesion posed by unsuitable footwear and must be encouraged to accept a certain type of footwear that may not necessarily coincide with personal taste.

In the discussion below, we first take a look at the various types of footwear most suitable for patients who do not have lesions, subdivided by category of risk. Subsequently we discuss the options available for patients who have active lesions, with a view to releasing the pressure overload at the point of ulceration.

Table 1
Risk Classes

Class	Definition
0: Low	Normal protective sensation
1: Medium	Loss of protective sensation, without foot deformities and without history of foot ulceration or previous amputation
2: High	Loss of protective sensation, with foot deformities but without history of foot ulceration and/or amputation
3: Very high	Loss of protective sensation, with foot deformities and with history of foot ulceration or amputation

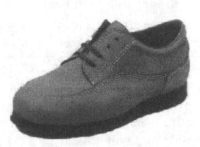

Fig. 1. A shoe with a soft sole and amply shaped soft upper that is available in different widths and is suitable for risk classes 0 and 1.

CATEGORIES OF RISK AND FOOTWEAR RECOMMENDATIONS

As outlined above, diabetic patients are at risk of foot ulceration not only because of diabetes but also because of diabetes complicated by neuropathy. It is clear that particular attention to footwear should be taken by these subjects at risk, insofar as suitable footwear is able to reduce abnormal pressure, reduce the formation of callus and ulcers, and protect from external trauma. Not all patients have the same level of risk, and a number of factors, including the presence/absence of protective sense perception, presence/absence of significant foot deformities, and presence/absence of previous ulcers, should be evaluated in determining risk categories and planning corrective means of prevention *(33)*. Four risk categories have been identified on the basis of these criteria (Table 1) *(33)*.

Category 0: Patients not at Risk of Ulceration
(Patients Without Active or Previous Lesions)

Diabetic patients without chronic complications and with a preserved protective sensation require adequate education but no real change to footwear for daily use. In general terms, given their diabetic status, they should be simply encouraged to evaluate a number of factors when selecting footwear, such as whether the shoe is well fitting and amply shaped, with soft uppers and a sole able to absorb vertical forces; they should avoid tight-fitting footwear with a narrow forefoot, tight toe box, or tight instep (Fig. 1).

Table 2
Suggestions for the Right Selection of Footwear

Both feet should be measured with an appropriate measuring device.

Both shoes should be fit while standing.

The position at the first metatarsophalangeal joint should be checked. It should be located in the widest portion of the shoe.

The right length of the shoe should be checked; additional volume should be considered at the top of the toes. Allow 3/8–1/2 inch between the end of the shoe and the longest toe.

The proper width should be tested; enough space should be present around the ball of the foot. A soft and moldable upper with extra space should be selected in the presence of foot deformities.

A firm heel counter for rearfoot stability with a soft padded collar is important.

Shoes with laces or straps should be selected because they allow a wider opening and an easier entry into the shoes; in addition, they allow better fit to the foot shape.

For every foot there is an ideal shape that avoids friction and the development of corns. It is important to consider not only shoe length but also width. Shoes made at least with different widths for each size should be preferred in order to fit the natural shape of the foot better without constriction. Education on selection of suitable footwear is very important (Table 2).

Category 1: Patients at Risk of Ulceration

The development of sensory neuropathy with an ensuing loss of protective sensation involves a subsequent risk of ulceration *(14,19–21)*. Education in patients with a loss of protective sensation assumes a very important role: above all, a number of behavioral traits need to be inculcated, such as never walking barefoot, avoiding mended socks, and learning to substitute the loss of sensation with alternative senses (e.g., eyesight or hand touch). These patients must learn to sample water temperature by hand before washing their feet in order to avoid burns, to detect foreign bodies such as pebbles before putting on their shoes, and to evaluate other dangerous signs (e.g., tacks or worn soles). They must be guided to an understanding that the selection of footwear cannot be based on the usual criteria, namely, the immediate sensation of comfort. Indeed, in the presence of sensory neuropathy, the patient perceives even tight shoes to be comfortable. Therefore, it is essential that the foot be measured in all its dimensions and that the footwear contain the foot without even the most minimal constriction. Education in the selection of the shoes is therefore very important in this category as well (Table 2). Soft, leather-laced oxfords of adequate size to accommodate pressure-dissipating accommodative insoles or foot orthoses are preferred (Figs. 2 and 3).

Category 2: Patients at High Risk of Ulceration

When the loss of protective sensation is complicated by foot deformities (e.g., bunion, clawtoe, hammertoe), whether independent of diabetes (e.g., idiopathic bunion) or more frequently secondary to motor neuropathy, the risk of ulceration is considerably increased.

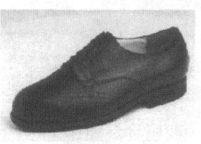

Fig. 2. A soft, flexible leather-laced oxford of adequate size to accommodate pressure-dissipating accommodative insoles.

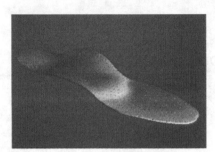

Fig. 3. A single-layer, pressure-dissipating accommodative insole.

Epidemiologic studies examining risk factors in ulceration always take foot deformities into consideration as a condition that increases the risk of ulceration *(18,34)*.

When foot deformities (e.g., of the toes) are accommodated in unsuitable footwear, the mechanism underlying the lesion involves friction caused by the upper part of the shoe, which first causes a superficial abrasion and later an outright ulcer. Ulcers associated with this sort of friction are usually localized on the top of the toes and on the lateral surfaces of the first and fifth toes. These cases necessitate a heightened awareness of the correct selection of footwear both in terms of shape, as the foot should not be constrained in any way, and from the point of view of materials used for the uppers. These materials should be soft and flexible, as well as adaptable to any surface irregularities in such a way as to guarantee perfect fitting and to avoid the threat of friction. Nonetheless, the increased risk associated with foot deformities is not exclusively owing to the difficulty in accommodating deformed toes, but above all to the biomechanical changes in gait pattern provoked by such deformities. In patients with motor neuropathy together with toe deformities associated with atrophy of the lumbrical and interosseous muscles *(35)*, it is evident that an alteration in the walking pattern could be related to atrophy of the frontal and rear muscles of the leg *(36,37)* and to modified control of the ankle joint; toe deformities involve a loss of walking function with a consequent appearance and persistence of overload at the metatarsal level in the propulsion and toe-off phases *(38)*.

Therefore a further pathogenic mechanism of ulceration involves the development of areas of overload; indeed, owing to motor neuropathy, some areas become overloaded and bear the brunt of altered biomechanics, with ensuing hyperkeratosis followed by

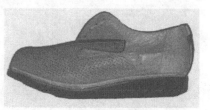

Fig. 4. Section of a shoe with "biomechanical properties": the recessed heel allows a soft impact at heel strike; the point of rolling inserted immediately behind the metatarsal heads allows a smooth transition from midstance to propulsion; the presence of a wider angle between the sole and the ground at the most anterior part of the shoe further reduces the stress at the level of the metatarsal heads during propulsion and toe-off.

Table 3
Tovey Suggestions for Correct Selection
of Shoes and Insoles in Diabetic Neuropathic Patients

Elastic insoles should ensure the right shock absorption.
Insoles should allow the spreading of plantar pressure on a wider area.
Shoes should be made with a rocker bottom.
Extra space should be provided in the anterior portion of the shoe to accommodate deformed toes and avoid undue hyperpressions from the shoe vamp.

ulceration *(39)*. Patients in this category benefit greatly from the use of footwear that corrects or at least mitigates these biomechanical defects *(40,41)*.

The aim underlying footwear recommendations in these patients is to offer an extra level of protection from the mechanical stress involved in walking, when there has been a loss of the capacity to perceive autonomously an excessive mechanical stress *(42,43)*. Shoes with "biomechanical properties" should allow the development of a protected walking pattern, with reduced plantar pressures. This may be guaranteed by the presence of a recessed heel that allows a soft impact at heel strike; by the presence of a point of rolling of the sole inserted immediately behind the metatarsal heads that allows a smooth transition from midstance to propulsion; and by the presence of a wider angle between the sole and the ground at the most anterior part of the shoe that further reduces stress at the level of the metatarsal heads during propulsion and toe-off (Fig. 4).

In 1984 Tovey *(44)* outlined the fundamental requisites for footwear designed for diabetic subjects (Table 3). These include the need for appropriate unloading absorbed by total contact, custom-fabricated, pressure-dissipating accommodative foot orthoses (Fig. 5), inserted in deep lacing shoes manufactured in soft leather with a frontal region designed to accommodate claw- or hammertoes suitably. Tovey also recommended footwear designed with a rocker bottom to reduce the load in the execution of the step in the rolling phase *(44)*. However, there are no prospective data to demonstrate the role of footwear in the primary prevention of ulceration in patients with peripheral neuropathy. Data reported in the literature refer either to clinical experience in secondary

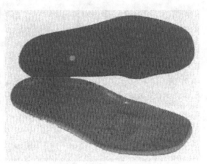

Fig. 5. Total contact, custom-fabricated, pressure-dissipating accommodative foot orthoses.

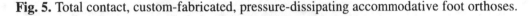

prevention or to studies in which the parameters evaluated were plantar pressures measured instrumentally and unloaded using different aids *(40–42)*.

Ashry and colleagues *(41)* have used insole sensors to measure peak plantar pressures to evaluate the effectiveness of five footwear-insole strategies. They found that, comparing extra-depth shoes with and without insoles, peak pressures were significantly reduced with insoles, whereas there was no significant difference between the different insole modifications. Using the same measuring device, Mueller and colleagues *(45)* have evaluated the peak plantar pressure in patients with diabetes and transmetatarsal amputation; they found that a full-length shoe with a total contact insert and a rigid rocker bottom sole was the most effective footwear combination in reducing peak plantar pressures on the distal residuum and the forefoot of the contralateral extremity in patients with diabetes and transmetatarsal amputation. Kästenbauer and colleagues *(40)* have shown that certain running shoes (Adidas Torsion Equipment Cushion) designed for maximal forefoot pressure relief are effective in decreasing plantar pressure, although the pressure relief obtained was not as great as that of the custom-made soft insole in an in-depth shoe *(40)*. Lavery and co-workers *(43)* compared the effectiveness of therapeutic, comfort, and athletic shoes with and without viscoelastic insoles. They concluded that when used in conjunction with a viscoelastic insole, both the comfort and athletic cross-trainer shoes were as effective as the commonly described therapeutic shoes and therefore viable options to prevent the development or recurrence of foot ulcers.

The measurement of plantar pressure inside footwear has allowed observation of significant differences (in terms of the reduction of pressure) between footwear with a rigid sole and that with a flexible sole *(43)*. An increased reduction in pressure is observed in the rigid model, as this type of sole minimizes the metatarsal-phalangeal joint articulation tension and maximizes foot contact area during the late stance phase (Fig. 6). This kind of shoe induces a modification in the walking pattern that is completely articulated at the ankle joint. (The patient, particularly when beginning to use this type of footwear, may complain about pain in the lower back muscles of the leg as these muscles begin to bear a greater load.) Indeed, it is important to consider the position of the axis of the roll of the step when designing this type of footwear. The characteristics of this type permit a significant reduction in overload. Footwear with a point of the roll of the step placed immediately behind the metatarsal heads is able to guarantee a reduction of peak pressure up to 30% *(46)* (Table 4). A further reduction is acquired by the

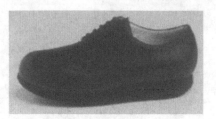

Fig. 6. Footwear with a rigid rocker sole. The rigid sole minimizes the metatarsophalangeal joint articulation tension and maximizes foot contact area during the late stance phase.

Table 4
Characteristics of a Suitable Footwear

Soft leather upper without sewings, preferably oxford type with laces

Rigid rocker sole with a roller axis immediately behind the metatarsal heads

Extra depth to ensure enough space for the deformed toes and the insertion of pressure-dissipating accommodative insoles or foot orthoses

Table 5
Characteristics of a Suitable Insert

Internal layer: soft material to relieve areas of hyperpression

Intermediate layer: elastic material, which helps in unloading and maximizes the contact area

External layer: less elastic material to support foot shape and function

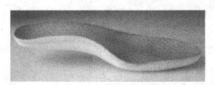

Fig. 7. Total contact inserts can reduce pressure peaks under the foot by maximizing the contact area and spreading the pressure over a larger plantar surface.

use of customized inserts; a reduction of a further 20% in peak pressure and peak time is possible depending on the materials used and the number of layers to realize the insert. Total contact inserts can reduce pressure peaks on the foot by maximizing contact area of the orthotic device to the foot and by spreading the plantar pressures over a larger plantar surface; these factors clearly have a positive impact on the risk of ulceration *(41,47,48)* (Table 5 and Fig. 7).

One of the most elementary rules of hygiene in these cases is simply never to use the same footwear for prolonged periods. Frequent change of footwear puts less stress on discrete areas of the skin and consequently reduces the risk of ulceration.

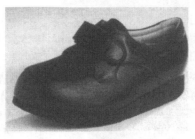

Fig. 8. Shoe with a rigid rocker sole and very high toe box to contain deformed toes and a multilayered customized insole.

Category 3: Patients at Very High Risk of Ulceration (Secondary Prevention)

This category includes patients who have already had an ulcer that has healed. Diabetic patients with a history of relapsing plantar ulcers or patients with a previous minor amputation have abnormally elevated pressures under their feet during walking *(50)*. Peak pressures most often occur under the metatarsal heads and correlate with sites of ulceration *(51)*. The reduction of peak pressure through the use of appropriate footwear represents an important aspect of an effective program of neuropathic foot treatment *(52)*. These patients present a very high risk of relapse. Statistical data demonstrate that this group of patients has a risk of up to 50% in a year *(53)*.

In terms of footwear recommendations, the principles outlined for patients with peripheral neuropathy hold true for this category as well. In particular, patients should be encouraged to select footwear with rigid rocker soles and a molded insert, preferably multilayered, as this type is most beneficial in reducing peak pressures *(48,49)* (Figs. 7 and 8).

In contrast to primary prevention, various studies have demonstrated the protective effect of footwear in secondary prevention, both in terms of made-to-measure solutions and prefabricated commercially designed models. Edmonds et al. *(54)* and Chanteleau and Haage *(55)* have evaluated the protective effectiveness of made-to-measure footwear, comparing the rate of relapse between subjects either wearing or not wearing the recommended and supplied footwear. The use of suitable footwear represented a significantly lower rate of relapse *(54,55)*. Our experience using commercial models has also demonstrated a lower rate of relapse *(53)*. That at 1-year follow-up has been 27.7% in the treated group versus 58.3% in the control group. Striesow *(56)*, who tested industrially produced special shoes realized according to Tovey guidelines, observed similar results.

The use of commercial footwear indeed offers a number of advantages. First of all, it is possible to standardize the type of intervention. It is important to highlight that Edmonds *(57)* in his review stresses the need to identify a single orthopedic procedure as a reference point in recommending corrective measures for the diabetic foot, given the general overall ignorance of the topic. The Consensus Development Conference on Diabetic Foot Wound Care reported that "Footwear should be prescribed, manufactured, and dispensed by individuals with experience in the care of diabetic foot"*(58)*. In addition, the Medicare guidelines related to the therapeutic shoe bill do not clearly define the qualifications of those who furnish therapeutic footwear. The only requirement with respect to footwear expertise states "The footwear must be fitted and furnished by a podiatrist or other qualified individual such as a pedorthist, orthotist or prosthetist." However, the guidelines do not specify standards for nonphysicians. Suppliers do not have to submit any evidence of their expertise to Medicare (59). It follows that in certain situations the physician is incapable of making recommendations and the orthopedic specialist is not sufficiently aware of the problem; in such cases the solutions offered may be ineffective at the least, if not overtly damaging.

Clearly the availability of commercial models with proven success expands the number of patients who can take advantage of beneficial corrective procedures in response to their clinical needs. In addition, other advantages may be related to the use of clinically tested prefabricated models, such as better availability, the possibility of producing stylish models (Fig. 1), and the significant reduction in cost.

Inserts and Bigger Shoes

A problem that often arises is that of using inserts in normal shoes. In general, if the footwear is not designed to offer extra space for the insert, the use of a correctly sized shoe will increase pressure on the foot, as the insert will naturally tighten the available space. The patient will try to resolve this problem by simply buying a bigger size. However, although this will ensure an extra length of 6.7 mm, it will offer only an increase of 4 mm at the circumference of the first and fifth metatarsal heads. The ensuing instability of the foot provokes blisters on the surface of the skin, on the heel, and on the surface of the back of the foot owing to the action of transversal forces on the foot as it slips backward and forward. It is important to measure the diameter of the foot at the level of the metatarsal heads, add the thickness of the insert to this measurement, and compare this with the diameter inside the footwear at that level. The suitability of the footwear depends on the availability of this extra space and not simply on shoe size. Ideally, the footwear should have soft, preferably heat-sensitive, uppers, which allows comfortable accommodation of the foot deformities, and the appropriately fitted insert.

Factors Involved in the General Risk of Ulceration

When one considers the general risk of ulceration in a patient, several variables need to be borne in mind that may influence the risk quite considerably. Beyond the structural configuration of the foot (that is, foot deformities, which we have seen represent a risk factor for increased plantar pressure—peak pressure—for example at the level of the prominent metatarsal heads), the function of the foot must be considered, that is, the cumulative amount of time of loading of these peak areas. (The risk of ulceration increases with the increase in the variable load peaks and overall time of overload).

Another parameter to consider is the protective function of footwear and inserts. This protective function may be effective and may consequently annul the risk of ulceration owing to overload and the time of application, which may be the case with suitable footwear and inserts. In other cases footwear may exercise no protective function whatsoever or may indeed be damaging.

A final consideration involves the lifestyle of patients. The level of activity is understood to be the cumulative load during daily activity, which will naturally be quite different in those with a sedentary lifestyle compared with an active one. It is fairly clear

Table 6
Options to Unload a Neuropathic Foot Ulcer

Total contact cast

Other casts/boots (air cast, walking cast)

Temporary shoes

Sandals

Felted foam dressings

that a neuropathic patient will not present ulcers if confined to bed all day, insofar as plantar overloads are not possible in such a situation *(60)*.

Aids for Patients with Active Lesions

As we have already highlighted, patients with peripheral neuropathy tend to develop ulcers at the point of maximum load. Often patients are not able to, and they should not, stay in bed for 4 or 6 weeks, which is ideally the time required to heal an ulcer in patients with normal arterial circulation and an absence of significant complications (e.g., overlapping infections). Often neuropathic ulcers do not heal owing to the continued load placed on the ulcer during walking. It is fundamental in these cases to provide for adequate unloading in order to favor healing *(61)*. Several options are available to ensure unloading in patients with active ulcers *(62)* (Table 6).

The total contact cast is the most extensively studied technique; it offers total unloading of the ulcer as well as rapid mobilization of the patient, who may resume normal activities immediately. Most experts believe that the total contact cast is the gold standard for the treatment of diabetic foot ulcers. It allows immobilization of the tissues of the ulcers, and it reduces pressure through distribution over a wide surface. However, use of the total contact cast must follow specific indications (neuropathic lesions in Wagner class 1 and 2 in the absolute absence of infections) and contraindications (ischemic lesions and infected lesions in Wagner class 3, 4, and 5). Furthermore, use of such casts is contraindicated in blind patients and in those with pathologic obesity or ataxia. The American literature shows excellent results using total contact plaster casts *(63–65)*. These plaster casts cover the lesion and are removed and substituted weekly to ensure a better fit as the edema subsides and to inspect the wound.

Alternatively, one may use the Scotch cast, a sort of removable boot made of stiff, light material padded with wadding in order to reduce pressure. This is suitable for elderly persons who do not tolerate the plaster cast or when ulcers are situated in difficult areas. Indeed, the Scotch cast is a sort of compromise between the plaster cast and other aids, as it is made to measure and easily removable *(62)*.

Other commercial techniques involve the use of stirrups or other pneumatic means of subpatellar unloading (air cast, walking cast) (Fig. 9). The high cost of these aids has prohibited their widespread use; moreover, their results do not seem to be more beneficial than those reported for the plaster cast *(43,66)*.

Nonetheless, the plaster cast is unsuitable in some conditions. Other aids must be used in these cases, namely, temporary shoes such as talus shoes, which allow unloading of

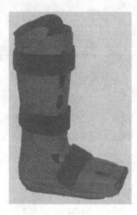

Fig. 9. Aircast: this device allows good control of high pressures at the ulcer site by means of subpatellar unloading.

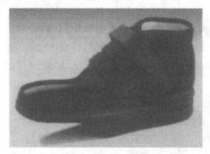

Fig. 10. Talus shoe, allowing unloading of a forefoot ulcer, because the patients walk by loading only the rearfoot.

the lesion in the forefoot owing to the absence of a sole in the front part of the shoe (Fig. 10). Using this healing device the patients walk by loading only the rearfoot. This type of footwear is particularly indicated in young persons who do not present problems of equilibrium. Other aids include temporary footwear with extra volume (extra deep 1/2 inch or super deep 3/4 inch) and a rigid rocker sole (Fig. 11). The extra space is necessary to contain a bigger foot because of the edema and infection that may be present; an insert can be grossly molded to form a depression in which the ulcerated area can be accommodated and unloaded (Fig. 12), and bandages can be different in volume according to the needs of the ulcer. The rigid sole guarantees immobilization of the metatarsal-phalangeal joint and a reduced load at the level of metatarso heads *(45)*. The foot ulcer unloading given by temporary footwear is not equivalent to that of the total contact cast or walking casts *(62)*; however, this kind of device may have other advantages such as wider usability because of the absence of adverse effects, better acceptance, and therefore better compliance: patients can experience quite a normal lifestyle, with the possibility of taking little walks and driving the car, while taking care of their foot ulcers.

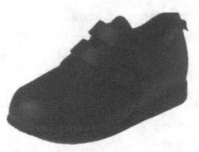

Fig. 11. Temporary footwear with extra volume and rigid rocker sole.

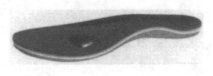

Fig. 12. Foot orthosis for temporary footwear.

Footwear in Charcot Foot

Charcot foot is characterized by complications of the bones and jonts of the foot in patients with diabetes and peripheral neuropathy. It may also occur in other forms of neuropathy such as syringomyelia, tabes dorsalis, and so on. A clear case of Charcot foot is characterized by complete involvement of the bones and joint structures and loss of the structural organization of the foot. In its most typical form, involving the tarsal bones, there is collapse of the plantar roof, with the foot becoming short and squat and the plantar surface assuming a rocking profile and the appearance of high pressure at the midfoot, an area that becomes at risk of ulceration *(67)*. Corrective intervention involves diverse phase-related options. In the less dramatic case, in which bone involvement is detected before bone collapse, the use of a plaster cast (followed by a corrective strategy involving the use of plantar support of the arch, which allows the stabilization of the lesion) can prevent structural damage to the foot. In other cases a diagnosis is made when the bone structure has already deteriorated and the tarsal bones have lost their articulation. A plaster cast is necessary in this case as well, at least until the lesion has been stabilized *(68)*. It should be borne in mind that the time frames for use of a plaster cast are fairly long (in some cases up to 6 months) and that such use is based on empirical observations of skin temperature, as there are no supporting scientific data. Subsequent corrective strategies will largely depend on the ensuing structural deformity; if the patient is able to wear shoes, albeit customized footwear, surgical intervention may not be necessary. Otherwise surgery is usually indicated. Corrective strategies aim at reducing high plantar pressures and the subsequent risk of ulceration *(69)*.

THE PRESCRIPTION AND USE OF SUITABLE FOOTWEAR

In a recent survey Pinzur and colleagues *(70)* observed that most diabetics and their physicians are aware of potential diabetic foot morbidity but that very few take advantage of prophylactic protective footwear. Considerable barriers exist to the use of these shoes. First of all, the reimbursement process for shoes and inserts can be complicated, and often no more than one pair of shoes is allowed every 12 months. Second, patients with foot problems often look for footwear that is presentable and fashionable as well as protective *(71)*. Third, patients often avoid wearing their prescribed footwear; Knowles and Boulton *(71)* found that only 22% of their subjects wore their prescribed footwear all day.

Many strategies need to be applied to encourage the use of protective shoes. In May 1993, the U.S. Congress passed legislation to add therapeutic shoe coverage to the benefits of diabetic Medicare patients at risk of foot disease as part of Medicare Part B coverage. This was done after a 3-year demonstration project found no evidence that such a benefit had increased overall Medicare costs *(72)*. However, the actual number of footwear beneficiaries in 1996 in respect to the potential number was reported to be <1 in 50 Medicare-aged diabetics *(73)*. This means that it is necessary to increase awareness of the benefit among eligible Medicare patients.

Another strategy would be to simplify the documentation and shorten the time necessary to obtain shoes and insoles. Finally, manufacturers should be encouraged to make shoes that are protective as well as fashionable.

CONCLUSIONS

Footwear clearly plays a vital role in prevention of foot lesions and their relapse. Health providers should be aware of this and should be able to make precise recommendations regarding the use of suitable footwear.

REFERENCES

1. Reiber GE, Boyko EJ, Smith DG. Lower extremity foot ulcers and amputations in diabetes, in *Diabetes in America*, 2nd ed. (Harris MI, Cowie CC, Stern MP, et al., eds.), Washington, DC, US Government Printing Office, 1995, pp. 232–238.
2. Centers for Disease Control. *Diabetes Surveillance, 1993*. US Department of Health and Human Services, Atlanta, GA, 1993.
3. Pecoraro RE, Reiber GE, Burgess EM. Pathways to diabetic limb amputation: basis for prevention. *Diabetes Care* 1990;13:513–521.
4. Moss SE, Klein BEK. The prevalence and incidence of lower extremity amputation in diabetic population. *Arch Intern Med* 1992;152:610–616.
5. Litzelman DK, Slemenda CW, Langefeld CD, et al. Reduction of lower extremity clinical abnormalities in patients with non-insulin-dependent diabetes mellitus. *Ann Intern Med* 1993;119:36–41.
6. Edmonds ME, Foster A, Watkins PJ. Can careful foot care in the diabetic patient prevent major amputation? in *Limb Salvage and Amputation for Vascular Disease* (Greenhalgh RM, Jamieson CW, Nicolaides AN, eds.), WB Saunders, Philadelphia, 1988, pp. 407–417.
7. Davidson JK, Alogna M, Goldsmith M, Borden J. Assessment of program effectiveness at Grady Memorial Hospital-Atlanta, in *Educating Diabetic Patients* (Steiner G, Lawrence PA, eds.), Springer, New York, 1981, pp. 329–348.
8. Runyan JW Jr, Vander Zwaag R, Joiner MB, Miller ST. The Memphis Diabetes Continuing Care Program. *Diabetes Care* 1980;3:382–386.
9. Assal JP, Muhlhauser I, Pernet A, Gfeller R, Jorgens V, Berger M. Patient education as the basis for diabetes care in clinical practice and research. *Diabetologia* 1985;28:602–613.
10. Boulton AJM, Kubrusly DB, Bowker JH, et al. Impaired vibratory perception and diabetic foot ulceration. *Diabet Med* 1986;3:335–337.

11. Sims DS Jr, Cavanagh PR, Ulbrecht JS. Risk factors in the diabetic foot. *J Am Phys Ther Assoc* 1988;68:1887–1902.

12. Lavery LA, Armstrong DG, Vela SA, Quebedeaux JL, Fleischli J. Practical criteria for screening patients at high risk for diabetic foot ulcerations. *Arch Intern Med* 1998;158:157–162.

13. McCabe CJ, Stevenson RC, Dolan AM. Evaluation of a diabetic foot screening and education program. *Diabet Med* 1998;15:80–84.

14. Young MJ, Breddly JL, Veves A, Boulton AJM. The prediction of diabetic neuropathic foot ulceration using vibration perception thresholds: a prospective study. *Diabetes Care* 1994;17:557–560.

15. McNeely MJ, Boyko EJ, Ahroni JH, et al. The independent contributions of diabetic neuropathy and vasculopathy in foot ulceration. *Diabetes Care* 1995;18:216–219.

16. Reiber GE, Vileikyte L, Boyko EJ, et al. Causal pathways for incident lower-extremity ulcers in patients with diabetes from two setting. *Diabetes Care* 1999;22:157–162.

17. Harris M, Eastman R, Cowie C. Symptoms of sensory neuropathy in adults with NIDDM in the U.S. population. *Diabetes Care* 1982;16:1446–1452.

18. Apelqvist J, Larsson J, Agardh CD. The influence of external precipitating factors and peripheral neuropathy on the development and outcome of diabetic foot ulcers. *J Diabetes Complications* 1990;4:21–25.

19. Litzelman DK, Marriott DJ, Vinicor F. Independent physiological predictors of foot lesions in patients with NIDDM. *Diabetes Care* 1997;20:1273–1278.

20. Birke JA, Sims DS. Plantar sensory threshold in ulcerative foot. *Lepr Rev* 1986;57:216–267.

21. Sosenko JM, Kato M, Soto R, Bild DE. Comparison of quantitative sensory-threshold measures for their association with foot ulceration in diabetic patients. *Diabetes Care* 1990;13:1057–1061.

22. Kumar S, Fernando DJS, Veves A, et al. Semmes Weinstein monofilaments: a simple, effective and inexpensive screening device for identifyng diabetic patients at risk of foot ulceration. *Diabetes Care* 1991;13:63–68.

23. Rith-Najarian SJ, Stolusky T, Gohdes DM. Identifying diabetic patients at high risk for lower-extremity amputation in a primary health care setting. *Diabetes Care* 1992;15:1386–1389.

24. Cavanagh PR, Simoneau GG, Ulbrecht JS. Ulceration, unsteadiness, and uncertainty: the biomechanical consequences of diabetes mellitus. *J Biomechanics* 1993;26:23–40.

25. Coughlin MS. Mallet toes, hammer toes, claw toes, and corns: causes and treatments of lesser toe deformities. *Postgrad Med* 1984;75:191–198.

26. Habershaw G, Donovan JC. Biomechanical considerations of the diabetic foot, in *Management of Diabetic Foot Problems* (Kozak GP, Hoar CS, Rowbotham JL, et al., eds.), WB Saunders, Philadelphia, 1984, pp. 32–44.

27. Ctercteko GC, Dhanendran M, Hutton WC, Lequesne LP. Vertical forces acting on the feet of diabetic patients with neuropathic ulceration. *Br J Surg* 1981;68:608–614.

28. Boulton AJM, Betts RP, Franks CI, Ward JD, Duckworth T. The natural history of foot pressure abnormalities in neuropathic diabetic subjects. *Diabet Res* 1987;5:73–77.

29. Gooding GAW, Stess RM, Graf PM. Sonography of the sole of the foot: evidence for loss of foot pad thickness in diabetes and its relationship to ulceration of the foot. *Invest Radiol* 1986;21:45–48.

30. Young MJ, Cavanagh PR, Thomas G, et al. The effect of callus removal on dynamic plantar foot pressures in diabetic patients. *Diabet Med Suppl* 1992;9:55–57.

31. Veves A, Murray HJ, Young MJ, Boulton AJM. The risk of foot ulceration in diabetic patients with high foot pressure: a prospective study. *Diabetologia* 1992;35:660–663.

32. Masson EA, Hay EM, Stockley I, et al. Abnormal foot pressures alone may not cause ulceration. *Diabet Med* 1989;6:426–428.

33. Lavery LA, Armstrong DG, Vela SA, Quebedeax TL, Fleischli JC. Practical criteria for screening patients at high risk for diabetic foot ulceration. *Arch Intern Med* 1998;158:157–162.

34. Mingardi R, Pasqualetti P, Strazzabosco M, et al. Risk factors for ulceration, amputation, death in a diabetic out-patients clinic. *Diabetologia* 2000;43(Suppl 1):A243.

35. Mayfield JA, Reiber GE, Sanders LJ, Janisse D, Pogach LM. Preventive foot care in people with diabetes. *Diabetes Care* 1999;21:2161–2177.

36. Andersen H, Gadeberg PC, Brock B, Jakobsen J. Muscular atrophy in diabetic neuropathy: a stereological magnetic resonance imaging study. *Diabetologia* 1997;40:1062–1069.

37. Andersen H, Poulsen PL, Mogensen CE, Jakobsen J. Isokinetic muscle strength in long-term IDDM patients in relation to diabetic complications. *Diabetes* 1996;45:440–445.

38. Payne CB. Biomechanics of the foot in diabetes mellitus. Some theoretical considerations. *J Am Podiatr Med Assoc* 1998;88:285–289 relief of plantar pressure in diabetic patients. *Diabet Med* 1998;15:518–522.

39. Delbrid L, Appleberg M, Reeve TS. Factors associated with development of foot lesions in the diabetic. *Surgery* 1983;93;1:78–82.

40. Kastenbauer T, Sokol G, Auinger M, Irsigler K. Running shoes for relief of plantar pressure in diabetic patients. *Diabet Med* 1998;15:518–522.

41. Ashry HR, Lavery LA, Murdoch DP, Frolich M, Lavery DC. Effectiveness of diabetic insoles to reduce foot pressures. *J Foot Ankle Surg* 1997;36:268–271.

42. Mueller MJ. Therapeutic footwear helps protect the diabetic foot. *J Am Podiatr Med Assoc* 1997;87:360–364.

43. Lavery LA, Vela SA, Fleischli JG, Armstrong DG, Lavery DC. Reducing plantar pressure in the neuropathic foot. A comparison of footwear. *Diabetes Care* 1997;20:1706–1710.

44. Tovey FI. The manufacture of diabetic footwear. *Diabet Med* 1984;1:69–71.

45. Mueller MJ, Strube MJ, Allen BT. Therapeutic footwear can reduce plantar pressure in patients with diabetes and transmetatarsal amputation. *Diabetes Care* 1997;20:637–641.

46. Cavanagh PR, Ulbrecht JS, Caput GM. Biomechanical aspects of diabetic foot desease: aetiology, treatment and prevention. *Diabet Med* 1996;13(Suppl):517–522.

47. Lord M, Riad H. Pressure redistribution by molded inserts in diabetic footwear: a pilot study. *J Rehabil Res Dev* 1994;31:214–221.

48. Mueller MJ. Application of plantar pressure assessment in footwear and insert design. *J Orthop Sports Phys Ther* 1999;29:745–755.

49. Foto JG, Birke J. Evaluation of multidensity orthotic materials used in footwear for patients with diabetes. *Foot Ankle Int* 1998;19:836–841.

50. Brand PW. Repetitive stress in the development of diabetic foot ulcers, in *The Diabetic Foot*, 4th ed. (Levin ME, Davidson JK, eds.), Mosby, St. Louis, MO, 1988, pp. 83–90.

51. Veves A, Murray HJ, Young MJ, Boulton AJM. The risk of foot ulceration in diabetic patients with high foot pressure: a prospective study. *Diabetologia* 1992;35:660–663.

52. Litzelman DK, Marriot DJ, Vinicor F. The role of footwear in the prevention of foot lesion in patients with NIDDH. *Diabetes Care* 1997;20:156–162.

53. Uccioli L, Faglia E, Monticone G, et al. Manufactured shoes in the prevention of diabetic foot ulcers. *Diabetes Care* 1995;18:1376–1378.

54. Edmonds ME, Blundell MP, Morris ME, et al. Improved survival of the diabetic foot: the role of a specialized foot clinic. *Q J Med* 1986;60:763–771.

55. Chantelau E, Haage P. An audit of cushioned diabetic footwear: relation to patient compliance. *Diabet Med* 1994;11:114–116.

56. Striesow F. Special manufactured shoes for prevention of recurrent ulcer in diabetic foot syndrome. *Med Klin* 1998;93:695–700.

57. Edmonds ME. Experience in a multidisciplinary diabetic foot clinic, in *The Foot in Diabetes: proceedings of the First National Conference on the Diabetic Foot, Malvern, England, May, 1986* (Connor H, Boulton AJM, Ward JD, eds.), John Wiley, Chichester, England, 1987, pp. 121–134.

58. American Diabetes Association: Consensus Development Conference on Diabetic Foot Wound Care. *Diabetes Care* 1999;22:1354–1360.

59. Department of Health and Human Services: Medicare payments for therapeutic shoes. August 1998 OEI-03-97-00300.
60. Cavanagh PR, Ulbrecht JS. Biomechanical aspects of foot problems in diabetes, in *The Foot in Diabetes*, 2nd ed. (Boulton AJM, Connor H, Cavanagh PR, eds.), John Wiley, New York, 1994, pp. 25–35.
61. Stess RM, Jensen SR, Mirmiran R. The role of dynamic plantar pressure in diabetic foot ulcers. *Diabetes Care* 1997;20:855–858.
62. Armstrong DG, Lavery LA. Evidence-based options for off-loading diabetic wounds. *Clin Podiatr Med Surg* 1998;15:95–104.
63. Caputo GM, Ulbrecht JS, Cavanagh PR. The total contact cast: a method for treating neuropathic diabetic ulcers. *Am Fam Physician* 1997;55:605–611.
64. Shaw JE, Hsi WL, Ulbrecht JS, et al. The mechanism of plantar unloading in total contact casts: implications for design and clinical use. *Foot Ankle Int* 1997;18:809–817.
65. Borssen B, Lithner F. Plaster casts in the management of advanced ischaemic and neuropathic diabetic foot lesions *Diabet Med* 1989;6:720–723.
66. Baumhauer JF, Wervey R, McWilliams J, Harris GF, Shereff MJ. A comparison study of plantar foot pressure in a standardized shoe, total contact cast, and prefabricated pneumatic walking brace. *Foot Ankle Int* 1997;18:26–33.
67. Armstrong DG, Todd WF, Lavery LA, Harkless LB, Bushman TR. The natural history of acute Charcot's arthropathy in a diabetic foot specialty clinic. *Diabet Med* 1997;14:357–363.
68. Armstrong DG, Lavery LA Elevated peak plantar pressures in patients who have Charcot arthropathy. *J Bone Joint Surg [Am]* 1998;80:365–369.
69. Lavery LA, Armstrong DG, Walker SC. Healing rates of diabetic foot ulcers associated with midfoot fracture due to Charcot's arthropathy. *Diabet Med* 1997;14:46–49.
70. Pinzur MS, Shields NN, Goelitz B, et al. American Orthopaedic Foot and Ankle Society shoe survey of diabetic patients. *Foot Ankle Int* 1999;20:703–707.
71. Knowles EA, Boulton AJ. Do people with diabetes wear their prescribed footwear? *Diabet Med* 1996;13:1064–1068.
72. Woolridge J, Moreno L. Evaluation of the costs to Medicare of covering therapeutic shoes for diabetic patients. *Diabetes Care* 1994;17:541–547.
73. Sugarman JR, Reiber GE, Baumgardner G, Prela CM, Lowery J. Use of the therapeutic footwear benefit among diabetic Medicare beneficiaries in three states, 1995. *Diabetes Care* 1998;21:777–781.

Index

Abciximab, 432
Abductor digit minimi, 367, 382
Abductor hallucis, 367, 382
Abscesses, 180, 190, 193
Acarbose, 21 table, 22
Acetylcholine, 104–105, 107
Achilles tendon, 156, 167, 168 figure, 242, 310,
    369, 374
Acinetobacter spp., 210, 211
Acute painful neuropathy of poor glycemic con-
    trol, 81–82
Acute painful neuropathy of rapid glycemic
    control, 82
Adductor muscles, 339
Adenosine diphosphate (ADP), 59–60
Advanced glycation end products (AGEs), 87
Aerobes, 210
Agency for Health Care Policy and Research
    (AHCPR), 250
Air cast, 157
Albuminaria, 100
Aldose reductase inhibitors (ARIs), 87
Alginate dressings, 261–265, 266
Allevyn, 260
Allodynia, 77, 81, 82
α-Lipoic acid, 94
American College of Radiology (ACR), 186
American Diabetes Association (ADA), 2, 16
Aminoglycosides, 213, 216
Aminoguanidine, 87
Amitriptyline, 93
Amoxicillin-clavulanate, 214–215
Ampicillin-sulbactam, 214–216
Amputation(s), 35. *See also* Surgery
    ambulation following, 340–341
    anesthesia, 322, 326
    assessment for, 170
    below-knee, 334, 336–337, 338
    blood pressure and, 47–49
    Boyd, 333
    Charcot foot and, 242, 244

Chopart, 330–333
claudication and, 46
cognitive considerations, 318
complications, 324, 329, 333, 334
costs, limb salvage and, 54
diabetes education and, 46
discharge status of amputees, 54–55
duration of diabetes and, 46
economic considerations, 51–55, 293
epidemiology of, 40–49
foot ulcer history and, 48
footwear and, 48
foot wounds and, 171–174
gangrene as cause, 118
gender differences, 43
geographic locations and, 42–45
glycemic control and, 48
Grade 5 foot, 289
of great toe, 224
guillotine, 213
healing parameters, 321–322
high-level, 168
hindfoot, 333–334
immunocompetence and, 321–322
levels of, 41
limb salvage vs., 318–322
Lisfranc, 324–330
load transfer and, 318–320
Medicare reimbursement, 54
metabolic cost, 318
mortality from, 49–51
nutrition and, 321–322
partial foot, 168
patient self-management education and, 48–49
perioperative considerations, 322
peripheral neuropathy and, 46
postoperative care, 323–324, 328–329, 333,
    334, 337, 340
prior, and ulcers, 40, 168–169
race and, 44–45
rates of, 40–42, 247, 293

From: *The Diabetic Foot: Medical and Surgical Management*
Edited by: A. Veves, J. M. Giurini, and F. W. LoGerfo © Humana Press Inc., Totowa, NJ